INTRODUCTION TO PATIENT CARE

a comprehensive approach to nursing

BEVERLY WITTER Du GAS

R.N., B.A. (University of British Columbia)
M.N. (University of Washington)
Ed.D. (University of British Columbia)
LL.D. (Hon., University of Windsor)

Health Science Educator, Pan American Health Organization, Barbados, Regional Allied Health Project; Formerly, Director, Health Manpower Planning Division, Department of National Health and Welfare, Ottawa; Nurse Educator, World Health Organization, University Nursing Education Project, India (Chandigarh); Associate Director of Nursing (Education), The Vancouver General Hospital School of Nursing, Vancouver, British Columbia

with special editorial assistance from
BARBARA MARIE Du GAS

B.A. (University of British Columbia)

Certificate (Simon Fraser University Professional Development Program, Department of Education, British Columbia)

Third Edition

1977

W. B. SAUNDERS COMPANY Philadelphia / London / Toronto

W. B. Saunders Company: West Washington Square
Philadelphia, PA   19105

1 St. Anne's Road
Eastbourne, East Sussex BN21 3UN, England

1 Goldthorne Avenue
Toronto, Ontario M8Z 5T9, Canada

Introduction to Patient Care   ISBN   0-7216-3226-2

Last digit is the print number: 9   8   7   6   5   4   3   2   1

DEDICATION

To my father,

Charles Edgar Witter,

for his constant encouragement
in my career
and in my personal life

PREFACE

In the 10 years since the first edition of this book was published, rapid social change has revolutionized the entire field of health care. Nursing has emerged from its dependence on other disciplines to become an independent health profession in its own right, with its own methodology and its own body of knowledge, firmly based on a sound scientific foundation.

The purpose of the present edition is therefore to provide students with an introduction to the practice of nursing as an integral component of total health care, and to help them to develop basic skills in utilizing the nursing process in their practice. With this purpose in mind, the book has been divided into four units. The first unit focuses on the role of the nurse in health care; the second is devoted to the nursing process. In the third unit, the nursing process is applied to helping people to meet their basic health needs, while the fourth unit carries the application further to the care of people with common problems the nurse will encounter in practice.

As in the previous edition, each chapter except the first one begins with a set of objectives for students to use in evaluating their own progress in learning. A guide for assessing the patient's status with regard to specific functional areas, and a guide for evaluating the effectiveness of nursing action, have been included at the end of each chapter wherever this is appropriate to the content. (In Unit III, guidance on planning and evaluating nursing care is included in the main text of the chapters.) In addition, a study vocabulary, a study situation, and suggested readings may be found at the end of each chapter. In this edition, the suggested reading list has been confined to basic references and to recent journal articles that students should be able to find in most nursing school libraries. References footnoted throughout each chapter provide an additional source of material for those who wish to pursue a particular topic more extensively. The appendix contains a list of prefixes and suffixes used in medical terminology, and a glossary of terms defined in the text.

BEVERLY WITTER DU GAS

ACKNOWLEDGMENTS

No textbook by a single author is ever written in isolation, and I would like to acknowledge with gratitude the assistance of the many people who contributed to the preparation of this third edition. I am especially grateful to the numerous nurse educators who helped with ideas and suggestions for the revision and reorganization of content. Special thanks are due Barbara Gillies, Senior Instructor and Clinical Coordinator of the Vancouver General Hospital School of Nursing, whose assistance as clinical consultant throughout the preparation of both the second and third edition has been most deeply appreciated. I am also indebted to Kay Turner, Long Beach City College, California, whose "marked up" copy, with notes and comments made while using the text in her teaching, was never far from my side during the many months it took to complete this revision. I would also like to thank Anna Curren, President of Wallcur Incorporated, for her helpful suggestions on the reorganization of the text.

My students in the Health Sciences Tutors' Course in Barbados also deserve thanks for their assistance in "pilot-testing" much of the new material developed for the third edition.

I am also very grateful to E. Apostolides for his advice on photography, and to Sven Fletcher-Berg for his assistance in taking pictures for the present edition, and to the patients, the graduate and student nurses, and other health team members who permitted their photographs to be used to illustrate the text.

Particular gratitude is owed to my daughter, Barbara Du Gas, for her editorial help throughout the work on this revision.

A special word of thanks is due, too, to Ina Brown, of the W. B. Saunders Company, for her invaluable assistance during the crucial stages of finalization of the manuscript.

Finally, I would like especially to express my appreciation to Robert E. Wright, Nursing Editor of the Saunders Company, for his patience, encouragement, and support over the years we have worked together since the first inception of the idea for this book through to its present edition.

CONTENTS

UNIT IV.   COMMON HEALTH PROBLEMS

UNIT I

THE
ROLE
OF
THE
NURSE
IN
HEALTH
CARE

1 INTRODUCTION

THE FOCUS ON HEALTH

The twentieth century has witnessed tremendous advances in medical science that have revolutionized health care in our Western societies. Most of the communicable diseases that necessitated lengthy hospitalization and took such a toll of human lives at the beginning of the century have been virtually eliminated by improvements in public health measures, coupled with the discovery and widespread utilization of specific immunity-producing agents. The "miracle drugs," the sulfonamides and antibiotics of the 1940s and 1950s, radically changed patterns of patient care by hastening recovery and lowering fatality rates from infections. The rapid advances in medical therapy and in surgical techniques during the 1960s and 1970s have also contributed significantly to increasing the life span of people in our society.

We can, and we should, be very proud of these accomplishments of Western medicine. At the same time, however, there has come a growing realization that the major portion of our efforts—and of our expenditures—on health care has been devoted to the relatively small proportion of the population who suffer major acute illnesses. Our health care, in other words, has been predominantly "sick" care. We are beginning to realize that the promotion and maintenance of health, and the prevention of disease by all known means, may be as important as and, in the long run, probably more economical than treating people after they have become ill.

We are witnessing an awakening (some say a reawakening) of interest in physical

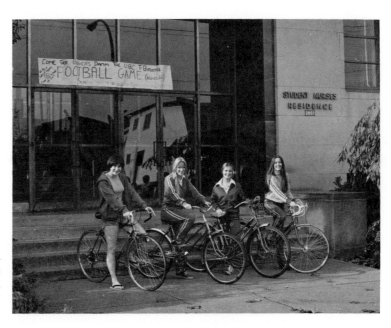

Nurses need exercise and recreation too. These students are combining both in an outing after classes are finished for the day.

fitness programs, in nutrition programs, and in programs to promote sound health practices as essential components of health care services. Nurses are seen as key figures in health promotion for several reasons. Health teaching has long been considered a major nursing responsibility, although it has not always received the emphasis it should in nursing education programs. Nurses have already earned their acceptance by the public as persons knowledgeable about health matters. Nurses are also more accessible than many other health professionals to people who want help and advice on health matters. Consider, for example, the nurse who is married and living in the community. Even if she is raising a family and is not actively engaged in nursing practice, her house soon becomes a neighborhood center for the care and treatment of minor illnesses, for first-stop emergency care in many cases, and for general counseling about health problems for the people in the neighborhood.

THE EMPHASIS ON COMMUNITY SERVICES

It is increasingly being recognized not only that acute care hospitals are the most expensive part of our health care system, but also that they are not always the most appropriate place for the care and treatment of many health problems. The emergency wards of acute hospitals are often crowded with nonemergency cases that could be looked after more efficiently and effectively if more primary care services were accessible to people on a 24-hour basis in the community. The "store front" and "free" clinics, the family practice units, the community (or neighborhood) health centers, and the Health Maintenance Organizations that have developed in recent years have all helped to ease some of the burden from the acute hospitals by providing more readily accessible services for people in the community.

As hospital care has become more expensive, and as the psychological and sociological benefits of being in one's own home for hastening recovery from illness have been increasingly recognized, there has been a major expansion of home care and other supplementary services for the sick and for people requiring help in maintaining their health. The provision of more home care services has meant that the necessity for hospitalization has been cut down in many cases, and that the length of stay in hospitals and other institutional facilities can be shortened for many others. In the field of mental health, for example, the huge

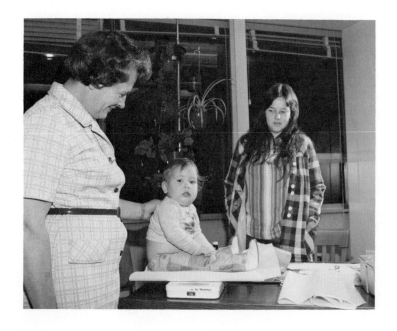

Healthy babies are happy babies. The nurse and this young man are renewing their acquaintance during one of his periodic visits to the health agency while mother looks on.

mental hospitals that were once a familiar landmark in many communities, and often had a population equal to that of a small town, are gradually being phased down with the development of more extensive community-based psychiatric services.

In the provision of home care and related services, nurses are playing an increasingly large role both in the identification of the need for such services and in the coordination of them, as well as in the provision of direct nursing care. Although many other types of services are frequently needed too, such as physiotherapy and occupational therapy, social services, homemaker services, and "meals-on-wheels," to name but a few, nursing is the one service that is most consistently required in home care.

THE INTEGRATION OF HEALTH CARE SERVICES

Despite the proliferation of workers in the health field and the increasing numbers and types of agencies providing services, it has become evident that there are still many deficiencies in the system and, at the same time, much duplication of effort. A person may go to one physician for treatment of a gastric disorder, to another for examination of his eyes, to the hospital emergency unit for a cut hand, and to a public health clinic for immunizations for his children, and may call in the visiting nurse service to give weekly liver injections to his aged aunt who is living with the family. Still, he may wonder to whom he should go with many of his health problems. The frustrations and delays in getting to the appropriate agency in our confusing health care maze result in many problems being left untreated, and referrals to agencies who could help being omitted. At times, the situation may be the reverse, with a plethora of agencies involved in assisting one family to resolve its problems.

Attempts are being made throughout the country to bring some order into the health care system. There is a major move toward the integration of services in order to eliminate some of the gaps and deficiencies of the present system and the duplication of services. Hospitals are becoming "hospitals without walls." In small communities, many hospitals have become community health care centers and offer a wide variety of services in addition to their traditional care of the bedridden sick. The local physician, for example, may have his office there, as may the community health nurse and the social worker. A community mental health center may also be housed in the same hospital building. Many city hospitals are providing a wide range of services these days also. Some offer home care services for the follow-up of discharged patients, and many have expanded their outpatient departments to provide more ambulatory care. A number also provide health promotion and health maintenance programs, such as prenatal and well-baby clinics, for people in the neighboring area. The development of multipurpose clinics and health centers with linkages to hospitals and other community agencies (such as a visiting nurse service) is another example of attempts to provide comprehensive and coordinated services to people.

At the state and provincial levels, there is a move toward the regionalization of services, that is, bringing all services in a geographical region under one administrative umbrella in order to ensure that all aspects of health care are covered and also to avoid duplication of services. In a regionalized plan, for example, one hospital might be designated as the center for care and treatment of people requiring highly sophisticated (and expensive) medical care. People needing heart surgery or specialized neurological treatment, for example, would be sent to this hospital, where the necessary specialists and the equipment would be centralized.

This movement toward the integration of health services means that nurses must become more versatile. Many feel that tomorrow's nurse should be able to work with equal ease in either the hospital or the community setting.[1] But there will also be a need for nurses with highly developed expertise in the complex skills

---

[1]*Community Health Nursing.* Report of a W.H.O. Expert Committee. Geneva, World Health Organization, 1974.

required to care for the acutely ill. There seems no doubt that hospitals in the future will be reserved for the care of the acutely ill.[2] Nurses working in these hospitals will require a high level of technical skill to cope with their responsibilities in regard to the care of these patients.

THE MULTIDISCIPLINARY HEALTH TEAM

The number of types of workers in the health care field has increased almost as rapidly as has the total number of persons in the field. A shortage of professional workers and the need for people with highly specialized skills have been two factors contributing to this trend. The "multidisciplinary health team" now encompasses a large and rapidly growing family of occupational groups who are involved in providing health care services. In the United States, over 600 health occupations (including primary and alternate or specialty job titles) have been identified in which people have education and training designed specifically to prepare them for work in the health care field.[3] The amount of education and training varies from a few weeks of on-the-job training, as for example a nurse's aide, to more than 10 years of post-high school preparation for a specialist physician.

In addition to the traditional health professions of medicine, nursing, dentistry, and pharmacy, a cadre of highly specialized workers has developed. Many of these people provide direct care services to patients that are complementary to medical and nursing care, such as physiotherapists and occupational therapists. Some are technologists whose occupations have evolved because of the need for people with specific skills in handling the complex machinery used in the care of the patients, such as the inhalation therapists and the renal dialysis (artificial kidney) technicians. Several of the newer groups have emerged as a result of the delegation of certain functions by the major professionals. These include the "physician's assistant" (such as Medex, Primex, and the like), licensed practical or vocational nurses (called nursing assistants in several provinces in Canada), dental hygienists, dental nurses, dental assistants, and pharmacy assistants.

Increasing awareness of the contribution that each discipline can make to health care has led to increased responsibility and autonomy for the allied health disciplines. The provision of comprehensive health care requires a multidisciplinary team approach; in the United States and Canada, we have seen the gradual evolvement of the team concept.

Although each discipline has its unique contribution to make and its own particular area of expertise, there are many areas of overlapping function. The same set of activities may be undertaken in one instance by a member of one discipline, and at other times by a member of another. For example, the physiotherapist may initiate a remedial exercise program for a person recovering from a stroke, but it may be up to the nurse to assist the patient with these exercises in between the physiotherapist's visits. In some cases, it may be the nurse who initiates the program. The nurse in her day-to-day work will have contact with the members of many other health disciplines. Nurses must be aware not only of the unique contribution nursing makes to health care, but also of the contributions made by other disciplines involved in the care of a particular patient or family. The various members of the health team with whom the nurse comes in frequent contact are discussed in Chapter 6.

CONSUMERISM IN HEALTH CARE

Increasing public awareness of health issues, increased knowledge about health

---

[2]Jessie Scott: Opening Remarks. *Report of the Conference on Redesigning Nursing Education for Public Health, May 23–25, 1973*. Rockville, Maryland, U.S. Department of Health, Education, and Welfare Publication No. (HRA) 75–75.

[3]U.S. Department of Health, Education, and Welfare: *Health Resources Statistics 1974*. A report prepared by the National Center for Health Statistics. Public Health Service Publication No. 1509. Washington, D.C., U.S. Government Printing Office, 1974, p. 3.

and illness, and the rising costs to the consumer of health services are three factors that have contributed to the rise of consumerism in the health field. The public is currently expressing many of its dissatisfactions with the present health system and demanding a voice in the type of care it feels it needs and should be provided with. The consensus that appears to be emerging is that the average citizen wants (1) better accessibility to services; (2) more comprehensive and coordinated services; (3) more personalized services; (4) the right to know what is being done for him and why; and (5) the right to monitor the quality of care he receives. Consumers' bills of rights have been developed and widely publicized in the United States, for example, by the American Hospital Association, and in Canada by the National Consumers' Association, as shown on pages 4 and 6.

CONSUMER RIGHTS IN HEALTH CARE

I Right to be informed
1 — about preventive health care including education on nutrition, birth control, drug use, appropriate exercise
2 — about the health care system, including the extent of government insurance coverage for services, supplementary insurance plans, and referral system to auxiliary health and social facilities and services in the community
3 — about the individual's own diagnosis and specific treatment program, including prescribed surgery and medication, options, effects and side effects
4 — about the specific costs of procedures, services and professional fees undertaken on behalf of the individual consumer

II Right to be respected as the individual with the major responsibility for his own health care

— right that confidentiality of his health records be maintained
— right to refuse experimentation, undue painful prolongation of his life or participation in teaching programs

— right of adult to refuse treatment, right to die with dignity

III Right to participate in decision making affecting his health

— through consumer representation at each level of government in planning and evaluating the system of health services,
— the types and qualities of service and the conditions under which health services are delivered
— with the health professionals and personnel involved in his direct health care

IV Right to equal access to health care (health education, prevention, treatment and rehabilitation) regardless of the individual's economic status, sex, age, creed, ethnic origin and location

— right to access to adequately qualified health personnel
— right to a second medical opinion
— right to prompt response in emergencies

Source: *Canadian Consumer, 41*, April 1974.

BILL OF RIGHTS FOR PATIENTS

In the interest of "more effective patient care and greater satisfaction for the patient, his physician, and the hospital organization," the American Hospital Association has adopted a "Patient's Bill of Rights" as a national policy statement and distributed it to its member hospitals throughout the country. Intended to "give the consumer something to go by," the 12 rights, in summary, are:

1. The patient has the right to considerate and respectful care.

2. The patient has the right to obtain from his physician complete current information concerning his diagnosis, treatment, and prognosis in terms the patient can be reasonably expected to understand.

3. The patient has the right to receive from his physician information necessary to give informed consent prior to the start of any procedure and/or treatment.

4. The patient has the right to refuse treatment to the extent permitted by law, and to be informed of the medical consequences of his action.

5. The patient has the right to every consideration of his privacy concerning his own medical care program.

6. The patient has the right to expect that all communications and records pertaining to his care should be treated as confidential.

7. The patient has the right to expect that within its capacity a hospital must make reasonable response to the request of a patient for services.

8. The patient has the right to obtain information as to any relationship of his hospital to other health care and education insitutions insofar as his care is concerned.

9. The patient has the right to be advised if the hospital proposes to engage in or perform human experimentation affecting his care or treatment.

10. The patient has the right to expect reasonable continuity of care.

11. The patient has the right to examine and receive an explanation of his bill regardless of source of payment.

12. The patient has the right to know what hospital rules and regulations apply to his conduct as a patient.

From: Bill of Rights for Patients. In *Nursing Outlook,* 21:82, February 1973. Adopted by American Hospitals Association as a national policy statement and distributed nationally to all member hospitals.

The implications of this trend for nursing are many, as they are for all health professions. Individuals representing the recipients of care are being appointed to the regulatory boards of many of the health disciplines, to committees concerned with the development of educational programs for health professionals, to advisory boards of health agencies that did not have them before, and to committees concerned with the quality of care in these agencies. There is increasing involvement of patients in the planning, implementation, and evaluation of health care. The consumer appears to be saying that he no longer wishes to be considered as simply an object of care but as a full participant in his health care.

ACCOUNTABILITY FOR PRACTICE

Health professionals have long been concerned over the need to maintain high standards of professional practice. Strict standards for entrance to each profession, for example, the registration examinations for nurses, have been established to ensure that candidates are well qualified and "safe" to practice that profession. Each profession also maintains a regulatory body to monitor the actions of its practitioners.

However, the growing rise of consumerism in the health field and the generally increased sophistication of the public in relation to health matters have put additional emphasis on the accountability of health professionals for the care they give to the public. No longer is it felt that the doctor and the nurse, or any other health professional, has a "divine right to knowledge" that is too far above their heads to be understood by the average citizens. The average citizen is much more knowledgeable about the complicated mechanisms of the human body and the things that can go wrong with it than his parents and grandparents ever were. He learns from the popular media about the latest advances in medical treatment and surgical procedures. He also feels that he has a right to question the treatment he is being given, to have a say in this treatment, and to be kept informed of his progress. Our elected representatives in government are also becoming increasingly concerned about the quality of health care, since more and more of that care is being paid for by public funds. They, too, are demanding that the work of health professionals be monitored to ensure that high quality standards are maintained. Nurses, as well as other health professionals, must carefully document the care they give to patients and be able to state the reasons for that care, and the care must be in line with accepted standards. The development of standards of nursing care and of criteria for evaluating care is, indeed, one of the major concerns of nursing associations today.

In order to carry out their own responsibilities within the health care system, nurses should also be knowledgeable about the structure of the health services within which they work. They should be aware, too, of the contributions made to these services by other members of the health team.

The role of nursing is constantly changing in response to societal needs. The scope of the professional nurse's practice today includes a much broader range of activities than is represented in the traditional image of the nurse at the bedside of the sick patient. The nurse still performs many of her time-honored functions in caring for the sick, but her role in all other aspects of health care continues to expand. Nurses should be aware of the scope of nursing practice as it exists today and, at the same time, be conscious of their responsibility to the public they serve.

SUGGESTED READINGS

A New Perspective on the Health of Canadians. A Working Document. Ottawa, Department of National Health and Welfare, 1974.

Community Health Nursing. Report of a W.H.O. Expert Committee. Geneva, World Health Organization, 1974.

Health United States 1975. Rockville, Maryland, U.S. Department of Health, Education and Welfare, Public Health Services, Publication No. (HRA) 76–1232. Health Resources Administration, National Center for Health Statistics, 1976.

Kelly, L. Y.: The Patient's Right to Know. *Nursing Outlook, 24:*26–32, January 1976.

Pasternak, S. B.: Care of the Well Child—Annual Well-Child Visits. *American Journal of Nursing, 74:*1471–1475, August 1974.

Redesigning Nursing Education for Public Health. Report of the Conference, May 23–25, 1973. Rockville, Maryland, U.S. Department of Health, Education and Welfare Publication No. (HRA) 75–75.

Steidl, Susan N.: Is There a Nurse in the Neighbourhood? *Canadian Nurse, 72:*35, July 1976.

2 HEALTH AND ILLNESS

The nurse should be able to:

Describe the health-illness continuum
Explain the concept of optimal health
Discuss the "holistic" approach to health care
Describe Maslow's theory of a hierarchy of human needs
List the stages of the human life cycle as identified by Erikson
Explain the concept of homeostasis as it applies to an individual's
   health
Explain the role of stress in the causation of illness
List and give examples of various types of stressors
Explain the general adaptation syndrome
Explain the local adaptation syndrome
Describe the flight-fight reaction of the body
List and give examples of commonly used psychological adaptive
   mechanisms

INTRODUCTION

Health and illness are matters of universal concern. In many languages, a polite form of greeting is an enquiry into the state of a person's health. We do not really expect a detailed answer to our query "How are you?" particularly if we have business matters to discuss, but it is considered only polite to ask. In the realm of social conversation, however, the state of one's health, one's ailments, and suggested remedies for those ailments that afflict others are said to be among our most common topics — and with little wonder! We are constantly being bombarded by radio and television commercials, by billboards, and by other forms of advertising to buy a myriad of patent medicines, each one guaranteed to be more effective than its competitors' products in curing our headache, our backache, or whatever else is wrong with us.

In the Western world today, we are a highly health-conscious people. The continuing popularity of the doctor-nurse novels and of medical books for the layman and the longevity of medically oriented television programs certainly attest to our interest in the subject. Yet, we are being told that we are not really healthy. We eat too much, we lead too sedentary lives, and we do not compare very well on international studies of physical fitness with some of our European counterparts.[1] Campaigns are currently being waged both by governmental agencies and other interested groups to remedy this situation. We are being exhorted to get out and jog, cycle, or even just walk to get some exercise, to eat nutritiously (while watching our caloric and cholesterol intake), and, above all, to cut out smoking. We are suddenly, it seems, being made aware of the need to improve our health.

THE HEALTH-ILLNESS CONTINUUM

Basic to the practice of all of the health professions is an understanding of the health-illness concept. Both health and illness are relative states, and the words themselves mean different things to different people. As a person gets older, he tends to accept a few aches and pains as a normal part of the aging process, whereas an athlete may feel that he is not in good health unless he can run five miles. Health and illness may indeed be viewed on a continuum that ranges from extreme poor health when death is imminent to peak or high-level wellness.[2]

Neither health nor illness is constant or absolute, but is an ever-changing state of being. A person may wake up in the morning, for example, with a headache. He may feel so ill, in fact, that he decides that he is not well enough to go to work, but he remembers that he has an important appointment at nine o'clock. After one or two cups of coffee and breakfast, he may begin to think that he is not so sick as he thought he was, and if his appointment goes well, he may feel in excellent health by lunch time.

[1] *A New Perspective on the Health of Canadians.* A Working Document. Ottawa, Department of National Health and Welfare, April 1974, p. 25.

[2] Hallburt L. Dunn: High-Level Wellness for Man and Society. In *A Sociological Framework for Patient Care* by Jeanette R. Folta and Edith S. Deck (eds.). New York, John Wiley and Sons, Inc., 1966, pp. 213–219.

THE HEALTH CONTINUUM

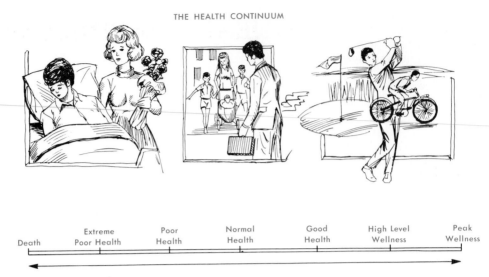

| Death | Extreme Poor Health | Poor Health | Normal Health | Good Health | High Level Wellness | Peak Wellness |

Health may be viewed as a continuum that ranges from extreme states of ill health to peak wellness.

What, then, constitutes health and illness? Extreme states of ill-health are usually fairly easy to identify, but a person who is carrying out his normal daily activities may have a serious illness according to his physician and yet appear healthy to other people. Some illnesses that are looked upon as serious deviations from health in our Western society may be highly desirable in other cultures. In some societies, for example, the person who sees visions or hears imaginary voices talking to him may be highly esteemed, whereas we might consider that this individual has a serious mental illness. Worm infestations are so common in some parts of the world that it is rare to see an individual who does not suffer from one.

THE TERMS: HEALTH, ILLNESS, AND DISEASE

At one time, health was defined as the absence of illness; a person was considered healthy as long as he was not sick. Statements in the literature of recent years, however, indicate that health is no longer looked upon simply as the absence of illness, but has a positive meaning of its own. In the preamble to the *Constitution of the World Health Organization*, health is defined as "a state of complete mental, physical and social well-being and not merely the absence of disease or infirmity."[3] Although this statement has been criticized by some on the basis that complete well-being for all is an unattainable goal, others feel that it should be looked upon as an ideal toward which we should consciously strive.

In a similar vein to the World Health Organization definition (although not quite so idealistically), the U.S. President's Commission on the Health Needs of the Nation stated that health means "optimum physical, mental and social efficiency."[4]

A working document prepared by the Department of Health and Welfare in Canada entitled *A New Perspective on the Health of Canadians* also discusses the goal of health care "to increase freedom

---

[3]From the *Constitution of the World Health Organization*, which came into force at Geneva, April 7, 1948.

[4]President's Commission on the Health Needs of the Nation: *Building America's Health: A Report to the President.* Washington, D.C., U.S. Government Printing Office, 1951.

from disability, as well as to promote a state of well-being sufficient to perform at adequate levels of physical, mental and social activity, taking age into consideration."[5]

Despite the difference in terms used to modify "well-being," these statements express essentially the same thought, that is, that health is a positive state of being that includes physical fitness, mental (or emotional) stability, and social ease.

As health has assumed a more positive meaning for us, the term "illness" has conversely taken on a more negative connotation. We are now inclined to talk of a person as having a "health problem" or a "health deficit," rather than say that he is ill. Illness in this context is looked upon as an interruption in the continuous process of health, manifested by abnormalities or disturbances of functioning.[6] When these abnormalities appear clustered together, they become recognizable as the signs and symptoms of a particular disease, for example, the high temperature, cough, and chest pain that are commonly seen in people with pneumonia.[6]

But definitions of the term "disease" are also changing. The following statement by McHugh is perhaps helpful in this regard:

The term "disease" is difficult to define, because it is a concept and not something given or concrete in nature. It is intended to convey that, among all the morbid physical changes in physical and mental health, it is possible to recognize groups of abnormalities as distinct entities or syndromes separable from one another and from the normal. . . .

All abnormalities can be viewed as quantitative changes merging imperceptibly into one another and into the normal.[7]

---

[5]*A New Perspective on the Health of Canadians,* op. cit., p. 8.

[6]*Ten Year Health Plan for the Americas.* Final Report of the III Special Meeting of Ministers of Health of the Americas (Santiago, Chile, 2–9 October, 1972). Official document No. 118, January 1973, P.A.H.O. Washington, D.C., Pan American Health Organization, Pan American Sanitary Bureau, p. 4.

[7]Paul R. McHugh: Psychological Illness in Medical Practice. In *Textbook of Medicine* (fourteenth edition) by Paul B. Beeson and Walsh McDermott. Philadelphia, W. B. Saunders Company, 1975, p. 562.

TWO BASIC CONCEPTS: OPTIMAL HEALTH AND HOLISM

Implicit in the definitions of health discussed previously are two basic concepts that underlie the framework on which modern health care is based. The first is the concept of optimal health, or optimal functioning, as the aim of health care for each individual. This concept is based on the premise that each individual has his own optimal level of functioning,[8] which represents the best state of well-being that is possible for him. Most people have some type of minor health deficit. They may have a minor physical problem, such as an allergy to certain foods, for example, or a small speech impediment. Or, they may be "shy" and have a problem in meeting people. Some people have an unreasonable fear of heights or of cats, which would be examples of problems in the psychological realm of functioning. The point here is that few people attain perfection in all aspects of their health—physical, mental, and social—and certainly do not achieve it all of the time, but each individual has his own unique optimum that is attainable for him.

Many people in our society have chronic health problems of a more serious nature than those described above, yet they manage to maintain a normal life-style as long as they take certain precautions and respect the limitations imposed by their illness. A person with a condition such as diabetes, for example, may consider himself to be in good health as long as his diabetes is under control and he can carry on with his usual activities. He may have to be careful with his diet and take more precautions than the average person does to guard against infection, but the majority of people with diabetes manage very well, with only occasional disturbances of total functioning. The optimal level of health for a diabetic would, of course, be different for each individual with diabetes, as well as be different from

---

[8]Sarah Ellen Archer and Ruth Fleshman: *Community Health Nursing: Patterns and Practices.* North Scituate, Massachusetts, Duxbury Press, 1975, p. 24.

that which is possible for a person without this problem.

To use another example, the person who has suffered a stroke and is paralyzed on one side of his body may not regain total functioning of his affected arm and leg, but he may be able to achieve independence in daily living activities and take an active functioning role in society again. Optimal level of health, in his case, would include the best possible restoration of physical, emotional, and social functioning compatible with his illness.

The second basic concept is the premise that an individual's health must be considered in terms of his total functioning. That is to say, man must be viewed as a whole; one cannot separate the physical, social, and emotional components of his health. This concept is frequently referred to as the "holistic" approach to health care. As one author has stated, "Basic to the discussion of measuring health is the functioning of the individual in terms of his family, his work, his recreation, and his position in society. . . . The real measure of health is the ability of the individual to function in a manner acceptable to himself and to the group of which he is a part."[9]

If we again take the example of the person who has had a stroke, it is easy to see that his physical disability will interfere with both his emotional and his social well-being. He will undoubtedly be very anxious and will probably be afraid that he is no longer the person that he was. His illness will perhaps require lengthy hospitalization and he will be cut off from normal social activities with his family and friends. This individual will need considerable help from nursing and other health personnel to regain optimal functioning in regard to all aspects of his health.

Even in the case of minor illnesses, such as a bout of influenza or a short-lived gastrointestinal upset, a person's mental

outlook and his interactions with other people are affected. Conversely, an emotional problem, such as anxiety over examinations or an unpleasant social encounter, will affect one's appetite, one's digestion, and perhaps other aspects of physical functioning. In considering a person's health, then, one must look at the whole person, not just his physical fitness, or his mental state, or his social functioning.

BASIC HUMAN NEEDS

If we accept the premise that good health is the ability to function at one's highest level physically, mentally, and socially, it seems appropriate to look next at the conditions that foster good health. What is needed for an individual to attain his optimal level of well-being? This leads us, then, quite logically, to a consideration of basic human needs.

There does not seem to be any doubt that there are certain basic needs that are common to all beings of the human species, and that these needs must be fulfilled if an individual is to attain his optimal level of well-being. The subject of basic needs has been studied in depth by people in the social sciences looking for primary motivating forces underlying human behavior, and by people in the health field seeking to identify factors causing health problems. At one point, it was felt that all human needs could be categorized under two headings, one physiological in derivation, and the other psychological. Another group of theorists classified needs on the basis of whether their origin was internal or external. Still others have identified long lists of human needs, all considered basic.

In recent years, Abraham Maslow's theory of a hierarchy of needs has received increasing attention as a conceptual framework for the consideration of human needs. Not everyone agrees with all aspects of his theory, and some have suggested modifications in his hierarchy, but the basic principles outlined in the theory appear to be fairly well accepted.

Maslow has suggested that there are five basic categories of human needs and

---

[9]J. G. Mills: Primary Health Care. Report of the Sub-committee on Primary Health Care, submitted to the Council of Medical Services of the Canadian Medical Association, 1973. (As reprinted in the *Report of the Alberta Task Force on Nursing Education.* Alberta, Department of Advanced Education and Manpower, September 1975.)

that these may be arranged in order of priority for satisfaction. According to Maslow's theory, lower level needs must be satisfied (or, at least, mostly so) before the individual attempts to satisfy needs of a higher order. The basic types of needs identified by Maslow, in order of priority, were:

1. Physiological needs
2. Safety and security needs
3. Needs for love and belonging
4. Esteem needs
5. Needs for self-actualization[10]

Physiological needs take precedence over all others because they are essential for survival. These include the need for water, for food, for air, for elimination, for rest and sleep, for temperature maintenance, and for the avoidance of pain.[11] For a person who is starving, for example, life revolves around the need to obtain food. Similarly, a person deprived of water for a long period of time can think of nothing else but his thirst. The fulfillment of certain of these basic needs is so essential that if there is interference with the attainment of them, immediate action must be taken to save the person's life. If there is interference with breathing, for example, and a person's air supply is cut off, prompt measures must be initiated to restore adequate respiration or the person will die within a matter of minutes. The relief of pain is another priority item. If pain is severe, a person cannot rest, he cannot sleep, and he can think of nothing else until he obtains relief from it.

Next in order of priority, according to Maslow, are the safety and security needs. These involve such fundamental components as adequate shelter and protection from harmful factors in the environment. But a person must also feel that he is secure and protected from real or imagined danger. People usually feel most secure in familiar surroundings, with accustomed routines, and with people

they can trust and things they know. Conversely, they feel threatened when they are in strange places, when their usual pattern of living is disturbed, or when they are with strangers or have no familiar objects around them. Often, inanimate objects assume a symbolism that represents safety and security for an individual. Linus' blanket, which he carries everywhere with him, has become a symbol of security that is recognized by most North Americans. Most children have a toy or other object that has become dear to them; they usually like to take it with them wherever they go and it helps to provide a feeling of security when they are in strange surroundings or unfamiliar situations. Many adults, too, have lucky charms or other objects that they feel give them some special form of protection against harm. Maslow has suggested that many of our religious rituals, our superstitions, and our traditions have their origins in this basic need for safety and security.

Following the security needs, Maslow places the needs for love and belonging as the next most important. There is little question that these are very basic needs. Infants deprived of love and affection just do not thrive, even if all their physiological and safety needs are met. But adults, too, need to have people who are close to them, to share their joys and sorrows, their anxieties, and their doubts. People who do not have close ties with other people often have pets — a cat, a dog, or a canary, for example — on which they lavish all the love and affection they do not have the opportunity to share with other people.

Next in Maslow's hierarchy are the esteem needs. A person must feel that he is worthwhile as a human being, that is, he must have self-esteem, and he must also feel that he is considered a person of worth and dignity by his family and by other people with whom he comes in contact. Maslow has suggested that many of the problems of people in our impersonalized society, particularly in the big cities, are due to failure to satisfy the two basic needs of love/belonging and esteem. If people do not have these needs satisfied, they come to have a low regard for themselves, and feelings of inadequacy, frus-

---

[10]A. H. Maslow: *Motivation and Personality.* Second edition. New York, Harper and Row, 1970.

[11]As discussed in Chapter One in the section on Man's Basic Needs in Joan Luckmann and Karen C. Sorensen: *Medical-Surgical Nursing: A Psychophysiologic Approach.* Philadelphia, W. B. Saunders Company, 1974, pp. 9–10.

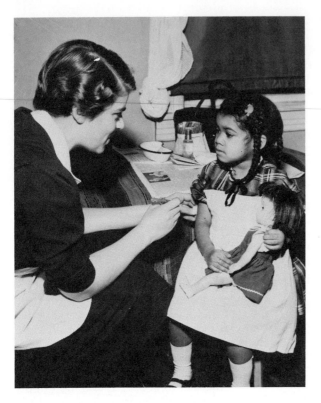

Most children have a favorite toy that provides them with a feeling of security when they are in strange surroundings or unfamiliar situations. This little girl has Dolly ready for her injection when the nurse has finished with hers.

tration, alienation, and hopelessness result.[12]

Finally in Maslow's hierarchy are the needs for self-actualization. These include the need to attain one's highest potential—to achieve one's ambitions in life. Maslow includes here also the need for knowledge and the aesthetic needs, that is, for something beautiful in one's life.

Kalish has suggested that the need for knowledge, as exemplified by man's curiosity, is a more fundamental need than Maslow has depicted in his hierarchy; he places it second, after physiological needs, and includes in this category sex, activity, exploration, and novelty.[13] Maslow's model of a hierarchy of human needs as adapted by Kalish is shown on page 17. Again, to use the example of infants, those who do not have sufficient opportunity to explore their surroundings and to manipulate objects or who have insufficient change in their environment do not attain their optimal development physiologically, emotionally, or socially. Older children, too—and adults—will often forget about safety and security in a desire to obtain stimulation or to satisfy their curiosity. The sex drive is also, of course, very fundamental and strong, although it is a drive that can be sublimated—that is, it can be channeled into other forms of activity, such as a career; or, its gratification can also be delayed indefinitely, for example, in the case of people in certain religious orders who take vows of chastity.

In Maslow's theory, the individual is seen as constantly striving to fulfill his basic needs. As one set of needs is gratified, others of a higher order emerge and become more powerful. A person who seemingly has all his needs fulfilled is still looking for something further. He may develop his aesthetic needs and hunt for rare art objects, or he may seek to increase his knowledge and become a scholarly authority on a particular subject.

The concept that is presented in Mas-

[12]Lyle E. Bourne, Jr., and Bruce R. Ekstrand: *Psychology: Its Principles and Meanings.* Hinsdale, Illinois, The Dryden Press, 1973, p. 179.

[13]R. A. Kalish: *The Psychology of Human Behavior.* Belmont, California, Wadsworth Publishing Company, 1966.

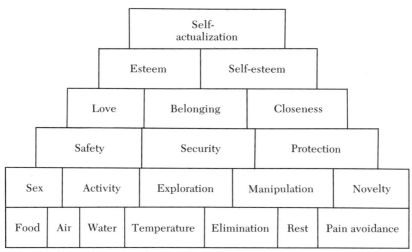

Maslow's hierarchy of needs, as adapted by Kalish. (From Kalish, R. A.: The Psychology of Human Behavior. *Belmont, California, Wadsworth Publishing Company, 1966).*

low's theory is not of man as a static entity, trying simply to maintain his equilibrium in a changing world, but of man as constantly reaching out for things beyond his immediate grasp. This concept embodies the idea of continuous growth and development of the human organism, which begins at the moment of birth and continues until death ensues.

THE STAGES OF MAN

Poets, dramatists, and theorists have long postulated that in his lifetime man goes through a series of definite stages. These stages are marked by changes in his physical being and by changes in his psychological and social makeup. While there is much uniformity of opinion concerning the physical changes that occur during the life span, since these are relatively easy to observe, there have been many theories proposed in regard to man's psychosocial development. Some of these are complementary, some contradictory and overlapping, since this information must be inferred by studying observable behaviors.

One of the most widely accepted theories at the present time is Erikson's theory of developmental tasks. Erikson has suggested that there are eight basic stages in the human life span; each stage carries with it certain tasks arising from the problems and conflicts encountered as one proceeds from infancy with its swaddling clothes to old age with its fond memories. The eight stages identified by Erikson are infancy, early childhood, preschool age, middle childhood, adolescence, early adulthood, the middle years, and the later years.

The eight stages in the life span identified by Erikson and the developmental tasks accompanying each stage are shown in the table on page 19.

These stages are poignantly illustrated in the poem on the following page.

Maintaining Equilibrium

As an individual progresses through the life cycle, he must continuously adjust to changes both within himself and in his relationships with the world around him. His basic needs must be met, and at the same time, he must maintain his equilibrium in a constantly changing world.

Physiological Homeostasis. As we go about the daily business of living, changes are constantly occurring within the body as it adjusts to the demands we make upon it. Our temperature rises, for example, during our waking hours and

what do you see, nurse?

What do you see nurse, what do you see?
What are you thinking when you look at me?
A crabbit old woman, not very wise,
Uncertain of habit, with far away eyes,
Who dribbles her food, and makes not reply,
When you say in a loud voice, "I do wish you'd try!"
Who seems not to notice the things that you do,
And forever is losing a stocking or shoe.
Who, unresisting or not, lets you do as you will
With bathing and feeding, the long day to fill.
Is that what your thinking, is that what you see?
Then open your eyes, you're not looking at me.
I'll tell you who I am as I sit here so still,
As I move at your bidding, as I eat at your will.
I am a small child of ten with a father and a mother,
Brothers and sisters who love one another.
A young girl at sixteen with wings at her feet
Dreaming that soon now a lover she'll meet.
A bride soon at twenty, my heart gives a leap,
Remembering the vows that I promised to keep.
At twenty-five now I have young of my own
Who need me to build a secure happy home.
A woman of thirty, my young now grow fast,
Bound to each other with ties that should last.
At forty my young now soon will be gone,
But my man stays beside me to see I don't mourn.
At fifty once more babies play around my knee,
Again we know children, my loved one and me.
Dark days are upon me, my husband is dead,
I look at the future, I shudder with dread,
For my young are all busy rearing young of their own
And I think of the years and the love I have known.
I'm an old lady now and nature is cruel,
'Tis her jest to make old age look like a fool.
The body it crumbles, grace and vigor depart,
And now there is a stone where I once had a heart.
But inside this old carcase a young girl still dwells,
And now and again my battered heart swells.
I remember the joys, I remember the pain,
And I am loving and living life over again.
I think of the years all too few, gone so fast,
And accept the stark fact that nothing can last.
So open your eyes, nurse, open and see,
Not a crabbit old woman, look closer, see Me.   Anonymous

It has been reported that this poem was found with the belongings of an elderly lady who died in a nursing home in Ireland.

(From *Journal of Gerontological Nursing*, 2:26, June 1976.)

STAGES IN THE HUMAN LIFE CYCLE, AS IDENTIFIED BY ERIKSON*

Age	Stage	Developmental Tasks

Birth–1½ years	Infancy	Mother-child adjustment
		Create experience:
		    learn to take solid foods
		    learn to walk
		    learn to talk

1½–3 years	Early childhood	Seek independence
		Acquire muscular and neuromuscular control
		Learn to control elimination
		Form concepts to describe reality
		Form conscience:
		    differentiate between right and wrong
		    acquire sense of modesty

3–6 years	Preschool age	Form basic concepts division: reality/fantasy Acquire muscular control Peer associations Establish social role
6–11 years	Middle childhood	Learn autonomy Develop and refine neuromuscular skills Acquire concepts distinction between inner and outer self and world Learn cooperation, self-control Acquire social role and skills Form values, judgment
11–18 years	Adolescence	Accept new physique Achieve independence from adults Achieve close peer relations Achieve social role based on sex Learn social responsibility Form abstract concepts Form system of moral values and ethics Prepare for marriage and family life Prepare for a career
18–35 years	Early adulthood	Choose a career Choose a mate Manage a home Start a family Raise children Assume social responsibility Adapt to new social life Form philosophy of life
35–65 years	Middle years	Adjust to physiological changes Assist children to independence Adjust to aging parents Attain satisfactory level of productivity Develop leisure activities
65 years–death	Later years	Adjust to aging process Adjust to invalidism Adjust to retirement Adjust to reduced income Adjust to death of spouse Adapt social role to new situation

*Erikson, Erik H.: *Childhood and Society.* New York, W. W. Norton and Company, 1963.

falls again during sleep. The heart beats faster when we exercise and returns to a lower rate when we rest. Our muscles alternately tense and relax as we engage in various activities. In fact, an infinite number of minor adjustments are continuously being made in the body during the normal process of daily living. However, these adjustments must be kept within certain limits if the individual is to survive.[14] As you proceed with your studies, you will notice that normal ranges have been established for body temperature, for blood pressure, for pulse rate, for the amount of sugar in the bloodstream—in fact, for all of the body processes that are measurable. Deviations outside the normal range usually indicate that the body's internal equilibrium, that is, its physiological homeostasis, has been disturbed.

Environmental Equilibrium. Just as the body must maintain a certain consistency in its internal environment, the human organism must also achieve a balance in its interactions with the surrounding environment. Man's environment is made up of two components: the physical environment, which consists of the natural elements as well as the structures that man has built upon the earth, and the social environment, that is, the people around him and the society in which he lives.

ECOLOGICAL EQUILIBRIUM. Man has learned both to adapt himself to the physical environment and to change that environment to suit his needs. In a cold climate, for example, his basal metabolic rate increases in order to maintain his body temperature at a constant level; he eats more energy-giving foods and he wears warm clothing to protect himself from the cold. But man also modifies the environment to meet his requirements. Depending on the climate, he either builds a well insulated home and installs central heating, so that immediate surroundings are suited to his needs, or designs a well ventilated house and puts in air conditioning (if he can afford to do so). In some climates, he may need central heating for the winter and air conditioning for the summer.

There are, however, many aspects of man's interaction with the physical environment that are currently giving cause for concern. There is renewed interest in the subject of *ecology*, as the study of man's relationship with the environment is called. Many people fear that the delicate balance between man and nature is being disturbed: for example, by nuclear

---

[14]Donald Oken: Stress—Our Friend, Our Foe. In *Blueprint for Health.* Vol. 25. Chicago, The Blue Cross Association, 1974.

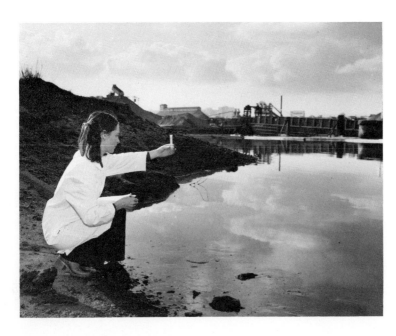

Good water is pure water. A sample of this water will be analyzed for pollutants that could endanger the health of people who will live in the housing development being built across the bay.

explosions, which alter atmospheric conditions, by the pollution of our lakes and rivers, which creates unsanitary living conditions, and by the rapid diminishment of many of our natural resources, to name but a few of the concerns of ecologists.

PSYCHOSOCIAL.   Then, there is the social environment. Man is a social animal and contact with other human beings is essential to his well-being. He is constantly interacting with his family, his friends, his neighbors, the people he meets at work or at school — in fact, with all of the people who inhabit his social world. Most of us have learned to achieve a balance in our relationships with other people, so that our psychosocial equilibrium remains intact. We have learned to use emotional outlets when stress becomes too great. We may use strenuous physical exercise, for example, to get rid of tensions caused by an unpleasant day with people at work. Or, we may go to a movie to forget our troubles with the family temporarily.

In discussing health and illness, it is impossible categorically to separate physiological homeostasis from ecological equilibrium or from psychosocial equilibrium. Each affects the others. A business executive, for example, may be under considerable pressure at work — in his psychosocial environment, if you like — but the ulcer he develops indicates a resultant disturbance in his physiological equilibrium. On the other hand, when a person is physically ill, his relationships with people undergo a change. You have probably found when you had a bad cold or the flu that you did not want to be bothered with other people. The physical environment, too, affects not only a person's physiological state but also his psychosocial equilibrium. A lack of adequate housing, for example, can be a major factor in both physical and mental illness.

STRESS AND STRESSORS

Stresses of any kind upset the delicate balance of the human organism, which reacts by altering certain structures, pro-

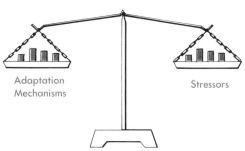

In homeostasis the body attempts to restore a state of equilibrium by counterbalancing the effect of stressors with adaptation mechanisms.

cesses, or behaviors to restore equilibrium. A person may perspire profusely on a very warm day, for example; he then becomes thirsty and increases his fluid intake to restore the fluids he has lost through sweating. The term "stressor" is used to designate any factor that disturbs the organism's equilibrium. There are a number of ways of categorizing stressors. They may be classified on the basis of whether they are internal or external, or as biological, psychosocial, or environmental (referring to the physical environment). Freeman has suggested four categories of stressors that would seem to be logical and to encompass all types of disturbances that may act as stressors:[15]

1. Deprivational stress
2. Stresses of excess
3. Stresses created by change
4. Stresses of intolerance

In *deprivational stress*, there is a lack of some essential factor for the well-being of the individual. Deprivational stressors, then, would include the lack of essential items needed to maintain the chemical balance of the body, such as the lack of water, of oxygen, of vitamins, or of food elements — in essence, a lack of any of the basic physiological needs mentioned earlier. Other types of deprivational stress might be psychological or sociological in nature. A person who is isolated from contact with other human beings suffers con-

[15]Victor J. Freeman: Human Aspects of Health and Illness: Beyond the Germ Theory. In *A Sociological Framework for Patient Care* by Jeanette R. Folta and Edith S. Deck (eds.). New York, John Wiley and Sons, Inc., 1966, pp. 83–89.

siderable stress. The lack of sufficient parental affection in infancy and early childhood is felt to be not only one of the causes of psychological disorders but also, as mentioned previously, a factor in an infant's failure to thrive. Lack of adequate housing, again a basic need, is an environmental factor that could be considered a deprivational stressor.

On the other hand, an *excess* of certain factors may also disturb the organism's equilibrium. Exposure to intense heat causes tissue damage in the form of a burn; intense cold causes frostbite. If a person eats excessively, he usually has disturbances of body functioning; he becomes obese and may suffer from gastrointestinal upsets and other types of physiological disturbances. His interpersonal relationships are affected, and he is usually unhappy because he is fat.

Excessive interpersonal contact may also be a source of stress, as in a family situation where individual members have no opportunity to get off by themselves

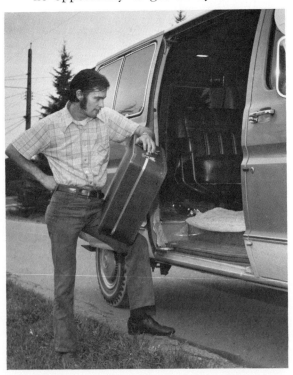

Stress wears many faces. As this young man wonders where to put all the luggage he is probably unaware of the many stressful situations yet to be encountered on the family vacation.

every once in a while, or in high density residential areas in a city where the neighbors seem to be constantly impinging on the privacy of one another. (The reverse is often quite true, of course, also; one can be very lonely in a crowded city if one does not have friends or close human contact.)

Changes of any sort may upset the physiological processes of the body as well as an individual's behavior. Even the time change exprienced by international travelers creates stress, and an individual may take several days to become adjusted to a different "time clock" for the normal body functions of eating, sleeping, and elimination. A number of studies in recent years have shown evidence of a positive relationship between the number of changes in a person's life and his subsequent development of illness. The amount of stress created by different types of change has been assessed for its impact on a person's health, and rating scales have been developed to calculate a person's vulnerability to illness on the basis of the number of major changes in his life in a one-year span of time. The death of a spouse is usually considered to be the change causing the greatest disturbance in a person's life. Other stressful events include losing one's job, changing jobs, moving from one part of the country to another, or even from one neighborhood to another, and changes in one's lifestyle. Happy events, such as marriages, getting a promotion, taking a vacation, and even Christmas, also bring their stresses. If a person has too many changes in his life in too short a period of time, he becomes a likely candidate for major illness.[16]

Stresses of intolerance are exemplified in the allergic reactions to certain foods, chemical substances, or pollens from which many people suffer. The body's reaction to poisons or toxins would also illustrate this point. If one eats food that has "gone bad," the body attempts to remove the substance, frequently by vomiting the stomach's contents. An intoler-

---

[16]Thomas H. Holmes and T. Stephenson Holmes: How Change Can Make Us Ill. In *Blueprint for Health.* Vol. 25. Chicago, The Blue Cross Association, 1974.

ance to psychological factors in the environment, such as an unhappy work situation, is also a source of stress. Moving to a different country where customs and social values are markedly different from those one has been accustomed to may cause stress sufficient to result in what is called cultural shock. Nurses working with minority groups in our own country or in poverty neighborhoods may experience some of this cultural shock when they encounter customs and ways of life that are different from their own.

THE BODY'S REACTION TO STRESS: ADAPTATION MECHANISMS

The nineteenth century French biologist Claude Bernard is credited with first pointing out the body's need to maintain a certain consistency in its internal environment. He described the process of physiological homeostasis, although he himself did not use the term. It was Walter Cannon, an American physiologist of the twentieth century, who coined the word "homeostasis." Cannon wrote of the "wisdom of the body" in bringing into play certain mechanisms if changes in its internal environment threaten to go beyond safe limits.[17] These are frequently referred to as "adaptation mechanisms"; they are the body's counterbalances, in other words.

For example, if body temperature threatens to go too high, the individual usually becomes very flushed and breaks out into a profuse sweat. Both of these reactions are attempts on the body's part to lower its internal temperature. Increased circulation to the tissues underlying the skin (which causes the appearance of flushing) helps to expose more blood to the cooling effects of the surrounding atmosphere. The perspiration from the profuse sweating evaporates on the surface of the skin and, in the process, also helps to carry heat away from the body. The body has a number of adaptation mechanisms, and

[17]Walter B. Cannon: *The Wisdom of the Body.* New York, W. W. Norton and Company, Inc., 1939.

we will be discussing many of these in later chapters of this text in conjunction with specific body processes.

The General Adaptation Syndrome

Hans Selye, a professor at the University of Montreal, was also interested in the body's reactions to disturbances in its equilibrium and pointed out that there is a general nonspecific response that occurs. He described this originally as the phenomenon of "just being sick" and later elaborated on it in his theory of the general adaptation syndrome (G.A.S.). This syndrome, he believed, is the response of the body to any agent that causes physiological stress. The response may be divided into three stages: the alarm reaction, in which the body's defense mechanisms are mobilized; the stage of resistance, when the battle for equilibrium is most active; and the stage of exhaustion, which occurs if the stressor is severe enough, or is present over a long enough period of time, to deplete the body's resources for adaptation.

The early signs and symptoms of disease are remarkably the same for many illnesses; this was Selye's original "just being sick" phenomenon. These symptoms usually include a slight rise in temperature, a loss of energy, a lack of interest in food, and a general feeling of malaise. It is in the second stage of the syndrome, the "stage of resistance," that the signs and symptoms of the body's reaction to specific disorders are seen: the rash erupts on the skin of the child with measles, or the localized pain in the chest and difficulty in breathing occur in pneumonia. If the stress is not relieved, or if it is of sufficient intensity to cause extensive damage to tissues, the body's adaptive mechanisms may not be able to restore equilibrium and exhaustion will set in.

The Local Adaptation Syndrome

In addition to the generalized reaction that occurs in the body as a result of stress, localized reactions occur when a specific part or organ is affected. Probably the most common example of a localized reaction is inflammation, which represents an attempt on the part of the body to barricade or "wall off" a particular section that has been damaged to prevent the spread of the harm-producing agent to other healthy sections of the body. Thus, if you prick your finger with an infected needle, you will probably soon have a swollen, painful finger. The finger may be very uncomfortable, but the localization of the inflammation is useful in that it helps to prevent the infection from entering the blood stream and traveling to other parts of the body.[18]

Selye called this local reaction the "local adaptation syndrome" (L.A.S.). It follows the same three-stage pattern as the G.A.S. First, there is a generalized reaction—the whole hand becomes slightly reddened and a little swollen. This is followed by a more localized reaction in the specific finger, which becomes very painful, reddened, and swollen. The inflammation will gradually subside unless the infection is sufficiently potent to overcome the defenses marshaled to stop it. In the latter case, it will surmount the "barricade" and travel up the arm, spreading to other parts of the body.

Reactions to Psychosocial Stressors

Although much of the early work on stress was related to the body's reactions to physiological stressors, there is now positive evidence that stress created by psychological or social factors will also cause physiological damage to the body, as in the case of the business executive discussed previously who developed an ulcer as a result of pressures at work.

One well-known response involving physiological reactions to psychological stress is the flight-fight reaction first described by Cannon. This reaction represents the body's response to immediate danger and is called forth whenever the

individual is frightened or feels threatened by harm. There is an emergency mobilization of the body's physiological defense mechanisms as the body prepares for instant action (either fight or flight). This, too, is an alarm reaction, but of a different sort from that described by Selye in his G.A.S. When a person is frightened, his heart beats more forcefully and faster; his breathing is increased in rate and depth; blood is withdrawn from surface vessels and the viscera and is shunted to the muscles; the unneeded gastrointestinal tract goes into a temporary slow-down; blood pressure increases, and the muscles become tense in preparation for action. This is the body's emergency mechanism, designed to protect the individual from real or imagined danger. Anxiety, which is a modified form of fear, usually accompanies people to a health agency, and the nurse will often note manifestations of the flight-fight reactions in her patients. She will probably also note them in herself, particularly when she is in new and unfamiliar surroundings or has to do a treatment for the first time. Helping the patient to become familiar with the physical surroundings and providing him with an explanation of routines and procedures in the particular agency will help to allay many of his fears. Fear of the unknown is one of the main sources of anxiety for most people. Nurses tend to become so accustomed to the environment of the agency in which they work that they often forget that everything may be strange and frightening for the patient. (The subject of anxiety is discussed in Chapter 12.)

PSYCHOLOGICAL DEFENSE MECHANISMS

Another level of response to stress is seen in the adaptive defense mechanisms we use to maintain psychosocial equilibrium. These are often referred to as "mental mechanisms" because they represent intellectual processes, or changes, in thought behavior; we use them to protect ourselves from stressors that threaten our self-esteem. If a person is frustrated in his attempts to fulfill his basic needs, he

---

[18] Hans Selye: Stress and the Nation's Health. In the *Proceedings of the National Conference on Fitness and Health, Ottawa, December 4, 5 and 6, 1972.* Department of National Health and Welfare, Canada.

usually becomes angry and may retaliate with aggression toward the person or object that is thwarting his goal-attainment. Open aggression toward other people is not generally acceptable in our society, and by the time a person has reached adulthood, he has usually learned to control his hostility. Adults seldom attack people in a physical sense, as children often do, but they resort to more subtle forms of aggression (such as verbal attacks) against the person or group of persons blocking their goal-attainment.

If a person fails to gain his objective on the first attempt, he may try again, fighting a little harder this time or seeking alternative means to achieve the same goal. A person who wants to be an executive in his company, for example, may not get the coveted job on first application. He may then decide that he needs to prepare himself better and enrolls in night classes to improve his chances the next time. Or, he may decide to use every means at his disposal, fair or unfair, to make sure that he gets promoted the next time there is an opening in the executive ranks. Alternatively, of course, he may decide to quit the field and move to a different company, or else to settle for a less prestigious position in the same company.

If a person has used socially unacceptable means to achieve his goals—for example, the executive who has ridden roughshod over others to reach the top—or if he has failed to achieve his goals either by withdrawing from the field completely or by accepting a lesser, more achievable goal, he must somehow protect his self-esteem so that he can continue to live with himself. In order to make his behavior acceptable to himself and to others, he frequently makes use of defense mechanisms.

One of the most commonly used defense mechanisms is *rationalization,* in which a person gives socially acceptable reasons for his behavior. A student who goes to a movie, for example, instead of staying in to study for exams, may rationalize his behavior by explaining to himself (and to others) that, after all, everyone needs a little relaxation. If he later gets angry at the teacher for not giving him what he considers a high enough grade,

he may not be able to express his hostility directly at the teacher. Instead, he may become annoyed with his best friend, or go home and take his anger out on his parents. This is a form of *displacement,* in which aggressive feelings are not directed at the offending person (or object), but are shifted to a substitute; it has often been called the "kick the cat" phenomenon. Another example to illustrate this very common defense mechanism is the man who has had a frustrating day at the office and is angry with his boss. He may, on arriving home, yell at his wife for not having dinner ready, or swear at a child's tricycle that is in his path. If the hostility is frequently directed at one particular person or group of people, it is called *scapegoating.* In a family situation, there is often one member, child or adult, who usually bears the brunt of the other members' anger. He, or she, is the family scapegoat.

Oftentimes, we ascribe our own unacceptable feelings or attitudes to other peo-

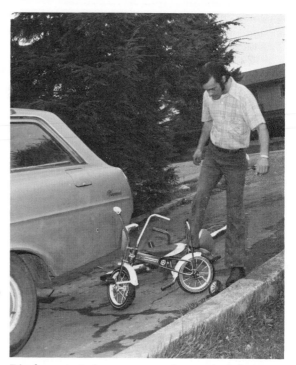

Displacement is a commonly used defense mechanism. A child's tricycle becomes the object on which this young father vents the anger and hostility he would probably like to direct at his employer after a frustrating day at work.

ple. A person may say that so and so is very ambitious or doesn't want any members of such and such a minority group in his neighborhood, when in actual fact these are his own feelings that he dares not admit to himself. This is called *projection* and is another form of defense mechanism by which we protect our feelings of self-worth.

When people cannot achieve their own goals, they may tend to identify themselves with someone who has. They may adopt his form of dress or his mannerisms and suffer acute distress when their idol is attacked. Children, of course, identify with parents of the same sex as themselves, and this is a necessary part of their development. Students, too, on their way to goal achievement, will frequently select one particular teacher or practitioner in their field as an example of the person they want to become when they graduate, and they try to model themselves upon the image they have of this person. *Identification*, like the other defense mechanisms we use, is not necessarily a bad thing; it is often a help in goal achievement, as long as it is not carried to extreme.

Compensation can also be a constructive defense mechanism. In this mechanism we attempt to make up for real or imagined inferiorities by becoming highly competent in a sphere of endeavor different from the one in which we feel we are not good, or sometimes in the same sphere. The child who has poor motor coordination and does badly at sports in his early school years, perhaps because of his growth pattern, may compensate by becoming a "bookworm" and subsequently a high achiever in the academic field. Alternatively, he may feel that he has to make good at sports whatever the cost in time and energy, and he will then practice night and day until he overcomes his physical problems and becomes skilled at some form of sports. He may choose a highly individualized sport where he can develop his skills at his own rate, and become an expert tennis player, Ping-Pong champion, or long distance runner, for example. Or he may become a physical education teacher with an unconscious (or expressed) desire to help children with problems similar to the ones he had.

When we have feelings or desires that we cannot accept consciously, or when we encounter problems that we do not feel capable of resolving, there are a number of defense mechanisms we use to deal with the situation. We may deny that we have the forbidden motive or problem and unconsciously refuse to acknowledge that it is there, in which case we are using *denial.* We may state, for example, "I would never do that sort of thing," when we may subconsciously be tempted to do just that (whatever it is). A person's first reaction on learning that he has a serious health problem may be to deny that the words he is hearing are true. He does not have venereal disease—he could not possibly—the laboratory has mixed up the test results. Sometimes the denial persists for a long time, and the person has to work through his acceptance of the diagnosis before he will undergo treatment.

At times, a person may attempt to remove a subconscious, and forbidden, motive or desire by vigorously attacking it. Witness the ex-smoker who soundly denounces the evils of smoking to those who still indulge. Then there is the person who jokes about unacceptable feelings, for example, fear, thereby giving the impression that only the weak are afraid—he certainly is not. Such behaviors as proclaiming too loudly against other people's sins and temptations and joking about unacceptable feelings or actions are termed *reaction formation.*

Socially unacceptable motives are, however, often channeled into acceptable forms of behavior. This is called *sublimation,* and we have mentioned it already in connection with the basic sex drive, which may be sublimated by an individual channeling all his energies into career advancement, to use one example. A person may sublimate his strong aggressive feelings by participating in sports where these feelings are acceptable; he can kick the football as hard as he likes and attack his opponents physically, within the rules of the game, of course.

When we have problems that we cannot resolve or experiences we would prefer to forget, we may unconsciously put them out of our mind; this is called *repression.* We forget all about the appointment we do not want to keep, or completely, and without knowing we are doing so, eliminate from our minds all memory of unpleasant events. This has sometimes been called the "old oaken bucket" phenomenon, from the lyrics in which the songwriter describes the fond memories of his childhood; the unpleasant ones for most of us are fortunately removed from our memory by the subconscious mechanism of repression. If, however, we consciously decide to forget about something, the behavior is called *suppression.* Like Scarlett O'Hara in *Gone With the Wind,* we decide that we will not think about that unpleasant thing until tomorrow.

Most of us also use *fantasy* in the form of daydreaming to escape temporarily from the realities of our everyday problems. In fantasy we can indulge our secret desires, achieve our goals, and forget our troubles. Daydreaming can, of course, be very productive. When lost in reverie, we may work out the solution to an impossible problem, or develop long-range plans to achieve our goals; sometimes it is very difficult to separate thoughtful reverie from daydreaming.

On occasion, in attempting to reach our goals, we may revert to a form of behavior that was acceptable at one stage of our development but is no longer considered appropriate. The expression "you are acting like a child" succinctly describes this type of mental mechanism, which is called *regression* in technical terminology. People, when they are ill, are often forced to sacrifice their independence in regard to caring for themselves; having to have someone else do for them the things they are accustomed to doing, such as feeding or bathing themselves, is often seen as a form of regression to an earlier dependent stage of their development.

Psychological defense mechanisms serve a useful purpose. They help to reduce the anxieties caused by conflicts or frustration in our attempts to fulfill basic needs; they help us to maintain our equilibrium. It is only when they are overused, or used inappropriately, that illness ensues. As with other disturbances of functioning, abnormalities in the use of defense mechanisms may be viewed as quantitative changes that blend imperceptibly into one another and into the normal as discussed earlier on page 20.

STUDY VOCABULARY		
Adaptation mechanism	Illness	
Basic need	Inflammation	
Compensation	Local adaptation syndrome	
Cultural shock	Optimal health	
Denial	Physiological homeostasis	
Deprivational stress	Projection	
Developmental tasks	Psychological defense mechanism	
Disease	Psychosocial equilibrium	
Displacement	Rationalization	
Ecology	Reaction formation	
Environmental equilibrium	Regression	
Fantasy	Repression	
Flight-fight reaction	Scapegoating	
General adaptation syndrome	Self-esteem	
Health	Stressor	
Holism	Sublimation	
Homeostasis	Suppression	
Identification		

STUDY SITUATION   Mr. Albert is a 45 year old clerk in a large department store. He has suffered from asthma since early childhood. He and his wife live in a modest bungalow in a working class neighborhood. They have no children, but keep two budgies as pets. Mr. Albert's hobby is growing roses, which he exhibits at the local Horticultural Society's annual show. He has won second prize the last two years in succession. The next show is in June this year. Mrs. Albert is a thin, nervous woman who does not work outside the home. She is an immaculate housekeeper and appears to be a devoted wife, catering to her husband's every whim. Mr. Albert is frequently off work because of his asthma.

Mr. Albert arrived at the Community Health Center one afternoon toward the end of May, saying that he was too ill to work and wanted to see the doctor immediately. He appeared agitated and his breathing was labored. On being told that the doctor was busy and he would have to wait, Mr. Albert became very hostile to the nurse, telling her that he was a very sick man and needed to see the doctor right away, whereupon he collapsed at the nurse's feet.

1. What factors would you take into consideration in determining Mr. Albert's optimal level of health?
2. Which, if any, of Mr. Albert's basic needs do you think are not being met?
3. What factors do you think might be causing stress to Mr. Albert?
4. How would you categorize these factors?
5. Is Mr. Albert showing any signs of the general adaptation syndrome?
6. Is Mr. Albert exhibiting any defense mechanisms? If so, what are they?
7. Can you identify any signs of the flight-fight reaction in Mr. Albert?

SUGGESTED READINGS

Andersen, M. D., and J. M. Pleticha: Emergency Unit Patients' Perceptions of Stressful Life Events. *Nursing Research, 23*:378–383, September/October, 1974.

A New Perspective on the Health of Canadians. A Working Document. Ottawa, Department of National Health and Welfare, April, 1974.

Archer, S. E., and R. Fleshman: *Community Health Nursing: Patterns and Practices.* North Scituate, Massachusetts, Duxbury Press, 1975.

Bourne, Lyle E., Jr., and Bruce R. Ekstrand: *Psychology: Its Principles and Meanings.* Hinsdale, Illionis, The Dryden Press, 1973.

Cannon, Walter B.: *The Wisdom of the Body.* New York, W. W. Norton and Company, Inc., 1939.

Dunn, Halburt L.: High Level Wellness for Man and Society. In *A Sociological Framework for Patient Care* by Jeanette R. Folta and Edith S. Deck (eds). New York, John Wiley and Sons, Inc., 1965, pp. 213–219.

Erikson, Erik H.: *Childhood and Society.* New York, W. W. Norton and Company, 1963.

Freman, Victor J.: Human Aspects of Health and Illness: Beyond the Germ Theory. In *A Sociological Framework for Patient Care* by Jeanette R. Folta and Edith S. Deck (eds.). New York, John Wiley and Sons, Inc., 1965, pp. 83–89.

Havighurst, Robert J.: *Developmental Tasks and Education.* New York, David McKay Company, Inc., 1972.

Holmes, Thomas H., and T. Stephenson Holmes: How Change Can Make Us Ill. In *Bluprint for Health.* Vol. 25. Chicago, The Blue Cross Association, 1974.

Kalish, R. A.: *The Psychology of Human Behavior.* Belmont, California, Wadsworth Publishing Company, 1966.

Levine, M. E.: Holistic Nursing. *Nursing Clinics of North America, 6*:253–264, June, 1971.

Luckmann, Joan, and Karen C. Sorensen: *Medical-Surgical Nursing: A Psychophysiologic Approach.* Philadelphia, W. B. Saunders Company, 1974.

Marlow, Dorothy R.: *Textbook of Pediatric Nursing.* Fourth edition. Philadelphia, W. B. Saunders Company, 1973.

McHugh, Paul R.: Psychological Illness in Medical Practice. In *Textbook of Medicine* (fourteenth edition) by Paul B. Beeson and Walsh McDermott. Philadelphia, W. B. Saunders Company, 1975, p. 562.

Michaels, D. R.: Too Much in Need of Support to Give Any? *American Journal of Nursing,* 71:1932–1935, October, 1971.

Mills, J. G.: Primary Health Care. Report of the Sub-committee on Primary Health Care, submitted to the Council of Medical Services of the Canadian Medical Association, 1973. (As reprinted in the *Report of the Alberta Task Force on Nursing Education.* Alberta, Department of Advanced Education and Manpower, September, 1975.)

Munsinger, Harry: *Fundamentals of Child Development.* New York, Holt, Rinehart and Winston, Inc., 1975.

Murray, Ruth, and Judith Zentner: *Nursing Assessment and Health Promotion Through the Lifespan.* Englewood Cliffs, N.J., Prentice-Hall, 1975.

Oelbaum, Cynthia H.: Hallmarks of Adult Wellness. *American Journal of Nursing,* 74:1623–1625, September, 1974.

Oken, Donald: Stress—Our Friend, Our Foe. In *Blueprint for Health.* Vol. 25. Chicago, The Blue Cross Association, 1974.

Peterson, M. H.: Understanding Defense Mechanisms. Programmed Instruction. *American Journal of Nursing,* 72:1651–1674, September, 1972.

Robinson, Lisa: Adjustment and Defense Mechanisms. In *Psychiatric Nursing as a Human Experience.* Philadelphia, W. B. Saunders Company, 1972, pp. 47–56.

Selye, Hans: Stress and the Nation's Health. In the *Proceedings of the National Conference on Fitness and Health, Ottawa, December 4, 5 and 6, 1972.* Ottawa, Department of National Health and Welfare, Canada.

Spring, Faye, E.: *Man: A Holistic Conception for Nursing.* Pilot project final report. Published by the Frances Payne Bolton School of Nursing, Case Western Reserve University, 1969.

Sutterley, Doris C., and Gloria F. Donnelly: *Perspectives in Human Development: Nursing Throughout the Lifecycle.* Philadelphia, J. B. Lippincott Company, 1973.

3 THE PERCEPTION OF HEALTH AND ILLNESS

The nurse should be able to:

Describe differences in the way people view health and illness
Explain factors influencing a person's perception of his health
    status
Discuss the role of folk medicine in health care in North America
    today
Name the three stages of illness
Describe reactions of patients in each of these three stages
Identify some of the needs of patients during each of these stages
Describe ways in which the nurse may help to meet these needs
Describe the impact of illness on the family

INTRODUCTION

People, of course, do not usually think of their health in the scientific terms we have used in the previous chapter. Most people are aware, however, when they are functioning at their highest level mentally, physically, and socially, and they usually know when they are sick—by standards they have established for themselves. Because every person is a unique individual, each interprets his health and illness status according to his or her own particular perspective.

These personal perspectives are, however, considerably influenced by social and cultural factors, and in assessing an individual's health, it is important to understand the social context in which he lives. All societies, as well as subgroups within these societies, have certain norms, or standards, with regard to health and illness. In some cultures, for example, obesity is considered a healthy and desirable state, whereas in others it is regarded as an affliction.

The customs, traditions, and mores of a society also dictate acceptable behaviors in regard to health and illness. Individuals are expected to take all measures necessary, as approved by that society, to promote and protect their health. In most developed countries, for example, parents are expected to take their infants to the physician or to a well-baby clinic for regular checkups and to see that their children have all of the recommended immunizations to protect their health. We frown on parents who fail to have their children inoculated against typhoid fever, whooping cough, measles, poliomyelitis, and the other communicable diseases for which there are known immunity-producing agents.

When a person is ill, there are also acceptable and unacceptable standards of behaviors laid down by society. The sick person is expected to seek "appropriate" care to restore himself to a healthy state—be it witch doctor, shaman, nurse practitioner, or specialist physician. While ill, he is also expected to cooperate with those who are caring for him.

CRITERIA FOR JUDGING HEALTH AND ILLNESS

Everyone has his own standards for assessing the state of his health. In a study to determine differences in the attitudes of people toward health and illness, Baumann identified three distinct ways in which people establish criteria to judge their health status.[1] One was related to the presence or absence of symptoms. Pain is, of course, one of the most common symptoms by which people judge the state of their health. If a person has pain, particularly of a severe or persistent nature, he usually considers himself ill. Vomiting and fever are two other common symptoms that people usually consider indicative of illness.

A second method by which people judge the state of their health is by the way they feel: they feel "good," "on top

---

[1]Barbara Baumann: Diversities in Conceptions of Health and Physical Fitness. In *Social Interaction and Patient Care* by James K. Skipper, Jr., and Robert C. Leonard (eds.). Philadelphia, J. B. Lippincott Company, 1965, pp. 206–210.

of the world," or in "top form," as the British say; or they feel "so-so," they "don't feel well," they "feel poorly," or as Selye put it, they just "feel sick."

A third way of establishing the state of one's health is on the basis of performance. Often, the criteria used relate to the individual's ability to carry out his daily activities. One person may feel that his health is good if he can work all day and still have enough energy to play a round of golf or enjoy a game of bowling in the evening. Another may decide he is ill when he finds he cannot walk up a flight of stairs without experiencing acute distress in breathing.

Recently, another set of performance criteria for assessing health status has been gaining popularity in the Western world; these criteria relate to physical fitness testing. An individual can compare his results on certain tests of physical fitness with established norms for his age, sex, and body frame. He can, for example, find out from these tests whether he is carrying too much fatty tissue, whether his heart beat responds normally to exercise, whether his respiratory functioning is as good as it should be, and whether the strength of his muscles is above average, below average, or normal for his age, sex, and body build. Physical fitness

testing is also being used in conjunction with lifestyle information (such as alcohol consumption, smoking habits, and the like) to assess a person's vulnerability to such illnesses as heart trouble and respiratory problems.[2]

FACTORS INFLUENCING THE PERCEPTION OF HEALTH

The way a person views his health status tends to vary with a number of factors. Sociologists tell us that our norms for health and illness are determined as much by social and cultural factors as they are by clinical investigation.[3] A person's socioeconomic status influences the way he perceives his health, as does his level of educational attainment. The people who are making use of the physical fitness testing centers (and those who are out jog-

[2]H. N. Colburn and P. M. Baker: Health Hazard Appraisal—A Possible Tool in Health Protection and Promotion. *Canadian Journal of Public Health*, September/October, 1973. See also: Lewis C. Robbins and Jack H. Hall: *How to Practice Prospective Medicine*. Indianapolis, Indiana, Methodist Hospital of Indiana, 1970.

[3]E. Gartly Jaco (ed.): *Patients, Physicians and Illness*. Part III: Socio-cultural Aspects of Medical Care and Treatment. New York, The Free Press, 1967.

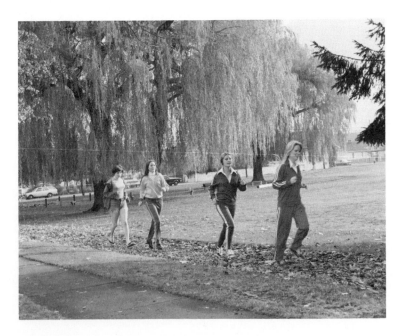

Nurses, like many other professionals, are concerned about the need to improve their own health. These young nurses are taking advantage of the recreational facilities of a park near their residence to improve their physical fitness.

ging around the park in the early morning hours) are, for the most part, the business executives and the professionals, the college professors and other teachers, and the well educated housewives. These people, too, are much more knowledgeable about the signs and symptoms of illness and are more inclined to seek the help of a health professional on the basis of symptoms than are people in lower socioeconomic brackets. Studies have shown that poor people are just as concerned over their health as people in higher socioeconomic brackets, but often poverty is associated with a lack of knowledge about health matters as well as, in some instances, a lack of accessibility to health care and, sometimes, a lack of trust in the prevailing health care system.[4]

Ethnic orientation is also a factor in how a person views his health. In both the United States and Canada, with their rich multicultural backgrounds, it is important to remember that beliefs about health and about ways of preventing and treating illness in other cultures do not always coincide with those of westernized medicine. One example, described in the report of a study on Chinese Americans, is the traditional Chinese belief in the forces of Yin and Yang, which are said to control nature and to control the body. Foods have inherent Yin and Yang properties, too, and may be used in the treatment of illness. Traditional Chinese medicine also makes extensive use of herb treatment and acupuncture.

Traditional cultural beliefs often persist through the first and second generations of new Americans or new Canadians. Thus, the grandmother who emigrated from a remote village in China some forty years ago may have completely different ideas about the care and feeding of children, and the treatment of childhood illnesses, from those of her well educated granddaughter who has gone to prospective parenthood classes in Vancouver or San Francisco (or in any other North American community).[5]

Another important factor to be considered is the individual's religious affiliation. Some religious sects believe in the total efficacy of prayer and do not believe in intervention by physicians or other health practitioners. One very common belief about the cause of illness is that the individual is being punished for his sins. This belief will, of course, affect a person's reaction to illness. He may feel guilty about being sick, or feel that he has to atone for his sins through suffering, and sometimes may feel that he does not deserve to get better.

Other factors also affect an individual's perception of his health status. Age, for example, has a great deal to do with it. Older people usually value health as one of the most important assets in life, but they do not expect to enjoy the same level of health as they did when they were younger. The community health nurse may have to persuade them to join in exercise programs designed to improve their physical fitness, because they may think they are too old to derive benefit from them. Many adolescents appear to be particularly concerned with their health and worry over every blemish on their skin.

In our stoical Western culture, men are not supposed to complain about pain as much as women are permitted to; hence, they may tend to negate the early signs and symptoms of illness. On the other hand, men are usually more concerned about maintaining their physical fitness than women are. They also appear to be more realistic in assessing their cardiovascular and respiratory functioning than do women.[6]

Situational factors also play a role in the perception of health. The mother in a family, for example, frequently does not become ill, even though one after another of the children, and father, take to their beds with a cold or influenza; she is too

---

[4]Margaret C. Olendzki: Concerns of the Consumer. Paper presented at the Conference on Education of Nurses for Public Health, May 23–25, 1973. In *Redesigning Nursing Education for Public Health, Report of the Conference, May 23–25, 1973.* Bethesda, Maryland, U.S. Department of Health, Education, and Welfare Publication No. (HRA) 75–75.

[5]T. Campbell and B. Chang: Health Care of the Chinese in America. *Nursing Outlook,* 21:245–249, April 1973.

[6]D. A. Bailey et al.: A Current View of Canadian Cardiorespiratory Fitness. *Journal of the Canadian Medical Association,* Vol. III, July 6, 1974.

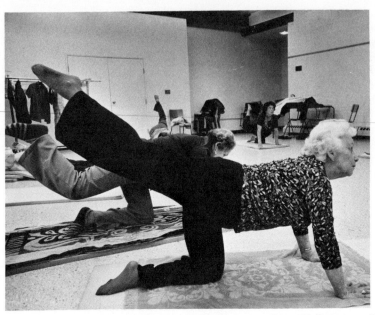

Physical fitness programs are available for people of all ages. These ladies are taking part in an exercise program for senior citizens at their local community center. Vancouver Sun photo. Used with permission.

busy looking after everyone else. Often, it is after a crisis is past that a person succumbs to illness, when the stresses and strains have subsided and the individual has time to rest.

THE LEGACY OF FOLK MEDICINE

The way a person views health and illness determines to a large extent the measures he will take to protect and improve his health and the type of care he seeks when he is ill. He is also influenced in this regard by the advice of his family and his friends. Studies in communication have shown that people are influenced more by the people around them, their friends, their family and individuals whose opinions they respect, than by any other means of communication. The person who feels in need of health care usually receives much advice on where to obtain it. He may elect to go to a physician or to a community health center, but he may also choose to seek help from any one of a number of nonmedical practitioners of the healing arts, such as herbalists, naturopaths, or spiritiual healers.

Although we pride ourselves on our sci-entific approach to health care in the Western World, the astounding sales record of numerous long-standing patent medicines attests to the prevalence of many widely held unscientific beliefs about the causes of illness and the methods of preventing and treating disease. If an individual is "liverish," has "tired blood," or has kidneys that need "flushing out," he can purchase a medicine in the drugstore professing to cure these conditions. Many women used to rely (and, indeed, a number still do) on tonics containing iron to cure their "women's ailments." While there may be some value in this, since women are more prone to be anemic than men are, it can hardly be considered a cure for everything that ails them.

Often, people attribute their illnesses to disturbances of the gastrointestinal tract; constipation, for example, has been cited as the cause of numerous illnesses, diabetes among them. Many people believe in the value of a good weekly purging of the gastrointestinal tract by means of a strong laxative. Currently, we seem to be in the midst of a cycle of food fads. A number of people are turning to vegetarianism, for instance, or the eating of a "macrobiotic" diet, while others subscribe to a belief in eating only organically grown foods.

The old wives' tales and guaranteed home remedies are still not far from the surface in scientific North America. One still sees the copper bracelet used to ward off rheumatism, or a clove of garlic worn around the neck to prevent colds.

THE STATE OF ILLNESS

Some people seek the advice of health professionals while believing or hoping that they are not ill, but the majority of people seeking such advice are concerned about their health and are aware that they are sick. Once a person makes the decision to obtain help he becomes a patient. As a patient he may or may not be restricted in his activities. Many people continue to carry on with their normal daily work and recreational activities even though they have an illness that requires medical supervision. People with hypertension (high blood pressure) or mild diabetes, for example, may only need to come into the physician's office or to the clinic for periodic checkups and consultation about their health problems unless complications develop. Other people who are ill may have to give up some of their usual activities but do not require hospitalization. They may, instead, be cared for in their own homes. Many sick people, however, do require the specialized care and services that are available in hospitals and other institutions on an inpatient basis.

In most cases, a person is considered to be sick by his family and friends when there is some restriction in his activities or when his illness necessitates taking precautions that interfere with a normal lifestyle. The individual may not be able to go to work or to school; he may be confined to bed; or he may not be able to undertake certain activities. There are certain expectations that go along with being sick. There is an implicit assumption on the part of others that the person who is ill requires care and cannot be expected to get better merely by an act of will. The sick person is usually excused from work while he is ill; he is not expected to fulfill all his social obligations, or even to carry out his normal functions within the family. However, the patient also has certain obligations. The state of being ill is considered undesirable in most cultures and the patient therefore has an obligation to want to get well. He is also expected to seek competent help to assist him in doing so, and to cooperate with those who provide this help.[7]

THE STAGES OF ILLNESS

In order to be able to provide the ill patient with the competent care and support he needs, the nurse should have an understanding of the various stages of illness. The patient, during the early stages of his illness, may require a considerable amount of psychological support to help him to accept his illness. When he is acutely ill, his physical needs and the therapeutic aspects of his care may predominate. As he is getting better, he may need the help of various members of the health team to assist him in his return to an active life insofar as he is able within the limitations imposed by his illness. Some patients, of course, do not get better, and they require comfort and supportive measures of a different nature (see Chapter 18).

It has been generally accepted that the experience of illness, insofar as the types of illness in which recovery is expected are concerned, consists of three stages: the initial, or transition, stage when the individual moves gradually (or sometimes abruptly) from a stage of health to a state of illness; the stage of "accepted" illness, when he may be acutely ill; and convalescence.[8]

---

[7]T. Parsons: Definitions of Health and Illness in the Light of American Values and Social Structure. In *Patients, Physicians and Illness* by E. G. Jaco. Glencoe, Illinois, The Free Press, 1958, pp. 165–187.

[8]Henry D. Lederer: How the Sick View Their World. In *Social Interaction and Patient Care* by James K. Skipper, Jr., and Robert C. Leonard. Philadelphia, J. B. Lippincott Company, 1965, pp. 155–167. Reprinted from the *Journal of Social Issues*, 8:4–15, 1952.

THE INITIAL STAGE OF ILLNESS

During the initial stage, the patient frequently remains in his home, although many people are admitted to hospital for investigation and undergo a series of diagnostic examinations as inpatients. During this period, the patient may experience many of the discomforts that Selye described as "just being sick" (see Chapter 2). He usually does not feel well; he may have distressing symptoms; and he often finds that he cannot keep up with his normal work load without tiring or, perhaps, cannot enjoy his usual leisure-time activities. He may not feel up to going bowling with his friends or participating in the Saturday night bridge game. People are usually irritable when they do not feel well. In women, this irritability may show itself in easy tears, which seem to come at the slightest provocation.

People react to the early signs of illness in a variety of ways. Some attempt to deny that they are ill and "keep going" despite their fatigue, or they may even try to do more than usual to prove to themselves that they are not really sick. Some people respond to the threat of illness with anger; others become very quiet and withdrawn. A few seem to enjoy their symptoms and the attention they receive from other people. If the individual subscribes to the belief that illness is a punishment, or knows that he has been transgressing some of the laws of health, he may feel guilty. Cigarette smokers, for example, are usually very self-conscious and guilt-ridden if they develop a cough or a chest condition. Often, people will try all the preventive measures they have heard of, and many of their family and friends' home remedies as well, before they seek professional advice.

By the time an individual has made a decision to seek professional help, he is usually quite worried. His first appointment in the office or the clinic is fraught with anxiety. He wants to know what is wrong with him, and he doesn't want to know. He would like to begin treatment, yet he may be afraid of what "they" are going to do to him. If he has to undergo diagnostic tests or be referred to a specialist for further examinations, his anxiety mounts and he awaits the final verdict with great trepidation. His fears are usually multiplied if he is told that his condition requires surgery or that he needs to be hospitalized for medical therapy. The hospital for most people is an unknown place; many people think of it as a place to die.

The attitude of the nurse in the physician's office or the clinic, and the initial contacts the patient has with the nurse who receives him in an inpatient facility, can do much to ease the patient through this difficult initial period of illness. Kindness and patience are essential. The patients who are most demanding and critical are usually the most frightened ones. Helping to allay their fears is a large part of the nurse's responsibility. The nurse who takes a personal interest in the patient and shows respect for him as an individual does a great deal to offset the depersonalization the patient so often feels in a busy health agency. Explaining treatments and procedures in simple terms, telling him the reason for them and what is going to be done, can take away much of his fear of the unknown. A knowledge of the routines and the physical environment of the agency will help the patient to feel more comfortable in his new situation (see Chapter 15).

THE STAGE OF ACCEPTED ILLNESS

In the second stage of illness, when a diagnosis (or a tentative one) has been made and therapy has been started, the patient begins to focus his attention and his energies on his illness. He is usually much concerned with his symptoms and wants to know what his temperature is and his blood pressure, and he anxiously awaits the outcome of tests and examinations. The interests of the sick person are usually narrowed; he is much more concerned with himself and with his immediate environment than with anything that goes on outside the sickroom.

The traditional patient role has been essentially a passive-dependent role; for example, the patient was expected to undergo prescribed treatments, often with

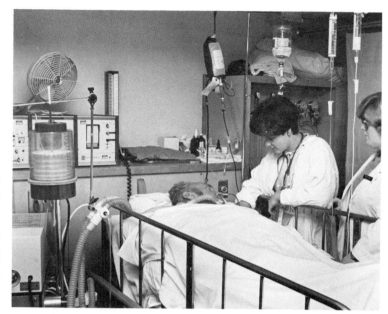

The acutely ill patient is often highly dependent on nursing personnel. This patient's recovery from anesthesia is being carefully monitored by nurses in the Postanesthetic Recovery Room of a large metropolitan hospital. (Courtesy of Vancouver General Hospital.)

little question. Such acceptance can be particularly difficult for the independent or aggressive person. The patient who has a minor illness may have less need to be dependent and may become critical and demanding.

Three factors contribute to the passive dependency of the patient. First, a person is usually weakened physically when he is ill; often he simply does not have the strength to carry out his normal activities. Second, the patient is under psychological stress (as well as physical) and so may be less able to cope with situations. The third factor comprises the expectations of health personnel, including nurses. Nurses usually expect a patient to act in a certain way and they communicate their expectations verbally and nonverbally. For example, the patient may be expected to accept a medicine without question.

Today there is much more emphasis on the participation of the patient as a member of the therapeutic team. He is being encouraged to participate in planning his care and in implementing the plan. It is important to create a climate in which this is possible. The patient needs to feel free to express his needs and wants, and to feel that his opinions are respected. When a person participates in planning his care and everything is done, not for him, but rather with him, he assumes more of the responsibility for the outcome. The degree and the type of active participation of a patient vary according to his needs. During the acute stage of an illness, the patient may be highly dependent on the nurse. He may need to be bathed or to have his position or dressing changed, or he may even need her help in maintaining vital body functions such as breathing, and the nurse is concerned with meeting the patient's dependency needs. It is important that each patient become increasingly independent and participate actively in his own care as he is able and as his need for dependence is decreased.

CONVALESCENCE

During the convalescent stage, the patient gradually leaves the sickroom and once again begins to move back into the ordinary everyday world. This is again a transition period and for many a difficult adjustment. The irritability of the conva-

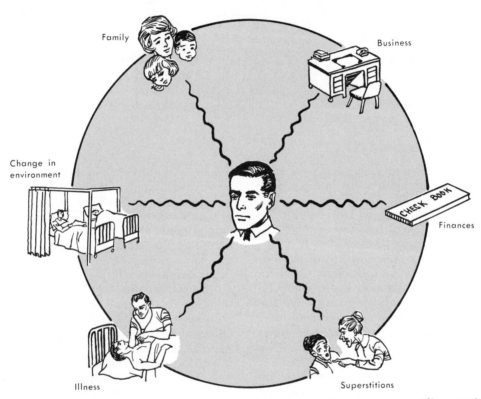

Anxiety usually accompanies illness; it is therefore a major consideration in providing nursing care.

lescent is well known. The attitude of nursing and other health personnel is important in providing the patient with the support and encouragement he requires at this time. Often the patient's family can be of much assistance. Convalescence may be prolonged in some people because they do not feel able to reassume the normal responsibilities from which illness excused them. They are often fearful of their ability to resume normal activities. Clear directions on how to care for themselves and simple explanations of what they may expect, combined with the reassurance that help is available if they need it, will often serve to relieve some of the anxiety attendant upon going home from a health agency.

THE IMPACT OF ILLNESS ON THE FAMILY

The illness of a family member has an impact on the total family. If the person who is sick is the breadwinner there is a natural concern about loss of his ability to maintain financial responsibility for the family; both he and the other family members may worry about how long he will be unable to work and the using up of sick leave from his place of employment. There may be additional concern over the costs of illness, the payment of medical and hospital bills, and the charges for diagnostic and therapeutic services. The head of the household may not be in a position to make decisions about family matters while he is ill; someone else may have to take over the responsibility for this.

When the mother in the family is sick, household routine is disrupted and other family members must take over the shopping, the planning and cooking of meals, the washing and the ironing. In our small nuclear families, the relatives who might have done this are often thousands of miles away, and the family may have to rely on friends or "homemaker services" to provide help.

If it is an older member of the family who is ill, there is usually much concern.

It may be the first member of the household to be seriously ill, and the family is reminded of the mortality of human life. There may be additional worries over who will care for the patient, and again the costs, particularly of prolonged illness, may be a matter to cause considerable concern.

When one of the children is sick, parents are usually very anxious. They may feel guilty of being in some way responsible for the child's illness. Often they feel helpless, and their anxiety and feelings of helplessness may be expressed in hostility and criticism directed toward those who are caring for the child. Many hospitals today permit open visiting on children's wards and encourage parents to share in the care of their children. If the nurse understands some of the reasons behind the parents' behavior and that of family members, and also realizes her own feelings about this behavior are normal, she is better able to accept hostility and criticism without showing anger and hostility in return.

When a person is hospitalized, his admission has many meanings for him and for his family. While he was ill at home, his care and the responsibility for it probably fell to other family members. After he enters a hospital, the responsibility for his care is transferred from the family to hospital personnel. This transfer of responsibility often produces emotions of mixed relief and guilt on the part of the family: relief because trained people will now provide professional care, and perhaps guilt because members of the family feel that the patient would be happier at home or that they have passed on responsibilities that they should be accepting as a family. These feelings are sometimes expressed verbally to hospital personnel or they may be expressed in activities such as bringing food to the patient or by criticizing the personnel and the institution. If the nurse recognizes the needs of family members and solicits their help in appropriate areas of patient care, such as assisting the patient to eat, the family will feel more comfortable and will be better able to assist in the patient's recovery.

STUDY VOCABULARY

Acute	Hypertension	Patient
Convalescence	Mortality	Transition
Dependency		

STUDY SITUATION

Mr. Lopez is a 34 year old man who emigrated from Mexico to California 15 years ago. He was born and raised in a small village, where he attended a school run by Catholic Sisters until the age of 13. He then worked as a migrant farm laborer until the time of his emigration. He now works as a truck driver for a large intercontinental van line. He has come to the doctor's office because his back has been bothering him and he finds it difficult to lift the heavy crates he carries in his truck. He also has pain when he drives for long periods. Mr. Lopez is married and has three small children. He asks whether he will have to go to the hospital.

1. What factors should be considered in assessing Mr. Lopez's perception of his health status?
2. For what reasons might Mr. Lopez be anxious?
3. What factors might affect how Mr. Lopez reacts to his illness if surgery is needed?
4. What are some of the implications of his illness and how might they affect his family?
5. What can the nurse do to help Mr. Lopez?

SUGGESTED READINGS

Anderson, G., and B. Tighe: Gypsy Culture and Health Care. *The American Journal of Nursing*, 73:282–285, February, 1973.

Bailey, D. A., et al.: A Current View of Canadian Cardiorespiratory Fitness. *Journal of the Canadian Medical Association*, Vol. III, July 6, 1974.

Baumann, Barbara: Diversities in Conceptions of Health and Physical Fitness. In *Social Interation and Patient Care* by James K. Skipper, Jr., and Robert C. Leonard (eds.): Philadelphia, J. B. Lippincott Company, 1965, pp. 206–210.

Brodnax, Suzanne: The Health of Young Adults in the Counterculture. *Nursing Clinics of North America*, 8:15–23, March, 1973.

Campbell, T., and B. Chang: Health Care of the Chinese in America. *Nursing Outlook*, 21:245–249, April, 1973.

Colburn, H. N., and P. M. Baker: Health Hazard Appraisal—A Possible Tool in Health Protection and Promotion. *Canadian Journal of Public Health*, September/October, 1973.

Folta, Jeanette R., and Edith S. Deck: *A Sociological Framework for Patient Care.* New York, John Wiley and Sons, Inc., 1966.

Jaco, E. Gartly (ed.): *Patients, Physicians and Illness.* New York, The Free Press, 1967. (Also see 1958 edition.)

LaFargue, J. P.: Role of Prejudice in Rejection of Health Care. *Nursing Research*, 21:53–58, January/February, 1972.

Lederer, Henry D.: How the Sick View Their World. In *Social Interaction and Patient Care* by James K. Skipper, Jr., and Robert C. Leonard (eds.). Philadelphia, J. B. Lippincott Company, 1965. Reprinted from the *Journal of Social Issues*, 8:4–15, 1952.

Perkins, Sister Mary Rose: Does Availability of Health Services Ensure Their Use? *Nursing Outlook,* 22:496–498, August, 1974.

Tyron, Phyllis, and Robert C. Leonard: Giving the Patient an Active Role. In *Social Interaction and Patient Care* by James K. Skipper, Jr., and Robert C. Leonard (eds.). Philadelphia, J. B. Lippincott Company, 1965, pp. 120–127.

Williams, F.: The Crisis of Hospitalization. *Nursing Clinics of North America,* 9:37–45, March, 1974.

4 HEALTH AND HEALTH PROBLEMS

The nurse should be able to:

Compare the nature of health problems in North America today
     with those at the beginning of the century
Discuss the biological, environmental, lifestyle, and health care
     factors affecting health
List the four principal health status indicators used in
     international comparisons
Explain the significance of these in assessing health conditions in
     a country
List the five leading causes of death in North America today
Discuss major causes of death and disability throughout the life
     span of people in North America.
Compare trends in mortality and morbidity in Middle and South
     America with those in North America
Identify sources of information the nurse may use to learn about
     factors affecting health and the principal health problems in a
     community
Describe how the nurse can go about gathering this information

HEALTH AND HEALTH PROBLEMS 4

INTRODUCTION

Good health is the bedrock on which social progress is built. A nation of healthy people can do those things which make life worthwhile and, as the level of health increases, so does the potential for happiness.[1]

So far, we have been talking about health as it pertains to the individual and, to a certain extent, the family. Nursing students at all levels, however, as well as students in the other health disciplines, need to be aware of the health status and the major health problems of people in the society in which they intend to practice.[2]

In all of the *developed* countries of the world, including the United States and Canada, there has been a marked improvement in health conditions since the turn of this century. Longevity has been increased dramatically, death rates have been drastically reduced, particularly among mothers and children, and the infectious diseases, with the exception of influenza/pneumonia and certain diseases of early infancy, have disappeared entirely from the lists of major causes of death.

Still, a large number of problems remain, and others have emerged, many as a result of the longer life span and the changing lifestyles of people in our society. Because people are living longer, more of them suffer from chronic and degenerative disorders that impose limitations on their way of life. Industrialization, increasing urbanization, and affluence have also contributed their share of health problems. The heightened tempo of life in our fast-moving world, alterations in family structure, and changing social values have created new stresses that affect our health. We are concerned, for example, about the alarming incidence of mental illness, of alcoholism and drug addiction, particularly among our young people, and of the premature loss of life resulting from accidents, suicide, and other acts of violence. We are also concerned about the respiratory problems aggravated by environmental pollution and by smoking, and about obesity and lack of exercise as contributing factors in many illnesses. Nor have we entirely eliminated the communicable diseases; the resurgence of the venereal diseases is currently a matter of major concern.

In many of the *developing* countries, longevity and mortality rates are still at about the same level as they were in the developed countries some 75 years ago. Infectious diseases continue to be a major problem in a large part of the world, and maternal and child death rates remain excessively high in the developing countries. Although remarkable progress has been made in many countries, the gap between the rich and the poor nations continues to be a matter of international concern. Even in countries where improvements in health have been considerable, such as our own, there is still a great difference in the health status of different segments of the population — between the rich and the poor, and between majority and minority ethnic groups.

The difference in health status between

---

[1] *A New Perspective on the Health of Canadians.* A Working Document. Ottawa, Department of National Health and Welfare, 1974, p. 5.

[2] Ruth R. Puffer and Carlos V. Serano: *Patterns of Mortality in Childhood.* Washington, D.C., Pan American Health Organization, 1973, p. 352.

43

people in the *developed* countries and people in the *developing* countries of the world is illustrated by comparisons between the various regions of the Americas, where we have countries at different stages of development. In this chapter, we will look at some of these differences and also at some of the differences that exist among different segments of the population in North America. First, however, we will look at the major factors affecting health. Later, we will explore ways the nurse can learn about the health status of people and the factors affecting health in the community in which she is going to work.

THE MAJOR FACTORS AFFECTING HEALTH

The four principal factors affecting both individual and group health are said to be human biology, environment, lifestyle, and health care organization.[3,4] (See figure below.)

Human Biology

The element of human biology includes an individual's genetic inheritance and the processes of maturation and aging

---

[3]*Community Health Nursing.* Report of a W.H.O. Expert Committee. Technical Report Series 558. Geneva, World Health Organization, 1974.

[4]*A New Perspective on the Health of Canadians,* op. cit., p. 31.

(which affect us all), as well as the complex network of structures and systems that compose the human body. We often hear it said that someone has inherited the strong constitution of his father's side of the family, or that another person has the same weak eyes as his aunt. Certainly, we inherit our physical structure, our skin texture and pigmentation, and some say our native intelligence, through the genes we receive from our parents.

A number of specific diseases are known to be passed down through families. One example is Huntington's chorea, a progressive degenerative disorder of the nervous system, which is transmitted through a single, dominant gene and may affect both males and females in the family. Another is hemophilia, the so-called bleeder's disease, which has afflicted several generations of males in the Hapsburg family and other royal families.

The more common disease of diabetes also has an inherited component, although its exact mode of transmission is still not well understood. Then, there are the congenital problems, that is, those present at birth. Although many are caused by difficulties encountered by the unborn infant in utero or by difficulties during delivery, in many congenital problems the genetic factor is clear and has been well documented. The underlying cause of Down's syndrome (mongolism), for example, is considered to be a defective chromosome.

In many other disorders that affect human beings, the effect of genetic inheritance is suspected, but the relationship

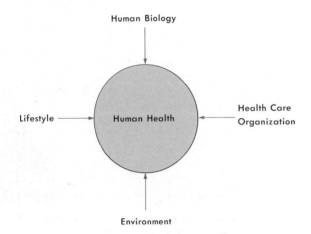

Factors affecting health. (Source: Community Health Nursing. Report of a W.H.O. Expert Committee. Technical Report Series 558. Geneva, World Health Organization, 1974, p. 8.)

has not yet been fully established. We do not know for certain at this point in time, for example, the extent of the role of heredity as a causative factor in heart trouble, or in hypertension, or in a number of other health problems. Nor do we know why some diseases seem to afflict people of one ethnic group more than another, as, for example, the high prevalence of diabetes among Jewish women, or of glaucoma (increased tension within the eyeball) among people in many of the West Indian ethnic groups.

The processes of maturation and aging also affect an individual's health in many ways. Each stage of development, from conception through maturity to old age, involves changes in the human body and, also, changes in the interactions of the individual with the world around him. Many things can go wrong during the process of change. During the period of growth, for example, the bones or other structures may not develop as they should, and disturbances may occur in the functioning of the endocrine glands. Emotional problems frequently result from the psychosocial stresses on an individual as he moves from childhood to adulthood, to parenthood, to middle age and then to old age. The number and types of problems related to difficulties associated with the processes of maturation and aging are numerous, and at the present time, we know far too little about many of them.

Then, too, there are all the disturbances that can occur in the complicated systems of the human body, such as the skeletal system, the nervous system, the digestive system, and the like. As you proceed through your nursing course, you will learn about a good many of the systemic disorders that can occur in the human body; we will be touching on some of these in later chapters of this text in connection with common health problems.

The Environment

The environment, as we have mentioned earlier, includes both the physical world that surrounds us and the people who inhabit that world. Man has learned to control many aspects of his physical environment to make it more conducive to healthy living. One of the major factors in the improvement of health in North America in the past 75 years has been the reduction of environmental hazards through the application of known public health measures. These have included such basic measures as standards for housing, provisions to ensure safe water, food and milk supplies, safety standards for places where people work, and the control of communicable disease.

In many of the developing countries, the lack of a pure water supply, of adequate sanitation, and of measures to effectively control communicable disease is held responsible for the continuing prevalence of many health problems, as, for example, the water-borne diseases such as cholera and typhoid fever, the fecally transmitted infectious diarrheas, and the air-borne communicable diseases such as tuberculosis, diphtheria, whooping cough, and the like.

Although we have greatly reduced the effect of environmental factors on health

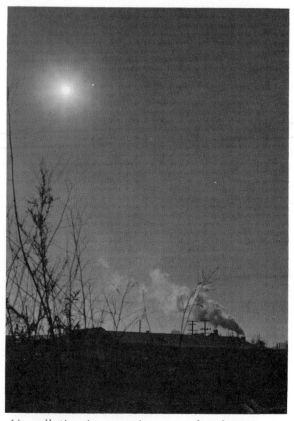

Air pollution is a growing cause for alarm in most major urban centers today.

in North America, there is still much lack of uniformity in the application of basic public health measures across the country. Housing for many people is still far from adequate, or even safe. Access to a safe water supply is not guaranteed to all. In some homes, there is still no running water or indoor plumbing. Raw sewage still pours into many of our lakes and rivers, and insects, rats, and other disease-carrying pests infest many poverty neighborhoods.

Then, too, other environmental problems have emerged in recent years, many as a result of industrialization and increasing urbanization. The contamination of our waterways by industrial pollutants is currently a matter of major concern. There is also growing alarm about the potential threat to health of air pollution, particularly in our large urban centers. Many cities have installed monitoring devices and instituted controls to curb industrial activity when air pollution reaches a level considered harmful to health.

The effect of increasing urbanization on both the physical and social environment is also causing considerable concern to people in the health field. In many instances, cities and new communities have grown too rapidly to cope with the housing, sewage, and other basic services needed by the population. Overcrowding,

lack of recreational facilities, excessive noise, violence, and solitude are among the social factors resulting from urbanization that contribute to the health problems of city-dwellers.

In looking at factors in the social environment that affect health, we must also take into consideration all of the personal relationships that occur in the family, the home, the work, and the school setting, as well as in the religious and recreational activities in which people engage. These relationships are important in the satisfaction, or lack of satisfaction, of basic human needs, and as such, they contribute positively or negatively to a person's health.[5]

Lifestyle

The ways of life of people in a community, and their individual lifestyles, also have a significant impact on health. Lifestyle is determined in part by circumstance, and in part by the decisions made, consciously or unconsciously, by people about the way they choose to live. A child born into a poor family in a ghetto neigh-

---

[5]*The Report of the Alberta Task Force on Nursing Education.* Alberta, Advanced Education and Manpower, September 1975, p. 15.

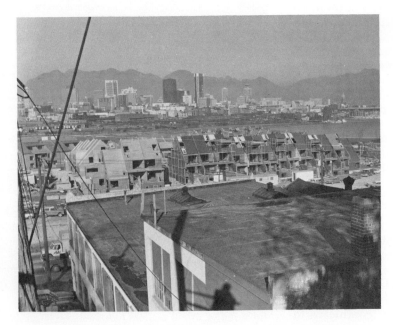

Increasing urbanization is another concern of health workers. New housing developments such as the one in this picture are rapidly being constructed in attempts to meet the needs of the ever-increasing influx of people to metropolitan areas.

borhood in a city in North America, for example, or into a poor family in a remote village in Central America, has little to say in the matter of his lifestyle—during his early years, at any rate. Lifestyle depends to a large extent on the occupation of the head of the household, the income level of the family, and the things that income can purchase in the way of housing, food, clothing, recreation, and even education and health care. Another major factor contributing to better health for North Americans in this century (in addition to improved public health measures) has been the general overall raising of income levels of the population with its concomitant raising of standards of living, perhaps one of the good things that has come from industrialization.

In much of the developing world, many health problems are directly attributable to a lack of the basic essentials of life, such as adequate nutrition and housing, resulting from widespread poverty among large segments of the population in many countries. Nor is North America entirely exempt from the influence of poverty on the health of its people. The effects of income level on health stand out in startling relief when we look at differences among socioeconomic groups in relation to infant mortality and maternal death rates in both the United States and Canada, as we shall

do later in this chapter. The poor are obviously at a disadvantage, healthwise.

In addition to circumstantial factors, there is also the element of personal decision-making that enters into an individual or family lifestyle, regardless of income. One of the byproducts of affluence has been obesity, which is considered a major health problem in North American society. Although other factors contribute to obesity—and we do not know about all of its causes yet—certainly individual choice of diet has a great deal to do with it. Obesity is felt to be a major contributing factor in many of the diseases that afflict large numbers of North Americans today, such as heart conditions, hypertension, diabetes, and the like. Nor should we forget that malnutrition can occur even in the midst of a plentiful food supply, as evidenced by recent studies on nutrition in both the United States and Canada. Malnutrition is most usually associated with poverty, but it may also result from poor choice in the foods eaten, as, for example, the eating of too many snack foods and sweets instead of regular, well balanced meals.

Our sedentary way of life in North America (and among people in higher socioeconomic groups in many parts of Central and South America as well) must also be considered as a lifestyle factor af-

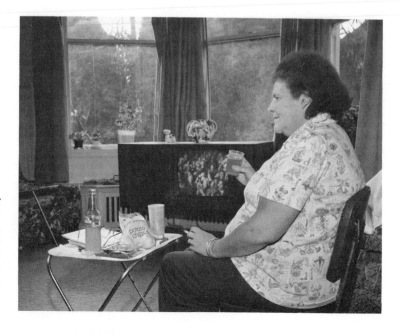

Obesity is considered a major health problem in North America. This individual, who has already lost 50 pounds under her doctor's supervision, shows, for the benefit of this photograph, the kinds of foods that formerly made up her diet.

fecting health. It, too, is a product of our affluent society, with its motor cars for transportation and television sets for entertainment. Many people believe that a lack of exercise has contributed to a generally lowered state of physical fitness among American and Canadian men and women as evidenced by the results of tests of physical fitness in comparison with Swedish adults, for example.[6]

In discussing health problems resulting from lifestyle factors, we should also mention the terrible toll in human lives from excessive speed and careless driving on the highways, and the heavy burden put on our health care system for the care, treatment, and rehabilitation of countless victims of automobile accidents. The lowering of the speed limit on U.S. highways and in several Canadian provinces that resulted from the energy crisis of 1974, it has been said, probably saved more lives and eliminated more hospital days than any other single factor in recent years.

Numerous other major problems that are causes of increasing concern in the health field today can also be attributed to lifestyle factors. These include alcoholism, drug addiction, the venereal diseases, and mental health problems, including suicide. It is especially troubling that these are affecting increasing numbers of young people.

Health Care Organization

Health care organization is the fourth and last on our list of major factors affecting health. Improvements in health care have been given as one of the main reasons for the reduction in maternal and childhood deaths in North America, and have contributed to increases in the life span in many ways. Yet, many problems remain in the equitable distribution of health care services. We discussed some of the problems in our health care systems in Chapter 1, and we will be going into this topic in more detail in Chapter 5. Suffice it to say here, then, that it is necessary to have comprehensive and accessible care for all, with a full range of services—promotional and preventive, as well as curative—if the highest level of health is to be attained for all of our people. And, these services must be acceptable to people, or they will not be utilized.

HEALTH STATUS INDICATORS

The individual health of people and their major health problems are reflected in the statistical information collected and compiled by governments about illness and death in the country. The kinds of statistical information usually compiled on an annual basis by national governments include:

1. the average life span of people in the country (life expectancy)
2. the number of deaths relative to the population (mortality rates)
3. the reasons for these deaths (causes of death)
4. the incidence of illness (morbidity data)

These four sets of statistical information are considered the main health status indicators for a given population. They provide a base for identifying major health problems, that is, those problems responsible for the most number of deaths and those causing the greatest amount of disability to people. They also help to give some insight into the principal factors affecting the health of the population.

Because virtually every country in the world collects information related to these four indicators, it is possible to look at differences between countries, and where statistical information has accumulated over a number of years, to look at trends over time.

Life Expectancy

Life expectancy is said to reflect the total effect on health programs and socioeconomic developments in a given country.[7] In the developed countries of

[6]D. A. Bailey et al.: A Current View of Canadian Cardiorespiratory Fitness. *Journal of the Canadian Medical Association*, Vol. III, July 6, 1974, pp. 25–30.

[7]*Health Conditions in the Americas 1969–1972.* Washington, D.C., Pan American Health Organization. Pan American Sanitary Bureau, Regional Office of the World Health Organization, 1974, p. 12.

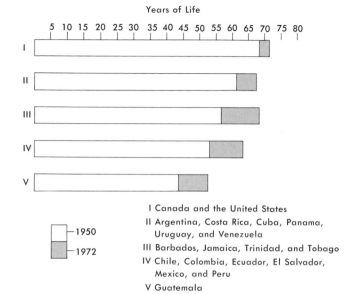

Years of Life

| 5 10 15 20 25 30 35 40 45 50 55 60 65 70 75 80 |

I

II

III

IV

V

I Canada and the United States

II Argentina, Costa Rica, Cuba, Panama,
  Uruguay, and Venezuela

1950

1972

III Barbados, Jamaica, Trinidad, and Tobago

IV Chile, Colombia, Ecuador, El Salvador,
  Mexico, and Peru

V Guatemala

Life expectancy at birth in five groups of American countries, 1950–1972. (Source: Health Conditions in the Americas 1969–1972. Washington, D.C., Pan American Health Organization. Pan American Sanitary Bureau, Regional Office of the World Health Organization, 1974, p. 12.)

the world, such as the United States and Canada, life expectancy has increased dramatically since the turn of the century—from a little under 50 years in 1900 to over 70 years in the 1970s. The biggest changes in the life span occurred during the first half of the century, with smaller but still significant gains since 1950, as shown in the data for North America in the figure above.

The reason for the remarkable extension in the life span in North America during this century has been attributed to a constellation of factors. These include the general overall raising of standards of living, improved sanitation, the development and widespread use of immunity-producing agents to protect people from communicable disease, improvements in health care services, and advances in medical science and technology.

One trend that should be noted in the statistics on life expectancy in North America particularly is the widening gap between men and women. In 1900, women outlived men by an average of approximately 2 years in both the United States and Canada. By 1970, this figure had increased to approximately 8 years in the United States, and 7 years in Canada. The resulting imbalance between the sexes, particularly in the older age group, has brought about changes in the structure of our society. The population pyra-

mids shown in Chapter 5 (page 64) graphically illustrate the increasing number of older women in our North American society. One of the unfortunate results of this trend is that widowhood and loneliness all too often contribute to the health problems of many of our senior citizens.

The figure above also shows the improvements in life expectancy in four other regions of the Americas. Even in the region with the lowest life expectancy (Guatemala), considerable progress has been made in lengthening the life span over the past two decades.

Mortality Rates

A major factor in the lengthening of the average life span in North America has been a dramatic reduction in the number of infant and maternal deaths. Relatively few women in either the United States or Canada die as a result of childbirth these days; the *maternal mortality rate* is now approximately 2 per 10,000 live births in both countries.[8]

In Middle and South America, the rates were approximately seven to ten times

---

[8]Reported maternal death rate in Canada was 1.6 per 10,000 live births in 1972, 1.9 for the United States in 1971. Provisional data for 1972 showed a slight upward trend in the U.S. for that year.

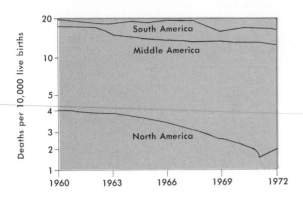

Maternal deaths per 10,000 live births in the three regions of the Americas, 1960–1972. (Source: Health Conditions in the Americas 1969–1972. Washington, D.C., Pan American Health Organization. Pan American Sanitary Bureau, Regional Office of the World Health Organization, 1974, p. 26.)

greater than in North America for the year 1972. Trends in maternal death rates in three regions of the Americas, as seen in the figure above, show the continuing decline in maternal death rates in North America and the progress made in Central and South America over the period 1960 to 1972.

Maternal deaths are considered to be largely preventable. They occur mainly as a result of toxemias in pregnancy, hemorrhagic accidents, infections, and clandestine abortions.[9] The importance of early and adequate prenatal care, therefore, cannot be overstressed. The reduction in maternal death rates in both the United States and Canada is attributed mainly to improved prenatal care for pregnant women and to hospitalization for the mothers during delivery.

Although the record in North America is very good, there are still differences in the extent of care received by women in different socioeconomic groups. It has been estimated that *early prenatal care*, that is, care during the first three months of pregnancy, is received by approximately three-quarters of white women in the United States and by only one-half of the women of other races, and by far more women with education beyond high school than by those who left school in the primary grades.[10]

Infant mortality is considered one of the most sensitive indicators of a nation's health status. In both the United States and Canada, major accomplishments are reflected in the significant drop in infant mortality rates, from slightly over 100 deaths per 1000 live births in the early 1920s to under 17 in 1974.[11] There is, however, still room for improvement, as can be seen when these figures are compared with Sweden's rate of 9.6 per 1000 live births in 1973, and with Finland's rate of 10.1 for the same year. In 1973, Canada ranked twelfth and the U.S. fifteenth in international comparisons of infant mortality. (See figure on page 51). The grounds for hope of further improvement in the reduction of infant deaths in North America are evident when one looks at the differences between segments of the population divided on socioeconomic and geographic lines. In the United States, for example, the mortality rate is considerably higher for black than white infants. The rates are higher among the poor, among the poorly educated, among the illegitimate births, and when the mother is under 20 or over 35 years of

---

[9] *Ten Year Health Plan for the Americas.* Washington, D.C., Pan American Health Organization. Pan American Sanitary Bureau, Regional Office of the World Health Organization, January 1973, p. 9.

[10] *Health United States 1975.* Rockville, Maryland, U.S. Department of Health, Education and Welfare Publication No. (HRA) 76–1232. Public Health Service. Health Resources Administration, National Center for Health Statistics, 1976, p. 158.

---

[11] Although American and Canadian infant mortality rates are not identical, over the years the differences have been slight, and progress in both countries has followed a similar pattern. The following statistics give some indication of trends in North America. In 1921, Canada reported an infant mortality rate of 102 per 1000 live births. In 1949, the rate in the U. S. was reported as 47 per 1000 live births. In the late 1950s and early 1960s, it remained stationary at about 25 deaths per 1000 live births in both countries, but has continued to decline from around 1965 to the present. In 1973, Canada's infant mortality rate was reported as 16.8 per 1000 live births; in 1974, that of the U.S. was provisionally reported at 16.5.

age.[12] In Canada, infant mortality rates vary from as low as 11 per 1000 live births in a wealthy Canadian suburb to as high as 40 in Canada's northlands.[13]

The majority of early infant deaths (neonatal) are associated with the status of the infant at birth. Later infant deaths (postnatal), with the exception of those caused by congenital anomalies, are more likely to be associated with environmental factors.[14] In the United States and Canada, the decrease in infant mortality has shown a continuous decline in both neonatal and postnatal deaths. In other words, babies are getting a better start in life (an important factor here would be better prenatal care for mothers), and the infant's chances of survival through the first year are better owing to less danger from environmental factors (including, in this instance, improved nutrition and better infant health care).

In both Middle and South America, infant deaths remain excessively high, although considerable improvement has been made since 1960. Rates were reduced in Middle America, for example, from an average of 70 deaths per 1000 live births in 1960 to 56 in 1972, and in South America from close to 85 in 1960 to 63 in 1972.

It is felt that a large number of these deaths could be prevented by further improvements in disease prevention, environmental sanitation, and better programs of maternal-child health care.[15]

---

[12]Health United States 1975, op. cit., p. 158.
[13]A New Perspective on the Health of Canadians, op. cit., p. 38.
[14]Health Conditions in the Americas 1969–1972, op. cit., p. 28.

Rank	Country	Rate
1	Sweden	9.6
2	Finland	10.1
3	Norway (1972)	11.3
4	Netherlands	°11.6
5	Japan (1972)[1]	11.7
6	Switzerland	°12.8
7	Denmark (1971)	13.5
8	France (1972)[2]	°16.0
9	German Democratic Republic	16.0
10	New Zealand	16.2
11	Australia (1972)	°16.7
12	Canada	16.8
13	Belgium	°17.0
14	United Kingdom (1972)	17.5
15	United States	17.7
16	Ireland	°17.8
17	Federal Republic of Germany (1972)	°20.4
18	Singapore	°20.4
19	Czechoslovakia	°21.2
20	Israel	22.1
21	Austria	°23.7
22	Spain (1971)[2]	°25.2
23	Italy	°25.7
24	Bulgaria	°25.9
25	Jamaica	26.2
26	Trinidad and Tobago (1972)	26.2

°Provisional
[1]Excludes data for Okinawa.
[2]The 1973 rates of 12.9 for France and 15.1 for Spain were not used because they exclude live-born infants dying before registration of birth.

Infant mortality rates: selected countries, 1973. (Source: Health United States 1975. Rockville, Maryland, U.S. Department of Health, Education, and Welfare Publication No. (HRA) 76–1232. Public Health Service. Health Resources Administration, National Center for Health Statistics, 1976, p. 38.)

Principal Causes of Death and Disability

Statistical data on the leading causes of death and the prevalence of illness (morbidity data) also help to identify the major health problems in a country. The pattern in leading causes of death in North America has changed considerably since the turn of this century. In 1900, deaths from infectious diseases headed the list. These included pneumonia/influenza, tuberculosis, and diarrhea/enteritis, in that order. Also on the list of major killers at that time were nephritis (for the most part, postinfectious) and diphtheria. By 1940, the three leading causes of death had become the noninfectious disorders of heart disease, cancer, and cerebrovascular accidents, although tuberculosis, pneumonia, and nephritis were still listed among the major causes. By 1970, influenza/pneumonia was the only infectious disease remaining on the list of major causes of death in both the United States and Canada.[16]

---

[15]Health Conditions in the Americas 1969–1972, op. cit., p. 29.
[16]J. H. Dingle: The Ills of Man. Scientific American, 229:77–84, September 1973.

The five leading causes of death in North America, as shown in the figure below, are now diseases of the heart, malignant neoplasms, cerebrovascular disease, accidents, and influenza/pneumonia, in that order.

Diseases of the heart are responsible for over one-third of all deaths each year. Although the number of early deaths from heart conditions has been declining in recent years, owing principally to a lowered incidence of rheumatic heart disease among young people, heart disease is still the leading cause of death in the population as a whole. It also accounts for the greatest amount of acute illness and major disability among the total population.

Malignant neoplasms (cancer) cause almost one-fifth of all the total number of deaths each year. Cancer strikes people of all ages and becomes a principal cause of death and disability among people from the latter half of the young adult years onward.

Cerebrovascular disease is primarily a problem of aging. It is a leading cause of death and of both acute and chronic conditions in people over 65 years of age. The fact that cerebrovascular disease now accounts for more than one-tenth of all deaths each year in North America is a reflection of the lengthening life span of people in our country.

Accidents have become the fourth leading cause of death in North America (accounting for more than 6 per cent of the total annual death toll each year). They are also the second leading cause of acute hospitalization, surpassed only by heart disease. The residual effects of accidents in the form of long-term disability also constitute a very major health problem.

Despite our progress in the control of other infectious diseases, influenza/pneumonia continues to be a major health problem in North America. It is a principal cause of death in infants under one year of age and remains an important cause of death and a major cause of acute illness throughout the life span. The proportion of total deaths in North America attributed to influenza/pneumonia each year is approximately 3 per cent.

MAJOR HEALTH PROBLEMS THROUGHOUT THE LIFE SPAN

The list of the five leading causes of death, taken alone, does not give us a full picture of all the major health problems in North America today. From the vast amount of statistical data gathered in both

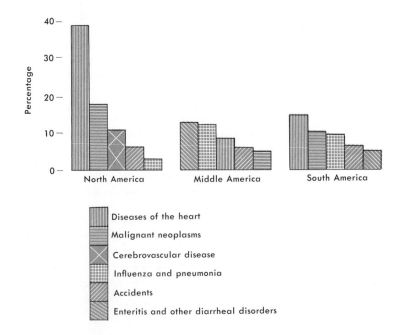

Diseases of the heart

Malignant neoplasms

Cerebrovascular disease

Influenza and pneumonia

Accidents

Enteritis and other diarrheal disorders

Five principal causes of death as a percentage of total deaths in three regions of the Americas, 1970–1972. (Source: Health Conditions in the Americas 1969–1972. Washington, D.C., Pan American Health Organization. Pan American Sanitary Bureau, Regional Office of the World Health Organization, 1974, p. 17.)

the United States and Canada on the causes of death and the prevalence of illness, it is possible to gain further insight into the nature of these problems, and to look at them from the point of view of the principal age groups affected.

The Childhood Years (Birth to 14 Years)

The period during and immediately after birth is the most critical time for infants. Most of the deaths at this time result from problems in regard to the infant's supply of oxygen or from abnormalities of the placenta (afterbirth), or from both.[17] After the first week of life, congenital abnormalities become the leading cause of infant deaths, and they account for a major portion of the conditions requiring care in acute hospitals. During the first year of life, the infant is particularly susceptible to infections of the respiratory and gastrointestinal tracts. These, together with accidents and nutritional disorders, account for the largest number of remaining deaths as well as acute illnesses in infants.

Once a child has passed his first birthday, his chances of survival are much greater. The age group of 1 to 14 years now has the lowest overall death rate of any period in the life span in North America. The common childhood illnesses continue to be a problem, but the number of deaths resulting from them has been markedly reduced. The only infectious disease that remains a major killer in this age group is influenza/pneumonia, which is the second most common cause of death and the principal cause of hospitalization in children. The leading cause of death in this age group is now accidents, with motor vehicle accidents responsible for approximately one-half of these. Accidents are also the second most common cause of acute illness in children and a major cause of long-term disability as well. The most common chronic conditions in children are the respiratory dis-

orders of bronchitis and asthma. Other problems in this age group include the developmental defects and the residual effects of congenital abnormalities, which account for a major portion of both acute and chronic conditions in children.

The Young Adult Years (15 to 44 Years)

More young people lose their lives each year from accidents, suicides, and homicides than from any other cause in North America today, with more premature deaths resulting from these among young men rather than among women. Suicide has become an important cause of death in people as young as 15 years, according to both U.S. and Canadian statistics. In the U.S., it has been estimated that deaths from motor vehicle accidents have increased by one-third in the 15 to 24 year age group, and deaths from homicide and suicide have more than doubled since 1950[18] Combined, these three causes now account for almost half of all deaths in the 15 to 44 year age group. Accidents are also the principal cause of acute illness, with their resultant head injuries, fractures, burns, and complicating disorders. Probably the most unfortunate aspect of these statistics is that so many accident victims are left with residual long-term disability as well. In the United States, it is estimated that over 1.6 million young adults (aged 15 to 24 years) and 3.7 million people in the 25 to 44 year age group suffer from permanent disability resulting from accidents occurring during these age periods or earlier.[19]

The second leading acute condition in young adults is mental illness, which has shown an alarming increase in this age group in recent years. Associated with mental illness are the problems of alcoholism and drug addiction. The rising incidence of alcoholism among very young teenagers, where it appears to be replacing the drug problem, is currently causing a considerable amount of concern.

The widespread prevalence of venereal

---

[17]*Health Field Indicators for Policy Planning.* Ottawa, Department of National Health and Welfare, 1974, p. 15.

[18]*Health United States 1975*, op. cit., p. 161.
[19]Ibid.

disease is also an alarming problem in adolescents and young adults. Currently, an estimated 2.7 million cases of gonorrhea and over 80,000 new cases of syphilis are reported each year in the U.S.

In the latter half of the early adult years, heart disease begins to assume importance, both as a leading cause of death and as a cause of acute and chronic illness. Although the chronic illnesses are not so prevalent among the younger members of this age group (the 15 to 25 year olds), hypertension and arthritis begin to show up as major disablers in the 25 to 44 year age group.

Obesity has been mentioned several times before as a factor in many acute and chronic conditions. It is of particular concern in young adults because it contributes another risk factor to health in later years. Diabetes, for example, in which the relationship to obesity is currently under considerable study, becomes a principal cause of death and disability in the 15 to 44 year age group (it is one of the leading causes of death in the 25 to 44 year age group).

Cancer also begins to attack a large number of people in the latter half of the young adult years, striking women at an earlier age than it does men.

The Middle Years (45 to 64 Years)

By the middle years of the life span, the chronic diseases have become, and remain, the principal causes of death and disability. Diseases of the heart are by far the most common of these. Other leading causes of death and of acute and long-term illness in this age group include cancer, cirrhosis of the liver (associated with alcoholism), and the chronic respiratory disorders such as emphysema, bronchitis, and asthma. These problems, together with mental illness and accidents, are among the principal disorders requiring hospital care in people during the middle years. Other common causes of hospitalization in this age group are disorders of the reproductive system (in women particularly), disorders of the nervous system, cholelithiasis (stones in the gallbladder), ulcers, hypertension and arteriosclerosis, diabetes, and hernia.

	10	20	30	40	50	60	70	80	90	100
Arthritis	92.9
Hearing impairments	71.6
Hypertensive disease	60.1
Heart conditions	50.4
Visual impairment	47.4
Chronic bronchitis	32.7
Diabetes	20.4

Prevalence of selected chronic conditions per 1000 persons in the United States, all ages. (Source: Adapted from Health United States 1975. Rockville, Maryland, U.S. Department of Health, Education, and Welfare Publication No. (HRA) 76-1232. Public Health Service. Health Resources Administration, National Center for Health Statistics, 1976, p. 247.)

The Older Age Group (65 Years and on)

Among the older age group, it is not surprising to find that the chronic and degenerative disorders are by far the principal causes of death, with heart conditions, cerebrovascular accidents (strokes), and cancer being the most common. These conditions, together with accidents, are also responsible for the largest amount of acute illness in the elderly.

The number of older people being cared for in acute care hospitals is very high in proportion to their numbers in the population. The majority of reasons for their hospitalization usually involve chronic problems or conditions that require a lengthy hospital stay. An increasingly large number of older people are receiving care in nursing homes and extended care facilities, and the residents of these homes usually have multiple chronic problems.

It is important to remember that the

chronic disorders have a cumulative effect. As people grow older, more of them tend to suffer from chronic and degenerative diseases, and their numbers add to those in whom chronic conditions began to appear at an earlier age, thus accumulating and increasing the proportionate number of people with long-term disability in the older age group. The most common causes of long-term disability among the total population in the U.S. are shown in the figure on page 54.

The picture is, of course, not entirely bleak for our senior citizens. The vast majority of them are not residents of institutions; only about 5 per cent are. A number of innovative programs are being developed to assist older people to maintain as independent a lifestyle as possible; some of these were discussed in Chapter 1 (page 00).

TRENDS IN MIDDLE AND SOUTH AMERICA

In the developing countries of the Americas, infective and parasitic diseases continue to be a major problem, and they rank high on the lists of major causes of death in Middle and South America. In contrast to North America, childhood deaths remain disproportionately high in the rest of the Americas, where the communicable diseases, malnutrition, diarrhea, and other infections of the gastrointestinal tract continue to take a heavy toll (see figure on page 52). Although malnutrition is not always listed as the principal cause of death, the relationship between it and infections in children has been well documented.[20]

Maternal deaths, as mentioned earlier, are also a major concern in most regions of Middle and South America. Other problems ranking among the leading causes of death are similar to those in North America, that is, conditions of the heart, cancer, accidents, influenza/pneumonia, and cerebrovascular accidents. The proportion of deaths attributed to the

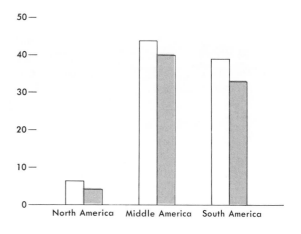

1964

1972

Percentage of deaths under five years of age in three regions of the Americas, 1964–1972. (Source: Health Conditions in the Americas 1969–1972. Washington, D.C., Pan American Health Organization. Pan American Sanitary Bureau, Regional Office of the World Health Organization, 1974, p. 26.)

five leading causes in North, Middle, and South America is shown in the figure on page 52.

THE NURSE AND HEALTH PROBLEMS IN THE COMMUNITY

It is important for the nurse to be aware of the major health problems in her country. National statistics and national averages, however, do not necessarily give a representative picture of the problems she will encounter in the community in which she is working. Each community will have its own unique set of problems, and the factors affecting health in each community will vary. The problems will be different, for example, in rural as opposed to urban settings, or between affluent neighborhoods and poor ones, and will also vary with the inhabitants of each community and their lifestyles.

In order to play her part in the promo-

[20] Ruth R. Puffer and Carlos V. Serrano: *Patterns of Mortality in Childhood.* Scientific Publication No. 262. Washington, D. C., Pan American Health Organization, 1973, pp. v–vi.

tion and protection of health, the care of the ill, and the restoration of health, the nurse should become knowledgeable about the particular health problems and the factors affecting health in the community in which she is going to practice.

A good first step in learning about a community is to find out what has been written about it. The nurse can often get quite a bit of information about the people who live and work there by reviewing the statistical data published by government agencies. Census data, for example, provide basic information about a given population, such as total number of people, age and sex distribution, ethnic origin of the inhabitants, population density (number of people per square mile), and birth rates. Government health departments—federal, state (provincial), and municipal—usually collect and publish basic health statistics such as life expectancy rates, infant mortality rates, leading causes of death, and major illnesses. These statistics often go down to the county or municipal level. Information about the nature of health services in a community and the financing and utilization of these services is also frequently available in the publications of governmental and other health agencies.

Other written material that the nurse can usually find in a library to increase her knowledge about a community includes maps, encyclopedias, informational brochures (such as those put out by government tourist bureaus), and local newspapers. From these sources the nurse can often learn much about environmental factors affecting health, such as the geographic location of the community, climatic conditions, and the community's transportation and communication systems, and major industries in the area, as well as something about recreational and educational facilities and churches. The community's concerns about health matters, such as health care financing and environmental pollution, are often discussed in articles in the local newspapers.

The information obtained from written material can be supplemented by talking with knowledgeable and informed people in the community, such as the medical officer of health and his staff, public health nurses in the area, social workers, clergymen, and teachers. Sometimes, too, the local law enforcement officer may be the best informed person in a community with regard to the assets and liabilities of its health status.

Direct observation, such as that made while walking about the community, gives the nurse who is new to the area an opportunity to note the location of health agencies, particularly in relation to

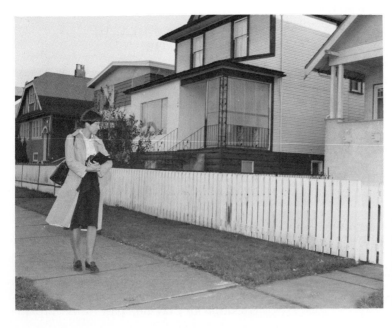

The nurse can learn much about factors affecting health through observations made while walking about the community. Here, the nurse explores the neighborhood in which she is to work.

FACTORS AFFECTING HEALTH IN A COMMUNITY

Human Biology	Environment	Lifestyles	Health Care System
Population Data	Geographic Data	Occupational character-	Preventive health services
Number of people	Climate	istics of population	Health maintenance services
Age distribution	Location (accessibility)	Average income level	Agencies for diagnosis, treatment and
Density/square mile	Transportation	Recreational facilities	rehabilitation of the sick
Ethnic origins	Communication	Educational facilities	Physician population
	Water supply	Churches	Nursing services available
Health Data	Food quality control	Health care financing	Attitudes toward health and
Life expectancy rates	Sewage disposal		health care
Probable birth rates	Environmental pollution		Utilization of services
Major causes of death	Housing		
Major illnesses	Major industries		

schools, shopping areas, and residential accommodation. It also helps the nurse to gain an insight into local housing conditions, the presence or absence of parks and other recreational facilities, the number of churches, and the general appearance of the community.

The nurse, in her appraisal of a community, might also talk with individuals who live there in order to gain an appreciation of their knowledge about health care services available in the community, their attitudes toward health and health care, and their utilization of health services.

Some of the types of information that are useful in assessing health problems and the factors affecting health in a community are detailed in the table above at the top of this page.

Looking at health problems from the point of view of major causative factors, it is apparent that we have not yet conquered all of the biological causes of ill health. There is still much more work to be done, particularly in the area of congenital problems, cancer, and the problems associated with aging. Nor have we eliminated all of the hazards in the physical environment; although many have been controlled, many new ones have emerged. Of increasing importance, too, are factors in the social environment and in the lifestyles of people in our North American society. Many people feel that it is in these last-named areas, the social environment and lifestyles, that our major problems, and our hope for further improvements in health, now lie.

STUDY VOCABULARY

Congenital problems	Human biology	Morbidity data
Diabetes	Huntington's chorea	Mortality rate
Environment	Infant mortality	Neonatal mortality
Glaucoma	Life expectancy	Postnatal mortality
Health status indicators	Lifestyle	Placenta
Hemophilia	Maternal mortality	Population density

STUDY SITUATION   You have been offered a summer job in a Neighborhood Health Center in an area of the city with which you are not familiar. In preparation for this assignment, you want to find out something about the factors affecting health and the health problems of the people in the neighborhood.

Outline a plan for obtaining the information you feel would be helpful to you. The following questions are suggested to help you to organize your plan for looking at biological, environmental, lifestyle, and health care organization factors.

Suggested Items to Be Considered Under Biological Factors

1. How many people live in the community?
2. What is the approximate age distribution of the population?
3. What is the population density?
4. What are the predominant ethnic groups?
5. What are the common illnesses of the people who live in the community?
    among infants
    among the children
    among the adults
    among old people

Suggested Items to Be Considered Under Environmental Factors

1. What is the general description of the community, e.g., housing, neighborhood conditions, and the like?
2. Is the housing adequate? Safe?
3. What is the state of sanitation in regard to:
    water supply
    sewage
    garbage disposal
    food handling in local stores and markets
    control of animals, insects and other vectors of disease, e.g., dogs, rats, mice, insects, cows, goats.
4. How would you describe the social environment of the community?
5. Are there parks or recreational areas in the community?

Suggested Items to Be Considered Under Lifestyle Factors

1. What are the principal occupations of people who live in this community?
2. Where do they work?
3. What is the approximate average yearly income?
4. Do people live in single family dwellings? Multiple family dwellings?
5. What do people do in their leisure time?
    children
    youth
    young adults
    middle aged adults
    older people

Suggested Items to Be Considered Under Health Care Organization

1. What health services are available in the community?
    health promotion services
    hospitals, health centers, or clinics
    physicians' offices
    nursing services
    preventive health services
    rehabilitation services
2. Where do people go when thay are sick?
3. How do they feel about the health services that are available?
4. How do they pay for their health services?

SUGGESTED READINGS

Ahern, C.: I Think I Have V. D. *Nursing Clinics of North America,* 8:77–89, March, 1973.

A New Perspective on the Health of Canadians. A Working Document. Ottawa, Department of National Health and Welfare, April, 1974.

Atwater, J. B.: Adapting the V. D. Clinic to Today's Problem. *American Journal of Public Health,* 64:433–437, May, 1974.

Brown, M. A.: Adolescents and Venereal Disease. *Nursing Outlook, 21*:99–103, February, 1973.

Chase, H. C.: The Position of the United States in International Comparisons of Health Status. *American Journal of Public Health,* 62:581–589, April, 1972.

Dingle, John H.: The Ills of Man. *Scientific American, 229*:77–84, September, 1973.

Erhardt, Carl L., and Joyce E. Berlin (eds.): *Mortality and Morbidity in the United States.* Cambridge, Massachusetts., Harvard University Press, 1974.

Ferrari, H. E.: The Nurse and V. D. Control. *Canadian Nurse,* 67:18–30, July, 1971.

Finnegan, L. P., et al.: Care of the Addicted Infant. *American Journal of Nursing,* 74:685–693, April, 1974.

Fort, Joel: *Alcohol: Our Biggest Drug Problem.* New York, McGraw-Hill Book Company, 1973.

Furnass, S. B.: *The Australian National University Report on Some Aspects of Drug Consumption in Canada, the U. K., Sweden, Denmark, U. S. A. and Australia.* Canberra, November, 1970.

Health Field Indicators for Policy Planning, Canada and the Provinces. Part I Mortality and Hospitalization. Ottawa, Department of National Health and Welfare, December, 1974.

Health United States 1975. Rockville, Maryland, U. S. Department of Health, Education, and Welfare Publication No. (HRA)76–1232. Public Health Service. Health Resources Administration, National Center for Health Statistics, 1976.

Interim Report of the Commission of Inquiry into the Non-Medical Use of Drugs. Ottawa, Department of National Health and Welfare, 1973.

Jamann, J. S.: Health is a Function of Ecology. *American Journal of Nursing,* 71:970–973, May, 1971.

Kandel, D., et al.: The Epidemiology of Drug Use Among New York State High School Students: Distribution, Trends, and Change in Rates of Use. *American Journal of Public Health,* 66:43–53, January, 1976.

Kitagawa, Evelyn, M., and Philip M. Hauser: *Differential Mortality in the United States: A Study in Socioeconomic Epidemiology.* Cambridge, Massachusetts, Harvard University Press, 1973.

Krepick, D. S., et al.: Heroin Addiction: A Treatable Disease. *Nursing Clinics of North America,* 8:41–52, March, 1973.

Lave, L. B., and E. P. Seskin: Air Pollution, Climate and Home Heating: Their Effects on U. S. Mortality Rates. *American Journal of Public Health,* 62:909–916, July, 1972.

Levengood, R., et al.: Heroin Addiction in the Suburbs. *American Journal of Public Health,* 63:209–214, March, 1973.

Lewis, L. W.: The Hidden Alcoholic: A Nursing Dilemma. *Nursing '75,* 5:20–27, July, 1975.

Long, B. L., et al.: New Perspectives on Drug Abuse. *Nursing Clinics of North America,* 8:25–40, March, 1973.

Louria, D. B.: A Critique of Some Current Approaches to the Problem of Drug Abuse. *American Journal of Public Health,* 65:581–583, June, 1975.

McGrath, P., et al.: Levels of Basic V. D. Knowledge Among Junior and Senior High School Nurses in Massachusetts. A Survey. *Nursing Research,* 23:31–37, January–February, 1974.

Pillari, G.: Physical Effects of Heroin Addiction. *American Journal of Nursing,* 73:2105–2108, December, 1973.

Proceedings of the National Conference on Fitness and Health, Ottawa, December 4, 5 and 6, 1972. Ottawa, Department of National Health and Welfare, 1973.

Puffer, Ruth R., and Carlos V. Serrano: *Patterns of Mortality in Childhood.* Scientific Publication No. 262. Washington, D. C., Pan American Health Organization, 1973.

Report of the Alberta Task Force on Nursing Education. Alberta, Department of Advanced Education and Manpower, September, 1975.

Resnik, H. L. P., and Berkley C. Hathorne (eds.): *Suicide Prevention in the 70's.* Washington, D. C., Department of Health, Education, and Welfare Publication No. (HSM)72–9054, 1973.

Rimm, Alfred A., et al.: Relationship of Obesity and Disease in 73,532 Weight-Conscious Women. *Public Health Reports,* 90:44–51, January–February, 1975.

Sims, Mary, et al.: Drug Overdoses in a Canadian City. *American Journal of Public Health,* 63:215–226, March, 1973.

5 HEALTH CARE AGENCIES

The nurse should be able to:

Discuss health care as social policy

Differentiate between explicit and implicit health policies

Discuss factors contributing to the increased demand for health services

Discuss the effects of escalating costs and increased demand on health care services

Compare and contrast the health care systems in the United States and in Canada

Describe the spectrum of health care services in a community

Describe the functions of official and voluntary agencies, with particular reference to their role in health promotion and protection

Discussion the principal providers of primary care services in a community

Explain the various functions of a hospital

Describe the functions of various departments within a hospital

Discuss the nature of home care programs

Discuss the nature of extended care facilities

Describe the nature of rehabilitation services

Discuss the role of the nurse in rehabilitation

Describe the usual procedure for admitting a patient to hospital

List principles relevant to the care of newly admitted patients

Describe measures the nurse can take to assist the patient to adjust to the hospital

Describe measures the nurse can take to assist the patient when he is being discharged from the hospital

INTRODUCTION

"Health is said to be a human right, that is, a condition to which everyone has a just claim. The very acceptance of the notion of human right implies that society assumes a responsibility and will give a high priority to carrying it out."[1] As discussed in the previous chapter, health is affected by a number of social and economic factors as well as health care per se. In order to develop and maintain good health, people must have adequate food, shelter, and a level of income sufficient to ensure these. It is indeed difficult to separate the social and economic components from health care, and in many national and state/provincial governments, the functions of social welfare and health have been brought together in one department. In the United States, for example, the Federal Department of Health, Education, and Welfare administers both the national health and the national social welfare programs, as does the Department of National Health and Welfare in Canada.

The provision of adequate health measures is viewed as an essential component of a country's overall social policies. In the United States and in Canada (and in many other countries too), we believe that society has a responsibility to look after its older people who have reached the age of retirement and may be unable to care for themselves financially. The assumption of this responsibility is a social policy to which both countries subscribe. The policy is evidenced in our social (income) security programs that ensure a basic minimum income for all senior citizens and in programs that provide health services for older people through public monies.

EXPLICIT AND IMPLICIT HEALTH POLICIES

The health programs for senior citizens illustrate national health policies that have been adopted in our countries. A policy is a plan of action that is used to guide and determine administrative decisions.

At every level of government, national, state/provincial, and municipal, health programs are based on certain policies that the prevailing government either initiated on its own or endorsed from a previous governmental policy. When policies are proclaimed in written statements, they are called "explicit" policies. It is not uncommon for a newly elected government, for example, to make a formal statement of the health policies it intends to follow during its term of office; indeed, these may have been planks in its election campaign, which are then made into explicit policy commitments after election. The following statements, taken from a speech made by one health minister in outlining his government's Ten Year Health Plan, are examples of explicit policy statements:

> "(development of) a Maternal Health Programme which would cover 75 per cent of the population"

and

> "decentralization and regionalization of the health services and the establishment of Community Health Advisory Boards made up of the people and the nursing personnel in the particular community."[2]

Health policies, once adopted, are frequently incorporated into legislation. In the United States, a major policy debate is currently in progress on the issue of na-

---

[1]Alexander Doronzynski: *Doctors and Healers.* Ottawa, Canada, International Development Research Centre, 1975, p. 5.

[2]Excerpted from an article in the *Guyana Sunday Chronicle* entitled "10 Year Health Plan Outlined," June 20, 1976.

tional health insurance. As soon as a consensus is reached on overall policy, and details for its implementation are worked through, appropriate legislation will no doubt be enacted. In Canada, a policy of universal prepaid medical and hospital insurance has been incorporated into national health insurance laws.

Sometimes, health policies are not explicitly expressed in formal statements, nor incorporated into legislation, but they may be inferred in the programs that are carried out by the department of government responsible for health. In this case, they are called "implicit" policies. An example here might be the policy of a municipal government to protect all children, insofar as possible, from the communicable diseases to which they are particularly vulnerable and for which there are known immunizations. Although the policy may not be explicitly stated, it would be demonstrated in citywide preschool and school immunization programs carried out by the municipal department of health.

HEALTH CARE FOR ALL: A MAJOR POLICY ISSUE

A major policy issue concerning most countries of the world at the present time is how to ensure that the services needed to promote and maintain health, to prevent disease, and to treat illness, as well as the rehabilitative services needed to restore the sick to an active functioning role in society, are made available to all persons in the country.

The importance attached to this concern is evidenced by the increasingly large portion of national budgets that is spent annually on health expenditures and by the rapidly growing number of people engaged in providing health care services. In 1969, the amount of money allocated for health expenditures in the Federal Budget of the United States was 16.7 billion dollars, or 9.1 per cent of all Federal outlays. By 1974, this figure had reached 32 billion dollars, approximately 11.6 per cent of Federal outlays for all purposes. Even after adjustments had been made for inflation, this represented

an increase of more than 40 per cent in Federal spending on health.[3] In Canada, there has been a comparable escalation in the amount of Federal Government monies allocated for health care services. For example, in 1969, Federal expenditures for health care in Canada by the Department of National Health and Welfare totaled 1.32 billion dollars; by 1974, this figure had increased to 2.44 billion dollars.[4]

The allocation of health monies by type of expenditure (United States figures) is shown in the figure on page 63.

The increased expenditure on health care has been accompanied by a marked increase in the number of people who provide health care services. Reports indicate that the number of people employed in the health field has been increasing at more than twice the rate of the number of employed persons in the total economy. It has been said that the "health care industry" now encompasses a combined manpower force larger than that of any other industry. In 1973, it was estimated that there were 4.4 million persons employed in health-related occupations in the United States, half of whom were in nursing or related services.[5] In Canada, in 1975, it was estimated that 500,000 persons were engaged in health and health-

[3]L. B. Russell et al.: *Federal Health Spending 1969–1974.* Washington, D.C., Center for Health Policy Studies, National Planning Association, 1974.

[4]It is difficult to compare Canadian figures with those of the United States because of the differences in responsibility for health expenditures of the two Federal Governments. The United States budgetary figures for health care expenditures include health resources, medical services, and prevention and control of health problems. The Canadian budgetary figures for the Department of National Health and Welfare include hospital care, general health, public health, and medical, dental, and allied services. Also, other Federal departments, such as the Department of Veterans' Affairs and the Department of National Defense, for example, allocate monies for health care services.

Statistics from *A New Perspective on the Health of Canadians.* A Working Document. Ottawa, Department of National Health and Welfare, 1974, p. 52.

[5]*Health United States 1975.* Rockville, Maryland, U. S. Department of Health, Education and Welfare Publication No. (HRA) 76–1232. Public Health Services. Health Resources Administration, National Center for Health Statistics, p. 103.

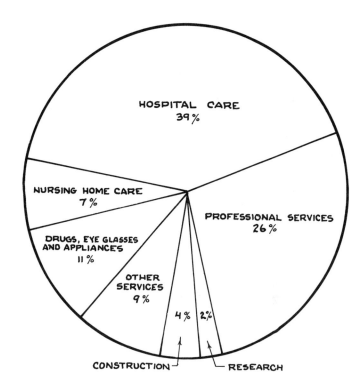

HOSPITAL CARE
39%

NURSING HOME CARE
7%

DRUGS, EYE GLASSES
AND APPLIANCES
11%

OTHER
SERVICES
9%

PROFESSIONAL SERVICES
26%

4% 2%

CONSTRUCTION   RESEARCH

Types of health expenditures, fiscal year 1974. (Source: Social Security Bulletin, Vol. 38, February 1975. Reprinted from Health United States 1975. Rockville, Maryland, U.S. Department of Health, Education, and Welfare Publication No. (HRA) 76–1232. Public Health Service. Health Resources Administration, National Center for Health Statistics, p. 65.)

related occupations, again, over half in nursing and related services.[6]

INCREASED DEMAND FOR HEALTH SERVICES

The fundamental reason for the increased expenditures on health care and the expansion in numbers of health care workers has been attributed to an increased demand for health services. Several powerful forces have contributed to this demand, including large population growth, greater public awareness of the value of health care, expansion of health care insurance and the provision of services for low income groups, government subsidies for the construction of health care facilities, and enlargement of the scope of health care services through research and technological progress.[7]

One of the most powerful forces contributing to the increased demand for health services has been the rapid rate of growth of our population. Both the United States and Canada have experienced tremendous population increases, particularly since World War II. In 1940, the total population of the United States was estimated at 132 million people; by 1974, this figure had jumped to 211 million.[8] Comparable figures for Canada were 11.5 million, according to the 1941 census, and 22.7 million for the estimated population on January 1, 1975.[9] Although the rates of population increase have slowed down considerably in both countries as a result of record low fertility rates in the 1970s, we have still not caught up with the increased demands put on our health services by the rapid population growth that started in the late 1940s and continued on through the better part of the 1960s.

The two groups in the population requiring the most health services are our youngest and our oldest citizens. Although the number of children propor-

[6]Ottawa, Department of National Health and Welfare, Manpower Planning Division, 1975.

[7]*Manpower Report of the President.* Prepared by the Department of Labor and transmitted to the United States Congress, March 1970, p. 174.

[8]*Health United States 1975.* op. cit., p. 175.

[9]*Census of Canada 1941*, Volume III, and *Estimated Population of Canada, by Provinces by Quarterly Periods.* Ottawa, Statistics Canada. Catalogue 91–001.

tionate to the total population has been decreasing in recent years (due to the low fertility rates), there were still 45 million children under the age of 15 years in the United States in 1973[10] — a sizable number when one considers their health care needs. (In Canada, there was a total of 6.2 million children under the age of 15 years in 1973.)[11] Children need a great deal of health supervision to promote their optimal growth and development and to protect them against the numerous diseases to which they are particularly vulnerable, in addition to the curative and restorative services required when they are sick.

[10]*Health United States 1975*, op. cit., p. 183.
[11]*Estimated Population by Sex and Age Group for Canada and Provinces*. Ottawa, Statistics Canada. Catalogue 91–202.

Much of the preventive and health promotional care is provided by physicians, nurses, and other health care workers in child care clinics across the nation. In many parts of the United States and Canada, community health nurses or specially prepared nurse practitioners are taking increasing responsibility for supervising the health care of children.

In the mid 1970s, the major "bulge" in our population pyramids (shown on pages 64 and 65) is in the adolescent and young adult age groups. When we consider future health care needs, we must not forget that these people are just beginning to produce children of their own (or will be soon). We can anticipate, therefore, increased demands on our maternal and child health care services during the next decade.

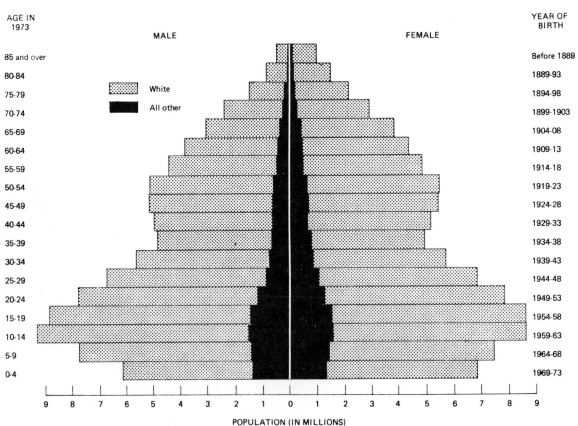

AGE-SEX DISTRIBUTION OF POPULATION BY COLOR: UNITED STATES, JULY 1, 1973

(Source: U.S. Bureau of the Census: Current Population Reports, Series P–25, No. 519. Reprinted from Health United States 1975. Rockville, Maryland, U.S. Department of Health, Education, and Welfare Publication No. (HRA) 76–1232. Public Health Service. Health Resources Administration, National Center for Health Statistics, p. 183.)

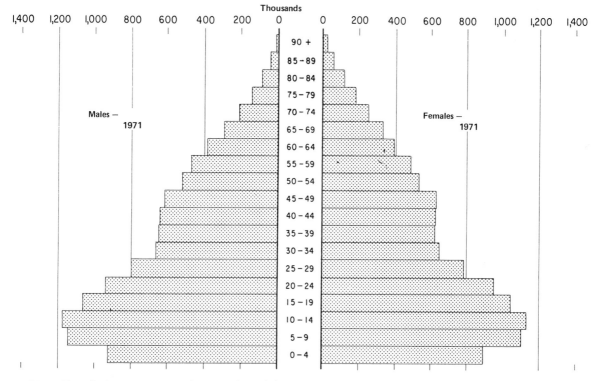

(From Population Projections for Canada and the Provinces. *Ottawa, Information Canada, June 1974,* p. 70.)

Then, too, if we look at the opposite end of the population pyramids, it is clear that the average age of people of North America is gradually increasing. Because of increases in life span, we have proportionately more older people in our society than we did a generation ago. The total number of people over the age of 65 years in the United States in 1973 was estimated at 21.4 million.[12] By the year 2000, it is expected that this figure will reach approximately 30 million.[13] In Canada, it is anticipated that the number of senior citizens will grow from an estimated 1.7 million in 1971[14] to approximately 3.3 million by the year 2001.[15] Older people have more

health needs than people in the middle years of the health spectrum. Because of their longer life span, they tend to suffer from more chronic and degenerative diseases. The needs for hospital, nursing home, home care, and other services to care for our senior citizens have put a strain on existing services and increased the demand for both facilities and personnel. There has been a major expansion in both the numbers and capacities of nursing homes to care for the sick among our aged population. This has meant additional requirements for trained workers in general and a heightened demand for professional nurses in particular to carry the major responsibility for supervising care in these homes.

Increasingly, too, it is being recognized that the provision of health promotion, health maintenance, and home care services for older people in the community can help to reduce the numbers needing

[12]*Health United States 1975*, op. cit., p. 181.
[13]Ibid., p. 195.
[14]*Population Projections for Canada and the Provinces 1972–2001*, p. 74.
[15]*A New Perspective on the Health of Canadians.* A Working Document. Ottawa, Department of National Health and Welfare, 1974, p. 60.

to be cared for in hospitals and other institutional facilities. Many innovative programs are being tried, with nurses becoming increasingly involved in the development and implementation of health clinics, health counseling, visiting nurse services, and the like for our senior citizens.

Another major factor contributing to the increased demand for health services has been a growing public awareness of the value of health care. Health is no longer considered a privilege, but rather a right. People have been made aware, through educational programs in the schools and through radio, television, newspapers, and the popular magazines, of the importance of periodic health checkups and the value of seeking professional help promptly in the event of suspected illness.

Then, too, an increased awareness of social need by the public has led to more extensive government involvement in health care and to the rapid expansion of health care programs to cover all segments of the population, rich and poor. In the United States, as we have mentioned, some form of national health insurance appears to be pending. Meanwhile, there has been a rapid expansion of private prepaid health insurance plans and increased outlays on both Medicare and Medicaid, two programs set up by the Federal Government to provide care for persons over 65 and the poor, respectively. In Canada, all provinces participate in a system of government-sponsored health insurance that covers almost 100 per cent of the population.

Government subsidies for the construction of hospitals, clinics, and health centers in both the United States and Canada have also contributed to the rapid growth in demand for both health care services and workers.

Although we seem to be catching up somewhat in meeting this demand, there are still many parts of the country where there are shortages of physicians and other highly trained professional people to care for the health needs of the population. This is particularly true of rural and isolated areas, but it is also true of low-income neighborhoods in our big cities. Many nurses are discovering challenging

careers as community or family nurse practitioners in underserviced areas.

Last, but by no means least, on the list of factors contributing to the increased demand for health services has been the explosion of scientific knowledge that has characterized the latter half of this century. It has been said that the total amount of new information stemming from research in the biomedical sciences in the past 30 years has more than doubled the total amount of knowledge in the field. Rapid advances in medical science have made possible surgery and medical treatment that could not have been contemplated at midcentury. More complex surgery, the development of complicated machines for the diagnosis and treatment of disease, and radical changes in therapy have intensified the need for people with highly specialized skills in the health care field. An ever increasing number of workers are engaged in research to promote still better methods of preventing and treating disease and newer and better ways of delivering health care services.

THE ESCALATING COSTS OF HEALTH CARE

Considerable concern has been expressed in both the United States and Canada over the rapidly escalating costs of health care. In Canada, the annual rate of cost escalation has been between 12 and 16 per cent in recent years;[16] in the United States, the average rate of change in national health expenditures has been running around 10 to 13 per cent during the past decade.[17] In both countries, these rates are far in excess of the rate of economic growth. Many people feel that if left unchecked, health care costs may soon be beyond the capacity of society to finance them.[18]

While population growth and factors such as increased utilization of services and quality changes account for a goodly proportion of the increased expenditures

[16]A New Perspective on the Health of Canadians, op. cit., p. 28.
[17]Health United States 1975, op. cit., p. 1.
[18]A New Perspective on the Health of Canadians, op. cit., p. 28.

on health care, price increases accounted for approximately half of the total increase. These price increases have been mainly in the increased cost of physician services and in increased hospital costs.[19]

Pressures created by the increased demand for health care services and the escalating costs of providing these services have forced a re-examination of our health care resources. Despite the huge sums of money being spent on health care and the growing numbers of people engaged in the health field, gaps and deficiencies in our present system of health care delivery have been pointed out in numerous study findings and conference reports of recent years. If we are to provide adequate health services to all of our citizens at a price we can afford to pay, it is apparent that we must utilize our resources as efficiently and effectively as possible.

At the present time, there is considerable turmoil in the field of health care. Existing arrangements for providing health services are being critically examined, and new approaches to the delivery of health care are being tried in many parts of the country.

HEALTH CARE SYSTEMS

The set of arrangements for the provision of health care in a country is usually referred to as its "health care system." Systems vary considerably from one country to another, both in the extent of responsibility assumed by government for the provision of health care services and in the administrative control of services. At one extreme is the completely free enterprise system, in which all services are bought and paid for by the consumer on an open market basis, in accordance with his perceived needs and his ability to pay. At the other extreme is the completely socialized system in which the government assumes full responsibility for the health care of all its citizens. In some countries the system is centrally controlled, that is, all services are administered by one central agency; in others, a multiplicity of agencies provide services. In between the extremes there are a wide variety of systems. The American and the Canadian health care systems both lie between the extremes. Although they differ in the extent of government sponsorship of programs, in both countries a wide variety of agencies provide services. The types of agencies providing services are similar in the two countries.

HEALTH CARE IN THE UNITED STATES AND IN CANADA

It is principally in the financing of personal health care services that differences currently exist in the American and the Canadian health care systems. The term "personal health care" refers to "services received by individuals and provided by health agencies and health professionals."[20] Personal health care expenditures are usually taken to include hospital services and those of related institutions, the services of medical and other health practitioners, nursing services, drugs, eyeglasses and appliances (such as artificial limbs), equipment, and supplies.[21]

In the United States at the present time, personal health care is paid for in a variety of ways. Government-sponsored programs include Medicare and Medicaid for senior citizens and the medically indigent, respectively. A large proportion of the remainder of the population is covered for personal health care expenses through private insurance plans. A number of industrial firms and mining, agricultural, and commercial enterprises also help people to meet the costs of personal health care through employer-employee cost-shared insurance plans or, in some instances, through the direct provision of health services for their workers as, for example, in a company hospital. Philanthropic (charitable) organizations also finance health services, particularly for specific groups in the population, such as the Shriners' hospitals for children, and the charitable clinics and hospitals run for the poor. Finally, there is the direct pay-

---

[19]*Health United States 1975*, op. cit., p. 10.

[20]*A New Perspective on the Health of Canadians*, op. cit., p. 27.

[21]*Health United States 1975*, op. cit., p. 16.

ment method of financing, whereby the individual pays for services directly out of his own pocket.

An increasingly large proportion of personal health care in the United States is being financed through public monies. In 1950, it was estimated that only one-fifth of the nation's expenditures for personal health care was paid for by the government. By 1970, nearly 38 per cent of these expenses were covered by government-sponsored programs, chiefly Medicare and Medicaid. There has also been a considerable increase in the amount paid for by private health insurance plans — from 8.5 per cent in 1950 to 25.6 per cent in 1970. It is estimated that approximately three-quarters of the American public now have some form of health insurance that covers major hospital and medical-surgical expenses. The out-of-pocket expenses borne by the individual consumer have decreased proportionately with the increase in public financing of health care and the expansion of private insurance plans, as shown in the figure below.[22]

In Canada, the major portion of personal health care expenditures is taken care of for the consumer of health services through a system of universal prepaid health insurance. The costs are borne almost entirely by the federal and provincial governments and indirectly by the consumer. The Federal Government's share of the costs is derived from general tax revenues. The provinces raise their share in different ways. Some finance the program entirely out of general tax monies. Others require the individual to pay a premium. In provinces where a premium is required, it is waived for people who would have difficulty in paying it, such as senior citizens and people on low incomes, and it is waived or reduced for students.

The range of services covered by the government-sponsored program varies from one province to another. All provincial plans must provide basic hospital and medical care services. Some include additional benefits, such as pharmaceutical services, foot care services, and eye care services. A number of people supplement the government program with private insurance plans to cover additional ex-

---

[22]*Health United States 1975*, op. cit., p. 40.

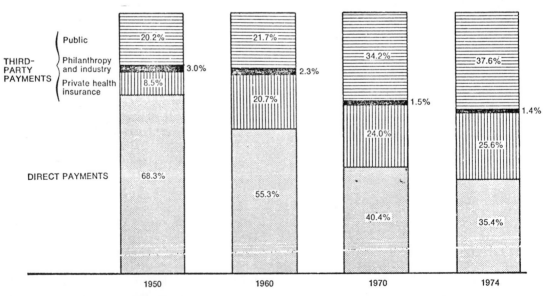

Distribution of personal health care expenditures, by source of funds, selected fiscal years 1950–1974. (Source: Social Security Bulletin, *February 1975, p. 17. Reprinted from* Health United States 1975. *Rockville, Maryland, U.S. Department of Health, Education, and Welfare Publication No. (HRA) 76–1232. Public Health Service. Health Resources Administration, National Center for Health Statistics, p. 41.)*

penses they might incur, such as the costs for private or semiprivate accommodations in hospital, or else to provide income security in the event of illness. In addition, industrial and commercial firms frequently offer supplementary benefits, such as dental insurance, to their employees on an employer-employee cost-shared basis. As in the United States, industrial firms also share in the financing of health clinics and hospitals in some instances.[23]

THE SPECTRUM OF HEALTH CARE SERVICES IN THE COMMUNITY

People seek the help of health services for a multiplicity of reasons. The new mother may take her infant to the physician's office or to a "well-baby" clinic to make sure that he is developing normally, to obtain advice on caring for him in order to promote his optimal growth and development, and to receive immunizations to protect him from disease. In our health-oriented society, a number of people go to their physicians for periodic health checkups, not because they are ill, but to be reassured that they are well. A great many people, however, do not seek the help of health professionals unless they are worried about their health. The majority of these people receive diagnostic services and are treated in physicians' offices, in clinics, or in outpatient departments of hospitals. Many who are ill, however, need to be hospitalized. They may later require rehabilitation services in specialized agencies. People with chronic or prolonged illnesses often need to be cared for in nursing homes or other extended care facilities over a long period of time.

The spectrum of health services in a community ranges from health promotion and protection services, through primary care facilities, to inpatient services and home care for the sick and rehabilitation services for those who require them. A wide variety of agencies provide these services, and many agencies combine a

number of them. Hospitals, for example, often have outpatient services for the detection and treatment of illness, as well as inpatient services for the acutely ill and home care programs for the convalescent. In many instances, two or more agencies combine to provide a more complete range of services for individuals and families. A city health department, for example, may work in combination with a visiting nurse service to provide nursing care in the home. Nurses in their practice work in all phases of the health care spectrum and are employed in a wide variety of health agencies.

THE PROVIDERS OF HEALTH CARE

In both the United States and Canada, health care services are provided by a wide variety of health agencies and health professionals. We will discuss these in regard to their roles in the provision of services in the various areas of the health care spectrum. It may be helpful, however, for the student to keep in mind the major headings under which the providers of health care may be categorized. These include:
1. Government agencies
2. Private, non–profit-making agencies
3. Private, profit-making (or proprietary) agencies
4. Private practitioners.

AGENCIES PROVIDING HEALTH PROMOTION AND HEALTH PROTECTION SERVICES

The nurse's role in the promotion of health and the prevention of disease is an expanding one. At the present time, most nurses whose work is primarily concerned with these aspects of health care are employed in official or voluntary agencies. Official agencies are agencies of the government; voluntary agencies are supported by contributions from people within the community and are operated as private, non-profit-making agencies. The specific services provided by official and voluntary agencies in any community de-

[23]*External Affairs Reference Paper No. 94.* Prepared in the Department of National Health and Welfare, Ottawa, 1975 (revised).

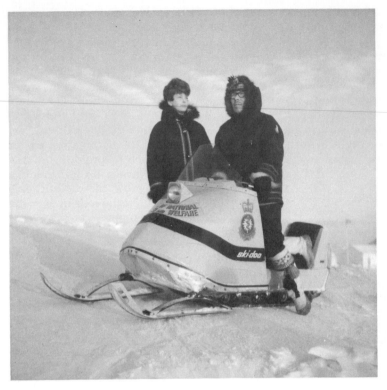

In some rural and remote parts of the country, the public health nurse is the chief source of health care. Here, the nurse and a native community health worker set off from a northern outpost nursing station to make their rounds.

pend to a large extent on the apparent needs of the people. In some communities, most health services may be provided through private physicians and private agencies; in others, official health agencies may offer more extensive programs.

Official Agencies

Official health agencies have been established at the local, state/provincial, and federal levels. At all levels, these agencies are concerned with the prevention of illness and the promotion of health. They often provide services of a curative and rehabilitative nature as well.

The local government agency is usually a city or a county health department, although other branches of a local government may also provide health services as, for example, the welfare department of the school board. The health department of a city or a county usually develops its own health program, based on the needs of the people in the community and the

resources available to meet these needs.[24] The general community program usually includes preventive measures, such as communicable disease control, the control of pollution, the safeguarding of water, milk, and other food supplies, and the maintenance of cleanliness of public beaches and swimming pools. Health education is also a large part of the program of most local community agencies.

Many official agencies at the local level provide a number of specialized health services in addition to the general community program. These frequently include maternal and child care services; immunization clinics; and often diagnostic, treatment, and rehabilitative services, particularly for people in low income groups. The school health program usually consists of health supervision of the students and counselling and consultative services for teachers and parents, as well as the supervision of environmental

[24]Ruth B. Freeman: *Community Health Nursing Practice.* Philadelphia, W. B. Saunders Company, 1970, pp. 89–93.

sanitation. School nurses may also participate in classroom teaching activities that relate to health matters.

The local government may also be responsible for the operation of hospitals and related facilities for the care of the sick. These are discussed later in this chapter under inpatient services.

State and provincial health departments, for the most part, assume leadership and advisory roles to local health agencies, but they may also provide direct services such as the operation of laboratories, the licensure of individuals and agencies, the dissemination of information, and the provision of financial assistance. In some states (and provinces), community health agencies serving centers outside the large metropolitan areas may be organized directly by the state department of health. State governments also operate hospitals, particularly tuberculosis hospitals and psychiatric facilities. Community mental health clinics may be directly operated by a state or provincial agency, as for example, are mental hospitals, schools for the mentally retarded, and other related psychiatric facilities.

Federal health agencies are concerned with promoting the general health of the nation. In both the United States and Canada, health is primarily the responsibility of the individual states (or provinces). National health policies are therefore initiated at the Federal level, but are implemented by the states. The Federal Government contributes a large share of the monies required to carry out various health programs at the state and community levels, as, for example, the Medicare and Medicaid programs in the United States and the National Health Insurance programs in Canada. The Federal Government, through its numerous agencies, provides advisory and consultative services for local and state health agencies. Another Federal responsibility is the maintenance of a national information service about health matters. Federal agencies, for example, collect vital statistics and statistics relative to the prevalence of disease, health facilities, and health manpower. The Federal Government's role in research in all aspects of health care is also highly significant.

At the direct services level, the Federal Government is concerned with the control of interstate hazards such as pollution, with the control of communicable disease, and the setting of standards for food and drug control. The Federal Government is also directly responsible for the provision of health care services to certain segments of the population such as Armed Services personnel and their families, war veterans, and the members of the native Indian and Inuit populations.

Voluntary Agencies

Voluntary agencies are established by the people in a community in response to a particular need that is felt in that community. They are usually supported by donations, and the services they provide serve to supplement or augment the functions performed by official agencies. Voluntary agencies usually provide services of a specific nature. They may be concerned with the preventive, curative, and rehabilitative aspects of one disease, as for example, heart disease, tuberculosis, diabetes, or arthritis. Some agencies confine their attention to a particular segment of the population, such as handicapped children or the mentally retarded. A number of voluntary groups are presently concerned with environmental programs such as pollution control. The visiting nurse agencies that provide care for the sick in the home are organized in many communities by voluntary associations. Voluntary agencies may develop at a strictly local level, at a state level, or they may be national in scope. In the United States, most visiting nurse services are locally organized; in Canada, on the other hand, the major visiting nurse service is the Victorian Order of Nurses, which is a national organization.[25]

PRIMARY CARE SERVICES

Although many health professionals tend to think of the hospital as the prin-

---

[25] For additional material on the organization and functions of official and voluntary agencies, the nurse is referred to Ruth B. Freeman, op. cit.

cipal place where sick people receive care, in actual fact, it has been estimated that approximately 95 per cent of this care is given outside of hospitals.[26] Most of the health service that people receive is provided in physicians' offices, in clinics, or in other community agencies. The term "primary care" is used to designate the initial health care given, that is, the point at which an individual enters the health care system.

The area of primary care has been singled out as one of the most pressing problems in the health field today. A shortage of physicians has been given as one of the principal reasons for the inadequacy of primary care services, particularly in rural areas and in low income neighborhoods in urban centers. Many hospitals have found their emergency wards overtaxed with nonemergency health problems, because people have been coming to them for care that was not available elsewhere. Because of this problem, a number of alternative methods of providing needed health services are being tried. The principal providers of primary care services in the community at the present time are private physicians, the clinics operated by community health agencies, the outpatient departments of hospitals, and other, newly emerging agencies such as Health Maintenance Organizations (HMOs), Neighborhood and Community Health Centers, and "free" or storefront clinics.

Private Physicians' Services

A large number of nurses are employed in physicians' offices. They may work with one physician who is in "solo" practice or with a group of physicians. Although the majority of physicians in the United States and Canada are still in individual practice, group practice is becoming more common. In this type of practice, several physicians may work together to provide more comprehensive care for individuals and families. For example, there may be one or two family practitioners in the group, an obstetrician, a pediatrician, and a surgeon. Frequently, there is also a psychiatrist, and there may be other specialists as well. Some group practices are small; others are quite extensive. In a large group practice, several nurses may be employed as well as other supportive personnel.

_____

[26]D. Curiel et al.: _Trends in the Study of Morbidity and Mortality._ (Public Health Paper No. 27.) Geneva, World Health Organization, 1965.

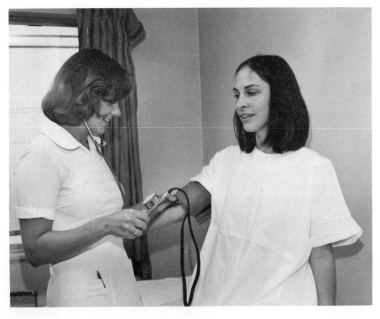

Many nurses who work in physicians' offices now undertake the initial assessment of patients.

The nurse's role in a "solo" physician's office or in a group practice setting varies. The traditional "office nurse" role included receiving patients in the office, making appointments and referrals for the patient, and assisting the physician with physical examinations and treatments. Increasingly, however, nurses are assuming a much more independent and expanded role in working with physicians in community practice. Many nurses these days undertake the initial assessment of patients, including history-taking and physical examination. They frequently do a considerable amount of health counselling, advising people and helping them to promote and maintain their health. Some nurses working as associates to physicians make home or hospital visits; some carry a caseload of patients, consulting with the physician about their care and referring to him (or her) those problems that he (or she) alone is qualified to handle.

Health Maintenance Organizations

Health Maintenance Organizations (HMOs) have been developing in increasing numbers in the United States in recent years. Their development has been encouraged by passage of the 1972 Social Security Amendments, which facilitated the use of HMOs by Medicare and Medicaid recipients, and the Health Maintenance Organization Act of 1973, which spelled out guidelines for HMOs seeking to be federally qualified.

The HMO is essentially a form of prepaid group practice. It provides a comprehensive range of services on a fixed contract basis, which is paid for in advance by people enrolling in the organization. The emphasis in the HMOs is on health promotion and the prevention of illness. The range of services provided by HMOs covers both preventive and curative care and includes physician services, health counselling, inpatient and outpatient hospital services, and diagnostic and therapeutic services, including home care. Many nurses are employed in HMOs, where they often work as associates to the physicians in an expanding role such as that described previously.

Clinic and Outpatient Services

The term "clinic" may be applied to a group practice of private physicians such as that just described or may be used to designate the services provided by a community agency for care and treatment of the sick on an ambulatory basis. In ambulatory care, the patient remains at home but comes into the agency for care and treatment. When community agencies operate clinic services, these usually are provided free of charge to the patient, or a nominal charge may be made. Outpatient services, also of an ambulatory nature, are provided by many hospitals. Again, these may be offered on a charitable basis, or the patient may pay a small fee. In the clinics and outpatient departments, diagnostic and treatment services are provided and often rehabilitative services as well. The nurse working in a clinic or outpatient service is frequently responsible for the day-to-day management of the clinic, and she assists the physicians with physical examinations and with treatments. She may also perform laboratory tests. The nurse is often involved in health teaching activities in the clinic and in health counselling for individuals and families.

Neighborhood Health Centers

A recent development in the area of primary health services for the people in a community has been the establishment of Neighborhood Health Centers. Originally these centers were set up by the Office of Economic Opportunity in the United States to provide health care services in poverty and ghetto areas. The centers provide comprehensive health services (exclusive of inpatient services) for the residents of a given community in their own neighborhood. They employ a clinic type of approach but are concerned with both health and social problems. They frequently utilize people who live in the community as adjunctive health workers. The concept of the Neighborhood Health Center is rapidly gaining wide acceptance as one possible solution to the problem of providing adequate primary care services in the community to other groups of residents besides the poor.[27]

Community Health Centers

The Community Health Centers that have been developing in Canada are similar in concept to the Neighborhood Health Centers in the United States. They are not, however, intended for any specific segment of the population, such as the poor, but rather for the use of all residents in a community. Community participation is encouraged on the advisory boards of the centers, which are usually government agencies, and a comprehensive range of services is offered, including social as well as health services.

"Free Clinics"

The so-called free, or storefront, clinics that have sprung up in both the United States and Canada in the past few years offer another example of innovation in the field of primary health care. These clinics have been set up in poverty or ghetto neighborhoods to provide health services

---

[27]Patterns of Care. *American Journal of Public Health, 60*:1723, September 1970.

for people who, because of an inability to pay, or a reluctance to use traditional agencies, were not receiving the care they needed. They offer a readily accessible, usually 24-hour, day care on a free or minimal charge basis in a setting that is as devoid of "red tape" as possible. The clinics have been staffed for the most part by health professionals, young doctors, nurses, and social workers (often students), or retired professionals, who work on a voluntary basis to provide needed health care. Although there are many problems associated with this type of agency, as, for example, the legal implications of who does what, the provision of personalized, accessible, and nonjudgmental care with a minimum of bureaucratic structure appears to be meeting an otherwise unmet need in many communities.

AGENCIES PROVIDING INPATIENT SERVICES FOR THE CARE OF THE SICK

The majority of registered nurses in both the United States and Canada are employed in hospitals or related institutions that provide inpatient services for the care of the sick. In addition, a large proportion of the clinical experience of

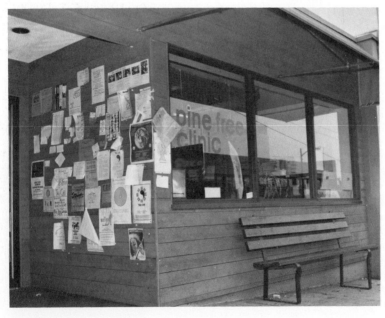

"Free clinics" offer easily accessible primary care to many who would otherwise not obtain needed health services.

nursing students takes place in hospitals. The nurse should therefore be familiar with the functions of hospitals, the kinds of hospitals and related institutions in her community, and the various departments within a hospital.

The Hospital

The hospital is an institution whose chief purpose is the care of sick and injured people. Although not the only agencies concerned with health, hospitals are the centers in which a wide range of specialized functions are brought to bear on health problems. People who are acutely ill generally come to a hospital to avail themselves of the services of the professional people and the facilities necessary for their care.

Hospitals, like other community health agencies, perform curative, preventive, and rehabilitative functions, and are also involved in two additional areas of commitment: research and education. The emphasis placed upon any of the three areas varies with the agency. Generally, the policies of agencies in this regard are determined by the following factors:

1. The cultural, religious, and social groups within the community
2. The nature of the health problems of the patients admitted to the hospital
3. The availability of medical and related personnel
4. The specific needs of the particular community and the facilities that are already available
5. The money available to provide these facilities
6. The existence of nearby institutions, for example, a university
7. The size of the community that the hospital serves.

Hospital policies are usually set by the hospital board of directors. Although the membership varies from hospital to hospital, the board usually consists chiefly of people representative of the community served by the hospital. There is usually also one or more representatives of the medical department on the board and, in hospitals operated or financed by government agencies, a member representative of government interests. The hospital administrator almost invariably attends board meetings and frequently serves as secretary to the board. In some hospitals, the director of nursing also attends board meetings, on either a regular or an occasional basis; in others, she does not. Sometimes she is a full-fledged member of the board.

In performing its basic function, the care of the sick and injured, the hospital usually renders emergency care as well as diagnostic, therapeutic, and rehabilitative services. Many hospitals also provide facilities for research so that members of the health disciplines avail themselves of the clinical resources of the hospital. Education, the third function of most hospitals, includes the in-service education of institutional personnel and programs for medical students, nursing students, laboratory technicians, dietetic interns, and a variety of other students in the health disciplines.

Kinds of Hospitals. There are many kinds of hospitals; they can be described according to their size, ownership, control, services, or the length of stay of the patients. Usually a hospital is described in terms of its available beds. The small community might have a hospital of 10 beds; a large metropolitan area might have one of 2000 beds. Often, smaller hospitals offer limited services, but they may have an arrangement with larger hospitals for the prompt transfer of patients in need of specialized facilities.

Hospitals may be owned or controlled by the government, by private groups, or by a single individual. Government ownership of hospitals may be at the federal, state, or local level. Often these institutions are governed jointly by representatives of the government and representatives of the community in which the hospital is situated. This arrangement is usually true of the county or municipal hospital. Private groups also own hospitals; for example, it is not unusual for religious organizations to have their own health institutions. An individual or a group of individuals may also operate a hospital or clinic. Physicians in particular often own and operate their own hospitals.

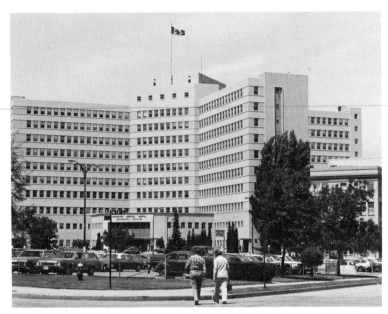

The hospital provides a center where a wide variety of specialized functions are available to combat health problems.

The services offered are another way of describing a hospital. Thus, a hospital may be a general hospital; that is, one that offers a diversity of services, such as surgery, medicine, psychiatry, obstetrics, and pediatrics. Or it may be a special hospital, admitting only patients of one sex, people with a particular type of illness, or children of a specific age group. In years past, psychiatric hospitals were the most obvious special hospitals, and often they were situated in rural areas. Today, however, there is a trend to incorporate a psychiatric nursing unit into the general hospital rather than isolate the mentally ill from the community. There has also been a considerable expansion of psychiatric outpatient facilities that enable people to carry on their normal activities while receiving care on an ambulatory basis.

The length of stay of the patient is also a basis upon which to classify an institution. Generally speaking, there are acute care hospitals, extended care hospitals, and day care hospitals. The acute care hospital has restrictions upon the length of stay of patients; some permit patients to stay 30 days at the maximum, after which they are transferred to an extended care insitution. The extended care hospital, as its name implies, is for long-term patients. Often its accent is upon the retraining and rehabilitating of patients over a period of

months. Nursing homes also provide long-term care for the sick who require nursing services over an extended period of time.

The day care hospital is a relatively new addition to hospital services. Originally intended for psychiatric patients, it now offers services to patients with various other illnesses. The patient stays at the hospital during the day and returns to his home at night. This arrangement has the obvious advantage of lowering hospital expenses as well as maintaining the home orientation of the patient. Many hospitals also operate day-surgery units for people requiring minor operations who do not need to be hospitalized for more than a few hours.

Standards for the quality of service in the hospital have been established by the Joint Commission on Accreditation of Hospitals. Instituted in 1952, the commission is composed of representatives of the American College of Surgeons, the American College of Physicians, the American Hospital Association, and the American Medical Association. The commission can accredit a hospital, provisionally accredit it, or not accredit it at all. A similar commission accredits hospitals in Canada.

The Departments Within the Hospital. The many services available within the hospital can be classified as direct or indirect with respect to the patient. These services can be divided into three groups: patient care services, institutional services, and financial services. The services correspond roughly with the departments of the hospital.

Usually, however, the number of separate departments in a hospital is dependent upon its size. The larger the hospital, the greater is the number of departments. The patient is usually aware of the medical department, the x-ray department, and the nursing department. He may be less aware of the maintenance department and the purchasing department, yet their services are also important to his comfort and welfare. The following departments are commonly found in the average hospital.

THE MEDICAL DEPARTMENT. The medical department includes the members of the medical staff who are responsible for the care of the patients. Often this department designates a board whose members keep watch on the quality of medical care given by the physicians attending the patients.

THE NURSING DEPARTMENT. The nursing department includes registered nurses, practical nurses, nursing orderlies, and nurse's aides. These people usually give direct care to the patients under the guidance of the head of the department and according to the policies of the hospital administration. The head of the nursing department is usually the director of nursing; she may have an assistant director as well as supervisors and head nurses to carry out administrative duties.

If a hospital has a school of nursing, it may be included within the department of nursing. However, a school of nursing can affiliate with a hospital and yet be a separate entity financially and administratively.

THE DIETARY DEPARTMENT. The dietary department includes dietitians as well as cooks, kitchen maids, tray girls, and dishwashers. The chief responsibility of this department is to supply food to the patients, and sometimes to the staff of the hospital. This responsibility usually includes the preparation of therapeutic diets for many patients.

THE LABORATORY DEPARTMENT. The function of the laboratory department is to perform laboratory tests ordered by the physician. These tests include blood serology and chemistry tests, urinalyses, bacteriological tests, and analyses of specimens for pathological diagnosis. The laboratory technologist collects some specimens; the nursing staff is responsible for the collection of others.

THE X-RAY DEPARTMENT. One of the obvious functions of the x-ray department is to take x-rays of patients as ordered by medical practitioners. In addition to the x-ray technologists who work in the department, many hospitals employ physicians who are specialists in interpreting x-rays and can aid other physicians in their diagnostic work. The use of x-ray equipment, radium, and the like for therapeutic purposes is also an important function of many x-ray departments.

THE MAINTENANCE DEPARTMENT. The number of services provided by the maintenance department varies from hospital to hospital. The department often performs carpentry, plumbing, and electrical services, as well as cleaning, heating, and possibly laundry services.

THE PHARMACY DEPARTMENT. The pharmacy department provides pharmaceutical supplies that are ordered by physicians for their patients. The pharmacist prepares some of the medications himself, while others are purchased commercially and are dispensed to the nursing units.

THE BUSINESS DEPARTMENT. This department is responsible for the financial business of the hospital. It prepares the patient's hospital bills, administers the hospital payroll, and is involved in budget preparation and general hospital business.

THE CENTRAL SUPPLY DEPARTMENT. The central supply department of the hospital is usually responsible for the cleaning, the sterilizing, and often the delivery of equipment used in the institution. It may also be responsible for the purchasing of supplies if the hospital has no purchasing department. In some hospitals, the central supply department is included in the nursing department.

THE PERSONNEL DEPARTMENT. This department is responsible for hiring personnel and for job placement within the hospital. Some nursing departments assume the responsibilities for hiring nurses, whereas at other hospitals this task is handled entirely by the personnel department.

THE SOCIAL SERVICE DEPARTMENT. Many hospitals have a separate department to provide welfare services for the patients. Among the concerns of the social worker are family finances and nursing home placement. Usually he maintains liaison between the hospital and other welfare agencies in the community.

OTHER DEPARTMENTS. Large hospitals may have many other departments. There may be separate departments for electrocardiography, physical therapy, public relations, and hairdressing. The services that hospitals supply vary considerably; however, no matter how many departments there may be, they have a common goal: to help meet the needs of the hospital patient and his family.

HOME CARE SERVICES

With the increasing emphasis today on early discharge of patients from hospital and on treating patients within their own home environment as much as possible, many nurses are being employed in home care programs. Home care programs are designed to provide nursing care and other services of a therapeutic nature to people in their own homes.

There are basically two types of home care programs: those that are community-based and those that are hospital-based. Community-based programs are administered by agencies other than a hospital. They may be operated by an official agency, for example, a city health department; by a voluntary agency such as a visiting nurse service; by a combination of agencies; or by a separately incorporated agency. Referrals are made to the agency by the physician who remains in charge of the patient's care. The patient may be admitted to the program either directly from the community or from a hospital where he has been receiving care.

Hospital-based home care programs are usually operated by a hospital in a manner similar to outpatient services. Nurses and other personnel involved in the home care program may be employed by the hospital, or the services of people attached to another agency may be utilized through a contractual arrangement. A hospital may enter into an agreement with a visiting nurse agency, for example, to provide home care services for its patients. The hospital programs are usually limited to patients who have been discharged from the hospital, or to those who would otherwise be admitted to the hospital as inpatients.

Home care programs frequently offer a wide variety of services, such as direct care nursing services, physical therapy, and occupational therapy. Sometimes specialized rehabilitative services or treatment are provided as well. Frequently, a "homemaker service" is a part of the total home care program.[28]

EXTENDED CARE SERVICES

A growing number of registered nurses and licensed practical nurses work in agencies whose primary purpose is the care of people with long-term illness. The majority of residents in these agencies are older people who require varying amounts of nursing care. With the rapidly growing numbers of older people in our society, there has been a great proliferation in both the number and types of extended care facilities. Included in this category are personal care homes, nursing homes, extended care units in hospitals, and hospitals solely for the care of long-term patients. A large-scale program to improve standards in all types of agencies providing long-term care is currently underway. Whereas many formerly operated with a minimal number of professionally qualified staff, regulations requiring adequate qualified nursing personnel are now being enforced. There has consequently been a considerably increased demand for registered nurses and licensed practical nurses to work in these agencies. The emphasis

---

[28]This material was based on a paper originally prepared by F. Catherine Maddaford: Organized Home Care Programs in Canada, at the School of Hygiene, University of Toronto, 1968.

in extended care agencies is changing, too, from a custodial type of care to one stressing the restoration of the individual to his optimal level of functioning, physically, mentally, and socially. Nurses specializing in the care of the long-term patient find the work rewarding and challenging. It demands a high level of nursing skill and, while perhaps not as dramatic as nursing in the acute care setting, offers considerable satisfaction.

REHABILITATION SERVICES

Rehabilitation is the restoration of an individual who has been ill, from whatever cause, to the most complete level of social, physical, and mental functioning that is possible for him. The concept of rehabilitation should permeate all health care, and should be a factor in the therapeutic plan of care for each patient. Rehabilitation does not commence when the patient is over the acute phase of an illness; nor is it the responsibility solely of specialized agencies. It begins with the patient's admission to whatever agency he comes to for the care and treatment of an illness; his restoration to an active, functioning role in society, insofar as this is possible, should be the aim of all who care for him.

In the past, the major health problems in our society were the acute infectious illnesses, which were usually of short duration; the patient either recovered quickly or succumbed to the infection and died. Today, with the increasing prevalence of the chronic and degenerative diseases, and the vast numbers of people suffering permanent injuries as a result of accidents, there is a growing need for long-term restorative services, and considerably more emphasis is being placed on rehabilitation.

For many people injured in accidents or crippled with degenerative disorders, restoration to their optimal level of functioning is a lengthy process that may take years of encouragement and require specialized care. Frequently these people need the help of members of a variety of health disciplines—physicians, nurses, therapists, clergymen, and social workers, among others—to assist in their rehabilitation. Often, they require facilities that are not usually provided in acute care hospitals, such as gymnasiums, swimming pools, and outdoor recreational areas, as well as nursing units especially adapted to facilitate increasing independence in the activities of daily living.

In response to the growing need for these types of services, specialized agencies have developed whose primary pur-

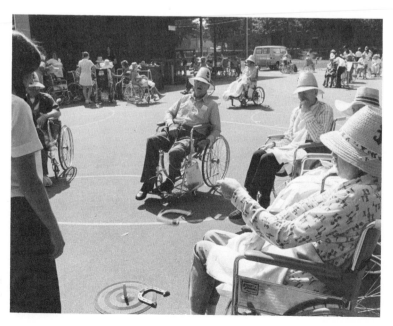

Outdoor recreational areas are important for people requiring long-term care.

pose is rehabilitation. Rehabilitation programs in independent centers in the community and as part of the programs of other health agencies and institutions offer comprehensive service to the disabled. A rehabilitation unit coordinates the efforts of many disciplines in order to plan an approach designed to meet individual needs. Generally, each patient follows an individual plan of therapy during his rehabilitation. The rehabilitation team meets regularly to discuss the patient's progress and revise the plan to meet his changing needs. In addition to the specialized agencies in the community, many acute care hospitals now have a rehabilitation unit to which the patient can be transferred when he is ready. At this time, the rehabilitation team assumes the major responsibility for his therapy.

Most people require physical and occupational therapy in order to restore maximum physical function. Learning to walk and regaining the use of various body muscles are important aspects of therapy. Most rehabilitation centers provide gymnasium facilities for corrective and preventive exercises for patients. Such exercises are conducted by a physical therapist both on an individual basis and in classes. Workshops, where patients relearn skill in utilizing muscles through using them in arts and crafts, are also an important part of most rehabilitation agen-

cies. These workshops are staffed by occupational therapists.

Relearning the activities that are necessary for daily living is most important to patients. To dress oneself, to prepare meals, and so on, represent areas of independence in which the handicapped person can maintain his self-respect. Rehabilitation programs teach the patient to carry out these activities for himself, often providing him with specially constructed tools, such as a fork with an enlarged handle, which a person with a partially paralyzed hand can grasp more easily.

Some patients require vocational education before they can obtain employment that is compatible with their limitations. Vocational counsellors can advise patients about fields in which they are likely to succeed and about the employment opportunities in these fields.

The psychologist and the psychiatrist are also important members of the rehabilitation team. Their professional help is often required to help patients cope with the psychological stresses accompanying illness and disability. Moreover, since rehabilitation services can be fully effective only when the patient is motivated to help himself and to cooperate in his plan of therapy, the guidance of the psychologist and the psychiatrist is often necessary to the success of the program.

Before a patient in an inpatient facility

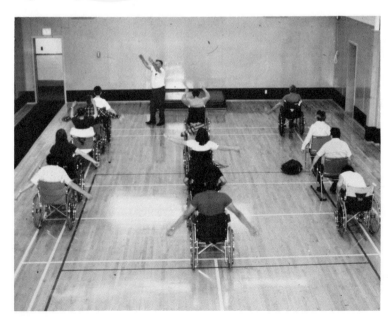

Rehabilitation centers usually have a gymnasium where patients learn corrective or preventive exercises individually or in groups.

is ready for discharge, he is visited by a member of a community health agency who assists him and his family in making arrangements for his return home. For example, if a patient cannot climb stairs, it may be necessary to change his sleeping arrangements in his home. Many community agencies provide nursing and rehabilitative services within the home. Encouragement and instruction carried on after discharge from a hospital help a person to continue to progress.

The Nurse's Role in Rehabilitation

Nurses play a key role in rehabilitation, both in the acute care setting and in the specialized rehabilitation agency. When the patient is acutely ill, good nursing care supports the patient's own resources in all areas of functioning and helps prevent the development of complications that can slow down or otherwise impede his fullest recovery. To illustrate this point, most people who are acutely ill—with a heart attack, a stroke, a fracture, or any other type of illness—are placed on bed rest. The patient's position in bed is important to maintain good body alignment and to prevent the development of deformities in joints, such as the wrist or the ankle, which the patient may not be able to move himself. Good skin care and frequent changes of position are essential to prevent the development of pressure sores that can take months to heal. Muscles that are not being used need to be exercised within the patient's level of tolerance, or they soon become weak and require considerable restorative treatment to regain their normal strength. The nursing care plan for every patient must take into consideration not only the immediate problems with which the patient needs help, but also the potential problems that can arise if good preventive care is not given.

Then, too, in both the acute care setting and in the specialized rehabilitation unit, nursing is the one constant in a variety of services that are needed to restore people to their optimal level of health. Nursing is *there,* on a 24 hours a day, seven days a week basis, whereas other health workers come and go, spending varying amounts of time with the patient. It is frequently up to the nurse, then, to ensure that all aspects of the rehabilitation plan for the patient are carried through, and that there is continuity and consistency in the approach used by all members of staff.

Because of her day-to-day contact with patients, the nurse is often the first person to recognize or become aware of many of the patient's needs. Patients often talk easily to a nurse whom they have come to know and who has helped them in the acute phase of their illnesses. Her observations, her understanding, and her knowledge, therefore, can be valuable assets to the rehabilitation team.

Another important responsibility of the nurse is to encourage and support the patient during the period of rehabilitation. Progress is not always steady; there are sometimes plateaus, and during these periods patients feel discouraged. An understanding nurse can help people through these periods of discouragement by reassuring them about their progress. In so doing, the nurse reinforces and supports the teaching of other members of the rehabilitation team.

Patients frequently find it necessary to relearn many skills of living. The nurse's role is vitally important in ensuring that all who care for him are aware of the patient's needs and support him in his relearning activities. She also helps him to plan his day's activities so that practice and learning sessions are well spaced in order to avoid fatigue.

Above all, the nurse is frequently responsible for coordinating the patient's care. Since she has contact with the various members of the rehabilitation team, the patient's family, and the patient, it is often the nurse who is in the best position to schedule the activities of the patient and to help interpret his needs to the various members of the team.

ADMISSION OF AN INDIVIDUAL TO A HEALTH AGENCY

Most people are anxious when they go to a health agency for the first time. Even if they are going for a routine checkup, there is always the nagging worry that something may be wrong. Minor irritations suddenly become magnified, and a person can imagine all sorts of horrible diseases that he may have. For example, the small rash on his arm may be the first sign of cancer—he had better remember to ask the doctor about that. Having to enter a hospital is especially traumatic for most people, and the transfer, if one is made, to an extended care facility frequently carries with it thoughts of being relegated to the "never going to get better" category. The admission of a patient to any type of health agency is therefore always a critical point in his care.

The patient is, as we have said, usually apprehensive, and the attitude and behavior of the nurses and other agency personnel concerned with his admission can do much to make him feel more comfortable. A sincere welcome and genuine interest in the patient help to reassure him that he is a person of worth and dignity. Many health agencies, particularly large ones, have been criticized for their impersonality. Much of the criticism stems from the fact that the agencies are busy places and the personnel are often rushed. But it does not take extra time to be kind or to convey to the patient that he is welcome.

Although each agency has its own admitting procedure, there are some commonalities that the nurse will find in all agencies. We have concentrated here on the admission of a patient to a hospital, because much of the experience a student will have is in a hospital setting, but it is important to remember that the principles are the same, regardless of the type of health agency to which the patient is being admitted.

When a patient comes to a hospital, he usually goes initially to the admitting office. Here he answers the questions of the admitting clerk or admitting nurse about his financial status, his age, his address, his next of kin, and his usual employment. Most hospitals supply an admission sheet for this purpose.

Often the patient's initial impression of a hospital is formed in the admitting department. Thus, the appearance of the area and the kind of reception provided by the staff are of utmost importance. If a patient is acutely ill, however, he may be admitted to the emergency department of the hospital. In this case it is often a member of the family of the patient who gives the needed information to the admitting clerk. Most hospitals ask patients to sign a consent form during the admitting procedure. This form gives the hospital staff permission to perform any diagnostic and treatment procedures that are considered necessary during the patient's stay.

After the patient has given the requested information to the receptionist in the admitting department, he is usually shown to a nursing unit. When the patient arrives at the nursing unit, a sincere welcome is again important in helping to ease the adjustment to his new environment. The patient should be greeted by name. His family or friends who have accompanied him to hospital should also be made welcome. The patient's room or his bed unit should be ready for him so that he feels expected and welcome. The nurse can help the patient by showing him where showers and bathrooms are located, also telephones and other facilities, and by explaining various routines such as mealtimes and visiting hours. In orienting the patient to his new situation, the following points are helpful to keep in mind:

1. The patient needs an introduction to nursing unit personnel and a brief explanation of their duties.

2. He needs an introduction to other patients in the room in which he will be staying.

3. He needs an explanation of pertinent hospital routines and policies. These assist the patient to become familiar with what is expected of him and what he may expect. Many hospitals have prepared patient information booklets, which are very helpful in this regard.

4. He needs to know how his call light or the intercom system at the patient unit is operated.

The nurse should also find out if the patient has any particular needs or desires that would make his stay in the hospital more comfortable. Some patients, because of their religious or cultural backgrounds,

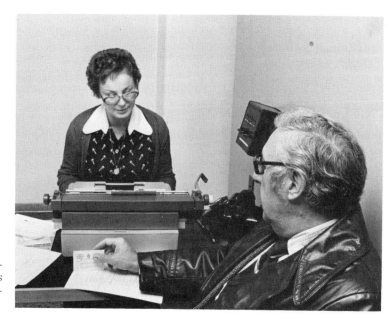

A patient's initial impression of a health agency is often formed in the admitting office.

have specific dietary requests, and the dietitian should be informed about these. The nurse should also find out from the patient if he has any allergies and if he has been on any medications at home, such as steroids. These observations should be noted on the patient's record and reported to the attending physician.

Once the initial orientation to the hospital has been completed, the patient is usually examined by the hospital physician. This examination includes a medical history, a physical examination, and routine screening tests. In most hospitals, all newly admitted patients have a urinalysis and a hemoglobin or hematocrit test. Many hospitals require a chest x-ray and a blood serology test for syphilis as part of the admission routine. Tests for pulmonary function and also tests for blood sugar are performed routinely for all newly admitted patients in some hospitals.

During her contact with the patient, the nurse's initial observations are of particular importance in identifying problems with which the patient needs help. The initial observations are an important part of the nursing assessment and provide a basis for the nursing care plan for the patient. (See Chapter 9.)

Basic Principles for the Care of the Patient Admitted to a Health Agency

Much has been written about the psychological effect of the admission procedure on the patient. Hospitals have been especially criticized for the impersonal manner in which this procedure is frequently carried out, and the depersonalization the individual feels as a result of the routines many hospitals have considered essential. From the patient's point of view, he is first asked a lot of personal questions—to which he is expected to give answers to a stranger. Then, he is given a number and "tagged" with an armband. He is taken to a nursing unit that is usually also designated with a number, not a name, and assigned to a room or a bed, likewise numbered. Once there, he is stripped of all of his clothes and most of his valuables that help to identify him as a person. A procession of strangers then begins to arrive at his bedside—to ask more personal questions and perform various examinations on his body. Sometimes, these people do not even introduce themselves, and the patient is left to guess who they are by the uniform they are wearing. If the patient is assigned to a room in which there are other patients, he often has to make their acquaintance himself.

The nurse can do a great deal to dispel the impression of agency impersonality and minimize the patient's feelings of depersonalization. The following basic principles are helpful in serving as guides to action for the nurse in admitting a new patient.

Strange Situations Can Elicit Fear. When people enter a hospital, for example, they encounter a new environment and a new set of behavior norms. A number of items that should be included in the new patient's orientation were mentioned on page 82. Most patients recognize their need to become familiar with the customs and the policies of the hospital. In fact, the patients themselves often provide the new patient with information about the hospital and nursing unit personnel, anticipating his need for information and allaying his fears by explanations.

Illness Can be a New Experience. Consequently, people need to have an understanding of their illness and an opportunity to come to terms with their new situation. Most people want to know what is wrong with them, and what is going to happen to them. The nurse can help by giving all the information she can about his condition to both the patient and the worried family or friends who accompanied him to the hospital. If the nurse is unable to furnish a sufficient amount of information to answer the patient's questions herself, and allay his and his family's anxiety, she has a responsibility to relay the questions to someone who can. The patient should be told in advance about the various examinations and procedures that are going to be performed and given an explanation of why they are being done.

Patterns of Response Are Learned. A person may fear a situation not because of the situation itself but because of conditioning through previous learning. Thus, a patient may have had a badly administered injection at some time and react with more than the usual amount of apprehension when he sees the nurse advancing toward him with a syringe and needle in her hand. The nurse's confidence in her own ability to give an injection competently, based on sufficient practice in the skill, will help her to reassure the patient and allay his fears. It is helpful for the nurse to find out from the patient about previous experiences he may have had with hospitals and with health personnel, and his feelings about these experiences. With this information, she is better able to anticipate his needs and reactions.

Maintaining Personal Identity is Important. A person's name, clothes, and valuables frequently serve as symbols of his identity. They also represent security to many people, since they serve as a link with the understood and the familiar. The nurse can help a patient to maintain his identity by making a point of calling him by name and by encouraging him to use his own clothes (when this is hospital policy) and personal possessions when he is admitted to the hospital.

Subgroups Within a Culture Tend to Develop Their Own Norms of Behavior. An understanding of the diversity of habits and modes of behavior and an endeavor to assist each patient to maintain his particular patterns whenever they do not jeopardize his health will help the patient to maintain his identity and will serve to acknowledge respect for him as an individual. Sometimes the behavior of a patient differs from what the nurse expects; however, acceptance of the patient as a person is basic to the kind of nursing care that enhances his confidence and security.

Specific Admitting Measures

Two nursing care measures that are concerned specifically with the admission of a patient to a hospital are the care of his clothes and the care of his valuables.

Care of the Patient's Clothes. The manner of caring for a patient's clothes upon his admission to a hospital is dependent upon the policy of the specific hospital. In some hospitals, the family is asked to take the patient's clothes home; in others, the clothes are stored in a central clothes room after each article of clothing is listed on a hospital form. An increasingly more common procedure is for the patient to keep his clothes in a closet that is provided in his room. In this case, a clothing list is usually not made; instead, the patient signs a form which states that he assumes responsibility for all the belongings that he brings to the hospital. Occasionally, a patient's clothes are infested with vermin; most hospitals provide facilities for sterilizing such clothes before they are returned to the patient.

Because clothes are so often important symbols of identity to a patient, some hospitals suggest that patients wear their own clothes while they are staying there. However, a more common practice is to provide each patient with a hospital gown or pajamas, particularly if he is to have an operation.

Care of the Patient's Valuables. If a patient is unconscious, very ill, or otherwise incompetent when he comes to the hospital, his valuables are often sent to the cashier's office for safe-keeping. The valuables of the patient usually include his money, jewelry, personal papers, and any other personal effects of value. Valuables that the patient usually wants to keep at his bedside include eyeglasses or contact lenses and dentures. If a patient is lucid and rational upon his admission to the hospital, he usually signs a statement in which he assumes responsibility for the valuables that he keeps at his bedside. Patients are often encouraged to ask their relatives to take home articles of great value rather than risk their theft or damage. Many hospitals routinely provide facilities for the safe storage of valuables.

DISCHARGE FROM A HEALTH AGENCY

Preparation for discharge should begin with the patient's admission to the hospital. The patient should be given every opportunity to gain increasing independence during his stay in an inpatient facility.

Hospitals provide a protective environment for their patients, and the world outside often becomes remote, threatening, and somewhat awesome to them. Thus, at discharge, the joy of being united with one's family and being restored to a state of good health are often mixed with fear and anxiety about the future.

Patients are genuinely concerned about their discharge. They wonder about how they will be able to manage, about being a burden to their families, and about their ability to contribute as a functioning member of the family and the community.

Many patients are anxious about the adjustments they must make in their life situations as a result of physical limitations. Changes in occupation and in a way of life are not easily accepted and are often looked upon with fear.

The psychological and physical needs of the patient at discharge can often be met by the patient himself with the support of his family and members of the health team. Some of the common needs of patients are:

1. The need to accept the limitations imposed by illness

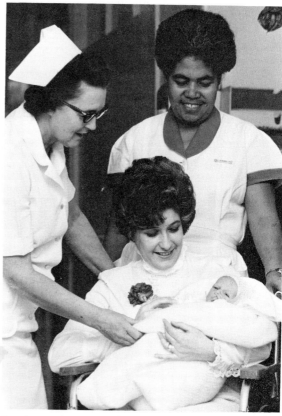

Discharge from a health agency may give rise to feelings both of joy and some degree of anxiety.

2. The need to learn to function effectively within these limitations

3. The need to be accepted as a member of the family and the community.

4. The need to learn specific skills and possess specific knowledge pertinent to healthful living.

Patients are usually discharged from the hospital, or other health agency, when they no longer require the services it offers. Occasionally, however, a patient leaves a hospital against the advice of the doctor. In such instances, most hospitals require the patient to sign a form that relieves the hospital and the physician of responsibility for any subsequent ill effects. If a person refuses to sign this release, the hospital administrator and physician are informed directly.

Should a patient require the services of another agency, the referral is made prior to his discharge. In a hospital, the business office must also be notified in order to prepare the patient's financial record so that the patient or his family can make the final business arrangements on the day of discharge.

On the day of discharge, the nurse assists the patient with his clothes and personal valuables. She also checks with the patient about any last minute questions he may have about his aftercare. New learning material should not be given to the patient just before he leaves the hospital, because patients find it difficult to remember instructions at this time. Moreover, last minute teaching never replaces a teaching plan that has extended over the time of the patient's stay in the hospital. Any final details are written down: for example, the date and time of his appointment with the physician.

When a patient leaves the hospital, he is escorted to the door of the hospital. Some hospitals have a policy that all patients are discharged in a wheelchair. In this way a patient does not overtax his strength while leaving the nursing unit.

In summary, the nurse has certain responsibilities in a patient's discharge from an agency.

1. Checking that the physician has signed the order for discharge

2. Helping the patient, as he requires, with his transportation, clothing, and personal effects

3. Clarifying any questions that the patient might have about aftercare

4. Notifying the business office and other related services in advance of the patient's discharge

5. Arranging the necessary referrals with the physician and the patient in cases in which the patient's aftercare is to be administered in a hospital department such as the outpatient department

6. Escorting the patient to the door of the hospital upon discharge.

An important part of any discharge procedure from a hospital is the entering of dismissal notes on the patient's record. It is general practice to include in the nurse's notes the general condition of the patient, the time of discharge, and any particular circumstances relevant to his discharge.

STUDY VOCABULARY		
	Clinic	Occupational therapist
	Community Health Center	Official health agency
	Dietitian	Personal health care
	Explicit policy	Physical therapist
	Extended care facility	Policy
	Free Clinic	Primary care
	Health Maintenance Organization	Rehabilitation
	Hospital	Social worker
	Implicit policy	Voluntary health agency
	Laboratory technologist	X-ray technologist
	Neighborhood Health Center	

STUDY SITUATION   The Parent-Teachers' Association of one of the schools in your district has asked you to talk to them about the health agencies in their community. In preparing your talk, you need to answer the following questions:

1. What health policies have been outlined by the local government that affect the people in this community?
2. What agencies provide health protection and health promotion services in your community?
3. What primary care services are located in the community?
4. What hospitals are located in the community? What services do they provide?
5. Are home care services available? Through which agencies?
6. Are extended care facilities available? If so, where are they located?
7. What services are available for rehabilitation in the community?

SUGGESTED
READINGS

A New Perspective on the Health of Canadians. A Working Document. Ottawa, Department of National Health and Welfare, 1974.

Bullough, Bonnie: The Medicare-Medicaid Amendments. *American Journal of Nursing,* 73:1926–1929, November, 1973.

Dorsey, Joseph L.: The Health Maintenance Organization Act of 1973 (P.L. 93–222) and Prepaid Group Practice Plans. *Medical Care, 13:*1–9, January, 1975.

Ellwood, Paul M., Jr.: Concept, Organization and Strategies of HMOs. *Journal of Nursing Administration, 4:*29–34, September-October, 1974.

Greenberg, B. G.: The Changing Scene in Public Health. *American Journal of Public Health, 64:*534–537, June, 1974.

Health Systems. Scientific Publication No. 234. Washington, D.C., Pan American Health Organization. Pan American Sanitary Bureau, Regional Office of the World Health Organization, 1972.

Health United States 1975. Rockville, Maryland, U. S. Department of Health, Education and Welfare Publication No. (HRA) 76–1232. Public Health Services. Health Resources Administration, National Center for Health Statistics.

Kibzey, H.: Health and Community Information Services. *Canadian Nurse,* 69:39–41, March, 1973.

Kisch, Arnold I.: Planning for a Sensible Health Care System. *Nursing Outlook,* 20:640–642, October, 1972.

Russell, L. B., et al.: *Federal Health Spending 1969–1974.* Washington, D.C., Center for Health Policy Studies, National Planning Association, 1974.

Skipper, James K., Jr., and Robert C. Leonard (eds.): *Social Interaction and Patient Care.* Philadelphia, J. B. Lippincott Company, 1965.

Wagner, Doris: Nursing in an HMO. *American Journal of Nursing,* 74:236–239, February, 1974.

6 NURSING PRACTICE, PART I

The nurse should be able to:

List the major fields in which nurses are currently employed
Distinguish between members of the nursing team on the basis of
    their preparation and major responsibilities
List other members of the health team with whom the nurse comes
    in frequent contact
Describe the principal functions of these team members
Explain the nurse's role in relation to its:
    care aspects
    curative aspects
    protective aspects
    teaching aspects
    coordinating aspects
    patient advocate aspects
Differentiate between independent, dependent, and interdepen-
    dent nursing functions
Describe the role of the nurse practitioner
Describe the role of the clinical nursing specialist
Explain the concept of primary nursing in a hospital setting

NURSING PRACTICE, 6
PART I

INTRODUCTION

"As each decade passes, nursing seems to become increasingly sensitive to health care needs, increasingly creative in meeting these needs, and more objective in analyzing its professional efforts and goals. Now, in this present decade of rapid change and intensified social need, we must intensify these efforts."[1]

Nursing is a dynamic profession and its practice is constantly changing. It is one of the helping professions, with a long and honorable tradition of service to humanity. Although we tend to date the emergence of modern nursing from the era of Florence Nightingale in the latter half of the last century, we should not forget that we owe much of our nursing heritage and, indeed, much of the high regard in which the nursing profession is held in our countries to the work of the nursing sisters who followed early in the wake of the first French colonists to the "New World." The Hotel Dieu Hospital of Quebec, for example, was established in 1639 by the Nursing Sisters of Dieppe in response to the request of the early colonists for help in ministering to the needs of the sick among both the new settlers and the native Indian population. Later, but still early in the development of the New World, the Order of Grey Nuns in 1738 organized district nursing services to assist in providing health care for residents of the rapidly growing community of Montreal. The work of the early French nursing sisters won them the respect and affection of settlers and Indians alike.[2]

Throughout our relatively short history in this part of the world, nurses have played an important role in bringing needed health services to the people, a role that has been continuously reshaped by the changing needs of our society. In the preceding few chapters, we have discussed some of the changes in health care needs that are affecting the current practice of nursing. Among those we have mentioned are the change in social thinking that has led us to view health as the right of every individual, with the resultant expansion of health services to ensure that right; a decided change of focus that is occurring, from a health care system that has been primarily illness-oriented to one stressing health promotion and the prevention of illness; a trend away from institutionalized and toward community-based services; the integration of services; an increased emphasis on a multidisciplinary approach to the delivery of health services; the rise of consumerism in health care; and a growing awareness of the accountability of health professionals to the public they serve.

These changes are having a profound effect on the practice of nursing. Nurses are being challenged to assume new roles, to work in new and different health care settings, and to accept increasing responsibility in the provision of comprehensive health care. As we discuss the practice of nursing as it exists currently, it

---

[1]Diane McGivern: Baccalaureate Preparation of the Nurse Practitioner. *Nursing Outlook*, 22:94, February 1974.

[2]J. M. Gibbon and M. S. Mathewson: *Three Centuries of Canadian Nursing.* Toronto, The Macmillan Company of Canada Limited, 1947, pp. 1–8.

is well to keep in mind that the "expanded" role that some nurses are pioneering today may well be the accepted practice role for all nurses in the future.[3]

NURSES AND THEIR CURRENT FIELDS OF PRACTICE

Nurses constitute the largest single group of workers in the health field in both the United States and Canada. In 1974, there were an estimated 857,000 nurses registered and actively practicing in the United States,[4] and 131,000 in Canada.[5] These figures, representing professional nurses alone, constitute over one-fifth (in Canada, almost one-fourth) the total number of persons employed in health care. When we add to these numbers the licensed practical nurses and the nursing aides, orderlies and attendants, nursing personnel account for roughly one in every two workers in the health field. To a large extent, then, the quality of our health care is dependent on the quality of the nursing component of that care.

The number of professional nurses has risen sharply in both the United States and Canada over the past few decades, both in absolute numbers and in proportion to the population, as can be seen in the table shown below. From the point of view of international comparisons, North America is in a very favorable position with regard to its nursing resources. Whereas our nurse-to-population ratios give us approximately one professionally qualified nurse for every 200 persons, in many countries of the world there is still only one professionally qualified nurse for every 5000 people.

Nursing is predominantly a women's profession in most countries of the world. The number of men in nursing has been increasing in both the United States and Canada in recent years; however, men still account for less than 2 per cent of the total number of registered nurses in both countries. Not too many years ago, the majority of nurses were young, unmarried women; today, more than two-thirds of all employed registered nurses are married, and their average age is now just under 40 years in the United States and 35 years in Canada. These last figures would tend to indicate that nurses, like women in other professions, are today engaging in longer careers, and this trend is evident in recent studies that have been undertaken on the career patterns of nurses.[6]

At the present time, the overwhelming majority of professional nurses are employed in hospitals, nursing homes, and

---

[3]Jessie M. Scott: The Changing Health Care Environment: Its Implications for Nursing. *American Journal of Public Health,* 64:364–369, April 1974.

[4]*Facts about Nursing 74–75*. Kansas City, American Nurses Association, 1976.

[5]Source: Health Manpower Planning Division, Department of National Health and Welfare, Ottawa, Canada, 1975.

[6]Lucille Knopf: Debunking a Myth. *American Journal of Nursing,* 8:1416–1421, August 1974.

NUMBER OF ACTIVE PROFESSIONAL NURSES AND NURSE–POPULATION RATIO, U.S. AND CANADA, SELECTED YEARS

	U.S.A.[°]			Canada[†]	
Year	No. of Active Professional Nurses	Nurses/100,000 Population	Year	No. of Active Professional Nurses	Nurses/100,000 Population
1930	214,292	175	1931	20,474	197
1940	284,159	216	1941	27,142	236
1950	374,584	249	1951	35,204	251
1960	525,374	293	1961	61,699	338
1970	722,000	356	1971	115,114	535
1974	857,000	407	1974	131,452	581

[°]Figures from *Facts about Nursing 74–75*. Kansas City, Missouri, American Nurses' Association, 1976, p. 3.
[†]Figures from Health Manpower Planning Division, Department of National Health and Welfare, Ottawa, Canada, December 1975.

other inpatient facilities for the care of the sick. Relatively few (approximately 7 per cent in the United States and 6 per cent in Canada, according to the latest figures available) are currently employed in the public health field. As discussed previously, however, there is a great deal of evidence to suggest that in the future more health care will be provided in the community, as, for example, in community health centers, clinics, and other types of health agencies offering ambulatory and home care services for people. The majority of nurses working in the field of "public health" currently are employed in governmental and voluntary agencies, as discussed in Chapter 5.

A growing number of nurses are also being employed in the field of occupational health. Many nurses today are working in factories, in industrial plants,

in department stores, and, in fact, in virtually any place where large numbers of people are employed. An important aspect of their work is participating in safety programs to protect the health of people in their work environment. Occupational health nurses are also often responsible for rendering emergency care to people who are injured or become ill on the job, as well as for providing health counseling and other health maintenance and health protection services for employees.

Another field that is attracting an increasing number of nurses is nursing education. With the rapid expansion of nursing schools that has taken place in the past decade in order to prepare the large numbers of nurses needed for our health services, more and more nurses are being recruited into this field; yet, we never

Fields of Employment	United States	Canada
Hospitals	66%	80%*
Nursing Homes	8%	3%
Public Health and School Health	7%	6%†
Occupational Health	3%	1%
Nursing Education	4%	3%
Private Duty	5%	—‡
Physician's Office and Other Fields	7%	7%

*Includes general, rehabilitation/convalescent, chronic/extended care, and psychiatric and other hospitals.
†Includes public health agency, home care/visiting care, and community health centers.
‡Included in other fields.

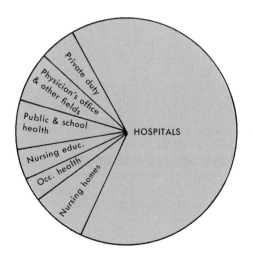

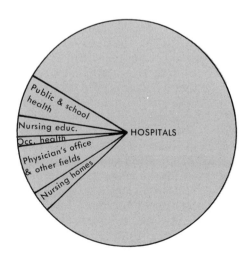

United States

Canada

Percentage of registered nurses in various fields of employment in the United States and Canada. (Sources: for United States: Source Book Nursing Personnel. Manpower References. Bethesda, Maryland, Department of Health, Education, and Welfare Publication No. (HRA) 75–43, 1975 [1972 data]; for Canada; Health Manpower Division, Statistics Canada, Ottawa, 1975 [1974 data].)

seem to have enough nursing teachers. Nursing education is a field that has been perennially short of qualified people.

We have mentioned earlier the nurses who work in association with physicians in solo or group practice in the community. This is also a major field of nursing practice. We can anticipate that an increasing number of nurses will be employed in physicians' offices in the future, as more nurses become prepared to function in an expanded role in both general and specialized practice.

One field that has declined in recent years is private duty nursing. Many acutely ill patients still require nursing care on a one nurse–one patient basis; but, increasingly, the type of care required for these patients demands highly skilled technical competence, and this care is usually provided by the nursing staff of a hospital's intensive care units. As the demand for the traditional type of private duty nurses has decreased, however, a few enterprising nurses have begun to establish themselves in private practice as independent nurse practitioners.[7]

THE NURSE AS A MEMBER OF THE HEALTH CARE TEAM

Regardless of where the nurse practices today, even if she has "hung up her shingle" and is engaged in independent practice, she functions as a member of the health care team. In Chapter 1, we discussed briefly the increasing emphasis that is being placed on a multidisciplinary approach to health care. The provision of comprehensive and continuous care to people requires the services of a number of different categories of health workers. The health team of today is composed of a variety of personnel representing professional disciplines concerned with the health and welfare of people.

In some instances, the team may consist of only three members—the physician, the nurse, and the patient; in others, there may be a dozen or more health professionals involved in the care of one individual, a family, or a community. Each member of the team possesses knowledge and skills unique to his discipline, and each contributes his special expertise to the care of the patient. There are also many areas of shared knowledge and skills. Students who have all or part of their educational program in the health sciences division of a community college, or in a university health sciences center, may find themselves sharing common core courses with the students in several other health disciplines. Most of the health professions require that their practitioners have a good foundation in the biophysical and the social sciences, and, frequently students from several health sciences programs take classes together in such subjects as anatomy, physiology, microbiology, psychology, and sociology.

Many skills are also shared among various members of the health team. Communication skills, for example, are needed by all health professionals, not only by those who work directly with patients. The nursing student and the medical student must both learn to give injections and to start intravenous infusions. The nurse must also learn to perform many of the common laboratory tests that are a part of the laboratory technologist's repertoire of skills.

The essence of the team concept is that all members work cooperatively with the patient, whether as an individual, a family, or a community. Together, they are able to make a concerted effort toward their common goal of attaining the highest level of health possible for that patient.

The Nursing Team

The nursing team is a component part of the overall health team. Essentially, the nursing team consists of registered nurses, licensed practical nurses (designated as licensed vocational nurses in some states and as nursing assistants in some provinces in Canada), nursing orderlies, nurse's aides, and attendants. The basic preparation of the registered nurse is a two to three year program of studies following high (secondary) school in a diploma school of nursing or in a tertiary edu-

---

[7]M. L. Kinlein: Independent Nurse Practitioner. *Nursing Outlook*, 20:22, January 1972.

cational institution, such as a community college. Preparation for initial registration as a professional nurse is also offered in baccalaureate programs, usually of four years' duration, in university schools of nursing. Many professional nurses undertake additional academic preparation in masters' and doctoral level programs in universities across the country.

The responsibilities of the various members of the nursing team vary according to the policies of the agency in which they are employed. In general, however, the registered nurse is responsible for coordinating and supervising the work of other members of the nursing team.

The licensed practical nurse, who has usually had a one year educational program in a community college or in a vocational school, may perform standardized nursing procedures and treatments, working under the direction of a registered nurse.

The nursing orderly's preparation varies from a few weeks of on-the-job training in some parts of the country to several months, or one year, in a program similar to that of the practical nurse. His responsibilities vary, depending on the amount of preparation he has had. He may assist in the personal care of male patients and undertake simple nursing tasks

or, if his preparatory program has been more extensive, undertake the same types of tasks performed by the licensed practical nurse.

The nurse's aide is frequently trained on the job, or in a course of a few weeks' duration. The nature of the tasks assigned to the nurse's aide varies considerably from one agency to another. In some agencies, nurse's aides perform tasks that are essentially housekeeping in nature, while in others they assist with the care of patients.

Other nursing attendants, designated by a variety of names (such as personal care attendant), may be employed to assist with such care as helping patients with their meals, helping them to dress and undress, and assisting them with personal hygiene. These attendants are usually given a short course of instruction by the agency that employs them.

Members of the Medical Team

Patients are admitted to a health agency in most instances under the care of their own private physician or a physician on the staff of the agency to whom they have been assigned. The physician is usually responsible for directing the diagnostic

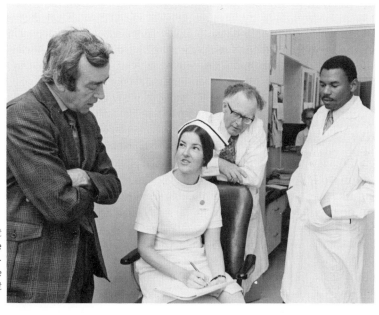

The nurse has frequent contact with various members of the medical team, such as the patient's private physician, the specialist, and the resident pictured here.

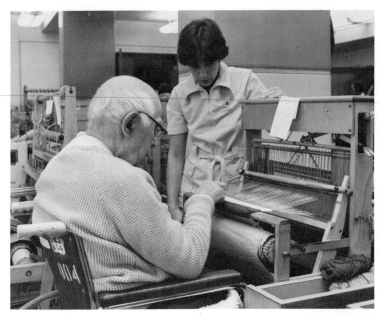

The occupational therapist helps patients with the restoration of function through specific tasks or skills.

and therapeutic plan of care for the patient. Most teaching hospitals and their related community agencies also have interns and resident physicians. Interns are recent graduates of medical school who have a planned program of clinical experience on the various services of these agencies in order to complete requirements for licensure as practicing physicians. Residents are qualified medical practitioners who are preparing for practice in a medical specialty. In some parts of the country, the internship year is no longer a basic requirement and may instead count toward specialization. If the agency is affiliated with a medical school, there will also be medical students receiving clinical instruction and experience in the various units of the agency.

Another member of the medical team who has recently arrived on the scene in the United States (and in a number of other countries) is the *physician's assistant.* Designated by various titles in various parts of the country, such as Medex, Primex, or simply Physician's Assistant, he or she is usually employed by a physician and performs, under the supervision of the physician, many tasks traditionally considered a part of medical practice. These tasks may include taking the medical history and undertaking the initial physical examination of a patient, assisting in primary care, and monitoring the progress of people under the care of the physician. Many physician's assistants work in rural areas with physicians in solo practice, where they help to extend the range of medical coverage in under-doctored areas. Many are former army corpsmen, some are nurses, and others enter the educational programs for preparation as physician's assistants without previous experience in the health field. The course of studies, which is usually offered in a university setting in conjunction with a medical school, ranges from one to five years in length, depending on the individual's previous training and experience in the health field.

Members of the Health Team Concerned Primarily with Health Promotion

With the trend toward the emphasis on health, as opposed to sickness-oriented care, the nurse should be aware of those in other disciplines who are working in the field of health promotion.

The *health educator,* for example, is a relatively new member of the health team. He or she (many health educators are women), is primarily responsible for the development of health education programs in the community. A large part of his or her work lies in community development—that is, in working with people in a community, assisting them in identifying their health needs and in taking steps to improve health conditions in the community, as well as the health status of the people who live there. The nurse will find the health educator an excellent resource person in her own work in health promotion. The health educator has usually had a university course of studies at the baccalaureate or higher degree level to prepare him for his work.

Also in the field of health promotion, the *recreation specialist* is increasingly being considered a member of the health team. His or her (again, many are women) responsibilities include the development of recreation, sports, and physical fitness programs in the community. The recreation specialist is usually a graduate of a baccalaureate program in physical education (or recreation).

The *family nutritionist* is rapidly becoming a familiar member of staff in many community health agencies. The special area of expertise for this member is food and its relationship to health. He or she advises people about good dietary habits, counsels them about their nutrition problems, and undertakes nutrition education programs for people in the community. The nutritionist has usually had a four to five year program of studies in a university, followed by a year of internship in various health agencies.

The nutritionist who works in a hospital, or other institutional setting, is called a *dietitian*. The dietitian is usually responsible for planning meal service for patients and staff, supervising other workers in the preparation of food, and counseling patients about their nutritional problems.

Members of the Health Team Concerned Primarily with Environmental Health

In working in the community, the nurse will also meet a number of workers whose primary concern is the improvement, con-

trol, and management of man's environment. The term "environmentalist" is increasingly being used in the United States, and "environmental technologist" in Canada, to refer to workers in this field.

The *sanitarian* (U.S.) and the *public health inspector* (Canada and some other countries) are traditional workers in this field. The responsibilities of these workers are principally the elimination or control of "nuisances," that is, factors in the environment that may endanger health (such as excessive noise, offensive odors, and the like); ensuring the safety of water, milk, and food supplies; ensuring that garbage and sewage disposal is properly carried out; enforcing public health laws with regard to sanitation; and assisting in the control of communicable diseases. The sanitarian in the United States usually has a baccalaureate degree in the biological, physical, and sanitary sciences; in Canada, programs for the preparation of public health inspectors are usually offered in institutes of technology or in community colleges.

A large number of new workers are emerging in this field of environmental health. Some are primarily concerned with the control of pollution, for example. Another relatively new worker in this field is the *industrial hygienist*, whose main concern is the detection and control of environmental hazards in the work environment.

Other Members of the Health Team

It is difficult to separate into discrete categories by area of primary interest all of the workers in the health field today. Like the nurse, many other health professionals have functions that include assisting people in all areas of the health care spectrum. Some of the other workers with whom the nurse will come in frequent contact are the social worker, the pharmacist, the physical therapist, the occupational therapist, the respiratory technologist, the medical laboratory technologist, and the radiology technologist.

The *social worker* assists in evaluating the psychosocial situation of the patient and helps people with their social prob-

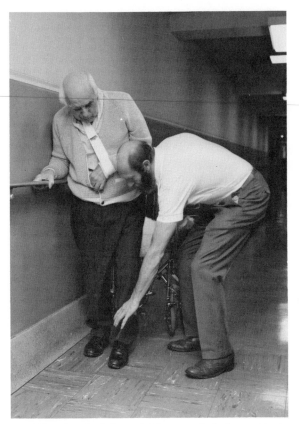

The physical therapist frequently helps patients with the difficult task of learning to walk again.

source of information for nurses on the nature of medications ordered for patients—their composition, mode of action, method of administration, dosage, and possible side-effects. Most pharmacists in North America receive their preparation in a four year course of studies at a university; a number of community colleges are developing courses for pharmacy assistants. In many countries of the world, new programs to prepare pharmacists (to replace the old apprentice type of training) are being located in community colleges and technological institutes as well as universities.

The *physical therapist* has specialized preparation in physical therapy in a three to four year program of studies, usually in a university setting. He assists in assessing the patient's functional ability, strength, and mobility; carries out therapeutic treatments, particularly those dealing with the musculoskeletal system; and teaches families and patients exercises and other measures that can contribute to the patient's recovery and rehabilitation.

The *occupational therapist* has a preparation similar to the physical therapist; many individuals, in fact, hold a combined degree (or certificate) in physical and occupational therapy. The occupational therapist, however, is primarily concerned with the restoration of bodily functions through specific tasks or skills, rather than exercises and treatments. Occupational therapists frequently play a large role in rehabilitation by helping people to develop new skills or to relearn skills lessened or lost through illness.

The *respiratory technologist (therapist)* is an expert in diagnostic procedures and therapeutic measures used in the care of patients with respiratory problems. He is skilled in handling oxygen therapy equipment, for example. Programs in respiratory technology are usually two to three years in duration and are offered in community colleges or other types of postsecondary educational institutions.

A large variety of clinical laboratory technologists also assist in patient care in both the institutional and the ambulatory care setting. The student has already probably come in contact with the *medical technologist* (medical laboratory technologist), for example, when she went to

lems. She (or he) usually has extensive knowledge of community agencies and frequently makes arrangements for the patient to be cared for by the appropriate agency, as, for example, to receive home care services and/or "Meals on Wheels," or to be admitted or transferred to a nursing home. The majority of social workers hold a bachelor's or master's degree in social work; many community colleges are now offering courses for the preparation of assistant social workers.

The *pharmacist* is an individual whose primary area of responsibility is the preparation and dispensing of drugs and other chemical substances used in the detection, prevention, and treatment of illness. The neighborhood "druggist" is a familiar person to many students. Because drug therapy is an important part of the treatment of many illnesses, most hospitals and other health agencies in the community usually employ a staff of pharmacists. The pharmacist is an excellent

the laboratory to have blood and other tests done in connection with her physical examination prior to entry to her school of nursing. The medical technologist is responsible for collecting many of the specimens needed for laboratory tests; he or she treats and analyzes these specimens and advises physicians and nurses on the results of these tests. The technologist is also helpful in advising nurses on the nature of tests and the specific procedure for carrying these out if the nurse is to do this task. In the United States, clinical laboratory technologists are usually required to have a baccalaureate degree in medical technology, chemistry, or a biological science. In Canada, courses in medical laboratory technology are offered in community colleges and technological institutes, and are generally two to three years in duration.

Most nursing students will have also met the *radiologic technologist* (x-ray technologist), again probably in connection with their pre-entry physical examination, since most schools of nursing require candidates to have a chest x-ray done, and it is the radiologic technologist who usually performs this task. He or she is specifically prepared to perform diagnostic and therapeutic measures involving the use of radiant energy. The radiologic technologist's preparation is usually a two to three year program of combined academic work and clinical experience. The programs are usually conducted by hospitals or post-secondary educational institutions, such as a community college or technological institute, with hospital affiliation.

THE UNIQUE ROLE OF THE NURSE

With the sometimes bewildering array of other workers in the health field, and the many changes that are taking place in health care today, the beginning student may well wonder just what it is that nurses do. Many of the nurse's traditional tasks have been delegated to other workers. Nurses have been relieved of most of the housekeeping chores that formerly occupied much of their time. Ward clerks and unit managers in many health agencies have taken over many of the clerical duties that nurses used to do. Auxiliary nursing personnel often look after a good deal of the patient's personal care and are now doing a number of treatments that were once carried out only by professional nurses.

The International Council of Nurses has stated that "the fundamental responsibility of the nurse is fourfold: to promote health, to prevent illness, to restore health, and to alleviate suffering.[8]

In carrying out their responsibilities, nurses assist individuals, families, and communities in the promotion of health and the prevention of illness; they minister to the needs of the sick, helping them to the fullest restoration of health compatible with their illness, or providing comfort and support in the event of incurable disease. In so doing, nurses work in close coordination with a growing number of other health disciplines to provide health services for people.

The scope of the professional nurse's practice, as outlined in this description of her role, implies a much broader spectrum of activities than is represented by the traditional image of the nurse as the ministering angel who soothed the patient's fevered brow, changed his linen, and dressed his wounds. The nurse still performs many of these activities, but today she is a skilled person who carries out a multiplicity of complex functions. She cares for the patient and about the patient. She participates in the detection and treatment of illness. She protects the patient from harmful factors that could endanger his health. She is an advisor and a teacher on health matters. She is expected to coordinate the activities of other members of the nursing team and to work with a variety of people in other disciplines as a cooperating member of the health team. She also acts as a spokesman, or advocate, for the patient.

The Care Aspects

From its earliest inception, nursing has had a nurturing quality, and this quality is

---

[8]Ethical Concepts Applied to Nursing 1973. *ICN News Release*, No. 6, September 1975.

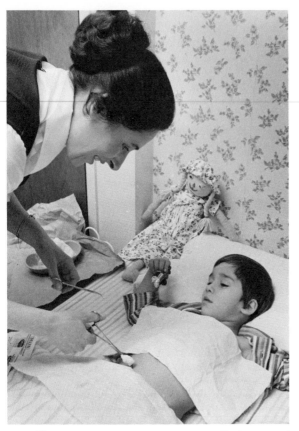

Nurses carry out many measures that are part of the patient's therapeutic plan of care.

and support, the nurse is concerned not only with his physical comfort but also with assisting him to cope with his health problems and the stress and anxiety that accompany even slight deviations from health. In all of these activities the nurse works with the patient, helping him to regain his independence as rapidly as possible and as much as he is able within the limitations imposed by illness.

In caring for the patient, the nurse also cares about him. To many patients these are seen as one and the same; that is, the person who cares for him is perceived as the person who cares about him.[10] Carrying out nursing activities with compassion, with empathetic understanding, and with respect for the patient as an individual of worth and dignity is caring about the patient. In this regard, a statement from the summary report of the National Commission for the Study of Nursing Education seems particularly relevant. In discussing trends in health care delivery and the problem of bringing about change while still retaining good practices from old patterns, the report states that, "It may well be that nursing, in particular, holds the key to maintenance of humane, individualistic concern for people and their health problems. And this capacity must be zealously enlarged."[11]

The Curative Aspects

Many of the nurse's activities involve participation in the detection and treatment of illness. The nurse's initial assessment of a patient, along with that made by other members of the health team, contributes to the identification of his health problems. (See Chapter 9.) The nurse is often responsible for carrying out many of the diagnostic tests that help to establish the exact nature of these problems. Although the diagnostic and therapeutic plans for an individual patient are usually the responsibility of the physician, nurs-

best evidenced in the care aspects of the nurse's role. In caring for the patient, the nurse assists him in carrying out those activities that he would normally do for himself if he were able. The caring aspects of nursing are perhaps most readily illustrated in the nurse's traditional function of care of the sick. Caring for the patient involves ministering to his needs and wants, providing comfort and support, protecting him from harm, and assisting him to regain his independence as rapidly as possible.[9] Much of nursing action is concerned with the daily living of the patient. Helping him to meet his needs for water, food, rest, and sleep and helping him to maintain normal body functioning are primary concerns of the nurse in caring for the patient. In providing comfort

---

[9]Frances Reiter Kreuter: What Is Good Nursing Care? *Nursing Outlook*, 5:302–304, May 1957.

[10]Ellen D. Davis: Giving a Bath? *American Journal of Nursing*, 70:2366–2367, November 1970.

[11]National Commission for the Study of Nursing and Nursing Education: Summary Report and Recommendations. *American Journal of Nursing*, 70:279–294, February 1970.

ing observations of the patient's condition and assessment of the need for medical or nursing intervention contribute significantly to the development of these plans.

Nurses also carry out a good many of the therapeutic measures that are part of the plan of care for each patient. The administration of medications and the carrying out of treatments are illustrative of some of the therapeutic measures undertaken by nurses. The nurse's skill in carrying out these measures, for example, in giving an intramuscular injection or in operating complicated monitoring equipment, is essential. In innumerable instances, the nurse must use her own judgment in initiating therapeutic action when she feels it is needed. For example, many medication orders are written "to be given as needed" (p.r.n.), and the nurse administers these when, in her judgment, the patient requires them.

The nurse also participates in evaluating the effectiveness of therapeutic measures. Nurses usually have more frequent contact with patients than do other members of the health team, and the immediacy of the nurse's presence (particularly in the hospital situation) provides her with a unique opportunity to observe the patient's reactions to therapy. These observations are of inestimable value in evaluating the patient's total plan of care and modifying it as needed.

The Protective Aspects

An important aspect of nursing care is assisting the patient to take those measures that will protect him from adverse influences in the environment and protecting and supporting his physiological defense capabilities. When the patient is unable to do this for himself, it is the nurse's responsibility to see that all protective measures are taken for his safety. In working in a community setting, the nurse must be alert to environmental factors that may endanger health and take steps to see that, insofar as possible, her patients' homes and the neighborhoods in which they live are conducive to healthy living. She also encourages people in the

development of good health habits, such as eating a balanced diet, developing and maintaining good hygiene practices, getting a sufficient amount of rest and relaxation—all of which help to reduce the individual's vulnerability to illness. She also encourages people to have all of the advised immunizations to further increase their resistance to specific diseases.

When an individual is ill, his protective capabilities and his resistance to other diseases are usually diminished. He may not be in a position to protect himself from environmental hazards and he is particularly vulnerable to infection. It then becomes the nurse's responsibility to see that the environment of the sick room is free from harmful (or potentially harmful) factors, and that all measures are taken to prevent the spread of infection.

The Teaching Aspects

Many of the teaching activities of the nurse have already been mentioned in the preceding section. Nurses both act as advisors to people on health matters—which is in essence teaching on a one-to-one basis—and engage in more formal teaching activities. Teaching functions are a very important part of nursing care. They may involve such diverse activities as advising new mothers on the care and feeding of babies, teaching hygiene measures to protect against illness, advising a patient about his diet, teaching deep-breathing exercises to patients before surgery to prevent postoperative complications, or helping a patient to cope with the activities of daily living when he has been handicapped by illness.

The nurse is also frequently involved in helping the patient to carry out activities that have been prescribed or in supervising him while he is doing them. For example, the visiting nurse may go into a patient's home to help him carry out exercises to strengthen his abdominal and leg muscles in preparation for learning to walk again. The nurse also helps the patient and his family to plan for his home care or to work through health problems and develop a plan for overcoming them.

The Coordinating Aspects

The delegation of many routine tasks to auxiliary personnel has freed the nurse for more specialized work, but it has also added to her responsibilities for the administration and coordination of the activities of others. The nurse plans and supervises the care given by such auxiliary nursing personnel as the licensed practical nurse, the nursing orderly, and the nurse's aide. In addition, she consults with other professional workers regarding the care given to the patient. She consults with the physician about his plan of therapy. She may need to talk with the dietitian about the foods the patient likes that are permissible on his diet; with the physical therapist about his exercise program; with the social worker and the community agency about plans for his home care. The nurse sees that appointments for the patient's laboratory tests and x-ray examinations are made and kept. If he is in hospital, she makes sure that the housekeeping staff have cleaned his room and that the aide has brought him drinking water. In most health agencies which have inpatient facilities, nursing is the only service that is provided on a 24 hour a day, seven day a week basis. Other workers come and go, usually during the daytime hours and not on weekends. It is the nurse, then, who establishes a plan for the patient's care and serves as the coordinator for all activities concerned with it. In this, she works cooperatively with the patient and his physician, with the patient's family, and with the other members of the health care team.

The Patient Advocate Aspects

As the health care system has become more complex, with a number of different agencies and an increasing variety of workers concerned with different aspects of the patient's care, the need for someone who can speak on the patient's behalf and intercede in his interest has become essential. This speaking for the patient and interceding on his behalf is an important aspect of nursing care.

The multitude of workers who do things for and to the patient, particularly in a hospital, seems never-ending. Some patients have reported that as many as 50 employees were in and out of their rooms in one day while they were in hospital. The patient needs some one person to whom he can relate in a meaningful way, and who can act as his spokesman with other members of the health team.

In the community setting, people often do not know about (or if they do know, have difficulty in contacting) the appropriate agency to help them with their health problems. The nurse, with her knowledge of the services offered by various community agencies, and by virtue of her professional contacts in these agencies, can facilitate the process of getting the patient to the appropriate people who can help him.

INDEPENDENT, DEPENDENT, AND INTERDEPENDENT NURSING FUNCTIONS

The terms "independent," "dependent," and "interdependent" are frequently used in connection with nursing functions. These terms refer to the extent of independent decision-making the nurse exercises in initiating and carrying out nursing activities. When a nurse makes a decision that certain actions should be taken in the care of a patient, and either takes that action herself or delegates this responsibility to another member of the nursing team, she is performing an *independent* nursing function.[12] The nurse may decide, for example, on assessing the condition of a patient's mouth, that he needs special mouth care that he is unable to do himself. She develops a plan for seeing that this care is given; for instance, she may write a directive on the nursing care plan to the effect that the patient is to have special mouth care every four hours. She then undertakes this care herself, or delegates it to another member of the nursing team.

---

[12]Betty Jane Anderson: Orderly Transfer of Procedural Responsibilities from Medical to Nursing Practice. *Nursing Clinics of North America,* 5:314, June 1970.

The nurse also carries out some of her responsibilities under the legal orders, or under the direction or supervision, of another health professional. The physician, for example, may order a medication for a patient. The decision that the individual should receive the medication is made by the physician. In giving the medication to the patient, the nurse is carrying out a *dependent* nursing function.

In other instances, decisions regarding the actions to be taken by nurses may be made jointly by two or more members of the health team. At a team conference concerned with the rehabilitation of a patient, for example, the nurse, the physician, the physical therapist, and perhaps other members of the team may together decide on a course of action to increase the patient's independence in the activities of daily living. Each member of the team may have specific responsibilities in this regard. The physician might order that the patient be up twice a day to sit in a chair. The physical therapist might start the patient on an exercise program to increase his muscle tone in limbs that have not been used while he was in bed. The nurse may include in her plan of care directives to other members of the nursing team to encourage the patient to feed and dress himself and to take increasing responsibility for his own hygiene. In carrying out these activities, the nurse functions *interdependently*, that is, on the basis of decisions made in consultation with other health personnel.

EXPANDED ROLES FOR NURSES

The distinctions between independent, dependent, and interdependent nursing functions are not always as clear-cut as the previous examples would indicate. Traditionally, the independent functions of the nurse have been principally in the care aspects of nursing and, to a certain extent, in the protective and teaching aspects. In all aspects of her role today, the scope of the nurse's independent functions, wherein she makes decisions and implements action on her own, is rapidly being expanded. Two examples of new nursing roles in which expansion of the nurse's realm of independent functioning are evi-

dent are the nurse practitioner role and the clinical specialist role.

The Nurse Practitioner

One definition of the term "nurse practitioner" reads:

The nurse practitioner is a nurse in an expanded role oriented to the provision of primary care as a member of a team of health professionals relating with families on a long-term basis.[13]

The role is seen as extending the present function of the nurse through the development and more effective utilization of her unique skills in the provision of health care, and through the assumption by the nurse of certain tasks that have traditionally been considered a part of medical practice.[14]

The nurse practitioner may be a generalist, that is, a family nurse practitioner, or a specialist, as, for example, a pediatric nurse practitioner. The concept of a family nurse practitioner, as viewed by the faculty of one educational program preparing this type of nurse practitioner, includes the following outline of her work:

As a primary care provider in ambulatory settings, she assesses the physical, emotional and developmental status of individuals and families; analyzes health behavior related to personality, life style, and culture; makes positive interventions to maintain, restore, or improve health; and critically evaluates the quality and effectiveness of her practice. By adding medical skills in diagnosis and patient management to her nursing knowledge and skills, she is able to expand her care to include all levels of prevention, that is, health promotion, specific disease protection, early recognition and prompt treatment, and disability limitation and rehabilitation.... The family nurse practitioner is able to provide care independently to many patients and works closely with physicians in the joint management of others.[15]

[13]Walter O. Spitzer and Dorothy J. Kergin: The Nurse Practitioner: Calling a Spade a Spade. *Ontario Medical Review*, 38:165–166, April 1971.
[14]*Report of the Committee on Nurse Practitioners.* Ottawa, Canada, Department of National Health and Welfare, p. 5, 1972.
[15]C. Januska, C. D. Davis, R. N. Knollmueller, and P. Wilson: Development of a Family Nurse Practitioner Curriculum. *Nursing Outlook*, 22:105, February 1974.

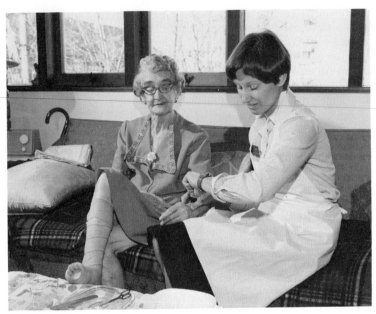

Many nurses employed in official and voluntary community health agencies are being given an opportunity to extend their scope of independent functioning.

Inherent in all descriptions of the role of the nurse practitioner is the premise that the nurse will exercise more independent judgment than has been permitted heretofore.

The concept of the nurse practitioner is not new. Many nurses working in rural and isolated areas in the United States and in Canada have been practicing in such an expanded role for a good many years, as have nurses in many other countries. Well-known examples that might be cited to illustrate this point are the Frontier Nurses of Kentucky, the Northern Nurses in Canada, the "Sick Nurse Dispensers" in the hinterlands of Guyana, the public health nurses in the outback in Australia, and also the nurses attached to the famous "Flying Doctor Service" in that country. What is new in the concept of the nurse practitioner is that nurses are now being given an opportunity to practice in this role in urban communities as well as in isolated areas, and in settings where their scope of independent functioning has previously been limited, as, for example, in official and voluntary community health agencies, in physicians' offices, in occupational health settings, and in the emergency departments of hospitals. Nurses are now being prepared to undertake this role through formal univer-

sity-based educational programs. In other words, the role is being legitimized. An ever-increasing number of nurse practitioners are being prepared in post-basic programs for registered nurses in universities across the country. A number of university schools of nursing are also including preparation for the nurse practitioner role in their basic baccalaureate programs. Graduates of these programs, both basic and post-basic, appear to be having no difficulty in finding employment in a wide variety of settings.

The Clinical Nursing Specialist

The clinical nursing specialist is a nurse who has expanded her nursing knowledge and skills in one particular branch of nursing. The term was coined by Frances Reiter in the early 1940s to describe the nurse who has achieved a high level of competence in her nursing practice, that is, as she saw it, in giving direct care to patients. Such a nurse would have increased her range of functions in regard to care, cure, and counseling (as Miss Reiter described the nurse's functions); she would have a broad knowledge base from which to operate; and she would be able to provide a more extensive scope of services than nurses heretofore.[16] At the time that Miss Reiter first outlined this concept, there was little opportunity for the nurse to increase her clinical competence except through experience in the field and through the preparation offered in a few hospital postgraduate courses of short duration. Career advancement, both academically and job-wise, was achieved by means of additional preparation (or demonstrated ability) in administration or teaching. Clinical competence was not rewarded — a complaint that has been noticed in other fields too, such as education, where the excellent teachers, it seems, must become administrators in order to advance their careers.

Although the clinical nursing specialist does not necessarily have to have an academic degree (a good many nurses have achieved clinical excellence by experience and self-instruction), the development of university programs at the master's degree level for preparation in a clinical specialty has advanced the concept considerably. The advent of the nurse practitioner programs has also furthered the idea, and in the United States particularly, the role of the clinical nursing specialist is rapidly becoming one with the role of the specialized nurse practitioner.

The clinical nursing specialist may work in a hospital setting or in ambulatory care in the community. In the institutional setting, at the present time, her responsibilities vary, depending on the agency in which she is working. The role is new, and many clinical nursing specialists have had to develop their own "job descriptions" as they worked and could see how they best fit into the existing nursing service structure of the agency. They often give direct care to patients, particularly those with multiple problems (or one especially difficult problem to resolve). They also function as a role model for other nurses, and provide consultative and advisory services for nursing personnel who are working in the specialist's particular area of expertise.

In the ambulatory care setting, the clinical nursing specialist functions in much the same manner as that described for the family nurse practitioner, except that her area of practice is limited to a clinical specialty. Thus, the clinical nursing specialist in an ambulatory care setting might, for example, be a pediatric nurse practitioner, a nurse midwife, or a medical, a surgical, or a psychiatric nurse practitioner.

PRIMARY NURSING IN THE HOSPITAL SETTING

The number of nurses practicing as clinical nursing specialists and as nurse practitioners is still relatively small. The vast majority of nurses at the present time are employed as "staff nurses" in a hospital setting. We have said that in this capacity, the registered nurse frequently acts as the leader of a nursing team, which may comprise a variety of nursing personnel. The team is usually responsible for the care of a group of patients. If the team is large, the number of patients, too, is likely to be quite large, and the nurse is often busy with the coordination of care and supervision of other members of the team.

A recent innovation in the method of allocating nursing responsibility for patient care is the concept of *primary nursing.* In primary nursing, each patient is assigned, on admission, to a specific nurse. This nurse is responsible for the patient's care throughout his hospital stay. She becomes "his" nurse, in other words. She admits the patient; orients him to the hospital; undertakes the nursing assessment; develops a plan of care for him, writing nursing directives that cover the 24 hours in the day; and gives direct care to that patient while she is on duty. When she is not on duty, other nurses carry out the care plan that she has made. The primary care nurse sees the patient with the physician when he makes his rounds and confers with him about her plan of care for the patient.

The usual "caseload" for the nurse is three to four patients, although she may

[16]Frances Reiter: The Nurse-Clinician. *American Journal of Nursing,* 66:274–280, February 1966.

assist with the care of patients assigned to other nurses. Nurses who have worked in settings where primary nursing is in effect are enthusiastic about it. It appears to be a very satisfying mode of practice for the nurse, who is able to individualize care and carry out nursing in the way she has envisioned it should be done.[17]

---

[17] K. Bakke: Primary Nursing; Perceptions of a Staff Nurse. *American Journal of Nursing*, 74:1432–1438, August 1974.

STUDY VOCABULARY

Attendant
Clinical nursing specialist
Dependent nursing function
Dietitian
Environmental technologist
Family nutritionist
Health educator
Independent nursing function
Industrial hygienist
Interdependent nursing function
Intern
Licensed practical nurse
Licensed vocational nurse
Medical laboratory technologist
Nurse practitioner
Nurse's aide
Nursing assistant
Nursing orderly
Occupational health nursing
Occupational therapist
Patient advocate
Pharmacist
Physical therapist
Physician
Physician's assistant
Primary nursing
Private duty nursing
Public health inspector
Radiologic technologist
Recreation specialist
Registered nurse
Resident
Respiratory technologist (therapist)
Social worker

STUDY SITUATION

You are a staff nurse on a surgical ward in a large city hospital. The head nurse has assigned you a new patient, Mrs. Marjorie Jones, who was admitted last night with acute pain in her upper abdomen, nausea, and vomiting. From her patient record you learn that Mrs. Jones is 35 years old, is 5'4" tall, weighs 180 pounds, and has had no serious illnesses previously. Her husband is an executive in a large national firm and they have three children, aged 12, 10, and 7 years. You note that she is allergic to penicillin and subject to hayfever. Her physician has left orders for bed rest, clear fluid diet, medication p.r.n. for pain, and instructions for x-ray examination and laboratory tests. His tentative diagnosis is cholecystitis (inflammation of the gallbladder).

You go down to talk with Mrs. Jones and find her sitting up in bed, smoking a cigarette. She tells you that she is hungry—they did not give her anything to eat for breakfast. She wants to know what they are going to do to her and if she will have to have surgery. She is anxious about her family, since they have recently moved to this city and have no relatives here. She says she hopes this doctor can do something about her weight problem. She is a compulsive eater and has tried several diets, but can never stay with them. She states that she smokes about a package of cigarettes a day to keep from eating. She does not have any interests outside the home. Now that the children are in school all day, she reads a lot, watches television, and usually takes a daily nap after lunch.

1. As Mrs. Jones' primary nurse, what would your responsibilities include?
2. Discuss the nursing care of Mrs. Jones under the following

headings: care aspects, curative aspects, protective aspects, teaching aspects, coordinating aspects, patient advocate aspects.

3. Name members of the health team currently involved in Mrs. Jones' care.

4. Identify other members of the health team who might be able to help in the resolution of Mrs. Jones' health problems.

SUGGESTED READINGS

Archer, S. E., and Fleshman, R. P.: Community Health Nursing: A Typology of Practice. *Nursing Outlook, 23*:358–364, June, 1975.

Bergstrom, Ingrid: Mary Berglund: Backwoods Nurse. *Canadian Nurse, 72*:44–49, September, 1976.

Bullough, Bonnie: Influences on Role Expansion. *American Journal of Nursing, 76*:1476–1481, September, 1976.

Colliere, M. F.: Thoughts on a New Approach to Public Health Nursing. *International Nursing Review, 22*:80–86, May-June, 1975.

Hayman, M. J.: The Occupational Health Nurse in the Work Environment. *The Canadian Nurse, 72*:36–41, July, 1976.

Henderson, N. E.: Nursing via Satellite. *The Canadian Nurse, 72*:31–33, January, 1976.

Manthey, Marie: Primary Nursing is Alive and Well in the Hospital. *American Journal of Nursing, 73*:83–87, January, 1973.

Martin, L. L.: I Like Being an FNP. *American Journal of Nursing, 75*:826–828, May, 1975.

Nurse Practitioner: A Journal of Primary Nursing Care (bimonthly). Seattle, Washington, Health Sciences Media and Research Services, Inc., Volume 1, 1975.

Splane, V. H. (Guest Editor): Symposium on Community Health Nursing in Canada. *Nursing Clinics of North America, 10*:687–778, December, 1975.

The Nurse Practitioner: Preparation and Practice. *Nursing Outlook, 22*:90–127, February, 1974.

Tirpak, Helen: The Frontier Nursing Service — Fifty Years in the Mountains. *Nursing Outlook, 23*:308–310, May, 1975.

Upcavage, A. T.: Individualized Nursing Care. *Nursing '75, 5*:64–66, January, 1975.

7 NURSING PRACTICE, PART II

ACCOUNTABILITY FOR
   PRACTICE
A CODE OF NURSING
   ETHICS
NURSING PRACTICE
   ACTS
AREAS OF NURSING
   FUNCTION

THE LEGAL STATUS OF THE
   NURSE
LEGAL ISSUES OF INTEREST
   TO THE NURSE
STUDY VOCABULARY
STUDY SITUATION
SUGGESTED READINGS

The nurse should be able to:

Discuss implications of the International Code of Nursing Ethics
   for nursing practice
State the purpose of nursing practice acts and certification
Differentiate between mandatory and permissive licensure for
   nurses
Compare the functions of the registered and the practical nurse
Discuss the legal status of the nurse
Define the following legal terms: tort, crime, negligence,
   malpractice, assault, battery, defamation of character, slander,
   libel, false imprisonment, invasion of privacy
Give examples of common types of incidents involving nurses
   leading to legal suits in which negligence is a factor
Discuss the status of the nurse in regard to confidential
   information
Discuss the nurse's responsibility if she is present at the scene of
   an accident or other emergency
Explain the legal implications of witnessing a will
Explain the implications on nursing practice of statutes controlling
   narcotic drugs

106

NURSING PRACTICE, 7
PART II

ACCOUNTABILITY FOR PRACTICE

People place a great deal of trust in the hands of health professionals. It therefore seems reasonable for individuals to expect that the people who provide health care are qualified to practice their profession and that they will be assured of safe and competent care in their hands. It also seems reasonable to assume that their basic rights as human beings will be respected by all who care for them.

Although nurses are not responsible for all aspects of health care, they have a responsibility to ensure that, insofar as the nursing component is concerned, the patient is assured of safe and competent care and that his fundamental rights, such as the right to courtesy, to privacy, and to information on his condition, will be safeguarded during the process of care.

Most of the developed countries of the world have laws which regulate the practice of health professionals; these laws are intended to protect the public from unqualified practitioners. In some cases, the laws also define the scope of professional practice—that is, they specify the functions which the qualified practitioner may undertake. In many instances, however, the law is vague in this respect, particularly in regard to the practice of nursing and medicine. Often it has been the professional associations that have undertaken to define the role and functions of the practitioner, based on currently accepted patterns of practice.

In most countries of the "free" world, an individual's basic human rights are protected, either in the constitution of the country or in its legally enacted laws. The Consumers' Bills of Rights, recently developed in both the United States and Canada, have sought to further clarify an individual's basic rights as these are applicable to health care (see Chapter 1, pages 7 and 8). Safeguarding the patient's rights is also an important aspect of the ethical codes adopted by each of the major health professions. These codes extend beyond the legal basis for practice and into the realm of social values to which members of the particular profession are committed.

The professional associations have also become increasingly concerned with the need to develop standards to ensure that patients will receive safe and competent care. Both the American and the Canadian Nurses' Associations, for example, have been developing statements regarding standards that must be maintained in various fields of nursing practice in order to assure the consumer of good quality nursing care.

The nurse should be familiar with the new International Code of Nursing Ethics, which describes social responsibilities considered important in nursing practice. She should also be familiar with the laws in her state concerning the provision of health care to the public, and particularly with the acts that control the practice of nursing. She should be aware of her functions and responsibilities, both as defined by law and as delineated by her professional nursing associations. It is important, also, for the nurse to be aware of how the law protects the patient and of her own legal status both as a student and as a graduate.

A CODE OF NURSING ETHICS

Every profession is based on a code of ethics that places positive values on the purposes and activities of the members of that profession.[1] This code commits the professional to certain social values which are above the selfish ones of income, power, and prestige. At its Congress in 1973, the International Council of Nurses adopted a new code of nursing ethics that focuses on the nurse's responsibilities in regard to people, to society, to practice, to co-workers, and to the nursing profession. Following is a statement of the Code in its entirety.

Code for Nurses—Ethical Concepts Applied to Nursing

The fundamental responsibility of the nurse is fourfold: to promote health, to prevent illness, to restore health, and to alleviate suffering. The need for nursing is universal. Inherent in nursing is respect for life, dignity, and the rights of man. It is unrestricted by considerations of nationality, race, creed, colour, age, sex, politics, or social status. Nurses render health services to the individual, the family, and the community and coordinate their services with those of related groups.

Nurses and People. The nurse's primary responsibility is to those people who require nursing care.

The nurse, in providing care, promotes an environment in which the values, customs, and spiritual beliefs of the individual are respected.

The nurse holds in confidence personal information and uses judgment in sharing this information.

Nursing and Society. The nurse shares with other citizens the responsibility for initiating and supporting action to meet the health and social needs of the public.

Nurses and Practice. The nurse carries personal responsibility for nursing practice and for maintaining competence through continual learning.

The nurse maintains the highest standards of nursing care possible within the reality of a specific situation.

The nurse uses judgment in relation to individual competence when accepting and delegating responsibility.

The nurse when acting in a professional capacity should at all times maintain standards of personal conduct which reflect credit upon the profession.

Nurses and Co-Workers. The nurse sustains a cooperative relationship with co-workers in nursing and other fields.

The nurse takes appropriate action to safeguard the individual when his care is endangered by a co-worker or another person.

Nurses and the Profession. The nurse plays the major role in determining and implementing desirable standards of nursing practice and nursing education.

The nurse is active in developing a core of professional knowledge.

The nurse, acting through the professional organization, participates in establishing and maintaining equitable social and economic working conditions in nursing.[2]

NURSING PRACTICE ACTS

The laws in both the United States and Canada derive from two main sources: the statutes passed by lawmaking bodies, such as Congress or Parliament, and the decisions of the courts. The latter are collectively known as common law. The law is a reflection of public opinion and of civic and social movements within a community. The law therefore is not static; rather, it is constantly changing. Changes in the statutes and the decisions of the courts in cases involving nursing reflect changes in public thinking about the development of nursing.

In recent years, there has been an increasing awareness by nurses and by the public of the need to standardize the laws concerning the practice of both the professional and the practical nurse. The authority to control nursing, together with various other professions and occupations concerned with health and welfare, has been vested in the states (or, in Canada, in the provinces). Thus, each state and province has enacted its own laws to control the practice of nursing. These laws

---

[1]Betty D. Pearson: Nursing Legislation: The International Dimension. *Nursing Clinics of North America*, 9:536, September 1974.

[2]*Code for Nurses.* Geneva, Switzerland. Copyright, International Council of Nurses, 1973. All rights reserved.

are generally termed "nursing practice acts," although the exact title of the statute varies in the different jurisdictions. Because each state and province has set up its own law, it is understandable that the statutes vary somewhat. Nevertheless, the purpose of these laws is the same — that is, to protect the health of the public through the establishment of minimum standards, which a qualified practitioner must meet in order to practice as a nurse.[3]

Licensure

In the past few years, there has been a considerable number of changes in licensing regulations in both the United States and Canada. All states and the District of Columbia now have legislation that requires mandatory licensure of professional nurses; the nurse must hold a valid, current license as a registered nurse in the state in which she is employed in order to be able to practice. In Canada, most of the provincial nursing acts are permissive in nature — that is, the nurse may or may not register, depending on whether she wishes to have the privileges that accompany registration. These privileges are, in general, that she may designate herself as a licensed nurse and that she may place the initials "R.N." after her name. There is a strong movement under way in Canada to make licensing compulsory in all provinces.

In addition to the laws controlling professional nurses, all states now have either mandatory or permissive licensing acts for practical nurses. In Canada, all provinces but one now have practical nursing laws.

Continuing Education Requirements

The rapidity with which new knowledge and technology are becoming available in nursing has created problems in keeping the practitioner up-to-date with the latest developments in her field. Many of the states and provinces are contemplating the inclusion of compulsory continuing education in their requirements for licensure. Should this occur, it would become necessary for the nurse to show that she had attended a specified number of continuing education classes in order to be able to renew her license each year. At least one state now has such legislation on its books, although the date for its implementation has been delayed to 1980.

Certification

The American Nurses' Association has recently introduced a program of certification for nurses specializing in particular fields of practice, such as geriatric nursing (the nursing care of older people), pediatric nursing, and the like. In order to be certified as a specialist, the nurse must demonstrate by examination that her knowledge of the field, is current and she must show evidence of excellence in practice. The certification program provides a mechanism for ensuring the quality of practitioners' competence at a level higher than simple licensure.[4]

AREAS OF NURSING FUNCTION

Nursing practice, as we have already noted, is constantly changing in response to societal needs. Eleanor Lambertsen has stated that "definitions of nursing practice have their origins in two domains: the law and societal demand or social sanction."[5]

Guidance on what constitutes nursing practice has come principally from two sources, the nursing practice acts and the statements of the professional nursing associations. Because of the interdependent nature of nursing and medical practice, it has become quite common too for joint statements to be made by nursing and medical associations on functions nurses

---

[3]*Principles of Legislation Relating to Nursing Practice* (revised). New York, American Nurses' Association, January 1958.

[4]Helen Creighton: *Law Every Nurse Should Know.* 3rd edition. Philadelphia, W. B. Saunders Company, 1975, pp. 13, 14.

[5]Eleanor C. Lambertsen: The Changing Role of Nursing and its Regulations. *Nursing Clinics of North America*, 9:401, September 1974.

may undertake. The opinions of state and provincial attorneys generally provide some additional assistance from the legal point of view, although these opinions are usually offered in response to requests from governmental agencies and pertain for the most part to specific situations.[6]

The Law and Nursing Functions

In their nursing practice acts, some states (and provinces) have specifically defined the functions of the professional nurse. Some protect the title of "Registered Nurse" and do not define her practice; some include a definition of both the professional and the practical nurse. Past statutes that have defined nursing practice for the most part have done so in very general terms, usually stating only that the nurse may carry out the physician's order, apply nursing skills, and supervise others less qualified than herself in the care of patients.

Most medical practice acts similarly have been written in broad general terms, giving to physicians the right to make diagnoses and to prescribe for and treat patients. The general nature of the wording in most medical and nursing practice acts has permitted both disciplines to enlarge the scope of their practices without the need for frequent changes in legislation. In many areas of professional practice, there is considerable overlap between nursing and medicine. The broad definitions contained in the statutes have also made possible the orderly transfer of many procedural functions from one discipline to another without changing the law each time. Not too many years ago, for example, only physicians were allowed to take blood pressures or to start intravenous infusions, yet today these are accepted nursing procedures.[7]

In recent years, however, there has been greater need for a more precise definition of nursing practice. One of the reasons for this has been the development of expanded roles for nurses, such as were described in the previous chapter. In some aspects of expanded role practice, as, for example, when the nurse initiates treatment on her own, the question of the legality of her actions has arisen. Another reason for the need felt by the nursing profession for clearly identified roles and functions for nurses has been the increasing concern by governments for legislation pertaining to all health manpower and governmental recommendations for changes in the existing laws. These two factors have led to an unprecedented number of changes in nursing practice acts in the past few years. In virtually every state in the United States, the nursing acts either have been changed since 1970, or plans are currently under way to change them.[8] In Canada, there is similar activity in regard to nursing legislation. Two provinces have just recently made major revisions in legislature pertaining to all health disciplines, including nursing. The nurse should familiarize herself with the particular laws concerning nursing in the state or province in which she intends to practice.

Statements by the Professional Nursing Associations

Statements issued by both national and state or provincial nursing associations have also helped to define the scope of nursing practice. The definitions of nursing practice suggested by the American Nurses' Association in 1955, for example, and its recommended new section of 1970, have provided a model for development of the definitions of nursing practice contained in many of the state nursing acts.[9] This definition reads as follows:

The practice of professional nursing means the performance for compensation of any act in the observation, care, and counsel of the ill, injured, or infirm, or in the maintenance of health or prevention of illness of others, or in the supervision and teaching of other personnel, or the administration of medications and treatments prescribed by a licensed physician or dentist; requiring substantial specialized

---

[6]Betty Jane Anderson: Orderly Transfer of Procedural Responsibilities from Medical to Nursing Practice. *Nursing Clinics of North America*, 5:313, June 1970.

[7]Ibid.

[8]Lucie Young Kelly: Nursing Practice Acts. *American Journal of Nursing*, 74:1310, July 1974.

[9]Ibid., pp. 1314–1315.

judgment and skill and based on knowledge and application of the principles of biological, physical, and social sciences. The foregoing shall not be deemed to include acts of diagnosis or prescription of therapeutic or corrective measures.

The suggested new section, advanced in 1970, was intended to encompass new areas of responsibility for nurses engaged in expanded role practice, without making these compulsory for all nurses. It reads:

A professional nurse may also perform such additional acts, under emergency or special conditions, which may include special training, as are recognized by the medical and nursing professions as proper to be performed by a professional nurse under such conditions, even though such acts might otherwise be considered diagnosis and prescription.[10]

In addition to the statements made by national nursing associations, most of the state boards of nursing and the provincial nursing associations have issued guidelines from time to time regarding the additional functions that may be performed by nurses when these are delegated by a physician. Increasingly common, also, have been joint statements issued by various professional groups, such as state nursing, medical, and sometimes hospital associations regarding the transfer of specific procedural functions from physicians to nurses. Although statements made by professional associations lack the authority of legally enacted laws, they are generally persuasive in that they reflect prevailing custom.[11]

Professional Versus Practical Nursing Functions

Creighton considers that "the essential difference between the registered professional nurse and the practical nurse is that by professional education and training and more refined skills, the registered professional nurse is obliged to evaluate and interpret facts in order to decide necessary action that may be required."[12] One would infer from this that the professional nurse's practice encompasses more independent nursing functions, whereas the practical nurse performs more dependent ones, and this is borne out in the statements regarding their functions.

The American Nurses' Association has issued the following statement of the practical nurse's role:

The work of the LPN is an integral part of nursing. The licensed practical nurse gives nursing care under the supervision of the registered nurse or physician to patients in simple nursing situations. In more complex situations the licensed practical nurse functions as an assistant to the registered professional nurse.

A simple nursing situation is one that is relatively free of scientific complexity. In a simple nursing situation the clinical state of the patient is relatively stable and the measures of care offered by the practical nurse require abilities based on a comparatively fixed and limited body of scientific facts and can be performed by following a defined procedure step by step. Measures of medical and personal care are not subject to continuously changing and complex modifications because of the clinical and behavioral state of the patient. The nursing that the patient requires is primarily of a physical character and not instructional.

In more complex situations, the licensed practical nurse facilitates patient care by meeting specific nursing requirements of patients as directed, such as preparing equipment, supplies, and facilities for patient care, helping the professional nurse to perform nursing measures, and communicating significant observations to the registered professional nurse.[13]

THE LEGAL STATUS OF THE NURSE

The nurse in her practice can be classed as either an independent contractor or an employee. Private duty nurses, that is, nurses who are engaged by the patient to perform nursing service, come under the category of independent contractors. Nurses who work in hospitals or clinics, in public health agencies, in in-

---

[10]American Nurses' Association: Memo to Executive Directors of State Nurses' Associations and State Boards of Nurses. April 3, 1970, as quoted in Lucie Young Kelly: Nursing Practice Acts. *American Journal of Nursing*, 74:1314–1315.

[11]Anderson, op. cit., p. 313.

[12]Creighton, op. cit., pp. 23–24.

[13]American Nurses' Association: Statement of Functions of the Licensed Practical Nurse. *American Journal of Nursing*, 64:93, March 1964.

dustry or for private physicians are considered employees. The distinction is a matter of control. On private duty, the nurse works independently; in the hospital, she works under the direction of the employing institution.

Student nurses, when assigned for clinical experience to a hospital or other health agency, are usually considered as employees since they are subject to the control of clinical instructors, head nurses and physicians.[14] In a school of nursing controlled by a hospital, students are generally held to be employees of the hospital insofar as they perform services for the hospital and are supervised by its staff. Students in collegiate or other independent schools of nursing may, however, be entirely under the supervision of the faculty of their school while in the practice area. Creighton considers that in these instances "the student would not seem to be an employee of the hospital, but might be held as an employee of the college."[15]

It is well for the student to remember, though, that even though she may be considered an employee, she is still responsible for her own actions. Anyone who gives nursing care, whether student or graduate, assumes certain duties, and it is expected that these will be carried out with "reasonable prudence" under the circumstances. "Reasonable prudence" is taken to mean that the individual acts with the care that any reasonable person with his or her knowledge, training, and experience would take.

The reason for the importance of determining the status of the nurse is that, under the law, not only is an individual liable for his own actions but also his employer is liable under the rule of respondeat superior (Let the master answer). Thus if a nurse is negligent and a patient is harmed, both the nurse and her employer can be sued by the patient.

In some states, charitable institutions and government hospitals, such as municipal or county hospitals, are exempt from the rule of respondeat superior and may not be sued; however, the employee of such an institution who performs a neg-

ligent act may still be sued. The law is somewhat different in various states in this regard.

Nor is the nurse absolved of responsibility for her actions simply because she is carrying out the orders of a physician. The law states that the nurse must understand the cause and effect of the treatment that she undertakes. If she carries out an order which she knows is wrong, she is guilty of negligence. At all times the patient's safety must be paramount.

If the nurse undertakes work that she knows is beyond the scope of her professional training—for example, if she performs some action or treatment which is defined as being within the province of medical practice—she may again be consider negligent or guilty of malpractice.[16]

LEGAL ISSUES OF INTEREST TO THE NURSE

Torts and Crimes

In addition to understanding her responsibilities as a professional nurse, the nurse should be aware of the types of legal proceedings in which she may become involved either as a witness or as a defendant. Generally speaking, there are two types of court actions in which a nurse can be involved. The first is called a tort. A tort is a legal wrong committed by one person against the person or property of another. The injured party may sue for damages and, if the suit is successful, he is usually awarded money to be paid by the other party. Sometimes this is spoken of as a civil suit, as opposed to a criminal suit.

A crime is also a legal wrong but, in general, it refers to a wrong committed against the public and punishable by the state. The punishment for a crime is either a fine or imprisonment. In a criminal action, the case is designated in the form The People versus Mary Jones, in a tort, John Doe versus James Jones, or Mary Doe versus the Blank Hospital. Acts such as murder, manslaughter, and robbery are

---

[14]Creighton, op. cit. pp. 59, 223.
[15]Ibid., p. 109.

[16]Kenneth G. Gray: Law and Nursing. *The Canadian Nurse,* *60*:546, June 1964.

considered criminal, whereas negligence and malpractice are usually torts.

Negligence and Malpractice

It has already been noted that each individual is responsible for his own actions and that a nurse can be held liable for her own negligent actions. Negligence on the part of nurses has been defined by the courts as "the failure to exercise that degree of skill, care, and diligence exercised by professional nurses in light of the present state of nursing science in comparable situations."[17] As a general rule, nursing negligence usually results when the nurse fails to take the appropriate action to protect the safety of the patient.[18] Thus, if the nurse does not carry out a physician's order correctly, as, for example, if she gives a wrong medication, she may be considered negligent. Similarly, failure to put up siderails on the bed of a confused patient could also be considered negligence on the nurse's part.

Malpractice has been defined as "any professional misconduct, unreasonable lack of skill or fidelity in professional or judiciary duties, evil practice, or illegal or immoral conduct."[19] Thus, it would appear that negligence implies more the failure to do something, whereas malpractice implies a more positive act of wrong-doing. A nurse who participates knowingly in an illegal operation could be considered to be guilty of malpractice.

In civil court actions, there appears to be little distinction made between willful wrong-doing, as opposed to negligence, with regard to damages or blame. Many courts use the terms "negligence" and "malpractice" interchangeably. Some courts have held that the term "malpractice" should be used in connection with only the two professions of medicine and the law.[20] The term is, however, being more widely applied now to other professional groups, including nurses.

Common Acts of Negligence. Profes-

sional nurses may be called upon to testify in a legal proceeding in regard to some matter pertaining to their work. The most common types of incidents leading to legal proceedings involving a patient and a nurse are those in which negligence is a factor. Some of the more common of such acts of negligence which have resulted in suits for damages are:

OVERLOOKED SPONGES. In any operative procedure care must be taken that no sponges are left inside the patient. Counting sponges is a nursing responsibility in most instances, and the nurse may be held liable if she fails to make a count when it has been ordered or if she makes an error in her count. Many hospitals now require that instruments and needles also be counted both before and after surgery.

BURNS. Hot water bottles, heating pads, inhalators, steam radiators, enemas, douches, and sitz baths are all items which can cause a patient to be burned. The nurse may be held responsible if she has neglected to take the usual safety precautions, such as taking the temperature of the water used in a solution administered to a patient or keeping articles that might burn the patient out of his reach.

FALLS. Another common type of accident which may result in injury to the patient and subsequently to a suit for damages is falling from bed. The usual safety precautions include the use of side rails and other restraints. Most health agencies have rules regarding the use of siderails for the beds of postoperative patients and patients under sedation. Many extend this ruling to include the beds of all irrational patients, patients over 70 years of age and children under a certain age.

WRONG MEDICINE, WRONG DOSAGE, WRONG PATIENT, WRONG CONCENTRATION. Another common area in which negligence occurs is in giving medications. Labels can be misread or may not be read at all. The nurse may fail to identify the patient correctly and consequently give a medication to the wrong person. Numerous errors are made in giving medicines. With the tremendous increase in the number of medications ordered for patients and the numerous trademarks commonly used for the various drugs, safety precautions assume

---

[17] Anderson, op. cit., p. 315.
[18] Ibid., p. 317.
[19] Ibid.
[20] Ibid.

know some talked about

greater importance in ensuring that the right patient gets the right drug in the proper concentration at the right time and in the proper manner.

5   **DEFECTS IN APPARATUS OR SUPPLIES.** Patients can be injured by the use of defective equipment. The nurse is not held responsible if the patient is injured as a result of a hidden defect, but if she uses equipment or supplies that she knows to be faulty, she may be held liable. The use of unsterile gauze for a surgical dressing could be an example of this.

6   **ABANDONMENT.** Instances in which patients have been left unattended and have injured themselves as a result have led to suits for negligence. For example, if the nurse leaves a baby on a table and the baby falls while she is absent, she can be held negligent.

7   **LOSS OR DAMAGE TO A PATIENT'S PROPERTY.** The nurse is held liable if a patient's property is lost when it has been entrusted to her care. Most hospitals now try to safeguard against suits for lost articles by asking the patient to sign a statement to the effect that he is responsible for items he retains in his possession while he is in hospital. Nevertheless, there are still many instances in which the care of a patient's property becomes of necessity the nurse's responsibility. For example, when the patient goes to the operating room for surgery, his valuables are placed in safekeeping. The property of the unconscious or irrational patient is also to be safeguarded. Perhaps the most commonly lost items are dentures, although diamond rings, watches and money also seem to disappear quite frequently.

8   **OTHER.** The above is by no means an exhaustive list of all of the acts of negligence which have resulted in suits for damages. In her book *Law Every Nurse Should Know,* Creighton discusses a number of others in which nurses have been involved, including the administration of injections, the administration of blood by nurses, failure to communicate important information, failure to exercise reasonable judgment, errors due to family assistance in patient care, infections, cardiac arrest, elopement (patient leaving the agency without notifying anyone), and pronouncing the patient dead.[21]

Reporting Accidents

The nurse has a moral and legal responsibility to report to the health agency any accidents, losses, or unusual occurrences. Most health agencies have special forms for this purpose. Filling out this report should not be interpreted as a punishment. The primary purpose is to ensure that there is a record of the details of the incident and the subsequent action taken, in the event that legal proceedings are instituted. Incident reports are also useful as a source of information in research to improve the quality of care and the effectiveness of policies.

Good Samaritan Laws

The majority of states (and some provinces) have enacted legislation designed to protect the professional practitioner from malpractice suits arising from care given to the injured at the scene of an accident or other emergency. Some of these statutes cover physicians only; others, all practitioners of the healing arts. These laws are usually referred to as "Good Samaritan" laws and are intended to encourage qualified people to give aid in an emergency. In general, these laws protect the individual who renders emergency care from civil liability for this care, unless he, or she, is guilty of gross negligence or extreme malpractice in giving the care.

In some states, there is specific legislation to the effect that no one may leave the scene of an automobile accident without first giving aid to those injured in the accident. In one state, a person is required to give first aid in any emergency; if he does not he can be criminally charged.[22] In the absence of such a

---

[21]Creighton, op. cit., pp. 122–137.
[22]Creighton, op. cit., p. 81.

law, there is no legal compulsion for the nurse, or anyone else for that matter, to give assistance in an emergency. If aid is given voluntarily, the person giving the aid is under an obligation to give the best care possible under the circumstances, commensurate with his knowledge, training, and experience. Most medical practice acts contain a waiver to the effect that, in an emergency, a volunteer who is not medically qualified may perform procedures to "save life or limb" that ordinarily lie within the scope of medical practice. In doing so, the volunteer is not considered guilty of practicing medicine without a license.

If a nurse is present at the scene of an accident, or finds herself in an emergency situation and feels morally obligated to give assistance, she should first of all ascertain that she is the best-qualified person there to give aid. She should also make sure that a state of emergency truly exists. The nurse should then render the care that is necessary and transfer the patient as soon as possible to a medically qualified practitioner for continued treatment. In such a situation, the nurse is expected to act as any other nurse of equal training and experience would act under the same or similar circumstances.[23]

Assault and Battery

In some instances, nurses have been involved in legal proceedings as a result of a charge of assault and battery by a patient. Assault refers to threats to do bodily harm to another. Battery is "the unlawful beating of another or the carrying out of threatened physical harm."[24] Assault and battery are considered criminal offenses as well as torts. The law protects every individual against bodily harm by another person and also against any form of assault due to interference with his person. Therefore a person cannot take a blood sample from a patient without his consent. Nor may a person be operated on for any condition unless he has given his consent to the procedure and understands the significance of the procedure. Autopsy without the consent of relatives may be considered assault and battery.

Most hospitals and other health agencies have standard forms which the patient signs to grant permission for treatment and operative procedures deemed necessary while he is under the care of the agency. The patient is usually asked to sign such a form on admission to the agency. Increasingly, however, the legality of a consent form signed on admission to cover all treatments and procedures which the patient may undergo is being questioned. It has been ruled by the courts that the patient must give *informed consent*. Informed consent is taken to mean that the patient has been given:

1. An explanation of the condition
2. A fair explanation of the procedures to be used and the consequences
3. A description of alternative treatments or procedures
4. A description of the benefits to be expected (not assured)

In order to lessen the likelihood of legal suits being filed between patients and health care agencies, nearly all agencies require the patient to sign various forms on admission. This is done (1) to absolve the agency of responsibility for loss or damages suffered by the patient while under care (which might give rise to patient-initiated suits), and (2) to ensure that financial obligations on the part of the patient will be met (which might otherwise result in agency-initiated suits to recover payment for charges).

Samples of some of the various forms used by agencies are shown on pages 117 to 120: (1) application for benefits under the Hospital Insurance Act (a legal requirement in most hospitals in Canada), (2) Responsibility for Retaining Personal Possessions Form, (3) a Patient Consent Form (general) covering authorization to perform medical acts, and (4) a Patient Consent Form pertaining to specific aspects of care.

---

[23]Harvey Sarner: *The Nurse and The Law.* Philadelphia, W. B. Saunders Company, 1968, pp. 86–88.

[24]Creighton, op. cit., p. 146.

5. An offer to answer the patient's inquiries

6. An understanding that the patient is not being coerced to agree and may withdraw if he changes his mind.[25]

Many health agencies are currently in the process of revising both their procedures for obtaining consent from patients and the forms that are used. The nurse should familiarize herself with those that are being used in the agency in which she will be working or having clinical experience.

In most hospitals, a separate consent form (in addition to the one the patient signs on admission) is used to obtain the patient's permission for surgical procedures, and often for other treatments as well. It should be noted that it is the attending surgeon's responsibility to explain the nature of the operative procedure to the patient; this is not a responsibility that can be delegated to the nurse. The nurse may, however, present the form to be signed.[26] This should be done before the patient is sedated for surgery, since consent obtained while the patient is under sedation can be questioned. Consent must be voluntary and the individual giving the consent must be rational. In an emergency, when treatment is a matter of life and death and the patient is unable to give permission, consent may be implied. In the case of children, either parent may give permission for treatments and operative procedures. In the case of mentally incompetent persons, it is necessary to obtain the consent of the patient's legal guardian.

Nurses have sometimes been involved in suits for assault and battery because of the use of restraints on patients. It is important to remember that, except in emergencies, restraints should not be used unless they are ordered by the physician. At all times, undue force is to be avoided in handling patients.

False Imprisonment

An individual who is unjustifiably detained, or confined against his will and without a legal warrant for his detention, may bring a charge of false imprisonment against the individual or the agency that has detained him.[27] Most instances in which nurses have been involved in court proceedings on charges of false imprisonment have been in relation to mental patients. United States and Canadian law does provide for the detention without a warrant of a person who is mentally disturbed and who may hurt himself or others, or destroy property, and also for the confinement of persons with communicable diseases, which present a danger to society. However, this covers only the length of time required to obtain legal authority for the person's restraint.[28]

A person cannot be prevented from leaving a health agency if he is of sound mind, even if it is advisable that he stay for additional care. If the patient insists on leaving, most agencies require that he sign a form stating that he will not hold the agency responsible for any harm resulting from his leaving.

The use of force to hold someone against his will, or even the threat of forcible restraint made in order to detain a person, is considered assault and/or battery. The nurse must therefore exercise caution in the use of restraints, as we have noted above.

Invasion of Privacy

Under both American and Canadian law, every individual has the right to withhold both himself and his property from public scrutiny. The right does not hold, however, if the individual has given consent for exposure; nor is there a tort when the person is a public figure or does acts of public interest.[29] A common instance in which the nurse must guard against invasion of a person's right to privacy is in the taking and use of photographs of patients. Consent must be obtained if these are to be used in any way not connected with the patient's medical treatment. Care must be taken by nurses also to avoid the exposure of patients to roommates, visitors, or others during the

[25] Lucie Young Kelly: The Patient's Right to Know. *Nursing Outlook*, 24:28, January 1976.
[26] Creighton, op. cit., pp. 147–148.
[27] Creighton, op. cit., pp. 155–157.
[28] Ibid.
[29] Creighton, op. cit., p. 158.

VANCOUVER GENERAL HOSPITAL | 101 | ADMISSION HISTORY | CLASS

1	ADMISSION No. 76	57123	DOE JANE	UNIT No. C1247	P
2	PREVIOUS ADMISSION	18.10.71	MAIDEN NAME BROWN	M.I. No.	
3	S.A. & No.	96245	ADM. AT (TIME) 1400	D/A 2 M/O 12 Y/R 77	
4	NURSING UNIT C9ˢ	STAND. 1 SEMI. 2 PRIV. 3 ✓ NURS. 4 TRANS. FROM			

ATTENDING PHYSICIAN DR. R.L. SMITH — DR. (PERSONAL/FAMILY) — PRIV. ✓ STAFF DES.

ADM. ON REQ. OF SAME — SERV. ON ADM. S — RELIGION R.C.

PT'S. RESID. B.C. PERM. YES — TRANS. D/ON M/A Y/O TO/R N.U. — TRANS. D/ON M/A Y/O TO/R N.U.

SEX M 1 F 2 ✓ | NBM MAT. 3 IMMAT. 4 | NBF MAT. 5 IMMAT. 6 | S. 1 | MAR. STAT. M. 2 WDS. 3 | D/B/A 10 M/O 8 Y/R 47 AGE 30

PAT'S ADDRESS 123 STATE ST — FROM MONTH | YEAR | TO: MONTH | YEAR

CITY OR MUNIC. VANCOUVER — S. IN. NO. 42346 — 8 | 70 | 12 | 77

MUNIC. ADDRESS SAME — POSTAL ZONE

PREVIOUS RESIDENCE 8961 - 275 ST SURREY BC 4 69 8 70

HEAD OF FAMILY JOHN DOE — RELAT. HUSBAND — SEPARATED FROM HOSPITAL

ADDRESS SAME — PHONE 232-9867

NEAREST RELATIVE SAME — RELAT. — PHONE

ADDRESS SAME — THIRD PARTY LIAB. INVOL.? YES NO

OCCUP'N EMPLR ARLINGTON BUSINESS MACHINE — FROM MONTH | YEAR | TO: MONTH | YEAR

EMPL'RS ADDRESS 922 WEST HOYT ST. VANCOUVER 5 71 12 77

PREVIOUS EMPL'T INCLDG. PERIODS OF UNEMP-LOYMENT

PREVIOUS RESIDENCE

B.C. 6 MOS. OR LESS | ARRIVED D/A M/O Y/R | PART PROV. | LEFT PART PROV. D/A M/O Y/R

RESPONS FOR PAY HIS 1 | WCB 2 | DVA 3 | FEDERAL OTHER 4 | SELF 5 | OTHER 6 | PROV. 7 | SPECIFY

W.C.B. No. — W.C.B. ACCID. (TIME) — D/A M/O Y/R

— STATE ON ADMISSION | ELECTIVE | URGENT | EMERG.

ADMIT DIAGNOSIS CHOLECYSTITIS

REFERENCES J. C. BROWN, MERCHANT

NAME ADDRESS & OCCUP. 72841 KARTON ST. VANCOUVER B.C. — RESPONS. FOR DR.

I HEREBY MAKE APPLICATION FOR BENEFITS UNDER THE "HOSPITAL INSURANCE ACT" ON BEHALF OF MYSELF OR THE ABOVE MENTIONED PATIENT, AND I CERTIFY THAT I HAVE READ THE STATEMENTS, EXCEPT DIAGNOSIS, ON THIS FORM OR HAVE HAD THEM READ TO ME AND THAT THE SAME ARE TRUE AND CORRECT.

WITNESS K. Smith DATE 12. 2. 77 | APPLICANT'S SIGNATURE Jane Doe RELAT. TO PAT.

APPLICANT RESIDED IN B.C. YRS. MOS. | APPLIC. ADDRESS

A MINIMUM FINE OF $100.00 OR NOT LESS THAN 10 DAYS IN JAIL OR BOTH IS THE PENALTY FOR MAKING A FALSE STATEMENT IN AN APPLICATION FOR BENEFITS OR FOR FAILING OR REFUSING TO COMPLETE SUCH AN APPLICATION WHEN REQUIRED TO DO SO BY AN OFFICER OF ANY HOSPITAL IN BRITISH COLUMBIA.

REMARKS:

B.C.C.I. YES NO V.L.I. | PAID ON ACCOUNT | ADMITTED BY

FORM M-1 - REV. 1-76
60010

Sample of the legal form required for a patient to receive benefits under the Hospital Insurance Act in one province of Canada. (Courtesy of Vancouver General Hospital.)

FORM A-166
REV. 3-67

VANCOUVER GENERAL HOSPITAL

Notice re PATIENTS' EFFECTS & VALUABLES

DATE   NURSING UNIT

MR., MISS, MRS.   UNIT NUMBER

SURNAME   GIVEN NAME

DOCTOR   PLEASE USE BLOCK CAPITALS

SEX   AGE

THE HOSPITAL WILL NOT BE RESPONSIBLE FOR ANY ITEM KEPT AT THE BEDSIDE.

Valuable articles and clothing should be returned home at the time of admission.

If you find it absolutely necessary to retain articles of value such as money, rings, watches, jewellery, please have them deposited with the Cashier for safe-keeping.

Patients may have radios or television sets, at the discretion of patient's physician or the Nurse in Charge of the Nursing Unit, subject to Hospital regulations in respect to electrical codes. The Hospital will in no way be responsible for loss or damage.

Articles left in hospital after discharge, if not claimed within 3 months, will be disposed of at the discretion of Hospital Administration.

DECLARATION

I   JANE DOE   fully understand that the Hospital
   NAME OF PATIENT

will not assume responsibility for any items of value which I have found

necessary to retain at the bedside and absolve the Hospital from any res-

ponsibility for their safekeeping.

K. Smith
WITNESS (HOSPITAL EMPLOYEE)

Jane Doe
SIGNATURE OF PATIENT

December 2, 1977
DATE

Sample of a form for assuming responsibility for retaining personal possessions. (Courtesy of Vancouver General Hospital.)

FORM M-IA
60015
20M - 11-71

VANCOUVER GENERAL HOSPITAL

MEDICAL AUTHORIZATION

Unit No. _C 1247_

I, the undersigned, do hereby authorize doctors, (including Active or Courtesy Staff doctors, and House Staff) and the Hospital staff and employees, and the staff and employees of such other institutions as may be requested by The Vancouver General Hospital, to carry out on my _self_
(SELF, SON, WIFE, ETC.)

Jane Doe
(NAME OF PATIENT)

such examinations, procedures, treatments, and operations as may be ordered by the doctors in attendance.

I also relieve the Vancouver General Hospital from any responsibility to provide or arrange any transportation from the hospital to or from any other hospital or institution upon referral for treatment or diagnosis, or any transportation from or to the hospital prior to or following my discharge, and from any liability arising in any manner in respect of such transportation.

Date _December 2, 1977_

Signed _Jane Doe_

Relationship
to Patient _____

Witness:

K. Smith

Sample of one type of patient's consent form from a hospital. (Courtesy of Vancouver General Hospital.)

AUTHORITY TO DIVULGE INFORMATION:

IF THIS HOSPITAL OR PHYSICIANS ACCOUNT IS TO BE PAID BY ANY FORM OF INSURANCE, OR IN THE CASE OF AN INDIGENT BY A MUNICIPALITY, I HEREBY AUTHORIZE THE RIVERSIDE HOSPITAL TO FURNISH TO SAID PARTIES SUCH INFORMATION AS MAY BE NECESSARY FOR THE SETTLEMENT OF ANY CLAIMS.

CONSENT TO TREATMENT - TRANSFER - OR REMOVAL

I HEREBY AUTHORIZE AND DIRECT THE ATTENDING PHYSICIAN, AND HOSPITAL STAFF TO CARRY OUT SUCH FORMS OF EXAMINATIONS, TESTS, AND TREATMENT AS THEY MAY DEEM NECESSARY FOR THE PHYSICAL IMPROVEMENT OF *James Doe* .SHOULD IT BE FOUND NECESSARY OR DEEMED ADVISABLE IN THEIR OPINION TO TRANSFER THE PATIENT TO ANOTHER HOSPITAL, I HEREBY CONSENT THERETO. I FURTHER AGREE TO LEAVE THE HOSPITAL OR REMOVE SAID PATIENT WHEN REQUESTED TO DO SO BY THE ADMINISTRATOR OR HIS ASSISTANT.

DATE *October 18 1977*   SIGNED *Mrs. John Doe*

WITNESS _____   RELATIONSHIP *Mother*
                                                    (IF OTHER THAN PATIENT)
RELATIONSHIP _____

OBSTETRICAL CONSENT:

I HEREBY AUTHORIZE AND DIRECT MY ATTENDING OBSTETRICIAN AND/OR HIS ASSOCIATES OR ASSISTANTS TO PROVIDE SUCH SERVICES FOR ME AS THEY MAY DEEM REASONABLE AND NECESSARY, INCLUDING, BUT NOT LIMITED TO, THE ADMINISTRATION OF ANAESTHESIA, AND THE PERFORMANCE OF SERVICES INVOLVING SURGERY, PATHOLOGY AND RADIOLOGY, AND I HEREBY CONSENT THERETO. I FURTHER CONSENT TO THE CIRCUMCISION OF MY BABY SHOULD IT BE DEEMED NECESSARY. THIS CONSENT FURTHER INCLUDES THE AUTHORITY TO DIVULGE INFORMATION AS NOTED TO ABOVE.

DATE _____   SIGNED _____

WITNESS _____   RELATIONSHIP _____
                                                    (IF OTHER THAN PATIENT)
RELATIONSHIP _____

CONSENT TO OPERATION AND ANAESTHESIA:

THE PHYSICAL CONDITION AND THE SURGICAL PROCEDURE CONTEMPLATED TO ALLEVIATE THIS CONDITION HAS BEEN EXPLAINED TO ME BY DR. *A Smith* AND I HEREBY AUTHORIZE AND DIRECT HIM AND/OR HIS ASSOCIATES OR ASSISTANTS TO OPERATE UPON *James Doe* FOR THIS CONDITION, AND/OR TO DO ANY OTHER THERAPEUTIC PROCEDURE HIS/THEIR JUDGEMENT MAY DICTATE TO BE ADVISABLE FOR THE PATIENTS WELL BEING. AND I FURTHER CONSENT TO SUCH ADDITIONAL SERVICES AS THEY MAY DEEM REASONABLE AND NECESSARY, INCLUDING, BUT NOT LIMITED TO THE ADMINISTRATION AND MAINTENANCE OF ANAESTHESIA AND THE PERFORMANCES OF SERVICES INVOLVING PATHOLOGY AND RADIOLOGY. THIS CONSENT FURTHER INCLUDES CONSENT TO TREATMENT AND AUTHORITY TO DIVULGE INFORMATION AS NOTED AT TOP OF PAGE.

DATE *October 18 1977*   SIGNED *Mrs. John Doe*

WITNESS *Mary Smith*   RELATIONSHIP *Mother*
                                                    (IF OTHER THAN PATIENT)
RELATIONSHIP _____

LEAVING HOSPITAL AGAINST ADVICE:

THIS IS TO CERTIFY THAT _____ AM/IS LEAVING THE RIVERSIDE HOSPITAL AGAINST THE ADVICE OF THE ATTENDING PHYSICIAN AND THE HOSPITAL ADMINISTRATION. I ACKNOWLEDGE THAT I HAVE BEEN INFORMED OF THE RISKS INVOLVED AND HEREBY RELEASE THE ATTENDING PHYSICIAN AND THE HOSPITAL FROM ALL RESPONSIBILITY OF ANY ILL EFFECTS WHICH MAY RESULT FROM THIS ACTION.

DATE _____   SIGNED _____
                                                    (PATIENT/OR PARENT/OR GUARDIAN)
WITNESS _____   RELATIONSHIP _____
                                                    (IF OTHER THAN PATIENT)
RELATIONSHIP _____

Sample of a patient's consent form. (Courtesy of the Riverside Hospital of Ottawa.)

process of nursing care or when the patient is being transported from one area to another in the health agency.

The right to privacy extends also to information about the patient. The patient's record contains confidential information; it should not be left where it might be read by unauthorized persons. In using information from patients' records (or information she has obtained from the patient) for case studies or other types of classroom work, the student should be careful not to reveal the patient's identity; nor should information about a patient be discussed carelessly with people who are not entitled to that information. The nurse should always be discreet in giving out information about patients. People have become increasingly aware of their right to privacy as a result of national publicity about prominent cases of wiretapping and subsequent legislation to safeguard the individual's rights in this regard. The use of tape recorders and Dictaphones without the patient's knowledge and consent could undoubtedly be taken as an invasion of privacy and should be avoided by the nurse.

Defamation of Character

Another area of the law of which the nurse should be aware is that of suits arising from defamation of character. The term "defamation of character" means that a person's reputation is damaged by written or spoken words which tend to lower his esteem in the eyes of other people. If written, as in a letter to a third party, or depicted in a cartoon which causes the person to be the subject of ridicule or contempt, the term "libel" is used to describe the action.[30] "Slander" is the term used for defamation of character through spoken words, as, for example, if one speaks badly of someone in conversation with another person. The nurse should always be careful not to discuss patients except with others who are concerned with their care. Not every mention of a patient is slander or libel, of course; these terms are used only when there is a threat to the individual's reputation. For example, most courts consider it defamatory to let other people know that an unmarried woman is pregnant, or that a patient has venereal disease. To state that a patient had a broken leg would not ordinarily be considered defamatory. If, however, one added that the broken leg resulted because the patient was intoxicated and fell down the stairs, this might be considered to be defamation of character.

The Nurse and Confidential Information

The question of whether confidential information entrusted to the nurse by the patient is considered to be a privileged communication and therefore inadmissible as evidence in court proceedings has not been definitely settled. A few states have enacted statutes which specifically state that the nurse-patient relationship is a privileged one, and therefore confidential information given to the nurse cannot be used in proceedings. In instances in which the doctor-patient communication is considered privileged, the ruling has been held to extend to nurses when they are acting as agents of the physician. In Canada, the rule of privilege for confidential information is not absolute. Although the nurse and the physician should not disclose confidential information entrusted to them, they may be directed to do so, if this is justified by public policy or if the law requires reporting of the matter.[31] In the United States, a witness cannot be required to give evidence which would tend to incriminate him, whereas in Canada the law requires that a witness answer all questions that are relevant whether or not the answer tends to incriminate him. He can, however, invoke the protection of the Canada Evidence Act in certain cases.

Malpractice Insurance

Because of the increase in the number of malpractice suits in general, and against

---

[30]Creighton, op. cit., p. 159.

[31]Creighton, op. cit., p. 229.

nurses in particular, many authorities now recommend that each nurse carry her own malpractice insurance to cover the cost of lawyers' fees and possible damages. The American Nurses' Association and several of the provincial nursing associations in Canada have made malpractice insurance available to their members at a reasonable cost.

Many nurses are under the mistaken belief that, because they are employees, their employer will carry the burden of responsibility for their negligent actions. This is not so; the nurse can be sued as an individual.

Wills

Nurses are often asked to witness a will for a patient. A will is a declaration of an individual's wishes regarding what is to be done with his property after his death.[32] The individual making the will is called the *testator*. A will must ordinarily be in writing and must be signed by the testator. The law usually requires the signature of two or three competent witnesses in addition. An individual who may expect to benefit from a will should not act as a witness to the signing of that will. The family and close friends of a patient are naturally reluctant, then, to be witnesses, and the nurse is frequently called upon to act in this capacity since she is a disinterested party. The nurse should not agree to act as a witness, however, if she is a minor. Minors, that is, persons under the legal age as defined by the law of the particular state or province, are not usually acceptable as witnesses.

In most jurisdictions, all witnesses are required to be present at the same time and to sign the will in the presence of the person making it. The witness should see the testator sign the will before signing it himself. If, however, the will has already been signed, the witness should either ask the testator to sign again or to declare that this is his will and he has signed it. In affixing his signature to a will, the witness indicates that he has either seen the person sign the document or

that the testator has declared to him that he has signed it, and that the testator was competent to sign.[33] It is not necessary for the witness to know the contents of the will, nor in most jurisdictions is it necessary for the witness to be told that the document is a will.

For a will to be valid, the person making it must be capable of understanding what he is doing. If the patient dies and the validity of the will is questioned, a nurse may be called upon to testify in court concerning the mental capacity of the individual at the time the will was made, whether or not she acted as a witness to the will. If the nurse is aware that a patient has made a will while in hospital, it is a good practice for her to note on the patient's record the fact that a will was made, the date and time that it was signed, and the nurse's observations regarding the mental state of the patient at the time the will was made.[34]

Narcotics Legislation

Another area of law in which the nurse is involved is the control and administration of narcotic drugs. In the United States, there are both federal and state laws controlling narcotics. Until recently the principal federal law was the Harrison Narcotic Act of 1914. However, in 1970 the Comprehensive Drug Abuse Prevention and Control Act was enacted, one section of which, the Controlled Substances Act, has replaced virtually all preexisting federal laws dealing with narcotics, stimulants, depressants, and hallucinogens. In addition, almost all the states also have their own laws regarding narcotics, and most have adopted the Uniform State Narcotic Act. Both federal and state laws affect the nurse in her nursing practice.

In Canada the control of narcotic drugs is under federal jurisdiction, the pertinent legislation being the Narcotic Control Act and the Narcotic Control Regulations. This legislation, which was enacted in

---

[32]Ibid., pp. 198–199.

[33]Sarner, op. cit., p. 108.
[34]For a more detailed discussion about wills, the nurse is referred to: Creighton, op. cit., pp. 198–205, and Sarner, op. cit., pp. 107–112.

1961, controls the use of opium, coca leaves (and their salts and derivatives), and a number of other drugs classified as narcotics, including cannabis. Certain other drugs, for example the barbiturates, have been designated as "controlled drugs." Regulations regarding these drugs are included in the Food and Drugs Act and Regulations of Canada (1961). A list of the "controlled drugs" appears in Schedule G of the Food and Drugs Act.

Under the Controlled Substances Act, the nurse can give narcotics under the direction or supervision of a duly licensed physician or dentist, but it is unlawful for her to have narcotic drugs in her possession. The attempt to obtain narcotic drugs by fraud or deceit is a violation of the law. Penalties for violation include fine or imprisonment or both. The nurse must be careful when handling narcotics to see that they have been ordered in writing by a duly licensed physician and that careful records are kept of their use.

STUDY VOCABULARY

Assault	Geriatric nursing	Negligence
Battery	Good Samaritan	Permissive licensure
Certification	Invasion of privacy	
Crime	Liability	Prudence
Defamation of character	Libel	Slander
	Licensure	Testator
Elopement	Malpractice	Tort
False imprisonment	Mandatory licensure	

STUDY SITUATION

As you are driving along a lonely country highway late one evening on your way home from a party, you and your escort notice skid marks on the pavement and a car overturned in the ditch at the side of the road. A young man, his clothes muddy and torn, waves his arms frantically to get you to stop. You think you hear a woman's voice moaning somewhere.

1. What would you do?
2. What are your legal responsibilities if you stop and find that the woman is badly injured?
3. Is there a Good Samaritan law in your state/province?
4. What protection do you have against possible charges of negligence or malpractice if you render first aid in this situation?

SUGGESTED READINGS

A Consumer Speaks out about Hospital Care. *American Journal of Nursing,* 76:1443–1444, September, 1976.

Continuing Education for Nurses: Vital for Effective Nursing Care, says ICN. *ICN News Release,* No. 7, September, 1975.

Creighton, H.: Law for the Nurse Supervisor. *Supervisor Nurse* (regular column).

Creighton, H. (Guest Editor): Symposium on Current Legal and Professional Problems. *Nursing Clinics of North America,* 9:391–589, September, 1974.

Lipman, M.: Defamation: a Rash Comment Could Get You Sued. *R.N.,* 38:48–51, February, 1975.

Rozovsky, L. E.: A Nurse is Sued. *Dimensions in Health Service,* May, 1975, pp. 8, 9.

Rozovsky, L. E.: Malpractice Insurance for Canadian Nurses. *Canadian Hospital,* 49:49–50, March, 1972.

COMMUNICATION; THE NURSING PROCESS; RECORDING

8 COMMUNICATION SKILLS

The nurse should be able to:

Explain the SMCR model of the communication process

Give examples of factors which can interfere with elements of the communication process

List factors the nurse should consider when she wants to convey a message

Discuss characteristics of language to be considered by the nurse in communications with patients

Give examples of various ways by which people communicate nonverbally

Discuss ways of fostering an open climate for nurse/patient communications

Develop beginning skills in listening to patients

Discuss the interview as a tool in nurse/patient communications

Give examples of various media used for information exchange between members of the health team

COMMUNICATION SKILLS 8

INTRODUCTION

The fundamental core of nursing is the relationship that is established between the nurse and the patient. This is a professional relationship, based on trust and mutual respect. An individual who comes to a health agency is there because he needs help in relation to his health; the nurse and other health professionals are there to provide the help he needs. In order to develop a relationship whereby she can help the patient, the nurse must develop skills in communicating, since, without communication, no relationship is possible.

Communication is the process by which one person conveys thoughts, feelings, and ideas to another. It is a tool which provides a means for one person to understand another, to accept and be accepted, to convey and receive information, to give and accept directions, to teach and to learn. The nurse communicates with the patient and the patient with her. Communication is always a two-way process. The nurse also communicates with the patient's family and friends, with visitors to the agency, with other members of the health team and other personnel, and with a host of other people during the course of a day. She should, then, know something about the process of communication.

THE BASIC ELEMENTS OF COMMUNICATION

Communication involves both the sending and the receiving of a message. If the message is not received, no com-munication has taken place. Five elements[1] are involved in the process:

1. A sender—someone who wishes to convey a message
2. A message—the thought, feeling, or idea that the sender wishes to convey
3. A channel—the means by which the message is conveyed
4. A receiver—the person for whom the message is intended
5. The effect on the receiver—behavior the intended receiver shows to indicate that he has received the message

Let us take an example. The nurse in a doctor's office wishes Mr. Brown to go into the examining room and tells him so. The sender is the nurse. The message is "Please go to the examining room." The channel is the spoken word. The intended receiver of the message is Mr. Brown. The desired effect on the receiver is that he gets up from his chair in the waiting room and proceeds to the examining room. If he does, the nurse will know that he received the message. If he does not, she will assume that the message was not received. The effect on the receiver provides the sender with *feedback*, since it enables the person who has sent the message to know if it was received or not; if it was not, communication has not taken place and the sender had best try again.

Because communication is such an essential component of most people's work, as well as a basic social process, it has received a great deal of study. Numerous models have been developed to illustrate

---

[1]James K. Skipper, Jr., and Robert C. Leonard (eds.): *Social Interaction and Patient Care.* Philadelphia, J. B. Lippincott Company, 1965, pp. 51–82.

the process. The Source, Message, Channel, Receiver (SMCR) model[2] of the communication process (shown below) is one that illustrates the process simply, contains all the basic elements and is easily understood.

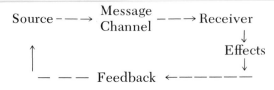

FACTORS AFFECTING COMMUNICATION

Effective communication means that the message the sender intended to convey reached the intended receiver, was received by him, was interpreted correctly, and that the receiver was able to respond in some meaningful way to indicate that he received the message. Difficulties can occur anywhere along the way in the communication process.

The Sender

The *sender* may have a problem in putting his message into a form that can be communicated. We communicate with words, both in speech and in writing, and with nonverbal behavior, such as facial expression, gestures, body postures, and touch. A person can sometimes communicate quite eloquently using nonverbal means, but, in order to convey many of the messages he wants to send, he needs to be able to attach symbolic meanings (in the form of words) to both living creatures and inanimate objects. He must also be able to arrange these symbols to form messages that can be understood by others, and he must be able to send his message clearly.

Consider the person who is in a foreign country, for example, and is unable to speak the language. He can get along to a

certain extent by pointing, using gestures, and pantomiming but, when it comes to asking directions or ordering a meal, he is unable to attach the right symbols to get his meaning across, and he will have difficulties. A person who has suffered brain damage and is unable to speak, or cannot put his thoughts into verbal expressions that can be understood by others, has similar problems. Difficulties in making vocal sounds also interfere with the ability to communicate.

Someone who has lost the use of his voice must depend on written forms of communication, on gestures, and other ways of expressing himself nonverbally in order to convey messages.

An individual's physical well-being and his emotional state also affect his ability to communicate. A person who is ill may find trying to communicate just too much of an effort, or his thought processes may not function well enough for him to put together a coherent message. A person's emotional state can make communication easier, may hinder his ability to express himself, or may put a stop to his communicating at all. When a person is at ease emotionally and feels comfortable with another person, he usually finds it much easier to talk and express himself. Nervousness and anxiety often interfere with a person's ability to put together a clear message and send it. The nervous applicant at a job interview, for example, frequently finds it difficult to say what he wants to say in the way it should be said, and comes out of the interview feeling that he has said all the wrong things.

All types of emotions can affect one's ability to communicate. A person can be so overwhelmed with happiness that he cannot find the words to express himself adequately. He can also be so angry that no suitable way of expressing his anger comes to him, or too frightened to say or do anything. In these cases, however, the person usually conveys his feelings in nonverbal ways. The look on a person's face can tell you that he is happy. The clenched fist, the pounding on the table, or the slamming of a door can convey anger as eloquently as words. The eyes and the taut facial expression often tell you that a person is frightened.

[2] Everett M. Rogers and Rekha A. Rogers: *Communication in Organizations*. New York, The Free Press, 1976.

The Message

The message itself may not be clear. Some people have a problem in getting the message they want to send clear in their own minds, let alone communicate it to others. Often, however, a person knows what he wants to communicate, but the way it comes out is not at all what he intended. Sometimes two conflicting messages are being sent simultaneously. For example, the nurse may say to a patient, "I am glad that you came, even if it is late," but the impatient tapping of her foot, or surreptitious glances at her watch, may convey an entirely different meaning to the patient. Noise or other distractions can also interfere with a message exchange. The child who is watching a television program may not hear his mother calling him to come to bed.

In order to convey the meaning intended by the sender, the message must be sent in a form the intended receiver can understand. If Mr. Brown does not speak English, the communication process breaks down, unless the nurse is able to put her message into a language he does understand, or can convey the intent of her message by nonverbal means. Even with someone who does speak the same language as the nurse, the words must be in terminology that the patient can understand, or again the message is unclear. If the intent of the message is not completely and explicitly stated, as, for example, if directions on how to get to the examining room are not included for the person who is unfamiliar with the physical layout of the office, the message is not complete.

The Channel

The channel chosen for sending a message must be appropriate. Basically, there are three main channels by which we communicate with other people: oral (speech), written, nonverbal communication.

For oral communication, we have a number of tools at our disposal: talking directly with a person in a face-to-face meeting, recording messages on tape, telephoning, or communicating by radio or television. All are media for the spoken word. There are also many forms of written communication: notes, letters, interoffice memos, records and forms, newspapers, books, and magazines all convey messages in written form. But we also convey messages nonverbally. It has often been said that a person communicates his true feelings more in his actions and his mannerisms than he does in words. A whole area of study in recent years has been on "body language"—that is, the interpretation of messages people send through their facial expressions, gestures, postures, ways of walking, and so forth.

The important point, here, however, is that the medium chosen must be appropriate for the message and must make the intent of the message clear to the intended receiver. Touch can sometimes convey more sympathetic understanding than words to someone who has suffered a loss. Direct face-to-face talking is often a more effective means of communication than telephoning, or writing a message. Some people have difficulty expressing themselves orally and can put their thoughts and feelings down on paper easier. When there is a long list of instructions for someone to follow, it is usually better if these are written down and supplemented with oral clarification as needed. At times the individual just needs time to think about the message, and thus, the written format serves as a future reference.

The Receiver

Problems in communication can also occur at the *receiving* end of the process. The message may reach someone other than the intended receiver. If Mr. Jones gets up and moves in the direction of the examining room while Mr. Brown continues to sit in his chair, the nurse knows that the wrong person received the message. An individual who is hard of hearing may have difficulty receiving spoken messages, unless he wears a hearing aid, or unless the message is given loudly enough and clearly enough for him to receive it. A person who cannot read or write is unable to receive communications sent in written form. The intended receiver must not only receive the message but also be able to interpret it.

A large number of physical and psychosocial factors can affect a person's ability to understand communications. Age, for example, must be taken into consideration. Children often do not understand messages that are directed to them by adults, either because the child's language skills have not developed sufficiently for him to be able to symbolize in the same terms as the adult, or because his intellectual development has not reached a level where he can comprehend the idea the adult is trying to convey. The integrity of the anatomical structures and physiological processes involved in interpreting messages must also be intact. When a person's mental faculties have been impaired by brain damage, or his ability to use his mental faculties is lessened by drowsiness, by alterations in his level of consciousness, or by alcohol or drugs, for example, his ability to receive and interpret messages is decreased.

A person's emotional state may also interfere with both his ability to receive messages and to interpet them. The frightened individual attends only to those messages that concern the object of his fear. He may not receive messages about anything else, or he may misinterpret messages sent by people who are trying to help him. The patient who is afraid that the injection he is about to receive will be painful may perceive the nurse's smile as sadistic rather than reassuring. Most people are at least a little bit afraid of injections; some people have a real phobia about them.

It has often been said that people hear only what they want to hear. Receiving and interpreting messages is an active process. A person who is told that he has inoperable cancer may not hear the message because he has "turned off" the sound of the doctor's voice. Nurses and other health professionals often do not receive messages sent by patients, simply because they are not attentive to what the person is trying to tell them.

Then again, because each person is a unique individual, who has his own personality traits, background of life experiences and set of values, each person may interpret a message differently. He will interpret it according to the way he *perceives* it. Therefore, the meaning he attaches to a message may be completely different from the one intended by the sender. The nurse may take the arm of an older person as he walks along the hall. The gesture by the nurse may be intended to convey her warmth of feeling for the older person, but he may interpret it as, "She thinks I can't walk by myself." He then sees it as a threat to his independence and brushes her hand aside.

Words, of course, do not have the same meaning for everyone. The meanings attached to symbols we use in our language differ, depending on the context in which the words were learned. In some countries, the examining room in a doctor's office is known as the doctor's surgery. Telling someone who is not used to this terminology to go to the doctor's surgery, then, might conjure up visions of a major operation about to take place, whereas the doctor may just want to put a simple dressing on the patient's injured hand.

Messages are received and interpreted on both an intellectual and an emotional level. Mr. Brown may be afraid to go into the examining room, particularly if the nurse calls it a "surgery," because of what he thinks may happen to him there, and he may not respond to the nurse's message. Or, he may react with hostility towards the nurse, perhaps because he did not like the tone of her voice, or the way she addressed him. He responds to the attitude that is conveyed nonverbally at the same time as the nurse's spoken words. He may think, "If that's the way she is going to treat me, I'm not going to do anything she wants me to do." This type of situation arises frequently with children, who will often do anything for someone they like and trust, but nothing for the person who has failed to win their confidence.

Source credibility is important, though, with adults too. That is to say, a person must believe that the other person is telling him the truth and that the person is a reliable source of information. In order to promote effective communication, the nurse must foster an atmosphere in which the patient feels that he is safe, that he is accepted as a person, and that he can trust the nurse.

THE NURSE AS A SENDER IN THE COMMUNICATION PROCESS

There is an old rhyme that goes, "I have six honest serving men who taught me all I know. Their names are Who and What and When, and Where and Why and How."

In thinking about communication and how to get a message conveyed to an intended receiver so that the message is received and correctly interpreted, the nurse may find it helpful to ask herself the six questions contained in the rhyme. We will start with the what, since the first thing to do is to get the message clear in your own mind, before you decide how to send it.

What Is to Be Communicated?

Is it directions, such as how to get somewhere or how to do something?

Is it information, such as explaining to a patient what is going to happen to him when he goes down to the x-ray department for a series of tests?

Is it an attitude, such as a feeling of warmth and acceptance?

Why Is This Message to Be Communicated?

Does the patient need to know something, in order to become oriented to the agency?

Does he need help to overcome his fear of surgery?

Does he need this message for his safety? To increase his independence?

How Should It Be Communicated?

Should I talk to the person, give him information (or directions) in writing, or

would nonverbal communication be best for this particular message?

Where Should the Communication Take Place?

In the patient's room, in the nursing station, in a classroom outside the nursing unit?

When Should It Be Communicated?

Is the person receptive to the message? Does he need the message now? Should it be delayed?

Who Is the Intended Receiver?

What is this person like as an individual? What is his background? What is likely to be his point of view?

The nurse will probably think of many more questions that could be asked, but, if she remembers the six basic ones, it will help her to keep in mind some of the fundamental elements of the communication process when she is in the position of being the sender in the process.

THE SPOKEN WORD AS A MEDIUM OF COMMUNICATION

In sending a message to anyone, either in speech or in writing, the language chosen for the message should be simple and clear. Some people have a tendency to overcommunicate. The message gets lost somewhere among the explanations, embellishments, or general extra wordage that the sender feels he should include. Some people undercommunicate, so that the message is incomplete, and the receiver has to ask for further clarification. If a person has something important to communicate, the message should be sent in the simplest language and with as few words as possible (but as many as are necessary to get the meaning across), if he wants to be sure his message will be interpreted correctly.

Then there is the choice of words. Although many people in our health-oriented society are quite knowledgeable about health matters, such as the causes and treatment of illness, they often do not understand the technical terms which health workers use. Each line of work has its own jargon—that is, technical terms which are used in that particular field but are not in common use outside the field. Health professionals have their own language and use a good many technical terms which are readily understood by other health workers but are incomprehensible to the average layman. The terminology which nurses learn in order to be able to communicate effectively with other health professionals is often not understood by patients. Effective communication with others depends on the use of a common language. It is important, then, that nurses talk to patients in terms that they can understand. The nurse must assess the patient's language level and use appropriate words to express her meaning clearly.

For example, the nurse might ask a sanitarian, or a medical officer of health, "What measures are taken for vector control?" and expect a satisfactory answer. If an average homeowner were asked the same question, he or she probably would not know what the nurse was talking about. On the other hand, if she were to say, "Do you have screens on the doors and windows to keep out bugs?" the person would be able to understand the question more clearly.

Health workers commonly use technical terms to refer to vital bodily functions. The words "void" and "defecate," for example, are used for urination and defecation, but terms like "pass water" and "bowel movement" are probably more readily understood by most people. In working with children, it is important to find out the particular terms that they have been taught.

NONVERBAL COMMUNICATION

Feelings and attitudes are conveyed not only in the words a person says, but also in his nonverbal behavior. Nurses should be aware that their facial expression, tone of voice, gestures, and posture all convey in subtle ways their regard and feeling for another person. At the same time, the nurse should be aware that clues about the patient's feelings, attitudes, and often his physical condition can be picked up through observations of his nonverbal behavior.

Facial expression is perhaps the most common way in which feelings are expressed by people nonverbally. One conveys feelings of happiness, fear, surprise, anger, disgust (contempt) and sadness by using the facial muscles. Facial expressions speak a universal language. In cross-cultural experiments, psychologists have found remarkable agreement in people from different countries in interpreting emotions expressed in photographs. Both literate and illiterate cultures have been tested, with remarkably similar results.[3]

Patients are very quick to note the expression on a nurse's face and to relate it to their own needs and anxieties. Conversely, the nurse can learn a great deal about people from their facial expressions. For example, the patient in pain has a typical facial grimace; the face of the fearful patient looks anxious; the worried patient usually wears a frown.

Humans, as opposed to the lower animals, can use the muscles around their eyes and mouths to express their feelings. Actors on the stage are aware of the impact of facial expression and learn to control their muscles to such an extent that the audience is able to tell, merely by looking at their faces, the emotions they wish to convey. Perhaps the nurse does not need as much skill in facial expression as the actor, but she does need to be able to control nonverbal expressions of dislike, hostility, and disgust. She can begin to accomplish this by examining her own motivations and feelings.

Body posture is also a means of communicating. An erect, upright posture usually indicates that a person has a feeling of self-esteem and a considerable degree of inner poise. Sadness, depression,

---

[3]Ekman, Paul: Face Muscles Talk Every Language. *Psychology Today,* 9:35, September 1975.

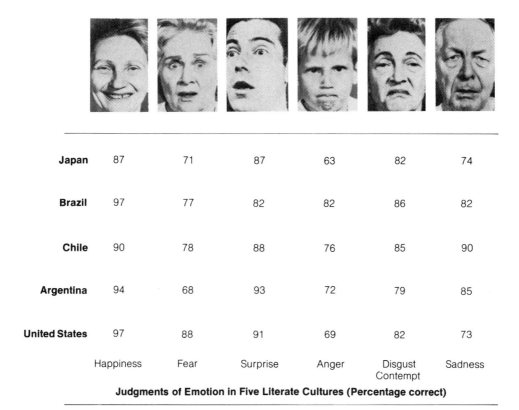

	Happiness	Fear	Surprise	Anger	Disgust Contempt	Sadness
Japan	87	71	87	63	82	74
Brazil	97	77	82	82	86	82
Chile	90	78	88	76	85	90
Argentina	94	68	93	72	79	85
United States	97	88	91	69	82	73

Judgments of Emotion in Five Literate Cultures (Percentage correct)

(From Ekman, P.: Facial Muscles Talk Every Language. Psychology Today, 9:36, September 1975.)

or a low regard for oneself usually makes a person stoop or slouch. It is not uncommon, for example, to see a severely depressed person sitting slumped over in a chair or shuffling along with his head down and shoulders rounded.

Grooming also conveys meaning. A neat, well-groomed look indicates that a person takes pride in his appearance. The attitude of the patient towards his grooming is often indicative of his state of well-being. Very ill people often do not have the strength or the desire to keep up their grooming. The request of a female patient for a mirror and her cosmetics has often been noted as an indication that she is feeling better.

People are often unaware of the *gestures* they use, but gestures play an important role in conveying thoughts and feelings. The welcoming gesture as you ask a person to sit down helps to put him at ease. A hurried manner with quick gestures on the part of the nurse evokes a feeling that the nurse does not have much time and, as a result, the patient becomes reluctant to ask questions or to confide his fears and worries. Significant, too, are the

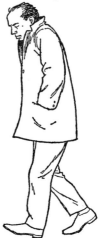

The dejected walker. (Reprinted from Nierenberg, G. I., and Calero, H. H.: How to Read a Person Like a Book. New York, Hawthorn Books, 1971.)

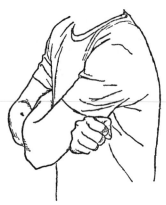

Tension indicated by the folded arms and clenched fists. (Reprinted from Nierenberg, G. I., and Calero, H. H.: How to Read a Person Like a Book. New York, Hawthorn Books, 1971.)

patient's gestures. Lowered eyes or an averted glance usually indicates a wish to avoid communication on a topic. A person who sits with his arms folded and his body occupying as little space as possible is often tense.

A wide variety of subtle meanings are conveyed by the *intonation of one's voice.* There is an adage that it is not so much what you say as how you say it. Small children in particular respond much more to the tone of a person's voice than to his words. Adult patients, however, are also sensitive to coldness or warmth as conveyed in the tone of the nurse's voice.

A person's tone of voice is often indicative of his feelings of well-being. An anxious person frequently has difficulty in expressing himself, as we have noted. A person who is ill usually speaks more slowly and in a lower tone than usual. With excitement, the voice often rises and is more highly pitched. A myriad of feelings may be expressed simply by changing the intonation of one's voice as, for example, in saying "Good morning." People are seldom aware of how their voice sounds to others. Listening to a tape recording of one's voice is often useful in helping to hear oneself as others do.

CREATING A CLIMATE FOR PATIENTS TO COMMUNICATE FREELY

In order to foster an atmosphere of openness in which the individual feels free to communicate, the nurse must convey a feeling of warmth and acceptance.

Warmth implies a genuine liking for people; *acceptance,* the ability to understand another person's point of view and to respect the right of each individual to be different. Acceptance means being nonjudgmental. This is not an easy task. Each person brings to his or her own work conscious and unconscious attitudes, biases, and prejudices that reflect his or her own social background and the learning and life experiences he or she has had. And, everyone tends to evaluate other people and events in the light of his/her own experiences. A member of one of the helping professions, however, must learn to understand other people in the light of *their* backgrounds and experiences. Learning to be nonjudgmental is a conscious undertaking for most people. It is helpful for the nurse to first become aware of her own attitudes, biases, and prejudices and to understand how they were acquired. Attitudes, biases, and prejudices are all learned; they can all, therefore, be unlearned or, at least, modified by additional learning and life experiences. Taking courses in psychology can help the nurse to gain an increased understanding of her own self and also greater insight into individual differences and the factors motivating behavior. Courses in sociology and anthropology help in developing an appreciation of cultural and social influences on behavior. Working with people from other cultures and from different social backgrounds, and getting to know them as individuals, also helps to change attitudes previously held, consciously or unconsciously.

LEARNING TO LISTEN

In any nurse/patient communication, the patient's problems, interests, feelings, and activities are the primary focus. In order to help the patient, the nurse must learn to listen. Most people will communicate quite readily if they have an attentive listener who is not going to impose his or her own values on them, nor proffer unwanted advice. The techniques of being a good listener can be learned. Many such techniques, developed in the behavioral sciences, are now being taught to students in the health professions. Although most beginners tend to feel a little self-conscious using them, the techniques soon become a habitual way of responding, particularly if the rationale for their use is understood, and practice is gained in using them.

One of the first things to learn is to listen attentively. To the patient, this conveys that someone is interested in him as a person and is willing to devote time and energy to hearing what he has to say. Listening attentively is an active process. The person must have the nurse's undivided attention. Some people feel that the nurse should not take notes when she is talking to a patient to obtain information; others, however, feel that taking notes does not hinder the communication process. Certainly, if a lot of information is needed from the patient, it is difficult to remember everything that has been said without the benefit of notes. It may be reassuring too for the patient to know that details of the things he likes and does not like, and his particular concerns, for example, have been noted and will not be forgotten.

Attentive listening is also indicated by the responses the nurse makes. Sometimes just a word or a nod of the head is sufficient to give the patient the feeling that the nurse is interested in what he is saying and would like him to continue. Words or utterances such as "Mmm . . . ," "Yes," "I understand," and so forth, have been termed "minimal responders" and are frequently used, although the nurse may find other words which she feels more comfortable in using.

Another way of indicating interest and attention is through the reflection of feelings the person has expressed. People sometimes express their feelings directly in words, as, for example, "I was so angry that I . . . ." Sometimes they describe their actions, and it is through this description that the nurse is able to identify the person's feelings. For instance, if the person says, "I couldn't stand it any longer, so I banged on the door," he is obviously expressing feelings of frustration and probably feelings of anger and hostility towards whoever was on the other side of the door. The nurse may also pick up clues about the patient's feelings from his nonverbal behavior, as discussed earlier in this chapter. The nurse might respond in words that acknowledge the feelings as, for example, by saying, "I understand that you were angry [or annoyed, or hurt]" or "You were upset by . . . [whatever it was he was describing]," or "I can see that this bothers you." Although it is sometimes useful to use the patient's own words in response, it is more important to reflect his feelings. Repeating the individual's words can make the nurse's response sound mechanical, as if she were parroting a learned response.

At times, though, it is helpful to repeat key words or phrases which the person has used, particularly if he has expressed a number of thoughts at one time. To use an example, a person might say, "Nothing seems to have gone right since I had that operation a year ago. I can't seem to work the way I used to. I haven't been able to go to the lodge either and I miss that. You know, the lodge folks are a mighty nice group of fellows." Here it might be useful for the nurse to pick up the key phrase "since I had that operation a year ago," rather than responding to the lodge item. Repeating a key word or phrase helps to keep the conversation focused on important issues rather than irrelevant items. It is helpful also if the nurse wishes to obtain more information about a specific point that may have been mentioned earlier. The nurse might say, "You said that you had an operation a year ago" (repeating the key phrase). "Perhaps you could tell me more about it."

Sometimes it is difficult to identify feelings or to understand the meaning of a person's words. The nurse may then want to ask for clarification. Phrases such as, "You mean that you were angry?" or "Am I right in thinking that you felt guilty [or depressed, or sad]?" are examples of responses the nurse could make to verify her impressions. Asking for clarification also helps to indicate to the patient that the nurse is trying to understand his point of view.

Sometimes the nurse can help an individual to explore possibilities in regard to resolving problems he has identified. She may be aware of factors in the situation which he has not mentioned, or she may help him to think about things he might want to take into consideration in working through his solution to these problems. She may then want to mention these factors in her responses to his statements or questions. She should be careful, however, not to give her own opinions on what he should do, but rather to help him consider all factors and possible alternatives in the situation.

Responses that hinder the flow of conversation can easily be made if the nurse is not thinking of the impact of her own words. The learned social responses, for example, are often said without thinking. "Don't worry, everything is going to be all right" may be said with the intention of reassurance, but may convey to the patient that the nurse is denying that he has a problem.

People who are anxious frequently react with anger and hostility to those around them. Nurses and other health workers often bear the brunt of this anger from patients and their families, and it is difficult not to be hostile in return. A hostile response made by a nurse, such as, "You shouldn't say things like that," can humiliate the individual and, most certainly, will hinder the progress of the nurse/patient relationship. The nurse should be careful not to impose her own values on the patient. "You shouldn't have done that," or "If I were you, I would have done this or that," are examples of evaluative responses which are best avoided. The nurse should also avoid asking probing questions. Silence is often preferable to asking direct questions, particularly if the individual appears to feel deeply about something.

The following example shows how the nurse can affect the patient's well-being through communication.

Mr. Angelo Niccolini is a 64 year old widower who was admitted to the hospital suffering from dyspnea and pain in his chest, left arm, and back. Mr. Niccolini emigrated from Italy 50 years ago and, although he is fluent in English, he speaks only Italian at home. He lives with his daughter and son-in-law and their four teenage children in a predominantly Italian neighborhood. He is a baker, head of the family business, which he runs with his three sons, who live in the same neighborhood. Mr. Niccolini's working day is usually from 0400 to 1800 hours, six days a week. He smokes about a package of cigarettes a day. He enjoys food and is overweight; he drinks what he considers a moderate amount of wine. He has never been hospitalized before and appears very anxious about being separated from his family.

Mr. Niccolini is sitting up in bed furiously playing solitaire and muttering to himself when the nurse walks in.

N: Good morning, Mr. Niccolini. How are you feeling this morning?

Mr. N.: What's good about it? I feel fine. Why can't I go home? I just sit here all day. Why can't I have a cigarette and some decent food? How can you expect me to eat these meals? Now, what I would like is some good pasta, some decent bread, and a little wine. I can't even taste the food you give me here.

N: I see you're upset, Mr. Niccolini.
(reflecting feeling)
You say you want to go home?
(picking up key words)

Mr. N.: Yes, I want to go home. Nobody's doing anything for me here. They just take my temperature and my blood pressure now and then, and expect me to lie around like this. I have better things to do with my time.

N: What sort of things do you feel you have to do, Mr. Niccolini?
(asking for clarification)

Mr. N.: Well, who's looking after the bakery, for example? They need me there.

N: Don't your sons work in the bakery with you?
(asking for clarification)

Mr. N.: Yes, yes, my sons. But they all have their jobs to do—who's going to make the bread? I always make it myself every morning. They need me.

N.: I'm sure they do need you, Mr. Niccolini. Is someone making the bread now while you are in the hospital?

(accepting the patient's feelings and helping him to explore situation)

Mr. N.: Yes, my oldest boy. But he has his jobs to do too. And who will mind the counter when everyone is so busy?

N.: You mind the counter as well as make the bread?

(picking up key phrase)

Mr. N.: My daughter does most of the time, but I help out when things get busy. Luigi comes in and helps on the weekends.

N.: Luigi?

(asking for clarification)

Mr. N.: Yes, he's my oldest grandson. He seems to like the bakery.

N.: Could Luigi come in and help after school?

(helping the patient to explore)

Mr. N.: That might be an idea. Luigi is 17 now and should know something about the business. I'll call my daughter and see about it.

When the nurse comes back a little later, Mr. Niccolini seems a little brighter after talking to his daughter.

N.: Well, Mr. Niccolini, do you feel better now that you have arranged things with your daughter?

(showing interest in patient)

Mr. N.: Yes, nurse, but I just remembered something.

N.: What's that Mr. Niccolini?

(encouraging patient to elaborate)

Mr. N.: I'm supposed to give a speech at the baker's association meeting next week. I've never missed a meeting. I guess that's how I became president. But now I can't go on the day I'm supposed to give my speech.

N.: Do the members of the association know you are in the hospital?

(picking up key words and helping patient to explore the situation)

Mr. N.: No. But my sons will tell them at the meeting tonight. Two meetings in a row I will have missed.

N.: Would you like to talk with one of the other members? The vice-president perhaps?

(helping patient to explore the possibilities to resolve problem)

Mr. N.: Yes, I would, but not until at least tomorrow. They might want to let someone else give my speech.

INTERVIEWING

The interview has been defined as a "talk with a purpose." It is a basic tool of communication that is used a great deal by health workers, although its use is not, of course, limited to the health field. Most nursing students will have had experience with interviews. If they have applied for a summer or full-time job, for example, they probably had an interview with their prospective employer. Prior to entering most schools of nursing, students are interviewed by a member of the school faculty as part of the admission procedure.

In the health field, the interview is used for a number of different purposes, and by most health professionals. The physician may interview an individual to obtain a medical history, to use a common example, or to assess the results of therapy.

Social workers use interviewing extensively in their work, as, for example, in discussing financial problems with a patient. The nutritionist, to use yet another example, may interview someone to find out his food preferences or to counsel a person about his special dietary needs. The psychologist uses the interview mainly as a therapeutic tool, as in helping a person to resolve his emotional problems.

Nurses, in their practice, may use interviewing for any or all of the purposes exemplified above—for gathering information or for verifying it, for assessing the results of nursing care, in counseling people about health matters, in planning with individuals about their care, and as a therapeutic tool.

When planning an interview, the nurse takes into account not only its purpose, but also the time and the setting for the interview. She should be familiar with some of the basic techniques of interviewing, such as those used in beginning and ending an interview, and in eliciting specific information. As with other skills, interviewing requires practice; one should

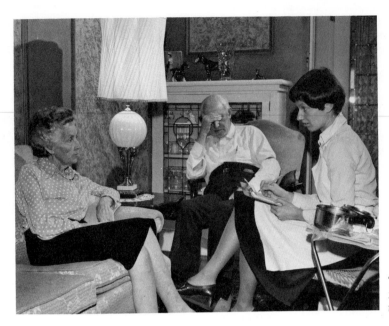

The nurse frequently uses the interview to gather information from a patient.

not expect to become an expert overnight, or in one easy lesson. The material presented here is intended simply as an introduction to the subject. Many textbooks and articles have been written on interviewing, and the nurse will probably want to supplement the material presented here with additional readings from the list of references suggested at the end of the chapter.

Setting the Time and Place for the Interview

An adequate amount of time should be set aside for the interview, the length depending on the purpose and nature of the interview. Judgment must be exercised on both the length of time allotted in the interview and the time at which it takes place. If the person is seriously ill and many new and frightening things are happening to him, for example, or if he has just been admitted to hospital and is having numerous tests and examinations, it may be best to delay an interview until the immediate crisis is over. Again, if the person appears to be becoming fatigued, it is wise to terminate an interview and complete the session at another time. Interviews should be scheduled for a time when both the patient and the nurse are free from other commitments. They should not conflict with appointments the patient has for x-rays, laboratory tests, treatments, or visiting hours. Nor should the nurse feel hurried or rushed because she has other things to do. In short, one strives for a relaxed, unhurried atmosphere.

It is always best to have a quiet and private room in which to interview an individual. This is, however, not always possible in our busy and often crowded health agencies. It is important, though, that the person being interviewed feel that he has the undivided attention of the nurse and that his confidentiality is being respected. A corner of a lounge or of an office can be used, or the curtains pulled around the patient's bed if he is in hospital and not in a private room.

Beginning the Interview

An interview is essentially a conversation between two people—and if the patient has just been admitted to the agency and the nurse has not met him before, between two strangers. The nurse, as the interviewer, has a responsibility to put the other person at ease. For the beginning

COMMUNICATION SKILLS **139**

student, who is perhaps a bit apprehensive about interviewing someone, it is helpful to remember that the patient, too, is probably anxious. Most people who seek the help of health professionals by coming to a health agency are either ill or in some way concerned about their health. Even those who are well and attending a health maintenance clinic usually have some minor worries. They are all, therefore, at least a little anxious. It helps if the nurse observes the common courtesies of greeting people by name, offering them a seat (in an ambulatory setting), or asking their permission to sit down and talk (if the person is in an inpatient facility). The nurse should also introduce herself by name. These courtesies convey a feeling of respect for the person who is being interviewed and help to put him at ease. The common ritual also helps the nurse to feel more comfortable.

The nurse should also state the purpose of the interview and the approximate amount of time it will take. This information helps to set the climate for the interview. The patient feels more comfortable when he knows what to expect and why the nurse is interviewing him. The nurse might say, for example, that the purpose is to learn something about the person so that his care can be planned to suit his individual needs and preferences if it is an initial assessment interview. Or she may say she would like to talk with him about plans for his going home.

Eliciting Specific Information

Although the nurse often has specific information that she wants to obtain from the individual during the interview, it should not be conducted as a question and answer session. It may be a structured interview in the sense that the nurse controls and directs the conversation, as when the nurse gathers information in her assessment interview, but the individual should feel free to discuss his feelings and concerns and the things that are important to him. Bernstein, Bernstein, and Dana, in their book, *Interviewing: A Guide for Health Professionals*, state that the patient will give all the in-

formation needed, and more, if an open climate is created.[4]

In this regard the section in this chapter on creating a climate in which the patient feels free to communicate and on learning to listen will be helpful.

When the nurse has specific information which she would like to obtain, some questions will have to be asked. In such cases it is probably a good idea to start with the person's immediate concerns, that is, his feelings and perceptions in regard to whatever the interview is about, without interjecting too many questions in the beginning. If the nurse does not do this, there is a possibility that important factors may be missed. It is usually considered best, in asking questions, to start from the general and then proceed to the specific details. Also, people usually respond much better to impersonal questions at first; the nurse should leave the more personal ones until the patient has had a chance to get to know the nurse a little during the course of the interview. In our computer-age society, most people are used to filling in forms and answering questions about their name, age, education, and place of employment; these are relatively impersonal items. An individual's likes and dislikes and his feelings are more personal; these should be left until after the general questions have been answered.

Ending an Interview

When the purpose of the interview has been accomplished, the nurse should take some time to ask the patient if he has any questions, or if there are other things that he is concerned about that were not discussed. Patients often feel that the nurse is busy and they are sometimes reluctant to take up her time. But taking a few minutes to listen to the patient's concerns often saves the nurse time in the long run, since patients are less apt to make frequent requests later if they are reas-

---

[4]Lewis Bernstein, Rosalyn S. Bernstein, and Richard H. Dana: *Interviewing: A Guide for Health Professionals.* 2nd edition. New York, Appleton-Century-Crofts, 1974.

sured that someone is concerned about them as a person.

In terminating an interview, it is again helpful to observe the social amenities. Thanking the person for his time, saying that you will see him again, and assuring him that he can call on you if he is concerned about anything are all ways of conveying to the patient that he is a person worthy of respect.

COMMUNICATING WITH OTHER MEMBERS OF THE HEALTH TEAM

Nurses very seldom work in complete isolation. Even in a remote nursing station where she may be the sole provider of health care for a community, the nurse almost always has at least radio contact with a base hospital where she can communicate with other members of the health team. Very few nurses work in isolated rural settings, of course. More usually, the nurse is employed in a busy, urban health agency where there are large numbers of nurses and a variety of other health personnel.

Communication with other members of the health team is an important part of the nurse's work. It is essential to facilitate the process of patient care. Information gathered by all team members provides the basis for planning comprehensive care for the patient. Sharing information helps to avoid duplication of effort in gathering data and also enables each team member to benefit from the information others have collected. Communication is essential too in the planning of patient care so that everyone shares the same goals for the patient; in that way, care is coordinated and people are not working at cross-purposes.

The actual implementation of health care today is also very much a team effort. The provision of comprehensive care requires the skills and talents of many different categories of workers. The physician and the nurse have always worked closely together in many aspects of patient care and continue to do so. With the number of specialized workers in the health field today, however, it is more

than ever essential that all coordinate their efforts in caring for patients. There must be adequate, effective communication channels for the achievement of this coordination.

Communication between members of the health team takes place in many ways. A great deal of information is exchanged informally, through face-to-face meetings and telephone conversations. But there are also more formal channels, both oral and written, which help to facilitate the exchange of information.

The patient's record is one very important tool which helps to keep all team members up-to-date on the latest information that has been gathered about a patient and the most recent developments regarding his progress. Patient records will be discussed in Chapter 11, so we will not go into them further at this point. Other commonly used communication media which the nurse will utilize frequently are reports, both oral and written, consultations, conferences, referrals, and patient rounds.

Reports

Reporting of information to other members of the health team is essential if they are to be briefed on events that have taken place (or are likely to take place), be told of developments that have occurred in regard to patients' progress, and be alerted to things to watch for in the care of specific patients. Reports may be given either orally or in writing. At the end of each shift, members of the nursing team usually report orally to the team leader on the progress of each patient they cared for during that shift. The team leader, in turn, reports to the head nurse, who uses this information to prepare her change of shift report for the nurses who are coming on duty.

The change of shift report is usually a fairly formal report, in which the nurse completing her tour of duty "hands over" the care of patients on the unit to those who will be responsible for their care on the next shift. At this time, the progress of each patient on the unit is reviewed, and the nurse who is leaving briefs the newly arrived staff on treatments or other activities that are still in progress, and on events that are likely to occur on the next shift. She may, for example, say that Dr. X is coming in to take out Mr. Smith's sutures this evening, or that the Admitting Department has called to say we are receiving a new patient, giving as many details as she has received herself.

As part of the change of shift report, the head nurse often makes rounds with the nurses coming on duty, and they exchange information about each patient in the process. Many agencies are now using tape recorders or Dictaphones to make the change of shift report less cumbersome. Each nurse who has been responsible for the care of a group of patients can dictate the report on her patients. Nurses coming on duty then need to receive only a minimal report from the head nurse going off duty and can obtain direct information about each patient from the nurse who cared for him during the previous tour of duty. In addition to patient care reports, most health agencies have a large number of other reports and forms which nurses utilize. These vary from agency to agency and the nurse must familiarize herself with those used in the agency in which she is working. There are usually forms for requesting laboratory, x-ray and other types of diagnostic tests, forms for recording the administration of narcotics and other controlled drugs (a count has to be kept of these), forms for ordering drugs and other supplies, and a good many others. We have already mentioned the accident (incident) report, which is completed whenever an unusual occurrence takes place (Chapter 7).

The head nurse on a nursing unit also reports to her supervisor about the patients on the unit. This is often a written report, supplemented by an oral report as needed.

Consultations

The nurse often feels the need to consult with another health practitioner about the care of her patients. She usually consults informally with her team leader, or with the head nurse, or with both. She also consults with the physician about the patient's plan of care and progress. If there is a clinical nursing specialist available, the nurse may want to consult with her about the patient's plan of care, or about unusual problems the patient has. She consults with the physical therapist frequently and with the nutritionist and the social worker—in fact, with all who may be involved with the patient's care.

Physicians consult with other physicians; they frequently call in specialists to see the patient and give opinions regarding diagnostic or therapeutic measures for that patient. The nurse will note the requests for specialist consultations and the specialist's report on the patient's record.

Conferences

Members of the nursing team usually meet daily in a team conference to exchange information about their patients and to review and revise their care plans. Increasingly common too are team conferences, at which various members of the health team meet to review their findings about a patient, to develop a combined plan of care or to review the patient's progress. Until very recently team conferences have been used most frequently in rehabilitation settings, in community health agencies, in psychiatric settings, and in agencies providing long-term care for people who are ill. However, they are becoming more common in all types of health care settings.

Referrals

Referrals are basically of two types, those requesting the services of another department within an agency in the care of a patient, and those referring a patient to another agency for care. In a multiservice ambulatory health care agency, such as a Health Maintenance Organization (HMO), a Community Health Center (CHC), or the Outpatient Department of a hospital, patients are frequently referred from one service to another for specialized care. A patient might be referred to the dental or eye clinic, for example, or to the nutritionist or social worker from a generalized service. In a hospital setting, a referral might be made to such departments as social service, physiotherapy, or inhalation therapy (respiratory technology) for their specialized services for the patient. Patients may also be referred from one agency to another. An HMO or CHC might refer an individual to a hospital if he needs inpatient care (he would be admitted under the care of his attending physician) or a hospital might refer a patient to an HMO or CHC. If a patient is being discharged from hospital and requires home care services, a referral would be made to the appropriate agency. Referrals may be made by a community health nurse (or a school nurse) for individuals to receive care from any number of agencies in the community.

A referral system is important to assure continuity of care. It is essential that the agency to whom the patient is being referred have sufficient information to assure that continuity. Most agencies have referral forms on which summary information about a patient is written; it is often the nurse who is responsible for completing these forms, although policies vary.

In a hospital, the patient's record would be available to the member of the department being called in to see a patient; therefore, the referral is usually simply a request for services.

Patient Rounds

Another means of communicating information about patients is through patient rounds. We have already mentioned one type, when nurses make the rounds on a nursing unit during the change of shift report. The nurse usually makes rounds with the physician when he visits his patients on a hospital nursing unit. A considerable amount of information exchange takes place at this time, as opinions are shared regarding the patient's progress and plans are discussed for his care. Often, nursing rounds are made by the head nurse on a unit with her supervisor, with the clinical nursing specialist, or with staff nurses on the unit. Teaching rounds are also made for the benefit of students; both medical and nursing schools use patient rounds as learning experiences for students.

STUDY VOCABULARY			
Acceptance	Initial assessment interview	Nonverbal communication	
Clarification	Interview	Personal information	
Evaluative responses	Jargon	Reflection of feelings	
Impersonal information	Minimal responders	Structured interview	
		Warmth	

STUDY SITUATION   With the help of your instructor select a patient in the clinical area in which you are gaining experience. Arrange a time for you to visit the patient for the purpose of getting acquainted with him (or her). By utilizing some of the techniques outlined in the section on learning to listen, see what you can find out about this patient as a person.

SUGGESTED READINGS

Hein, C.: Listening. *Nurses '75*, 5:93–102, March 1975.

Mezzanotte, E. J.: Getting it Together for End-of-Shift Report. *Nursing '76*, 6:21–22, April 1976.

O'Brien, M. J.: *Communications and Relationships in Nursing.* St. Louis, C. V. Mosby Co., 1974.

Paton, M.: I Told Them All. *American Journal of Nursing*, 76:113, January 1976.

Petrello, J.: Your Patients Hear You, But Do They Understand? *RN*, 39:37–39, February 1976.

Rosendahl, P. L.: The Verbal Side of Effective Communication. *Journal of Nursing Administration*, 4:41–44, September-October 1974.

Ross, R. S.: *Speech Communication: Fundamentals and Practice.* Third edition. Englewood Cliffs, N. J., Prentice-Hall, Inc., 1974.

Smiley, O. R., et al.: Interviewing Techniques for Nurses. *Canadian Journal of Public Health*, 65:281–283, July-August 1974.

Ujhely, G. B.: The Patient as an Equal Partner. *Canadian Nurse*, 69:21–23, June 1973.

Van Dersal, W. R.: How to Be a Good Communicator—And a Better Nurse. *Nursing '74*, 4:57–64, December 1974.

Weiss, B.: The Invisible Smile. *Psychology Today*, 9:38, September 1975.

Wiley, L.: Whadda Ya Say at Report? *Nursing '75*, 5:73, October 1975.

9 THE NURSING PROCESS, PART I

The nurse should be able to:

Define "nursing process"

Describe the circular nature of the four basic steps in the nursing process

List the types of information needed to plan nursing care

Identify sources of information available to the nurse to assist her in planning nursing care for an individual

Discuss the rationale for gathering information about a patient in each of the major content areas usually included in a nursing history

Describe methods and techniques the nurse uses in her clinical appraisal of a patient

Demonstrate skill in taking a patient's temperature (oral, rectal, and axillary)

Demonstrate skill in taking the pulse

Demonstrate skill in observing respirations

Demonstrate skill in taking blood pressure

Demonstrate beginning skill in observing deviations from the normal in a patient's functional abilities other than the vital signs

THE NURSING PROCESS, 9
PART I

INTRODUCTION

Nursing care may range from the simple act of cleansing and putting a bandage on a child's cut finger to the highly complex measures involved in caring for a patient in the intensive care unit of a hospital, or in helping a family with multiple problems to meet their health needs in a community setting. The process of nursing is the same, however, whether the nursing care given is a basic first aid measure or a sequence of complicated nursing activities.

The term "nursing process" has become widely accepted in recent years to designate the series of steps the nurse takes in planning and giving nursing care. Described by a number of authors as application of the problem-solving, or scientific, approach to nursing practice, the process provides a logical framework on which to base nursing care. The nursing process has a universality of application in that it may be used in working with an individual, a family, or a community, and in promoting health, in preventing illness, or in care and rehabilitation of the sick. Moreover, a terminology is evolving which can be readily understood by all nursing personnel, as well as by other members of the health team.

The essential elements of the process are that it is planned, it is patient-centered, it is problem-oriented, and it is goal-directed. The term "patient" is used here to denote the recipient of care and can mean an individual, a family, or a community. Four basic steps are involved in the process:

1. Assessment
2. Planning
3. Implementation
4. Evaluation

The focus of this text is on the care of the individual, since the fundamental basis of nursing practice is the one-to-one relationship of the nurse and the patient. In this chapter, then, we will discuss the nursing process in relation to the individual patient. It should be noted, however, that the process is the same, whether the patient is an individual, a family, or a community.

The steps in the process follow logically one after the other. As a basis for making decisions about actions that she will take, the nurse must first of all assess the need for such action. This assessment involves the gathering of all pertinent information, the analysis of the information, the synthesis of information from all sources, and the identification of problems which the nurse, by her actions, can help to resolve. Once problems are identified, expected outcomes are established and a plan of action developed to help the patient to attain these objectives. The next step is to implement the plan of action— that is, to carry out the specified measures (nursing interventions) outlined in the plan. The final step is to evaluate the results of the action taken, or, in other words, determine if the expected outcomes have been attained. The last step may result in new information that leads to modification in the problem list, changes in the plan of action, or a restatement of expected outcomes. Thus, the process becomes a circu-

145

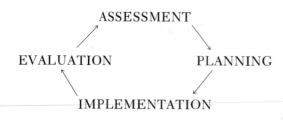

Diagram of the nursing process

lar one that involves a continuing dynamic set of activities on the nurse's part.

ASSESSMENT

In the past, much of nursing care was based on the nurse's intuitive assessment, which was often the result of her previous experience in similar situations. An experienced nurse could—and still can, for that matter—walk into a home to visit a new mother and baby and, within a few minutes, assess the situation and identify several problems. Although the baby seems to be thriving well, two year old Johnny has a cold that has persisted too long, mother is in dire need of rest, and is anxious and worried about how she is handling the baby. An experienced nurse in a hospital setting can enter the patient's room and immediately sense that he is uncomfortable, that his position needs changing, that he is having difficulty in breathing, and that he is worried and apprehensive. But nurses, even experienced nurses, have often found it difficult to explain how they arrived at their assessments.[1]

The development of a systematic method of nursing assessment and identification of the necessary tools to undertake it have only recently evolved. Today many health agencies use forms which they have developed to assist the nurse in her assessment and to provide a written record of the information she obtains. Although the format used and the specific items recorded vary in different agencies, they have a common purpose in that they help to guide the nurse in making a sys-

tematic appraisal of all relevant factors. The assessment is undertaken in an orderly manner; the nurse knows what to look for and there is less danger that important factors will be overlooked.

Systematic nursing assessment involves four sets of activities on the nurse's part: the collection of information, the analysis of that information, the synthesis of information from all sources, and the identification of problems.

THE COLLECTION OF INFORMATION

The systematic collection of information for a specific purpose is called "data gathering," and one uses the information collected to develop a "data base" which can be analyzed in a number of different ways, depending on the purpose for which the information was collected in the first place. In order to develop a solid data base for the planning and implementation of nursing care, the nurse needs to know (1) the purpose for which she is collecting information, (2) what information is needed, (3) what sources can be used to obtain data, (4) how these sources can be tapped, and (5) how to organize and utilize the information collected.

The Purpose of Collecting Information

The basic objective of the nurse in collecting information about a patient is to identify areas in which nursing intervention is required. The information that the nurse gathers in her initial assessment enables her to make a beginning plan of care for the patient. Information gathered by the nurse, however, may identify problems which require the intervention of other members of the health team, such as the physician, the social worker, or the physical therapist. The initial data collected by all members of the team provide a baseline for assessing an individual's health status, for identifying existing and potential health problems, and for developing a combined plan of action to assist the patient.

---

[1] R. Faye McCain: Nursing by Assessment—Not Intuition. *American Journal of Nursing*, 65:82–84, April 1965.

Information Needed by the Nurse

Virginia Henderson, in her well-known and often-quoted definition of nursing, has stated, "The unique function of the nurse is to assist the individual, sick or well, in the performance of those activities contributing to health or its recovery (or to peaceful death) that he would perform unaided if he had the necessary strength, will, or knowledge."[2]

We might rephrase this to say that the nursing care of an individual is primarily concerned with assisting him to cope with the activities of living in such a way as to promote his optimal level of functioning or, in the case of incurable disease, to cope with terminal illness.

In order to identify areas in which the individual requires nursing assistance to be able to cope with either of the above, the nurse needs to have information that will tell her:

1. Something about the individual as a person
2. His usual abilities (or lack of abilities) in coping with the activities of living
3. The nature of any health problems that are interfering with his abilities to cope
4. His current status in regard to these abilities
5. The physician's plan of care for the individual

Some of this information the nurse collects herself; some she gathers from other sources.

Sources of Information

The first, or "primary," source of information is always the patient. Other sources, termed "secondary sources," include other people, such as family members or "significant others" with whom the individual has a close relationship. In the case of a child or an unconscious or irrational patient, much of the information the nurse needs to know must be obtained from someone other than the patient.

The patient's health record is also a valuable source of data for the nurse, and today an increasing number of health team members contribute to it. If a record has already been started, or if old records are on file, the nurse should review these, if possible, prior to setting out to gather information herself. This review helps to avoid duplication in gathering information and also gives the nurse the benefit of data gathered by others. The physician, for example, is usually responsible for taking the patient's medical history, for identifying medical problems the patient has, and for developing diagnostic and therapeutic plans for the individual, if such are warranted. The results of the physician's findings and the medical plan of care are incorporated into the patient's record. In order to develop her plan of care for the patient, the nurse must be aware of the nature of the patient's medical problems and of the physician's plan of care.

Other members of the health team also contribute to the nurse's understanding of the patient and his health status. Observations and interpretations may be communicated by the social worker, the nutritionist (dietitian), the physical therapist, or the occupational therapist to name only a few, through written notes on a patient's record, in consultations with the nurse, or in conferences and other meetings of various members of the health team. Nor should the nurse overlook the importance, as sources of information, of the reports on x-ray findings and the results of laboratory tests performed on the patient. These reports are usually attached to the patient's record.

If the individual has a known medical problem, the nurse will probably want to increase her knowledge about it by reading available literature on the subject in the library and by reviewing notes she may have from classes that will contribute to her understanding of this particular patient's problem.

---

[2]Virginia Henderson: *The Nature of Nursing: A Definition and its Implications for Practice, Research and Education.* New York, Macmillan Company, 1966.

Methods of Collecting Information

The basic methods used by nurses to gather information about an individual pa-

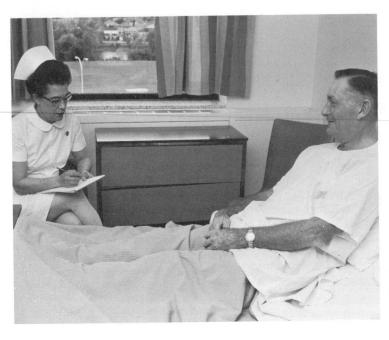

The nursing history provides much important information which the nurse uses in her assessment of the patient.

tient are the interview (talking with the patient), observation and examination, consultation (with other members of the health team), and review of records and other written material.

Essentially there are two types of information which the nurse gathers through interviewing the patient and through her observations and examination. One is information of a relatively *"constant"* nature that is not expected to change during the period of care. For example, the fact that an individual wears dentures or that he is right-handed would be considered data of a constant nature. This type of information is usually collected by talking with the individual, that is, through an interview. The second type of information the nurse collects is concerned with the current status of the patient; this may be expected to change and such facts are therefore called *"variable"* data. A person's temperature, for example, may change from day to day and even during the course of one day. Temperature recordings from individual patients, then, would be considered variable data. Variable data are obtained through the nurse's observations and/or examination of the patient.

Specific tools have been developed to assist the nurse in gathering the informa-

tion she needs to collect in interviewing and in observing the patient. Most health agencies now use a "nursing history" form to provide a written record of the information about a patient which the nurse gathers by interview. A number of agencies now use in addition a "clinical appraisal guide" (or an initial patient progress record) to record baseline information the nurse has gathered in her observations/examination of the patient's current functioning abilities.

The forms shown on pages 150 to 152 were developed during a project on nursing information systems sponsored by the Division of Nursing, U.S. Department of Health, Education, and Welfare.[3] The first form (p. 150), used in connection with the nursing history, is intended for gathering basic patient data of a constant nature, which can be obtained by interviewing the patient. The second form (p. 172), used in discussing the nurse's clinical appraisal of a patient, is for collecting baseline and reassessment data on factors that may vary

---

[3] Deane B. Taylor and Onalee H. Johnson: Systematic Nursing Assessment: A Step Toward Automation. DHEW Publication No. (HRA) 74–17. Washington, D. C., U. S. Government Printing Office, 1974.

in the patient's health/illness status. This particular form was developed for use with hospitalized patients. It is intended that these and other forms developed during the project be used with a manual of instructions that provides the nurse with guidelines for completing them.

THE NURSING HISTORY

The nursing history provides a guide for systematically obtaining information which can help the nurse to (1) plan and modify her care to suit the individual patient's preferences and usual living patterns, and (2) establish a baseline from which to evaluate the results of nursing action.

The history is taken as soon after the patient's admission to the agency as is feasible, preferably by the nurse who has primary responsibility for planning the patient's care. The technique for obtaining the history is a structured interview—that is, the nurse controls and directs the interview for the purpose of gathering specific information.

Generally the information gathered includes items which nurses in a particular agency have found helpful in assessing patients' needs and in planning care for the majority of patients.[4] Among the items frequently included are: events leading up to the patient's admission to the health agency, basic social data about the patient, basic physiological data (verbal information that can be obtained by interview), the person's usual patterns of daily living, environmental factors that may affect his health, the individual's understanding of his health and illness status, and the patient's concerns and his expectations of the care he will receive in the agency.[5] Not all nursing histories include all of these items. Some of the data (all of which is helpful to the nurse) may be obtained from other sources, as for example, the basic physiological data may be gathered by the physician during his initial examination of the patient.

[4]Eileen Pearlman: *Manual for the Use of the Nursing History Tool.* Gainesville, Fla., University of Florida College of Nursing, 1971, p. 15.
[5]Ibid.

Events Leading Up to the Patient's Admission

In order to know how she can help the individual, the nurse needs to be aware of the reasons for his admission to the health agency. In an ambulatory care setting, the individual may have come for any one of a number of reasons. He may want assistance in maintaining his health or in protecting himself from illness, or he may be worried and anxious about his health. He may or may not have a health problem. The person who has been admitted to the hospital has a recognized problem and has come for diagnosis or treatment, or both. The patient used here to illustrate the nursing process was admitted to a large city hospital following transfer from another agency. He had been injured in a car accident and suffered compressed fractures of three vertebrae. Details of events leading to his admission are recorded on page 150.

Basic Social Data

The basic social data gathered about an individual usually includes biographical information (or vital statistics), and information about the person's educational level and his employment status. Often included are items about his interests, hobbies, and community affiliations.

Vital statistics about an individual help to give the nurse some idea of what this patient is like. The name sometimes helps to identify ethnic origin, as does information about birthplace and citizenship. The person's address can give some indication of the type of neighborhood in which he lives. Information can be elicited about whether there are relatives who might be helpful, and whether they live nearby or far away. Knowledge of the language a person speaks is essential for communicating with him. Age, sex, and employment status are important in understanding a person's perceptions of his health and illness status. For example, a woman of 40 who is admitted to hospital for termination of her first pregnancy may be expected to react quite differently from the 30 year old woman who is in the hospital for a therapeutic abortion and already has four children. A singer who is to

HOSPITAL _North West General_

NURSING ASSESSMENT: BASIC PATIENT INFORMATION

ADMISSION TIME _16 00 HRS._ DATE: _16/9/77_

Sept. 16, 77

Jordan Paul
2465 Washington Ave. Shore City
_234-7566_
Smith James 1600 Surg. R.C.
SAME
_9-16-77_ PATIENT'S IDENTIFICATION

1. GENERAL ADMISSION INFORMATION

MODE:	ACCOMPANIED BY:	SOURCE OF DATA:
walking ☐	family ☐	patient ☑
wheelchair ☐	friend ☑	family ☐
stretcher ☑	no one ☐	
		other _____

PRIMARY LANGUAGE: (If not English) _____

DIFFICULTY WITH ENGLISH IN RELATION TO: comments: _____

speaking ☐ _____

understanding ☐ _____

2. PRESENT ILLNESS

Instructions: Check first box for single term or first double term, check second box for second term

Reason for present admission _CAR ACCIDENT - COMPRESSION FRACTURE 3 VERTEBRAE_

Primary signs/symptoms:

blurring/double vision ☐☐	fatigue/weakness ☐☐	pain ☑
chills/fever	heart burn/indigestion	pruritis
cough	incontinence	voiding difficulty ☑
		weight loss/gain
cyanosis ☐	injury/trauma ☑☑	L.M.P. _____
diarrhea/constipation	insomnia	Date
		Site of
dysphasia ☐	jaundice ☐	discharge _____
S.O.B./dyspnea	loss of appetite	bleeding _____
edema/swelling	nausea/emesis	

DURATION: _7_ hrs.; _____ days; _____ weeks; _____ mos.; _____ yrs.

LOCATION: _D11, D12, L1_

SEVERITY: _POSSIBLE NERVE DAMAGE   PAIN VERY SEVERE_

comments: _TRANSFERRED FROM NORTH COAST HOSPITAL - BY PLANE X-RAYS WITH PATIENT_

3. PREVIOUS HOSPITALIZATION(S)

NONE ☐   NUMBER _1_   LAST ADMISSION   reason and date _MOTORCYCLE ACCIDENT 1972_

PREVIOUS ADMISSION in this hospital: No ☐ Yes: ☑ reason/date _AS ABOVE_ _____

FEELINGS ABOUT NURSING CARE   strongly positive ☐   positive ☑   neutral ☐

negative ☐   strongly negative ☐   Why liked/disliked? _RECEIVED GOOD CARE_

comments:

4. ALLERGIES

NONE KNOWN ☑

	DRUGS	FOOD	OTHER
1.	_____	_____	_____
2.	_____	_____	_____
3.	_____	_____	_____
4.	_____	_____	_____

comments:

5. MEDICATION(S) HISTORY

MEDICATION(S) TAKEN ROUTINELY: None ☑

DRUG(S) WITH PATIENT?   No ☑

name or reason	freq.	last dose		
1. _____	_____	_____	sent home:	1 2 3
2. _____	_____	_____	given to staff:	1 2 3
3. _____	_____	_____	with patient:	1 2 3
comments:			other	1 2 3 (circle)

FORM 0001

HOSPITAL _____

NURSING ASSESSMENT: BASIC PATIENT INFORMATION

PATIENT'S IDENTIFICATION

6. CHRONIC HEALTH PROBLEMS

None known ☑

(a) Diabetes ☐	(d) Hypertension ☐	(g) Epilepsy ☐
(b) Heart Disease ☐	(e) Arthritis ☐	(h) Amputation ☐
(c) Emphysema ☐	(f) Ulcer ☐	(i) _____ other

RESTRICTED ACTIVITIES (specify) _____

Comments: *POSSIBLY HAD TB. AGE 12 YRS. ANNUAL CHEST X-RAYS*

7. RESPONSE TO ILLNESS(ES)

to indicate which disease(s) the information pertains (Sect.6), place the letter(s) of disease(s)
in the box(es) following statement(s). Place a check mark to indicate which information
pertains to present illness.

PERCEPTIONS OF SIGNS/SYMPTOMS:

denies presence of	
preoccupied with	✓
has misconceptions	
inadequate information	
_____ other	

Unable to evaluate ☐☐   comments: _____

PERCEPTIONS OF PROGNOSIS:

complete recovery	
partial recovery	
to die	
doesn't know	✓
no change	

8. SUPPORTIVE AIDS

PROSTHESES:

DENTURES   rt lt

upper ☐	leg ☐☐
lower ☐	arm ☐☐
partial ☐	breast ☐☐
	eye ☐☐
_____ other	

DOMINANT HAND:

Right	✓
Left	

AIDS TO MOBILITY:

crutches	☐
cane	☐
walker	☐
brace	☐
wheelchair	☐
other	

comments: _____

9. ELIMINATION

USUAL DEFECATION FREQUENCY

OD: (am)/pm   QOD: am/pm
        (circle)

impacted ☐
other _____
date of last BM *SEPT. 16, 1977*

AIDS USED AT HOME   (name & frequency)

dietary _____
laxative _____
suppository _____
enema _____

	URINATION:	INCONTINENCE:
Colostomy ☐	frequency ☐	total ☐
ileostomy ☐	urgency ☐	stress ☐
_____ duration	nocturia _____ no. of times	
No self care ☐		

Comments: _____

FORM 0001

HOSPITAL *NORTH WEST GENERAL*

NURSING ASSESSMENT: BASIC PATIENT INFORMATION

PATIENT'S IDENTIFICATION

---

10. SENSORY STATUS

VISION: rt lt   HEARING: rt lt   TASTE: SMELL:

uncorrected □ □   severe loss □ □   loss of taste □   loss of smell □

severely impaired □ □   deaf □ □   distorted □   distorted □

blind □ □   wears Aid □ □   circle: dec./inc. □   dec./inc. □

Uses Aid(s): _____   _____   comments: _____
(type)   (type)

Does not have glasses [✓]   Does **not** have hearing aid [✓]

SPEECH: COMMUNICATION: SENSE OF FEELING:

Slurring □   Unable to speak □   circle: dec.(inc) sensitivity to:

Stuttering □   Unable to write □   Heat □

Dysphasia □   Sign language □   Pressure [✓] Cold □

Other _____   Reads lips □   Locate *SACRAL AREA*
comments: *BRUISED, TENDER*

---

11. NUTRITION

HEIGHT *177.8 cm. (5'10")*   SPECIAL DIET AT HOME: RESPONSE TO DIET:

WEIGHT *61.4 kg. (135 lb.)*   diabetic □   Lack of understanding □

USUAL APPETITE: low salt □

anorectic □   bland □   Strong dislike □

voracious [✓]   soft □

_____   _____
other   other

comments:

---

12. USUAL REST AND SLEEP PATTERNS

SLEEPING PATTERNS: AIDS USED TO SLEEP   (name & frequency):

usual hours of sleep: (circle)   position in bed _____

extra pillows _____

from *11* p.m. to *5* a.m.   medication _____

food _____

insomnia □   Daily naps [✓]   other _____

comments:

---

13. SOCIAL HISTORY

WORK   HOUSING

OCCUPATION *FISHERMAN* INTERESTS/HOBBY

SHIFT   evening □ night □   radio □   patient lives with: nursing home □

Head of Household [✓]   T.V. □   no one □   institution □

Homemaker □   reading □   family □   single dwelling □

needlework □   friend [✓]   multiple dwelling [✓]

Retired □   crafts □   walk-up □

Dependent □   puzzles □   other _____   Floor *GROUND*

other *PLAYS GUITAR*   Bed & Bath on separate floor □

comments: *SELF-EMPLOYED*   Bath shared with other tenants □

COMMERCIAL FISHERMAN   other _____

comments:

---

14. VISITORS

NO VISITORS ANTICIPATED □   comments: _____

RESTRICTIONS DESIRED   _____

family only □   _____

no visitors □   _____

other _____

FORM 0001   3 of 3

have even a minor operation on his throat may be extremely anxious about the results of the surgery and its effects on his career. Knowing the individual's marital status and next of kin assists in the identification of significant family members and helps the nurse to assess the potential support of family and friends.

Knowledge of the individual's educational level is helpful both in adjusting the nurse's use of language for communicating with him, and also in assessing his ability to comprehend information about his health/illness status. Knowledge of his interests, hobbies, and community affiliations also helps to give the nurse insight into the person as an individual and some understanding of his inner resources.

An example of basic social data is given below.

NAME: Paul Jordan
SEX: Male
MARITAL STATUS: Single
BIRTHDATE: October 2, 1951
RELIGION: Roman Catholic
BIRTHPLACE: Philadelphia, Pennsylvania
CITIZENSHIP: U.S.
ADDRESS: 2465 Washington Avenue, Shore
    City
LANGUAGE: English
EDUCATION: 2 years university
EMPLOYMENT STATUS: Self-employed commercial fisherman. Works April-October, 7 days/week. Fishing trips average 8-10 days out; 1-3 days ashore. Hours: 0400–2300 during season.
INTERESTS: Plays guitar; skiing, hiking, camping
COMMUNITY AFFILIATIONS: None

Basic Physiological Data

The amount of basic physiological data included in the nursing history depends on the policy of the health agency. In some agencies, much of this type of data may be obtained during the initial physical examination of the patient. If this is the case, the information would not be duplicated in the nursing history. In many agencies, however, the nurse gathers basic physiological data about the individual in the course of taking the nursing history.

The type of information that is helpful

for the nurse to have about the patient's physiological status includes a general body description, which takes into account such constant factors as: height and weight (often both the "usual" weight and the present weight are noted), the individual's dominant hand, prostheses (artificial parts such as a limb, dentures, and the like), amputations the individual may have had, visual or auditory impairments of long standing, the person's ability to communicate, and his mobility status. Observations about the individual's current status in regard to these items are often noted as well as past history. In addition, chronic health problems the individual may have, as well as known allergies, are often noted. Many nursing histories also include information about medications the person is currently taking, and some include the person's immunization record.

This type of information helps to provide baseline data on which to assess the individual's current health status. It is also useful in the identification of nursing problems and in the establishment of realistic goals for nursing care.

Let us add the basic physiological data to our information about Mr. Jordan.

HEIGHT: 177.8 cm. (5 ft. 10 in.)
WEIGHT: 61.4 kg. (135 lb.)
DOMINANT HAND: Right
VISION ⎱ Normal
HEARING ⎰
COMMUNICATION: No problem
HEALTH HISTORY: No known allergies
    Possibly had tuberculosis when approximately 12 years
    No prostheses
    No medications
    Immunization: Had all recommended childhood ones
    Other: Has chest x-rays once/year
MOBILITY STATUS: Normally no problem
    Present mobility limited by injury
    Confined to bed rest
    Cannot life arms above head because of pain

Usual Patterns of Daily Living

Most nurses have found it helpful in planning care for an individual to have information about his usual habits of daily living. Information generally collected includes habits in regard to rest and sleep, eating, elimination, and hygiene practices. Habits relating to smoking and alcohol consumption are increasingly being included too as a part of the nursing history.

The person's usual time for going to bed, the number of hours he sleeps, and the aids he may use to get to sleep are particularly helpful if the person is ill and needs to be cared for in an inpatient facility. The individual's usual appetite and normal diet are important in assessing nutritional status, in identifying problems with regard to nutrition, and in planning this essential element of his care. If the person has been on a special diet at home, the nurse needs to be aware of this fact and also of his response to it. Does he understand his diet? Is he adhering to it? These are among the questions that should be asked. With regard to elimination, the usual time and frequency of defecation are noted, as well as aids the person uses regularly, such as foods or fluids which the person feels are helpful in maintaining regularity. If the individual is in the habit of taking laxatives regularly, or using suppositories or enemas to aid in elimination, it is helpful to have this information.

The nurse also needs information about the person's usual pattern of urination and any problems he has, such as frequency, urgency, or having to get up at night to void. Habits with regard to hygiene are also important to note. Particularly if the patient is ill, it is helpful for the nurse to know if he prefers a tub bath or a shower, for example, and the time of day he usually takes it.

The type of information gathered about usual habits of daily living is useful not only in planning care, but also in detecting existing and potential problems. It also provides a base for assessing the individual's present functional abilities.

Let us add the information about Mr. Jordan's usual patterns of daily living to the data we already have.

USUAL REST AND SLEEP PATTERNS: During fishing season, 5 to 6 hours a night and approximately 1 to 2 hours during day. No aids, no medications. Sleeps soundly.

NUTRITION: Three meals/day plus snacks when available. Healthy appetite. Well balanced meals: meat, potatoes, vegetables, fruits, and milk.
ELIMINATION: Daily bowel movement after breakfast. No problems, no laxatives.
No problems with urinary elimination. Never has to get up at night.
HYGIENE: On shore—daily shower and washes hair. On boat—daily wash and wash with disinfectant after cleaning fish (hands and face)
SMOKING: One to two packs since age 16
ALCOHOL: Socially with other fishermen and when on shore
Not a heavy drinker

Environmental Factors

Among the environmental factors which affect a person's health are his family, where he lives, and where he works. The amount of detail included about these factors in the nursing history is a matter of agency policy. Usually much more information is gathered in a community health agency than in a hospital about a person's family, his living accommodations, and the neighborhood in which he lives. If the individual is living with other family members, it is helpful to have basic social data about them and information about their health history and present health status.

In planning and adjusting care for the patient at home, or discharge care for the person who has been hospitalized, it is important to have information about the person's living accommodations. For example, if the bathroom is located on a different floor from the sleeping area, this may pose a problem for the person who becomes short of breath on climbing stairs. With older people, especially, it is important for the nurse to be aware of the location of shopping areas and other facilities in relation to the home. Knowledge of this type can be very helpful in identifying existing and potential problems, as well as in planning realistic care for people.

Knowing the environment in which a person works is important too. Again, it is helpful not only in identifying problems, but also in planning for the rehabilitation of the individual if he has a health problem.

Let us suppose that the community health nurse has made a visit to Mr. Jordan's home and work environment and has gathered the following information:

RESIDENCE: 2465 Washington Avenue, Shore City

NEIGHBORHOOD DESCRIPTION: Urban residential. Mainly apartments and multifamily dwellings

PROBLEMS: Noisy—on a main thoroughfare. Near beach. Good parks nearby.

LIVING ACCOMMODATIONS: Ground floor apartment (one bedroom)
Safety hazards: Old building—fire potential

FAMILY MEMBERS: Lives with fishing partner, Joe (James) Smith aged 21 years

SIGNIFICANT OTHERS: Family in Philadelphia (parents, 2 sisters, 5 brothers). Girl friend in city

WORK ENVIRONMENT: Fishing boat cabin clean but difficult to maintain; area where fish are cleaned is dirty and smelly

The Individual's Perceptions of His Health and Illness Status

In planning care for an individual, it is essential for the nurse to be aware of how the patient regards his health and illness status. People vary considerably in the way they view health and illness, as we discussed in Chapter 3. Although many people today are highly sophisticated in their knowledge of health matters, it is not uncommon to find mistakenly held views about the causes of illness and the significance of signs and symptoms. Then, too, illness is caused by a multiplicity of factors; it is helpful to know what the patient thinks is causing his health problem.

People vary also in their reactions to illness, as we discussed too in Chapter 3. Some people become very angry; some react by denying that it exists; some people can talk of nothing else but their signs and symptoms. Usually, if a person has been injured, or admitted to a health agency for emergency treatment of any kind, his physical well-being is the most important thing on his mind and he is naturally going to be preoccupied with his condition. Some people may realize the implications of their signs and symptoms;

others may be totally unrealistic about these or about their *prognosis,* that is, the expected outcome of their health problem. People often have some knowledge about the state of their health, but it may not be enough for them to be able to cope with a major health problem.

Knowing how a person views his current health and illness status enables the nurse to identify discrepancies between his perceptions and factual findings. This type of information is also helpful in identifying his learning needs and also in anticipating the amount of support the patient may need in accepting his health problem, if he has one, and its implications. For example, the person who has a stomach ulcer may need help in accepting the limitations imposed on his diet, particularly if he has had only a mild attack and is not convinced that there is anything seriously wrong with him.

Let us see how Mr. Jordan views his current health problem and what his anxieties are. Following are the nurse's notes in this regard:

> Mr. Jordan is in great pain. He knows that he has broken his back. He does not know how bad it is and is worried and anxious about whether he will have to have surgery. He guesses he's "going to be laid up for a long time." He is also anxious about his clothes and money, which have been lost during the transfer from North Coast Hospital.

Expectations of Care

An indication of the patient's expectations regarding his care, i.e., what he expects to happen to him and the care he anticipates from nursing personnel, helps the nurse to understand how much explanation the patient will require and may help to clarify some of his reactions to the care he receives. Asking the patients about these matters in itself indicates interest and helps to establish a trusting relationship between nurse and patient.

People usually have preconceived ideas of what they may expect from a health agency. These expectations are conditioned by their own previous experiences with the agency, if they have had any, and the accounts of care received by relatives and friends, as well as by information they have picked up from other sources, such as newspapers, books, and magazines, or radio and television programs.

Their expectations may or may not be realistic. In any case, it is helpful for the nurse to know just what these are.

Let us see what Mr. Jordan expects of his care.

> Mr. Jordan says he will be happy if they can just relieve his pain and fix his back. He was in the hospital four years ago following a motorcycle accident in which he suffered a head injury. He was released after observation because there was no apparent fracture or brain damage. He says he has positive feelings about the nursing care and the treatment he received at that time.

The Patient's Concerns

An indication of the things about which the patient is concerned is important for the nurse both in planning care and in establishing a trusting relationship with the patient. Knowing about the things that are worrying him helps to identify some sources of anxiety and provides the nurse with some guidance on what she can do to help the patient. The woman who is worried about how her husband and children are managing while she is in the hospital might be relieved by having a telephone at her bedside so she could call home, or the nurse might ask the social worker to see the patient, with a view to making arrangements for "homemaker" services while the mother is in the hospital.

An indication of what is important to the individual helps the nurse to attend to the small details which mean so much to patients. A woman patient may request the nurse to telephone her husband to bring in a clean nightgown and her makeup, for example. This may seem an unimportant detail to the nurse who is busy with medications and treatments, but it is important to the patient in contributing to her sense of well-being. Attention to such requests helps the patient to feel more secure and comfortable in a strange environment; it also helps maintain the patient's feelings of self-worth.

Asking the patient about his concerns in itself helps to make him feel that he is being treated as an individual—that someone cares. In following through and doing something about his concerns the nurse helps to establish a feeling of trust between herself and the patient, which is essential in any nurse-patient relationship.

Here are Mr. Jordan's expressed concerns:

> Mr. Jordan was primarily concerned with his excruciating pain. He wants to know if he has to have surgery and whether he will be OK. He is concerned about his clothes and money, which were lost in transit.

THE CLINICAL APPRAISAL

The ability to observe intelligently and systematically is a basic element of nursing practice. It is a fundamental requisite in nursing assessment and is also essential in all subsequent steps of the nursing process. Nurses should begin to develop skills in observation early in their educational programs and continue to refine and polish these skills throughout their professional careers.

Intelligent observations are based on the nurse's knowledge of the biological, physical, and social sciences. As the nurse's knowledge increases through education and experience, she develops increasing skill in observing significant factors in the patient's appearance, in his behavior, and in the environment. She learns what to look for in making observations and how to differentiate the normal from the abnormal. Skill in observing requires a knowledge of what is normal, the ability to identify and describe deviations from the normal, and the capacity to assess the significance of these deviations in relation to the patient's health status.

To be systematic, the nurse's observations must follow a logical and orderly plan. In recent years, a considerable amount of research has been undertaken and numerous articles and reports have appeared in the nursing literature on the development of systematic methodology for nursing observations. Most of the study reports and articles have included examples of forms (such as the nursing assessment forms shown in this chapter) and manuals which provide guidelines for the nurse in making observations. Although the format and specific items recorded vary in different agencies, there is a growing consensus on general content areas to be included in the initial appraisal of an individual patient. These content areas, for the most part, follow the functional abilities approach to nursing assessment outlined originally by R. Faye McCain in 1965 and described by her as "an orderly, precise method of collecting information about the physiological, psychological and social behavior of a patient."[6]

McCain identified 13 functional areas in which the individual's abilities should be assessed: "the patient's social, mental, emotional, body temperature, respiratory, circulatory, nutritional, elimination and reproductive status; state of rest and comfort; state of skin and appendages; sensory perception and motor ability."[7] It is essential that both abilities and disabilities be noted so that the nurse can identify both the individual's strengths and his weaknesses in all functional areas.

The concept of functional assessment provides a logical framework on which the student can begin to develop skills in observation of an individual patient. Some of the information needed for the assessment is obtained by interview. This constitutes the constant data about the individual's normal or usual status in regard to his functional abilities.

The observations described in this chapter do not require extensive skills in physical examination. They depend rather on the acquisition of the basic nursing skills of taking temperature, pulse, respirations and blood pressure, and utilization by the student of awareness of the structure and functioning of the human body (his or her own) to detect readily observable deviations from the normal.

In schools of nursing where preparation for an expanded role is incorporated in the basic curriculum, the student will learn additional skills in physical examination.

---

[6]R. Faye McCain: op. cit., p. 82.
[7]Ibid.

METHODS AND TECHNIQUES OF OBSERVATION

Some authorities call any information which the nurse acquires about an individual *observations.* The term is used here, however, to denote the information the nurse obtains about the patient through the use of her senses of *sight, hearing, smell,* and *touch.* The nurse *looks* at a child's face, for example, to inspect the rash on his cheek; she *listens* to the wheezing breath sounds of the asthmatic; she *smells* the fruity breath odor of children with high fevers; she *touches* a painful ankle to see how much swelling there is.

Visual examination for the detection of abnormalities is called *inspection.* The observations are detailed and focused on a particular area of the body. *Palpation* is the method of examining by using one's fingers. Size, texture, temperature, swelling, and hardness are qualities noted by palpation. *Auscultation* is the listening for sounds within the body. Direct auscultation, with the ear placed on the body, is seldom used; instruments to amplify the sounds are used instead, the most common example being the stethoscope.

The nurse's physical senses are augmented by tools such as the *clinical thermometer,* the *sphygmomanometer* (instrument used for measuring blood pressure) and the *stethoscope* (mentioned above), which have been developed to obtain measurements indicative of the functioning of various body processes. In addition to these commonly used tools, a wide variety of instruments and machines are now available to assist in the observation and measurement of vital body processes. The student will see, and later will probably use, cardiac monitoring machines, for example, in emergency rooms and in the intensive and coronary care units of most hospitals.

Observations reported by the nurse include both *objective* findings, that is, what the nurse observes, and the patient's *subjective* observations. To use an example, the nurse may observe that an individual is not moving his right arm; this is an *objective* observation made by the nurse. The individual may say, "My right arm is very painful." This is a *subjective* observation on the patient's part.

The Validation of Information

Information the nurse obtains from talking with the patient and from her observations should always be validated by checking with the patient as to whether the impressions she has gained are in line with his perceptions.

The Vital Signs

Temperature, pulse, and respirations have traditionally been referred to as the *vital,* or *cardinal,* signs of life. Together with blood pressure and heart beat, they indicate basic physiological functioning, specifically in the functional areas of temperature status, circulatory status, and respiratory status. In making observations about an individual's current functional abilities, the nurse frequently starts with the vital signs.

Although temperature, pulse, respirations, and blood pressure readings vary from individual to individual and at different times of the day in the same individual, there is a range that is generally considered to be normal for temperature, pulse, respirations, and blood pressure. The normal ranges are shown in the table at the bottom of this page.

Temperature. The surface temperature of the body fluctuates with the temperature of the surroundings. In a cool room, for example, exposed skin surfaces soon feel cold and are cold to the touch. The internal, or core, temperature of the body, on the other hand, is precisely regulated and maintained within a very narrow range. It is this internal temperature which is usually measured as an indicator of a person's temperature status. Under normal conditions it does not vary more than a degree or so from the mean, or average, for that person. Variances greater than that are usually indicative of disturbed functioning of the body's heat regulating system.

The temperature regulating system is one of the principal homeostatic mechanisms whereby the internal climate of the body is maintained at an optimal level for functioning. The center for controlling the internal temperature of the body is located in the hypothalamus, in the lower portion of the brain. In health this center maintains a fairly precise balance between heat production and heat loss. Heat is continually being produced in the body as a by-product of metabolism. It is also constantly being lost through *evaporation* (perspiration from the skin); *radiation* (the transfer of heat in the form of electromagnetic waves), e.g., from the body to cooler objects in the environment; *conduction* (the transfer of heat from a warmer to a cooler substance by direct contact), e.g., from the body to the surrounding air; and *convection* (movement of air), as currents around the body carry away heat that has been conducted to the air from the body surface. The factors affecting heat production and the processes by which heat is lost from the body are described in more detail in Chapter 25.

The *body temperature,* as measured by a clinical thermometer, reflects the balance between heat production and heat loss. It usually varies slightly during the course of a 24 hour period in any one individual, being lowest during the early morning hours before a person wakens and highest in the evening. This cycle may be reversed in persons who work at night and sleep during the day. Many people who are ill have an elevated temperature; it is often one of the first observable indications of disturbed body function. In addition, a temperature below normal may be indicative of illness.

Factors other than disease processes, however, can affect body temperature. The

RANGE OF VITAL SIGNS CONSIDERED NORMAL FOR AN AVERAGE, HEALTHY ADULT

Vital Sign	Normal Range
TEMPERATURE	36.1°C to 38.0°C (97.0°F to 100.4°F)
PULSE RATE	60 to 80 beats per minute
BLOOD PRESSURE	120 mm./80 to 90 mm.
RESPIRATIONS	12 to 18 respirations per minute

activity of the individual can make some difference, with the active person usually having a higher temperature than the sedentary person. Exercise can cause a marked, but temporary, elevation in body temperature. Age also affects temperature; the infant and the aged often have a body temperature of 0.6° C (1° F) higher than the young adult. Emotions and anxiety can increase the basal metabolic rate of an individual and thereby elevate temperature (see Chapter 25).

The normal range for body temperature in most adults is considered to be between 36.1° C and 38.0° C (97° F and 100.4° F) when taken orally. The rectal temperature is expected to be approximately 0.6° C (1° F) higher and the axillary temperature, 0.6° C (1° F) lower. *Pyrexia* and *fever* are two terms used to refer to an elevated temperature. The term *hypothermia* refers to a temperature that is below normal.

PROCEDURES FOR TAKING TEMPERATURE. Body temperature is usually measured with a clinical thermometer, which is an elongated glass tube calibrated in degrees Celsius (centigrade) or degrees Fahrenheit. Within the tube is a column of mercury which expands in response to the heat of the body. The scale on the thermometer generally starts at about 33° C (91.5° F) and terminates at 44° C (111° F). Calibrations beyond this scale are considered unnecessary, because temperatures above and below these limits rarely occur.

In addition to the standard clinical thermometer, a number of other devices have been developed in recent years to measure body temperature. An electrical thermometer, for example, is said to give an accurate temperature recording within a matter of seconds. Disposable thermometers also are available. A temperature monitoring probe has been developed for use with seriously ill patients when it is considered important to maintain a constant surveillance of the body temperature. An alarm, attached to the probe, is set to alert the person watching the monitor when the patient's temperature deviates from within a set range. Also commercially available is a temperature sensitive tape which is used in some health agencies for normal, full-term infants. The tape is usually applied to the abdomen of the infant and will change color if the temperature goes above or below the normal. A rectal temperature is taken if deviations are noted.

The most common site for obtaining a measure of internal body temperature is the mouth (*per os*). The small blood vessels on the underside of the tongue lie close to the surface. When the thermometer is placed under the tongue (in the sublingual pocket) and the mouth is closed, it is possible to obtain a reasonably accurate estimate of the body's internal temperature. The thermometer is wiped off, shaken down, and placed sublingually (under the tongue) for 7 to 10 minutes. The patient is instructed to hold

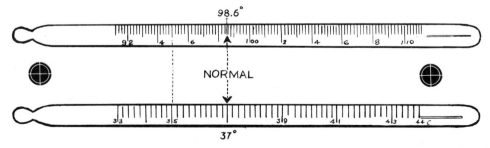

Fahrenheit and Celsius (centigrade) scales are used to measure body temperature. In order to convert Fahrenheit to Celsius, subtract 32 from the Fahrenheit reading and multiply by the fraction 5/9; thus C = 5/9 (F − 32). To convert Celsius to Fahrenheit, multiply the Celsius reading by 9/5 and add 32; thus F = 9/5C + 32.

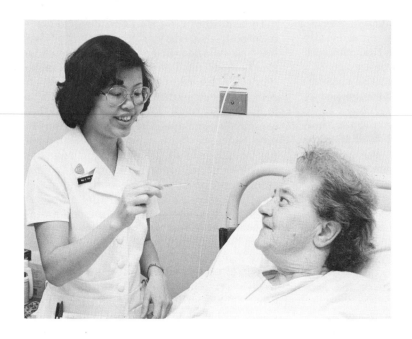

An elevated temperature is often one of the first indications of disturbed body functioning.

the thermometer between his lips and avoid biting it. After the thermometer is removed and the temperature noted, the thermometer is wiped off, shaken down, rinsed under cold running water and dried. In wiping a thermometer, a rotating or twisting motion is used. The thermometer is wiped starting from the tip and working downward to the mercury bulb, that is, from clean to dirty.

The conventional clinical thermometer is usually kept in a small vial containing a disinfectant. Various kinds of disinfectants are used to soak the thermometers; the synthetic phenols, isopropyl alcohol (70 per cent) and tincture of Zephiran (1:1000) are all considered suitable. Because thermometers are soaked in a disinfectant when not in use, they need to be washed or wiped off carefully before they are given to patients. The method of disinfecting thermometers varies in different agencies. However, the same basic steps are usually followed: wiping off the thermometer to remove mucus and secretions, shaking down the mercury, rinsing in cold water, drying, and soaking in a disinfecting agent.

It is frequently necessary to take a patient's temperature via the *rectum*. In most agencies, the temperature of infants is taken rectally. This method is also in-dicated for adults when it is considered either unsafe or inaccurate to take it by mouth, as when a patient is unconscious or irrational. It is customary in many agencies for a rectal temperature to be taken when a person is receiving oxygen therapy, when he has a Levin tube in place, or when he has had oral or nasal surgery. The rectal method should not be used for people with diseases of the rectum, those with diarrhea, or those who have had rectal surgery. The patient lies on his side for this measure. After the thermometer is wiped off and has been shaken down, it is lubricated with petrolatum or other lubricant. This facilitates the insertion of the thermometer into the rectum and lessens the danger of irritating the mucous membrane. The thermometer is inserted from 1 to 2 inches and held in place for at least 2 minutes. When it is removed, the temperature is noted, the thermometer is wiped, washed in cold soapy water, and gently shaken down then returned to its container. It is important to remove all fecal material and to wash the thermometer in cold or lukewarm water, since organic materials interfere with disinfection. The use of cool water prevents the coagulation of protein material. Hot water is never used because it may damage the thermometer.

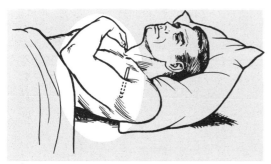

In order to obtain an axillary temperature the thermometer is placed in the patient's axilla, and then his arm is placed across his chest.

Rectal and oral thermometers are sometimes differentiated by the color of the bulb. Oral bulbs are often silver and rectal bulbs are blue. In addition, some rectal thermometers are more rounded at the ends, although many thermometers may be used for taking either rectal or oral temperatures.

Taking an axillary temperature is safer than taking an oral temperature for irrational or mentally disturbed patients. The thermometer is treated in the same manner as the oral thermometer. The axilla is dried before the thermometer is inserted because moisture conducts heat. The thermometer is placed between the inner surface of the patient's arm and his side while his arm is held across his chest. The thermometer is left in place for at least 10 minutes; then it is removed and the temperature is noted. The nurse can expect the axillary temperature to be approximately 0.6° C (1° F) lower than the oral temperature.

Pulse.[8] Pulse is the throbbing of an artery as it is felt over a bony prominence. When the left ventricle of the heart contracts, blood surges through the systemic arteries. This wave of blood is felt as the pulse.

At rest the heart is required to pump only 4 to 6 liters of blood per minute. This volume is increased as much as five times during exercise. Normally each ventricle pumps 70 ml. of blood with each contraction, although wide variations in the amount are compatible with life. This volume of output is reflected in the pulsations that can be felt where arteries pass over bones.

When taking a pulse, the rate, rhythm, size (volume), and tension of the pulse are noted. The *rate* of the pulse is the number of beats per minute. Deviations from the normal frequently are seen in illness. In addition, a number of factors other than disease processes also affect the pulse rate. Pulse rate varies according to age, sex, size, and physical and emotional activity, for example. The pulse rate decreases as a child grows and continues to decrease until extreme old age. Men generally have a slower pulse rate than women, and exercise increases the rate of cardiac contractions. When a person is experiencing strong emotions, such as anxiety, fear, or anger, the heart usually beats faster also (see Chapter 12). A pulse rate between 60 and 80 beats per minute is usually considered normal for most adults. If the pulse rate is greatly accelerated (for example, over 100 beats per minute), the condition is referred to as *tachycardia.* A very slow pulse rate (under 60 beats per minute) is called *bradycardia.*

The *rhythm* of the pulse refers to the pattern of the beats. In health the rhythm is *regular;* that is, the time between beats is essentially the same. The pulse is *irregular* when the beats follow each other at irregular intervals.

The *size,* or amplitude, of a pulse wave reflects the *volume* of blood pushed against the wall of the artery in the ventricular contraction. A *weak* pulse lacks a feeling of fullness and a definite beat; it may feel thready. When a pulse cannot be felt or heard, it is said to be *imperceptible.* A *bounding* pulse is one in which the volume reaches a higher level than normal, then disappears quickly.

The *tension* of the pulse refers to the compressibility of the arterial wall. If under slight pressure the pulse is obliterated, that is a pulse of low tension. A pulse that is obliterated only by relatively great pressure is a pulse of high pressure. The words *"soft"* and *"hard"* are used to describe pulse tension.

PROCEDURE FOR TAKING THE PULSE. Pulse is assessed by palpation, and there are numerous sites on the body at which a

---

[8] Terminology used here and on the following pages reflects current trends as exemplified by Taylor and Johnson, op. cit.

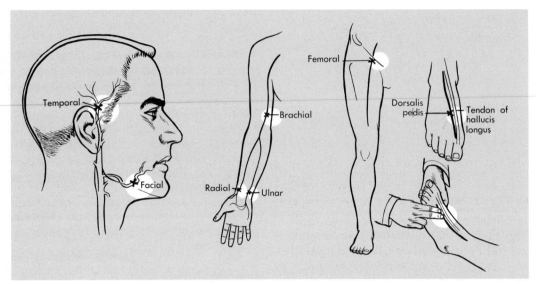

There are many sites on the body where the pulse may be taken; however, the radial pulse is taken most frequently. Other sites which are used, particularly when the radial pulse cannot be obtained, are the brachial, the temporal, the facial, the femoral, and the dorsalis pedis. Pulses are also taken at these points in order to assess arterial circulation to the specific area.

pulse may be obtained. In the assessment of a person's circulatory status, the peripheral pulses are commonly used. These are the pulses located in the head, the neck, and the extremities. Of these, the radial and the brachial pulses are the ones most frequently used by nurses. The radial site is used to assess the pulse, and the brachial site is used in taking the blood pressure. Other peripheral sites may be used for pulse assessment if the radial pulse is obscured, or if there is a need to test the circulation of blood to a specific area. The temporal, the femoral, and the dorsalis pedis pulses are three that are used most often.

The *radial pulse* is located on the inner aspect of the wrist on the thumb side where the radial artery passes over the radius. With slight pressure, the artery may be held against the radius so that the pulsations of blood may be felt. The *brachial pulse* is located on the anterior surface of the arm, just below the elbow, where the brachial artery passes over the ulna. The *temporal pulse* is felt anterior to the ear at the mandibular joint, where the temporal artery passes over the temporal bone. It can also be felt at the temple, that is, to the side of the eyebrow just in front of the hairline. The *femoral pulse* may be taken

at the point in the middle of the groin where the femoral artery passes over the pelvic bone. The *dorsalis pedis pulse* (usually taken to assess circulation in the foot) can be felt on the dorsum of the foot in a line between the first and second toes, just above the longitudinal arch.

When the nurse takes the patient's pulse, she places her second, third, and fourth fingers lightly on the skin at the place where the artery passes over the underlying bone. The thumb is not used because the nurse might feel the pulsations of the radial artery of her own thumb. Usually, counting the rate for 30 seconds and then multiplying by two gives an accurate record of beats per minute. Some people prefer to count the rate for 15 seconds and multiply by four. If the pulse is irregular in any way it is counted apically for a full minute.

Generally the patient should lie or sit quietly so that his pulse rate can be compared with previous observations. Exercise and anxiety accelerate the pulse rate to an extent that it does not reflect the normal rate at rest.

APICAL BEAT.   It is often necessary to determine the rate of the apical beat of the heart. The apical beat is the beat of the heart as felt at its apex. The apex is considered to be the point of maximal impulse. The apical beat can usually be heard in the fifth intercostal space, two to three inches to the left of the sternum, just below the left nipple. By reaching with the stethoscope in this area, the point of maximal sound can usually be found.

To determine the apical beat, the bell of the stethoscope is placed over the apex of the heart and the beats are counted for a full minute. A heart beat is heard as "lubb-dubb." The "lubb" represents the closure of the atrioventricular or tricuspid and mitral valves; it occurs at the onset of systole. The "dubb" represents the closure of the semilunar (aortic and pulmonic) valves at the end of systole. The rhythm of the heart beat can also be noted and recorded in the patient's chart.

An *apical-radial* pulse is ascertained by two nurses. One nurse counts the patient's radial pulse at the same time that the second nurse counts the apical beats of the heart with the same watch. Each is counted for a full minute. In health, the apical and radial rates are the same, but in illness they sometimes differ, as when some apical beats are not transmitted to the radial artery. The difference between the apical rate and the radial rate is the *pulse deficit.*

Blood Pressure. Blood pressure refers to the pressure of the blood within the arteries of the body. When the left ventricle of the heart contracts, blood is forced out into the aorta and travels through the large arteries to the smaller arteries, arterioles, and capillaries. The pulsations extend from the heart through the arteries and disappear in the arterioles. The *systolic pressure* is the arterial pressure at the height of the pulsations; it is normally 120 mm. of mercury in a young adult. The *diastolic pressure* is the arterial pressure at the lowest level of the pulsation, that is, during ventricular relaxation. It is normally 80 to 90 mm. of mercury. The difference between the systolic and diastolic pressure is the *pulse pressure.*

A number of variables affect the arterial blood pressure. It is dependent on the *force* of the ventricular contractions of the heart and on the amount of blood ejected from the heart with each ventricular contraction (cardiac output). The force of the contractions depends on the pumping ac-

tion of the heart. The greater the strength of the pumping action, the more blood is ejected with each contraction.

The amount of cardiac output is also affected by the total *volume of blood* circulating in the body. A decrease in blood volume, such as occurs in hemorrhaging, will result in a lowered blood pressure. Changes in the *elasticity* of the muscular walls of the blood vessels also affect the blood pressure. Aging, for example, decreases the elasticity of muscular tissue, and an older person's blood pressure is usually higher than a younger person's. Blood pressure is also affected by the *viscosity* (thickness) of the blood, which is dependent on the number of red blood cells and on the amount of plasma protein it contains. Viscosity may be altered by disturbances of fluid balance. Another factor which affects the blood pressure is the *resistance of the peripheral vessels* (peripheral resistance). Normally, the pressure in the large blood vessels is high, and the pressure in the smaller vessels (the arterioles and capillaries) is low. Blood, as any other liquid, tends to flow from areas of high pressure to areas of low pressure. Factors which decrease the lumen of the blood vessels affect the smaller vessels proportionately more than the larger ones, and increase the amount of pressure required to pump the blood through them. Any constriction of the vessels, e.g., as when deposits occur on the lining of the vessels, increases the peripheral resistance and, therefore, the blood pressure.

An individual's blood pressure varies from hour to hour and from day to day. It falls during sleep and may be strikingly elevated by strong emotions, such as fear and anger, and by exercise. When a person is lying down, his blood pressure is lower than when he is sitting or standing. Also, the pressure may differ in the two arms of the same patient. Therefore, before taking the blood pressure for a comparison value, the nurse should check (*a*) the time of day, (*b*) the arm used, and (*c*) the position the patient was in for previous readings.

An abnormal elevation of blood pressure is referred to as *hypertension. Hypotension* refers to abnormally low blood pressure.

PROCEDURE FOR TAKING THE BLOOD

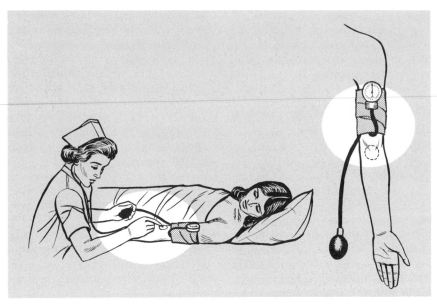

The blood pressure cuff is wrapped evenly around the upper arm so that the lower edge is 2.5 cm. (1 inch) above the antecubital space. The arm is positioned so that the cuff is at the level of the heart.

PRESSURE.   There are two practical clinical methods of taking an individual's arterial blood pressure: the auscultatory method and the palpatory method. In the auscultatory method, a stethoscope, a blood pressure cuff, and a sphygmomanometer are required. Mercury and aneroid sphygmomanometers are available commercially. The mercury instruments, which are less compact than the aneroid, are commonly used in physicians' offices.

In taking the blood pressure, the cuff is wrapped smoothly and firmly around the patient's upper arm so that the lower border of the cuff is 2.5 cm. (1 in.) above the antecubital space. The bell of the stethoscope is placed over the site of the brachial pulse and the cuff is pumped to 30 mm. of mercury above the pressure at which the pulsation in the brachial artery disappears. (The pulsation disappears when no sounds can be heard through the stethoscope.[9]) This means that the artery is collapsed by the pressure of the cuff and no blood is flowing through it. The pressure is then gradually released and, when the blood slips through the artery, sounds are heard in the stethoscope. At the same time, the manometer is watched closely. The reading when the first sounds are heard is the *systolic pressure*.

With the continual lowering of the pressure in the cuff, the sounds continue to be heard as the artery alternately collapses and fills. Eventually the sounds diminish in intensity as the artery no longer collapses; weakened beats are usually heard for a few seconds and then disappear altogether. The onset of muffling (point at which the sounds change) is used by many clinicians as the index of *diastolic pressure*, although some prefer to use the point at which the sounds disappear entirely. In some agencies, both points are recorded.

It usually takes practice to learn to distinguish the systolic and diastolic points of pressure with ease and accuracy, and in some patients, they are very difficult to discern. Care should be taken, however, to avoid repumping the sphygmomanometer repeatedly within a short space of time.

In the palpatory method of taking arterial blood pressure the blood pressure cuff and sphygmomanometer are used but the stethoscope is not; the radial pulse is palpated to ascertain the systolic blood pressure. The cuff is pumped up and the

[9]Jane Lancour: How to Avoid Pitfalls in Measuring Blood Pressure. *American Journal of Nursing,* 76:773–775, May 1976.

pressure is slowly released; the reading at the point at which the radial pulse is first felt is the systolic pressure. The diastolic pressure is determined by noting the change in the character of the radial pulsations; however, this reading is not generally considered to be sufficiently accurate.

Respirations. The term "respiration" is used either for the metabolic process of gas exchange with the environment or for the breathing movements an individual makes in inspiration and expiration. Respiration is the means by which gases are exchanged with the atmosphere. External respiration is the exchange of carbon dioxide and oxygen between the alveoli of the lungs and the blood, whereas internal respiration is the exchange of these gases between the blood and the body cells.

The two main types of external respiratory movements ("respirations") are thoracic (costal) and abdominal (diaphragmatic). Thoracic respirations are accomplished chiefly by the costal muscles of the chest; abdominal respirations are accomplished by the abdominal muscles. The respirations of women are chiefly thoracic, while those in men are abdominal.

Respirations are essentially controlled by the respiratory center in the medulla oblongata. This center is influenced by several factors, such as the carbon dioxide level of the blood and the expansion of the lungs (see Chapter 30). Respirations controlled in this manner are automatic. Their rate and depth are regulated within a range that meets the metabolic needs of the body for oxygen. Any activity that necessitates increased oxygen supply will result in more rapid and usually deeper respirations. It should be noted, too, that the rate and depth of respirations are to a certain extent under voluntary control. A person can take deep breaths or shallow breaths, or breathe quickly or slowly, within the limitations imposed by the body's need for oxygen. In assessing respirations, the nurse observes their rate, depth, rhythm, and character. Detailed procedures for making these observations are given below.

The normal *respiratory rate* for an adult is generally considered to be 12 to 18 respirations per minute. An abnormal increase in the respiratory rate is called *tachypnea* (polypnea), and an abnormal decrease is technically referred to as *bradypnea.* Normal breathing which is (effortless, regular, and noiseless) is called *eupnea.* An absence of breathing is termed *apnea.*

The *depth* of respirations refers to the amount of air inhaled and exhaled with each breath movement. A young adult normally inhales and exhales approximately 500 ml. of air with each breath. Normal respirations result in deep and even movements of the chest. In *shallow* respirations, the rise and fall of the chest and abdomen are minimal. If the respirations are shallow and rapid, the person is said to be *short of breath.* The term *air hunger* is frequently used to describe respirations that are abnormally deep and accompanied by an increased respiratory rate.

The *rhythm* of respirations refers to the regularity of inspirations and expirations. Normal respirations follow one another evenly, with little variation in the length of the pauses between inspiration and expiration. *Symmetry* refers to the synchronous movements of each side of the chest. The nurse may observe *asymmetrical* breathing in some individuals.

The *character of respirations* refers to digressions from normal, effortless breathing. *Labored breathing,* for example, involves active participation of accessory inspiratory and expiratory muscles. Difficult breathing accompanied by whistling sounds is called *wheezing.* If bubbling sounds can be heard in air cells (alveoli) or bronchial tubes, the term *rales* is used. Another descriptive term that is commonly used for noisy breathing is *stertorous* respirations.

PROCEDURE FOR OBSERVING RESPIRATIONS. The nurse observes respirations unobtrusively, often after taking the pulse. If a person is aware that his respirations are being observed, he usually finds it difficult to maintain his normal breathing pattern. In assessing respirations, the nurse counts their rate, watches the chest movements, and listens for breath sounds.

In calculating the respiratory *rate,* the nurse counts the respirations as she

A sample Clinical Chart. (Courtesy of Vancouver General Hospital.)

would for the pulse. Either the inspirations or the expirations are counted, but not both. Inspiration is the movement of air into the lungs; expiration is the movement of air out of the lungs. Sometimes it is impossible to see a person's chest movements or hear his breathing. By placing a hand on the person's chest the nurse can often detect these otherwise undetectable respirations.

The *depth* of respirations is determined by watching the chest movements. The depth of respirations may be characterized as shallow, normal, or deep. The *rhythm* and the *character* of respirations are both observed by watching the chest movements and by listening to the breath sounds. In observing the chest movements the nurse should not only watch the extent of rise and fall of the chest, but should also note if accessory muscles are used in breathing. In normal breathing the principal muscles concerned are the external and internal intercostal muscles and the diaphragm. If, for any reason, respiration becomes difficult, all the muscles attached to the thoracic cage are brought into play. These include the major and minor pectoral muscles, the sternomastoid, the scalene, and the subclavius.

Coughing is a means by which a person clears his respiratory tract of secretions and foreign material. A cough is almost always abnormal and should always be noted. The individual may tell the nurse that the cough has come on suddenly (*acute cough*) or that he has had it for a long time (*chronic cough*). By listening to the person cough, the nurse can usually ascribe certain qualities. Common descriptive terms include *hacking* (frequent, short cough), and *paroxysmal* (sudden, periodic attack of coughing). A cough may be termed *dry* or *nonproductive* if the individual does not bring up any *sputum* (secretions from the bronchi or lungs) with the cough. If the person does bring up sputum (cough is *productive*), the nurse needs to describe the appearance of these secretions since sputum varies in character. It may appear *watery* (thin and colorless), *frothy* (having the appearance of being light and aerated, containing bubbles), or *viscous* (containing a thick, tenacious mucoid exudate). Sputum may also be described according to its color; it

may be *green, yellow, blood-tinged* or *gray*. Sometimes sputum has a distinctive odor—it may have an offensive (*foul*) smell, for example, or sometimes a *sweetish* smell. In recording observations about sputum, the nurse indicates the amount: *scant* (small amount), *moderate*, or *copious* (large amount). Often a 24 hour specimen of sputum is collected to obtain a more accurate estimate of volume.

Nutritional Status

In assessing an individual's nutritional status, the nurse will have information about his *height,* his *usual weight,* and his *present weight* from the nursing history. She also observes his general appearance—does he look *obese, plump, average* in build, *thin,* or *emaciated?* She should be aware of the individual's usual eating habits. Does he usually have a small, average, or big appetite? The nurse should also know about special diets he has been following as well as any dietary restrictions he observes for cultural or religious reasons, or because of allergies. Observations can be made regarding the individual's *present response to food* and eating. Normally people enjoy food, although they do not always eat enough of the proper nutrients. Abnormalities that should be noted in the person's ability to eat or in his response to food include: *nausea* (a queasy feeling in the stomach); *anorexia* (loss of appetite); refusal to eat; difficulty in swallowing; *distention* (enlargement of the abdomen due to internal pressure of gas or liquid); or *distorted tastes.* The nurse should also note if the patient has any difficulty in swallowing (dysphagia). The nurse notes the amount of food or fluids that the individual takes. If he takes only small amounts of food or fluids, this also should be noted.

Elimination Status

Constant data collected about an individual's elimination status are usually included in the nursing history. In assessing the individual's current elimination status, the nurse makes observations about the following.

Emesis. Emesis is the vomiting of contents of the gastrointestinal tract through the mouth. Vomiting is always an abnormal condition. The nurse should make observations about the *amount* (it should be measured or approximated) and the *contents* of the emesis. Common terms used to describe the latter include: *bloody* (containing red blood); *liquid* (primarily liquid in consistency); *undigested food* (recognizable particles of food), or *bile* (a thick, viscid fluid varying in color from yellow to brown or green, and having a bitter taste).

Bowel Status. Significant observations about current bowel status include the date and time of the individual's last bowel movement, the color of the stools, and the frequency of bowel movements. Normal stool is brown, soft, and formed. Abnormal findings should be noted, such as *clay-colored* stools; *tarry* stools (black or blackish-brown viscous semi-liquid or liquid stools). Common problems with bowel functioning which the individual may report are *diarrhea* (frequent bowel movements; stools of more or less fluid consistency); *constipation* (infrequent passage of feces or difficult defecation; stools are unduly hard and dry); and *flatulence* (gas in the digestive tract). When the individual is unable to control the movement of his bowels, he is said to have *involuntary* bowel movements (incontinent). The term *impacted* bowel refers to a condition in which there is an accumulation of feces in the rectum pressed firmly together so as to be immovable.

Urinary Status. Normal urine is clear and straw colored, and observations must include its color, clarity, and amount. Common terms used to describe abnormalities are: *cloudy, dark orange, pink, red, frothy,* or *containing sediment.* Common problems in urinary functioning, which the individual may report, include: *frequency* (urinating at short intervals); *urgency* (the need to void suddenly with an inability to retain urine without acute distress); *burning* (a scalding sensation on voiding); *dribbling* (an intermittent flow of urine). A person is said to be *incontinent* of urine when he is unable to control urination.

Sensory Perception

The abilities to see, to hear, to feel, to taste, and to smell are vitally important in coping with the daily activities of living. In making observations relating to an individual's sensory perception, the nurse is concerned with the integrity of the anatomical structures needed for functioning in these areas: the eyes, the ears, the nose, the mouth and throat, and the skin, as well as their disturbances in functioning per se. Deviations from the individual's normal abilities, as indicated in the constant data collected about that person, should be noted in all sensory areas.

Vision. In assessing current visual status, the nurse makes observations about the condition of the eyes, the eyelids, and the pupils, as well as asking the person about visual disturbances he may be experiencing. When observing the individual's eyes, the nurse should look first at the condition of the eyelids. They may be *reddened* and look irritated, or they may appear *swollen* (puffy enlargement). The individual may complain of *itching* or *burning* of the eyes or lids; frequent rubbing of the eyes is often indicative of this feeling. The nurse should also look for *tearing* or *exudate* from the eyes. In addition, she should ask the individual if he has any visual disturbances such as *blurring* (seeing objects as vague or lacking in outline), or *diplopia* (double vision, seeing two objects when there is only one). In noting comments about the eyes the nurse should record which eye is affected—right, left, or both.

The nurse also observes the pupils of the eyes. The average normal pupil is 4 to 5 mm. in diameter. If the pupils are excessively large, they are said to be *dilated*; very small pupils are termed *pinpoint*. It is often important also to observe the reaction of the pupils to light. Normally an individual's pupils contract when exposed to a strong light. A flashing light directed at the eyes is used to observe this reaction. The nurse should note if both pupils react at the same time (consensually), as well as watch the separate reactions.

Hearing. The average individual can hear a normal conversation from a distance of approximately 15 feet. Hearing is one of the senses that become less acute as one grows older. Men lose the ability to hear high sounds first (women's voices, for example), whereas women find the low tones more difficult to hear as they grow older. Long-standing deficits in hearing are included in the constant data collected about an individual.

The nurse observes the condition of the ears. Normally, these are clean and free from discharge. Abnormalities that should be noted include the presence of *cerumen* (earwax), a sticky substance, usually brownish in color, and any discharge coming from the ear. These may be described as *watery* secretions, *purulent* (yellowish), or *bloody* (usually red in color). The amount of discharge should be noted as scant, moderate, or copious. The nurse always records which ear is affected (right, left, or both).

The nurse also asks if the individual has noticed any disturbances in hearing, such as a buzzing or ringing in the ears (*tinnitus*), or any *dizziness* or *loss of balance*.

Smell. The nose is not only instrumental in the ability to smell, but it is also an important part of a person's respiratory apparatus. Common abnormalities include *nasal discharge* (secretions from the nose), or bleeding (*nosebleed*). Disturbances in the sense of smell, such as an *absence of this sense*, or *distorted odors* (odors usually considered agreeable are unpleasant, and vice versa), should also be noted.

Taste. The condition of a person's mouth and throat is important not only to his sense of taste but also to his ability to take food and fluids, thereby affecting his nutritional status. Pertinent observations include noting if the mouth looks dry. A *dry mouth* is evidenced by a lack of saliva, and often one can see fine cracks in the surface of the lips or mucous membrane lining of the oral cavity. A mouth that is *not clean* has a collection of mucus and food particles around the teeth and gums or adhering to the mucous membranes. Sometimes the oral cavity appears *red* and inflamed. Any *bleeding* in the mouth should be noted; it usually occurs in the gums around the teeth.

The nurse also observes the condition of the tongue. The term *coated tongue* is used to describe the presence of a thick, furry covering which may be variously colored. The mouth may also have a *foul odor*. Another abnormality to look for is *lesions* in the mouth, such as sores or fever blisters. The nurse notes whether the individual's teeth are in good condition. *Dental caries* (decayed teeth) may be observed. If the individual wears dentures, the nurse should note this fact and also their condition. A person without teeth is said to be *edentulous*.

Disturbances in taste which the individual may describe include a *bad taste* in the mouth, an *absence of taste*, or *distorted taste* (misinterpretation of tastes). Or he may report that he has an *increased acuteness* of this sense or, conversely, *decreased ability* to distinguish tastes. When looking at the mouth, the nurse should observe the throat; it may appear *reddened* or *swollen*, and the individual may complain of a *sore throat*.

Touch and Feeling. Touch and feeling are subjective experiences, and the nurse must rely on the individual's observations regarding deviations from the normal in this sensory area. Disturbances in feeling, such as *numbness*, *prickling*, or *tingling*, are most commonly noted in the extremities or in the facial area. Sometimes there is a *heightened sensitivity* to touch (pressure), heat, or cold, or, conversely, a *decreased sensitivity*.

THE SKIN AND ITS APPENDAGES. The intact skin provides a protective covering for the body. Normal, healthy skin is clear (free from blemishes), intact (unbroken), warm to the touch, and has a characteristic color, depending on the person's ethnic background and inherited complexion tones. Although each individual's skin coloring varies to a certain extent, the nurse may observe common abnormalities such as *flushing* (redness of the skin, particularly noticeable in the face and neck), *pallor* (lack of color), *cyanosis* (bluish or grayish cast to the skin, particularly noticeable in the lips, earlobes, and nailbeds), and *jaundice* (yellow color of the skin or whites of the eyes).

The nurse should also look for blemishes and breaks in the skin. Common blemishes include *rashes* (eruption of the skin, usually reddish in color); *bruises* (superficial discolorations due to hemorrhage into the tissues from ruptured ves-

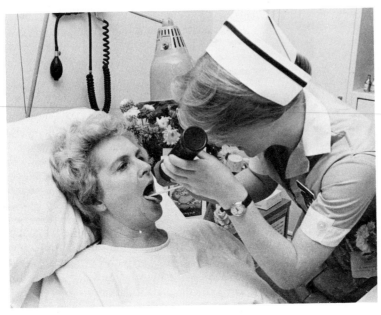

The nurse observes the condition of the patient's mouth and throat in her clinical appraisal.

sels); *reddened areas* (diffuse red discoloration); *weeping areas* (oozing a watery secretion); *dry, itching areas* (rough and scaly skin which the individual has a desire to scratch); and *mottled areas* (marked with blotches of different shades of color). *Scabs* (crust of a sore, wound, ulcer, or pustule) and *lesions* (open areas or breaks in the skin surface) should be noted, as well as scars on the body or incisions from surgical operations. The presence of *lumps* under the skin (abnormal masses that perform no physiological function) should also be observed. Both the location (specific area of the body on which the blemish or lesion appears) and its size should be recorded.

Other observations which the nurse may make about the skin are the presence of excessive perspiration, which may be seen on the forehead, upper lip, palms of the hands and/or soles of the feet, in the axillary area, or covering the entire body. If the entire body is bathed with perspiration, the term *diaphoresis* is used. The nurse may also notice abnormalities in the temperature of the skin. For example, it may feel *hot* (abnormally warm) or *cold* (abnormally cool) to the touch.

Motor Status

A normal individual can sit, stand, walk, and perform a great number of movements, provided that the bones and mus-cles, circulation, and nerve supply are intact. Limitations in mobility due to chronic health problems, as, for example, paralysis, weakness, or difficulty in movement of one or more limbs (or parts of limbs), should be including in the constant data collected about the individual. Nursing observations to gather variable data pertaining to present motor status usually focus on the integrity and functioning ability of the extremities. Abnormalities to which the nurse should be alert in the extremities include disturbances in circulation or sensory perception, limitation of movement, and abnormal muscular movements.

An important observation which the nurse should make relative to circulation is the *presence or absence of distal* (peripheral) *pulses* — that is, whether a pulse can or cannot be obtained by compressing the arteries at the points farthest from the heart in any of the extremities (see page 162). Other pertinent observations include the presence of *swelling* (abnormal localized enlargement) or *edema* (an excessive amount of tissue fluid) in any part or all of an extremity. Sensory disturbances which the individual may tell the nurse about include *parasthesia*, that is, an abnormal sensation without objective cause, such as *numbness, prickling,* or *tingling,* or a *heightened sensitivity* (to pressure, heat, or cold) in any part, or all of one or more limbs.

The nurse should also observe the

limbs for deficiencies in range of motion of a part or of the whole extremity (see Chapter 17, pp. 303–306). *Weakness* (that is, a lack of strength in any area) should be noted, especially a marked decrease in the ability to grasp an object (*weak hand grip).*

Abnormal muscular movements include: *contractures,* a permanent contracture of a muscle due to spasm or paralysis; *tremors,* a quivering or involuntary convulsive muscular contraction; and *muscle spasms,* involuntary convulsive muscular contractions. *Missing limbs,* or parts of a limb, absent as a result of a birth defect, trauma, or surgery, should be noted if not already reported in the constant data.

The nurse includes observations relating to the individual's response to activity. Some common terms that people use to describe abnormal responses to activity are: feelings of *dizziness,* a whirling sensation in the head with a tendency to fall; *faintness,* a feeling of weakness; *fatigue,* a feeling of tiredness or weariness; and *shortness of breath,* slow, rapid respirations on exertion. It should be noted that these observations are predominantly subjective. The nurse must ask the individual if he has noticed any of these symptoms in response to normal activities, such as walking, climbing stairs, and the like.

The individual's mobility should also be determined. Aids to mobility required at the present time, such as crutches, a cane, a walker, a wheelchair, or persons to assist the individual, are noted. If restrictions have been placed on his activities because of a current illness (such as bed rest or bathroom privileges only), these are included also.

State of Rest and Comfort

The individual's usual patterns of rest and sleep are noted in the constant data collected about him. Problems that the person is currently experiencing should be noted in the variable data, e.g., insomnia or excessive drowsiness. The nurse notes the presence of any pain, since it is one of the most common causes of disturbances in rest and sleep. Pain is, of course, a subjective experience and the nurse must rely on the patient's observations of the pain he feels. She records the exact location of the pain, if the patient is able to tell her, and also its nature. People use a variety of expressions to describe pain that they are experiencing. Common terms which the individual may use include: *sharp,* (acute or cutting); *aching* (dull, generalized, persistent); *cramp-like* (severe paroxysmal type); *throbbing* (pulsating); *constant* (continuous, unchanging); *intermittent* (coming and going at intervals). The nurse also notes if the pain reacts to therapy—the severity or intensity of the pain is, or is not, appreciably alleviated by the ministrations of the nurse or by the medication or treatment specified.

Reproductive Status

Age, sex, and marital status are vital statistics about the individual that are noted in the constant data. Other information about reproductive status that is collected in the nursing or medical history of a female patient includes data about usual menstrual pattern, and, if applicable, the age of menopause and of menarche, the number of pregnancies and of live births, the number and ages of children, and information about contraceptive methods used.

Variable data about an individual's reproductive status include the data of last menstrual period (if female) and the presence of any discharge from the genitals (both sexes). If the patient reports, or the nurse observes, discharges from the vagina or penis, it is important to note the color and amount of the discharge. Common types of discharge include *bloody, white,* or *yellow* discharges. An intermittent bloody discharge is termed *"spotting."* If a discharge has a *foul odor,* this also should be noted.

Mental Status

Normally, during his waking hours, a person is alert and responsive. In appraising the mental status of an individual, the nurse should observe his movements. If he is slow or sluggish in moving, or appears to suffer from abnormal drowsiness, he is said to be *lethargic.* If he appears bewildered and perplexed, and/or makes

NURSING ASSESSMENT: PATIENT PROGRESS

HOSPITAL NORTH WEST GENERAL

SEPT. 16, 77

JORDAN PAUL
2465 WASHINGTON AVE SHORE CITY
SMITH JAMES   234-7566
SAME   1600   SURG.   R.C.
9-16-77 PATIENT INFORMATION

DATE	9/16		
HOSPITAL/P.O. DAY	1		
TIME	1800		

DATE	9/16		
HOSPITAL/P.O. DAY	1		
TIME	1800		

1. VITAL SIGNS

BLOOD PRESSURE	Systolic	120		
	Diastolic	60		

TEMPERATURE (O) R A (circle) 37

PULSE/min.	radial	80		
	apical			

irregular		☐	☐	☐
bounding		✓	☐	☐
weak		☐	☐	☐
imperceptible		☐	☐	☐
other		☐	☐	☐

RESPIRATIONS/min. 16

non-rhythmic	☐	☐	☐
labored	☐	☐	☐
rales	☐	☐	☐
wheezing	☐	☐	☐
shallow	☐	☐	☐
short of breath	☐	☐	☐
other	☐	☐	☐

2. RESPIRATORY AIDS none ✓ ☐ ☐

OXYGEN	flow			
		l/min.	l/min.	l/min.
nasal		☐	☐	☐
mask		☐	☐	☐
tent		☐	☐	☐
trach collar		☐	☐	☐

TRACHEOSTOMY			
cuffed	☐	☐	☐
not cuffed	☐	☐	☐
mist	☐	☐	☐
suctioned	☐	☐	☐

VENTILATOR			
rate/min.	☐	☐	☐
controlled	☐	☐	☐
assisted	☐	☐	☐
other			

*AMOUNT/SEVERITY = 1 small/occasionally
2 moderate/frequently
3 copious/most of the time

3. EENT

R=right L=left		blurring	☐	☐	☐
		diplopia	☐	☐	☐

PUPILS	dilated	☐	☐	☐
	unequal	☐	☐	☐
	pinpoint	☐	☐	☐
	do not react to light	☐	☐	☐

	tinnitus	☐	☐	☐
	nasal discharge	☐	☐	☐
	nosebleed	☐	☐	☐
	throat irritation	☐	☐	☐
other				

MOUTH	dry	✓	☐	☐
	not clean	☐	☐	☐
	coated tongue	☐	☐	☐
	reddened	☐	☐	☐
	bleeding	☐	☐	☐
	foul odor	☐	☐	☐

4. COUGH*

	acute	☐	☐	☐
	chronic	☐	☐	☐
	hacking	☐	☐	☐
	non-productive	☐	☐	☐

SPUTUM	green	☐	☐	☐
	yellow	☐	☐	☐
	blood-tinged	☐	☐	☐
	gray	☐	☐	☐
	viscous	☐	☐	☐
	not deep-breathing	☐	☐	☐
other		☐	☐	☐

5. POSITION IN BED

PRESCRIBED POSITION	legs elevated	☐	☐	☐
	side only	☐	☐	☐
	semi-Fowlers	☐	☐	☐
	Trendelenberg	☐	☐	☐
other	BED FLAT	✓	☐	☐

FORM 0002

NURSING ASSESSMENT: PATIENT PROGRESS

HOSPITAL *NORTH WEST GENERAL*

DATE	9/16		
HOSPITAL/P.O. DAY	1		
TIME	1800		

DATE	9/16		
HOSPITAL/P.O. DAY	1		
TIME	1800		

6. SKIN*

flushed			
pale	✓		
cyanotic			
jaundiced			
perspiration			

LOCATION

rash			
bruise	✓		
reddened			
weeping			
dry/itching			
mottled			

LOCATION   *SACRAL AREA*

size/cm (approx.)			
depth/cm (approx.)			
other *SEVERAL BRUISED AREAS*			

7. EXTREMITIES*

R=right
L=left
B=both
A=arm
D=leg

NO distal pulses			
paresthesia			
limited movement	✓		
paralyzed			
swelling			
edema			
weakness			
hand grip weak			
contractures			
muscles spasms			
tremors			
missing			
other _____			

8. GENITALS*

L.M.P. DATE ___/___/___

DISCHARGE white			
yellow			
spotting			
foul odor			
other _____			

9. RESPONSE TO FOOD/EATING

WEIGHT			
nausea			
anorexia			
refuses to eat			
distention			
diff. swallowing			
distorted taste			

SPECIAL DIET _____

SMALL INTAKE OF: fluids			
food			
other *NPO*			

10.   ELIMINATION*

EMESIS	bile			
	undigested food			
	bloody			
	liquids			
	other			

BOWEL	bowel movement			
	constipated			
	diarrhea			
	involuntary			
	impacted			

URINARY	cloudy			
	dark orange			
	pink			
	red			
	bladder distended			
	scanty amount	✓		
	not voiding			
	dysuria	✓		
	incontinent			
	frequency			
	urgency			
	other _____			

*AMOUNT/SEVERITY = 1   small/occasionally
2   moderate/frequently
3   copious/most of the time

NURSING ASSESSMENT: PATIENT PROGRESS

HOSPITAL _NORTH WEST GENERAL_

JORDAN PAUL   SEPT. 16, 77
2465 WASHINGTON AVE SHORE CITY
SMITH JAMES   234-7566
SAME   1600   SURG.   R.C.
_9-16-77_ PATIENT INFORMATION

DATE	9/16		
(HOSPITAL)/P.O. DAY	1		
TIME	1800		

DATE	9/16		
(HOSPITAL) P.O. DAY	1		
TIME	1800		

11. WOUND*

inflamed			
hematoma			
gaping			
DRAINAGE serous			
sero-sanguineous			
sanguineous			
muco-purulent			
bile			
fecal matter			
urine			
_____ odor			
other _____			

12. CAST/TRACTION*

describe/locate _____

DRAINAGE sanguineous			
sero-sanguineous			
purulent			
odor			
pale			
cyanotic			
cold			
swelling			
other _____			

13. DRAINAGE TUBES*

A. N/G	B. Foley	C. H'vac	Use letters/tubes opposite
D.	E.	F.	related term(s).

not patent			
suction			
gravity			
irrigated			
cloudy			
pink			
red			
dark amber			
clots			
viscous			
other _____			

*AMOUNT/SEVERITY = 1 small/occasionally
2 moderate/frequently
3 copious/most of the time

FORM 0002

14. ACTIVITY LEVEL

bed only	✓		
dangles only			
chair only			
BRP only			
room only			
one level only			
ambulates			
other _____			

15. AIDS TO MOBILITY

crutches			
cane			
walker			
brace			
wheelchair			
person(s)			
other _____			

16. RESPONSE TO ACTIVITY*

dizziness			
faint	✓		
fatigued			
short of breath			
other _____			

17. PAIN*

R=right
L=left
B=both

incisional			
chest			
abdominal			
lower back	3		
calf of leg			
head			
sharp	3		
aching			
cramp-like			
throbbing			
constant	✓		
intermittent			
not relieved by therapy			
other _____			

NURSING ASSESSMENT: PATIENT PROGRESS

HOSPITAL *NORTH WEST GENERAL*

DATE	9/16		
HOSPITAL/P.O. DAY	1		
TIME	1800		

DATE	9/16		
HOSPITAL/P.O. DAY	1		
TIME	1800		

18. MENTAL STATUS*

lethargic			
confused			
disoriented			
inattentive	1		
forgetful			
unresponsive			
other _____			

19. SPEECH COMMUNICATION*

reticent			
evasive			
verbose			
stuttering			
slurring			
unable to speak			
other _____			

20. OBSERVED BEHAVIOR*

restless	2		
crying			
withdrawn			
underactive			
combative			
abusive			
noisy			
other _____			

21. SOCIAL RESPONSE*

wants to be alone	1		
doesn't want to be alone			
UPSET BY: family			
visitor(s)			
roommate(s)			
staff			
other _____			

*AMOUNT/SEVERITY = 1 small/occasionally
2 moderate/frequently
3 copious/most of the time

FORM 0002

22. FEELINGS EXPRESSED BY PATIENT*

depression			
nervousness	2		
anger			
fear			
wants to die			
undersired changes due to illness			
other _____			

23. PERCEPTIONS OF ILLNESS* - PATIENT

misconceptions			
inadequate information			
refuses to talk about illness			
preoccupied with illness	3		
denial			
other _____			

24. PERCEPTIONS OF PROGNOSIS* - PATIENT

complete recovery			
no change			
to die			
doesn't know	✔		
partial recovery			
other _____			

25. COMMENTS

Pt. in severe pain
Wants to know if he's going
to have surgery, will he be o.k.
Worried about clothes and
money lost in transit

26. SIGNATURES

Instructions: (1.) *J. Smith* R.N.
sign your name
under column of (2.) _____ R.N.
date you recorded.
(3.) _____ R.N.

page 4 of 4

inappropriate answers to questions, the term *confused* is commonly used to describe his mental state. The *disoriented* individual perceives himself and/or his environment incorrectly in relation to time, place, or person. He may not know who he is (or recognize familiar people), where he is, or what day it is. A person is said to be *inattentive* when he is unable to focus his mind on an idea or on some aspect of his surroundings or on reality. The term *forgetful* is used when a person has a temporary loss of memory, e.g., he cannot remember what you asked him a few minutes ago, or whether he has eaten lunch. When the individual makes no response to sensory stimulation, meaning that he does not answer or obey simple commands such as, "Please raise your hand, or nod your head," or he does not turn his head away from a bright light or react to touch, he is said to be *unresponsive*.

Emotional Status

People are not happy all the time. Most people experience a range of emotions in their day-to-day lives. These emotions are communicated to other people both by what the individual says and by his actions. In assessing an individual's emotional status, the nurse needs to identify both the individual's feelings as he expresses them in words and his observable behavior. These feelings include: *depression* (a feeling of sadness or melancholy); *nervousness* (easily excited, irritated, jumpy, uneasy, or disturbed); *anger* (strong feelings of displeasure or antagonism); and *fear* (unpleasant emotion caused by anticipation or awareness). The person may say that he *wants to die*. He may have feelings of *anxiety* concerning possible ill effects from his present state of health, or from surgery.

Some common types of observable *behavior* include: *restless* (continually moving the body or parts of the body); *crying* (weeping or lamenting); *withdrawn* (socially detached and unresponsive); *underactive* (not moving about as much as is desirable); *combative* (physically striking or attempting to strike others); *abusive* (harshly attacking others verbally); *and noisy* (talking loudly, shouting, or banging objects).

Social Status

People normally are gregarious; they enjoy the company of other people. The ability to make contact and to exchange communication with other members of the human race not only makes life more interesting and enjoyable, but is essential to daily living. People convey messages to other people by speaking, by writing, and through their behavior. Deviations from the normal in regard to an individual's social status may also be observed through these means.

Verbal Communication. Normally a person has the ability to carry on a conversation with another person and to respond to questions in such a way that his meaning is clear. This of course, assumes that there are no language problems. Two common abnormalities of speech which the nurse can identify by listening to a person talk are *stuttering* (stumbling and spasmodic repetition of the same syllable), and *slurring* (sliding or slipping over word sounds that would normally be heard). A person who is unable to make his meaning clear (provided everyone is speaking the same language) is said to be *incoherent*. When an individual who previously was able to speak normally is unable to speak at all, the term *aphasia* (or *aphasic*) is used. *Dysphasia* is a general term used to refer to difficulties in speaking.

In observing an individual's speech, the nurse should note his willingness to communicate. He may, for example, be *reticent* (inclined to be silent and uncommunicative); *evasive* (avoids answering people directly); or *verbose* (extremely talkative). If the individual is unable to write, this fact should be noted.

Social Response. People respond to other people in an infinite variety of ways. Behavior that is normal for one individual may be abnormal for another. If the individual is ill, however, the nurse should note his response to the presence of others.

It is important to note, for example, if the individual wants to be alone (to have minimal or no contact with *anyone*) or does not want to be left alone, but desires or needs constant companionship. The nurse should also record her observations if the patient becomes *upset by contact* with his family, friends, staff, visitors, or roommates.

STUDY VOCABULARY

Air hunger
Anorexia
Aphasia
Apical beat
Apical-radial pulse
Apnea
Assessment
Auscultation
Body temperature
Brachial pulse
Bradycardia
Bradypnea
Cerumen
Confused
Constant data
Constipation
Contractures
Cyanosis
Depression
Diaphoresis
Diarrhea
Diastolic pressure
Diplopia
Disoriented
Distention
Dorsalis pedis pulse
Dysphasia

Edentulous
Emesis
Eupnea
Evaluation
Femoral pulse
Fever
Flatulence
Flushing
Hypertension
Hypotension
Hypothermia
Implementation
Incontinent
Inspection
Jaundice
Labored breathing
Lesions
Lethargic
Muscle spasms
Nausea
Nursing history
Nursing process
Pallor
Palpation
Paresthesia
Planning
Pulse

Pulse deficit
Pulse pressure
Pulse rate
Pulse rhythm
Pyrexia
Radial pulse
Rales
Respiration
Scabs
Significant others
Slurring
Sphygmomanometer
Sputum
Stertorous respiration
Stuttering
Systolic pressure
Tachycardia
Tachypnea
Temporal pulse
Tinnitus
Tremors
Unresponsive
Variable data
Viscosity
Vital signs
Wheezing

SUGGESTED READINGS

Blainey, C. G.: Site Selection in Taking Body Temperature. *American Journal of Nursing,* 74:1859–1861, October 1974.

Browning, M. H., and P. L. Minehan (eds.): *The Nursing Process in Practice.* Contemporary Nursing Series. New York, The American Journal of Nursing Company, 1974.

Fuller, D., and Rosenauer, A.: Patient Assessment Guide. *Nursing Outlook,* 22:460–462, July 1974.

Gebbie, K., et al.: Classifying Nursing Diagnoses. *American Journal of Nursing,* 74:250–253, February 1974.

Gordon, M.: Nursing Diagnoses and the Diagnostic Process. *American Journal of Nursing,* 76:1298–1299, August 1976.

Graas, S.: Thermometer Sites and Oxygen. *American Journal of Nursing,* 74:1862–1863, October 1974.

Marriner, A.: *The Nursing Process: A Scientific Approach to Nursing Care.* St. Louis, C. V. Mosby Company, 1975.

Mundinger, M. O., and Jauron, G. D.: Developing a Nursing Diagnosis. *Nursing Outlook,* 23:94–98, February 1975.

Nicholls, M. E.: Quality Control in Patient Care. *American Journal of Nursing,* 74:456–459, March 1974.

Nichols, G. A., et al.: Taking Adult Temperatures: Oral Measurements. *American Journal of Nursing,* 72:1090–1091, June 1972.

Nichols, G. A., et al.,: Taking Adult Temperatures: Rectal Measurement. *American Journal of Nursing,* 72:1092–1093, June 1972.

Roberts, S. L.: Skin Assessment for Color and Temperature. *American Journal of Nursing,* 75:610, April 1975.

Roy, Sr. Callista: A Diagnostic Classification System for Nursing. *Nursing Outlook,* 23:90–94, February 1975.

Sparks, C.: Peripheral Pulses. *American Journal of Nursing,* 75:1132–1133, July 1975.

Yura, H., and Walsh, M. B.: *The Nursing Process: Assessing, Planning, Implementing, Evaluating.* 2nd edition. New York, Appleton-Century-Crofts, 1973.

10 THE NURSING PROCESS, PART II

The nurse should be able to:

Demonstrate beginning skill in analyzing data collected in the
    nursing history and clinical appraisal
Discuss the synthesis of information from all sources
Demonstrate beginning skill in
    (1) identifying and stating nursing problems
    (2) arranging a problem list in order of priorities for action
    (3) identifying relevant principles to assist in planning
        nursing care
    (4) developing goals in terms of expected patient outcomes
    (5) developing a nursing care plan
Discuss the use of flowsheets and other forms as aids in planning
    and implementing nursing care
Discuss methods of evaluating the effectiveness of nursing
    interventions

ANALYSIS OF INFORMATION

Once the nurse has gathered information about the patient through taking the nursing history and through her observations, her next step is to analyze that information. The question is, what does it all mean?

In order to critically examine the data she has collected, the nurse will find it helpful to group the information by categories. This helps to put it into some sort of logical order and to develop a structure, or framework, which not only makes the mass of data she has collected more meaningful, but also makes it much easier to manage. If her observations have been made on a basis of functional areas, for example, this already gives the nurse a framework on which to analyze the data logically and systematically.

When the data are organized (or grouped), the next step is to look at them from the point of view of significant deviations from the normal. What is unusual in the findings about this patient? In what way does the status of his functional abilities differ from normal functioning? How important are the deviations from normal that the nurse has found in this patient? In this analysis, the nurse is aided by: (1) her knowledge of normal functioning, which she has derived from her courses in the basic biophysical and social sciences; (2) her understanding of normal and abnormal factors that may affect functioning in a particular area; and (3) her awareness of common problems, signs, and symptoms that accompany various health problems.

At the beginning of her nursing program, the student will not, of course, have an extensive knowledge base from which to draw. She can, however, identify many deviations from the normal and can relate these to the knowledge she does have. As her knowledge increases, and her clinical experience grows, she will be able to assess the significance of her findings more readily and with a greater depth of understanding. At all times, however, it is important that the nurse communicate her findings and interpret them honestly at the level of her understanding.

In taking the nursing history, the nurse has noted the patient's usual functional abilities, and has gained some information about him as an individual. In her clinical appraisal, she has made observations about his current status in regard to his functional abilities and noted deviations from the normal. By comparing data from her observations with data from the history, she is able to note any changes that have occurred between the person's usual functioning and his present abilities. Now she separates the abnormal findings from those which appear to be normal and assesses the importance of these in relation to his current health status. A person may have a long-standing abnormality which may or may not be significant in the present situation. For example, the patient may have had an amputation of one of his little fingers a number of years ago. This is a deviation from the normal, but probably is not significant if he is in hospital to have surgery for removal of his appendix. On the other hand, the fact that a person has been confined to a wheelchair for years is significant in planning his care.

In Mr. Jordan's case (Chapter 9), the nurse will note deviations from the normal in regard to his rest and comfort status (he is in pain), to his mobility status (he cannot walk or lift his arms above his head, and movement aggravates the pain), to his elimination status (voiding is difficult), to his nutritional status (his weight is below normal for his height), to the status of his skin and appendages (he has several large bruised areas on his lower back). All of these findings would appear to be significant.

SYNTHESIS OF INFORMATION

When the nurse has analyzed the information she has collected from all sources and identified significant findings she has made, she then relates it to information she has obtained from other sources. From the admission notes she has learned that Mr. Jordan was in a car accident and suffered compression fractures of three vertebrae. She has noted the location of the injury, vertebrae D11, D12, and L1. The nature and location of the injury have been confirmed in the report of the x-rays taken on admission to this hospital. The laboratory reports of blood tests and urinalysis (telephoned to the ward) show normal findings. From the physician's notes, she learns that he has ruled out surgery at this time, that he suspects there may be internal injuries, and there is a possibility of nerve damage.

The physician's orders include:

Bed rest
Fracture board
Bed flat—pt. to maintain back-lying position, may turn on side for care
2 pillows under head—1 supporting shoulders
1 pillow under knees
NPO 48 hr
Dextrose—Saline 5% 1500 cc/d × 2
Vital signs q4h—48 hr
Intake and output
Demerol—100 mg IM q4h p.r.n. for pain

By putting this information together with the data she has collected, the nurse can begin to think about some of the things that will be important in Mr. Jordan's care. He is having severe pain—it will be important to relieve that. She will

have to be careful in helping him to move—he will probably need instructions on "log rolling" in turning and in maintaining his position as the doctor has ordered. NPO (nothing by mouth)—this might be a problem since Mr. Jordon normally has a voracious appetite. Watching the vital signs—that will help determine presence of internal injuries. Watching intake and output—that's to watch for signs of damage to the nerves innervating the bladder, also for possible internal injuries.

At this point the nurse is ready to begin organizing her initial impressions and identifying specific problems that require nursing intervention.

IDENTIFICATION OF NURSING PROBLEMS

A problem has been defined as "any condition or situation in which the patient needs help."[1] A nursing problem, then, is any condition or situation in which the patient needs the nurse's help. Nurses are frequently confused about *needs* versus *problems*. To illustrate the difference, the following example may be helpful. The patient is having difficulty in breathing and requires oxygen therapy. The *problem* is the difficulty in breathing. The *need* is for oxygen therapy. The problem identifies the difficulty which the person is having. The need spells out the type of intervention that the nurse feels would resolve the problem. There may be several possible alternatives, so the nurse has to decide which intervention is most appropriate for that problem. Changing the patient's position, for example, might relieve the difficulty in breathing; giving medication might be another possibility.

In order to plan nursing care and decide on the intervention that is most suitable for the situation, it is necessary first to identify the problems the patient is having. These may be either actual or potential problems. *Actual problems* are those which, in the nurses's opinion, are

[1]Rosemarian Berni and Helen Readey: *Problem-Oriented Medical Record Implementation.* St. Louis, C.V. Mosby Company, 1974, p. 2

causing the patient difficulty at the present time. For example, Mr. Jordan has an actual problem with pain (to select one problem). *Potential problems* are those which may arise because of the nature of the patient's health problem or because of the diagnostic or therapeutic plan of care. Mr. Jordan, for example, is not allowed out of bed, and he is restricted to a certain position in bed. He is thin and there is a potential problem of skin breakdown, particularly over bony prominences, such as the lower part of his back, his heels, and his elbows.

Problems should be identified systematically. Again, using the functional abilities approach helps the nurse to systematically check where the patient needs help with either actual or potential problems. In stating problems, the most important thing is that the nurse communicate the intent of her message so that it can be understood by others. Wherever possible, the nurse should state the cause of the problem as she understands it.

If we review the information we have about Mr. Jordan by functional area, we can identify several problems, some actual and some potential, with which he needs the nurse's help. Following each problem, there is a statement which gives some of the nurse's thinking in relation to that problem.[2]

Social Status: No actual problem: potential problem of feelings of isolation because family are in the East.

    Analysis: Mr. Jordan has mentioned his family. Would like them to be notified of his accident. His friends in the city are all working.

Mental Status: (1) Restlessness due to pain.

    Analysis: Pain relieved by medication, restlessness more noticeable as time approaches for medication.

    (2) Potential problem of disorientation and drowsiness due to medication for pain.

    Analysis: Patient will probably be kept sedated while pain is severe to ensure his safety from further injury.

Emotional Status: (1) Anxiety due to uncertainty about physician's plan of care and prognosis.

    Analysis: Physician has decided against surgery "at this time." Patient unsure as to just what this means

    (2) Anxiety over loss of clothes and money.

    Analysis: Patient admitted first to North Coast Hospital. Transferred by plane, then by ambulance. Money and valuables could have been left in any one of three places.

Temperature Status
Respiratory Status
Circulatory Status } No actual problems. Potential problems due to possibility of internal injuries.

    Analysis: Vital signs may change quickly if there is internal bleeding. Physician has ordered monitoring of vital signs q4h, or more often if changes are noted or if observations warrant it.

Nutritional Status: (1) Hunger, due to NPO.

    Analysis: Patient says he is hungry. Aware that he can have nothing to eat or drink for 48 hours; aware of reason for order. Normally has a big appetite.

    (2) Potential problem of maintaining nutritional status if NPO is continued.

Elimination Status: (1) Difficulty in voiding, possibly due to nerve damage.

    Analysis: Injury to vertebrae D11, D12, and L1 could have caused damage to nerves leading to bladder. There could also be a possibility of damage to kidneys as a result of trauma suffered in accident.

    (2) Potential problem of constipation due to bed rest and lack of solid food intake.

    Analysis: Immobility and lack of sufficient food and fluids may cause constipation. Possibility of

---

[2] Marlene Glover Mayers: *A Systematic Approach to the Nursing Care Plan.* New York. Appleton-Century-Crofts, 1972.

nerve damage may also cause interference with intestinal elimination.

(3) Potential anxiety about finances due to anticipated lengthy convalescence and possible need to change his line of work.

Analysis: People with the sort of back injury Mr. Jordan has usually require a long time to recover. He will probably be unable to work for several months. He may not even then be able to return to fishing as a career.

State of Rest and Comfort: (1) Severe pain in lower back due to injury, aggravated by movement.

Analysis: Pain relieved by medication. Pain causes restlessness, and increased movement when restless increases pain.

(2) Sensitivity to touch in area of injury and bruised area due to damaged tissues.

Analysis: Sensitivity confirmed by patient's facial expression and involuntary exclamations when back is touched.

State of Skin and Appendages: (1) Bruises in sacral area due to trauma.

Analysis: Area very sensitive to touch, as noted above.

(2) Potential problem of pressure areas developing over bony prominences because of bed rest and limited movement.

Analysis: Patient is thin; this will increase possibility of pressure areas developing. Restlessness increases rubbing of skin surfaces on bedclothes.

(3) Inability to maintain own hygiene due to limited mobility.

Analysis: Patient unable to raise arms to upper part of head; can reach mouth; unable to reach below thighs without pain. Cannot comb hair; hair is shoulder length and curly.

(4) Potential problem of poor oral health due to NPO.

Analysis: Patient says that his mouth feels dry. Teeth and gums in good condition at present.

Reproductive Status: No actual problems.

Motor Status: Limited mobility due to pain and restrictions on position.

Analysis: Patient is careful about moving; restricts movement because of pain. Physician has left specific instructions about position. Patient can turn on side for bed-making and back care. Patient will need assistance with exercises to maintain muscular strength and tone, and to prevent contractures if on extended bed rest.

Priority Setting

Once problems are identified, they are placed in order of importance. It is not possible to attend to all problems at the same time, nor is it possible to help the patient with all of his problems all of the time. It is necessary, then, to decide which problems the nurse can assist the patient in resolving and which of these should be attended to first.

In establishing priorities to assist in planning nursing intervention, a helpful guide is Maslow's hierarchy of human needs, which was described in Chapter 2 pp. 14 to 17. To review these briefly, the basic human needs, in order of priority according to Kalish's model, are:

1. Physiological needs
2. The need for knowledge
3. The need for safety and security
4. The need for love and belonging
5. The need for esteem and self-worth
6. The need for self-actualization.

It is perhaps useful at this time to state that it is not possible, even under the most favorable circumstances, for the nurse to help the patient to meet all of his needs. Through her awareness of basic human needs, however, she can direct her actions toward helping the patient to resolve problems that interfere with his ability to meet those needs that are essential to his well-being or to his recovery.

In Mr. Jordan's case, the nurse's problem list might be arranged in order of priority as given below. Note that the statements of problems have been shortened in some cases for ease of communication.

1. Pain, due to injury, aggravated by movement

2. (a) Limited mobility because of pain and prescribed position

   (b) Potential problem of loss of muscle tone

   (c) Potential problem of contractures of ankle joints

3. Sensitivity to touch in lower back area due to site of injury and bruised tissues

4. Potential deviations in vital signs because of possible internal injuries

5. Difficulty in voiding, possibily due to nerve damage or internal injuries

6. Anxiety because of uncertainty about physician's plan of care and prognosis

7. Anxiety due to loss of clothes and money

8. (a) Hunger due to NPO

   (b) Potential problem of maintaining nutritional status if NPO is continued

9. Decreased mental alertness due to sedation for pain

   (a) May fall from bed

   (b) May burn self or set fire to bed while smoking

10. Potential problem of maintaining good oral health status due to NPO

11. Potential pressure areas over bony prominences, sacral area, elbows and heels (see No. 2)

12. Potential problem of constipation due to bed rest and NPO

13. (a) Inability to look after own hygiene (see No. 2)

   (b) Potential problem of poor status of skin and appendages (see No. 13a)

14. Potential problem of feelings of isolation because family is far away and friends are working

15. Potential problem of anxiety about finances due to anticipated lengthy convalescence and possible need to change occupation

The student will note that this ordering does not follow exactly the priority listing of Maslow's hierarchy of human needs. The nurse uses her judgment in allocating priorities; the hierarchy only provides a base from which to start. The concerns that were causing Mr. Jordan anxiety were very important to him and the nurse felt they should be attended to as quickly as possible. Hence, his anxiety problems were given high priority. Also, the patient was smoking frequently; his safety was a matter of immediate concern.

When problems are resolved, they may be crossed off on the nurse's problem list, or they may be left on and the date of resolution recorded. Policies in this regard vary from one agency to another. (See Chapter 11 for discussion on resolved problems when the problem-oriented medical record is used). The statement of problems that have changed is modified. For example, constipation may become an actual problem rather than a potential one; this would necessitate a change in the problem statement. New problems that emerge are added to the list.

PLANNING

Planning is the second major step in the nursing process. It involves determining what the nurse can do to help the patient and selecting appropriate nursing interventions to accomplish this.

It has been said, and rightly so, that nurses have always planned the care of their patients. In the past, however, planning often was a mental process on the nurse's part, with minimal guidance in the form of written material developed to assist others in their care of the patient when that particular nurse was not on duty.

Taking time to sit down and write out a plan of care helps the nurse to organize her mental activities: to think through what she hopes to accomplish by nursing care; to take into account potential problems as well as those which are actually present; to review the possibilities of alternative nursing interventions; and to develop a plan of care that can be followed through by all nursing personnel concerned with the patient. A written plan of care helps to ensure: continuity and completeness of care; that everyone is using the same approach with the patient, and that nothing is left to the uncertainties of human memory.

Planning is a continuous process. The patient's problems change. Some are quickly resolved; some seemingly minor problems suddenly become acute; new ones arise. Sometimes a nursing intervention does not succeed in accomplishing its purpose and alternative approaches must be explored. The planning of nursing care, then, is constantly under revision.

Professional nursing care is based on

principles, rather than the application of routine or standard techniques. The body of scientific knowledge which is the foundation of nursing is constantly enlarging; techniques and routines of care are continuously being revised because new information has emerged. The nurse cannot depend on a learned repertoire of skills and procedures to carry her through a lifetime career; skills and techniques soon become obsolete. She must instead base her practice on relatively unchanging principles to guide her in modifying techniques she has learned or in acquiring new skills and techniques.

Many situations the nurse will encounter are unique. She may have never met this set of circumstances before. Indeed, because every person is a unique individual, nursing care must be adapted to suit each patient's particular needs. In order to help the patient in resolving his problems, the nurse must draw on principles rather than rely on rule-of-thumb techniques or standard procedures.

Planning involves basically two sets of activities on the nurse's part: setting goals for patient attainment and developing a plan of action to achieve these goals. Before the student sets out to undertake these activities, however, she will find it helpful to identify relevant principles applicable to the set of problems her patient has.

Identifying Relevant Principles

Nursing is an applied science. The theoretical basis of nursing draws from many areas, including the biophysical sciences, the medical sciences, pharmacology, nutrition, and the social sciences. The principles applied in nursing practice may be derived from any one of the science areas.

People's interpretations of the word "principle" vary, but it is used here to mean essentially one of four things: a concept, a scientific fact, a law of science, or a generally accepted theory.[3] Principles are used as guides in determining appropriate nursing action. For example, the holistic concept of man as an integrated being who functions as a whole (discussed in Chapter 2), leads the nurse to consider his social and psychological needs as well as his physical needs when planning care and deciding on specific nursing interventions.

Scientific facts derived from anatomy and physiology, for example, guide the nurse in many of her actions. The normal ranges for measurements of body processes, such as those for temperature, pulse, respirations, and blood pressure discussed in the previous chapter, are scientific facts which alert the nurse to take action when she observes deviations from the normal in her patients. The law of gravity finds its application many times over in nursing actions. From the physical sciences, the student will learn in body mechanics that pulling or sliding an object requires less effort than lifting it, since lifting necessitates moving against the force of gravity (see Chapter 17). We have just used the theory of a hierarchy of human needs (drawn from psychology) as a guide in setting priorities for nursing actions for solving patient problems.

Taking the case of Mr. Jordan, some principles applicable in his care would include:

1. The bony vertebral column protects and supports the spinal cord (Anatomy and Physiology).

There is not much space between the spinal cord and the bony structure supporting and protecting it. Injured vertebrae that are out of alignment or broken may press on or actually damage the cord and the roots of nerves innervating the part of the body below the site of the injury. Therefore, the injured vertebrae must be immobilized until the broken pieces of bone knit together sufficiently to maintain their normal structure and placement. This means that the physician's orders regarding Mr. Jordan's positioning must be followed exactly. Thus, in turning Mr. Jordan, when the nurse is changing the bed linen, it is important that his trunk be maintained in good alignment at all times. Later, when Mr. Jordan is allowed out of bed, he will have to learn to do such activities as getting up, walking, and picking things up without bending his back.

---

[3]Nordmark, Madelyn T., and Rohweder, Anne W.: *Scientific Foundations of Nursing.* 3rd edition. Philadelphia, J. B. Lippincott, 1975.

This principle is probably *the* most important one for the nurse to remember in caring for Mr. Jordan. His fractured vertebrae are, after all, the reason for his hospitalization.

2. The loss of blood volume causes a decrease in systemic blood pressure (Anatomy and Physiology).

When a person is bleeding heavily at any point in the circulatory system, his blood volume drops and his blood pressure is lowered. When this happens, the heart greatly increases its activity in an attempt to increase its output and maintain the amount of circulating blood; blood is withdrawn from surface areas and shunted to vital organs; the skin becomes cold (and clammy); temperature drops (to lessen demands for oxygen transported by the blood); and respirations become rapid and deep (to supply more oxygen for the body).

The physician suspects that Mr. Jordan may have internal injuries as a result of the trauma his body suffered in the accident. There is therefore a possibility of internal bleeding. Vital signs are monitored to watch for: decreased blood pressure, increased and/or irregular pulse, subnormal temperature, and rapid and deep respirations.

3. Adequate elimination of wastes is essential for efficient body functioning (Anatomy and Physiology).

Mr. Jordan is having difficulty voiding and the physician suspects that there may have been damage to the nerves innervating the urinary system. Monitoring of intake and output is therefore essential. This principle is also applicable in regard to intestinal elimination.

4. Demerol depresses the central nervous system (Pharmacology).

The physician has ordered Demerol for the relief of Mr. Jordan's pain. From pharmacology, the nurse knows that this drug causes drowsiness and dulling of mental faculties. It may also cause a person to experience a feeling of happy well-being (euphoria); Mr. Jordan described it as a feeling of "floating." The person may not be fully alert to his surroundings and his safety must be protected.

5. All body cells require adequate amounts of essential nutrients (Nutrition).

The physician has ordered NPO for 48 hours, and has prescribed intravenous feedings. If the NPO order is extended, maintaining adequate nutrition will be a problem.

6. The intact skin is the body's first line of defense against infection (Microbiology).

Because of his injury, Mr. Jordan is more vulnerable to infection than he normally would be. It is important therefore to maintain skin integrity and prevent the development of pressure areas.

7. Friction is caused by the rubbing together of two irregular surfaces (Physics).

The rubbing of the skin surfaces on bed sheets causes friction. The irregularities between the skin surfaces and the bedclothes can be minimized by keeping the sheets smooth and by separating the surfaces as, for example, by using a lubricant to coat the surface of the skin.

8. The need for knowledge is a basic human need, ranked by some theorists as second only to physiological needs (Psychology).

Mr. Jordan is very worried because of his lack of information about his therapy (is he going to have to have surgery?) and also about his prognosis. He is also worried about the loss of his clothes and valuables. Therefore, it is important that the nurse take action to see that he receives information about these matters.

9. One of the functions of the family is to support its members in times of crisis (Sociology).

Mr. Jordan has asked that his family be notified of his accident. It is important that the nurse take steps to see that this is done.

Determining Expected Outcomes

The identification of patient problems leads to the development of *objectives* or *expected outcomes* to be attained by the patient with the assistance of nursing action. These objectives should be realistic and attainable both in terms of the potentialities of the patient and the ability of the nurse to help him to meet these objectives. For example, to set as an objective that the patient regain normal motor functioning may be completely unrealistic for a patient who has been partially paralyzed by a stroke, but the patient may be able to achieve independence in feeding and dressing himself, and these are objectives which the nurse can help him to achieve.

Objectives are stated in terms of expected patient outcomes, rather than nursing activities. Nursing intervention is then planned to help the patient to achieve these. The *expected outcomes* describe the behavior the patient is expected to attain. For example, "The patient dresses himself each morning without help" might be one objective for the partially paralyzed patient. Behavioral objectives are usually written in sentence form and include: the subject (in this case, the patient), an action verb which describes the desired behavior (dresses himself), the conditions under which the activity is to take place (without help), and a criterion or standard for judging the action (each morning).[4]

Long-range general objectives such as "The patient will regain optimal motor functioning" are important to keep in mind, but for planning specific nursing intervention for one patient, it is helpful to have goals that are worded more specifically. Another objective for the partially paralyzed patient might be, "The patient maintains his right arm and leg [if these are the affected ones] in good anatomical position at all times." Objectives worded in terms of expected behavioral outcomes help to communicate to other personnel, to the patient, and to his family just what is to be attained.[5] They also provide scope for prescribing definitive nursing intervention, such as the use of a footboard and pillows to support the arm and leg, and the use of a roll in the patient's hand to maintain flexion of the fingers, in the case of the objective just stated. Stating the expected outcomes also provides the means for evaluating the patient's progress and the effects of nursing action.

Some agencies advocate the use of deadlines, or intervals, for checking on the progress the patient has made in relation to the expected outcomes.[6] Thus, in the case of the objective stated above, the patient would be checked at regular intervals (e.g., q4h) to ensure that his right arm and leg were being maintained in good position. One would expect that the nurse caring for the patient would, in the course of giving other care, check the positioning, but a designated deadline draws attention to this aspect of care, and ensures that it is not neglected or forgotten.

In Mr. Jordan's case, one expected outcome in relation to his problem of pain might be that he is quiet and comfortable at all times as evidenced by his relaxed facial expression, his decreased restlessness, and his statements that his pain is lessened.[7]

Expected outcomes in regard to Mr. Jordan's other problems are shown in the nursing care plan prepared for him (see pp. 188–189).

In the past few years there have been a number of articles and books in the nursing literature about the writing of behavioral objectives. Some of these are included in the list of suggested readings at the end of this chapter. For additional help, the nurse is directed to Mager's book, *Preparing Instructional Objectives.*[8] This book, although originally intended for teachers, is equally useful for nurses.

Developing a Plan of Action

Once objectives have been established in relation to the identified problems, the next step is to determine those nursing interventions which will best help the patient to attain the expected outcomes. This involves the exploration of possible courses of action and a decision to try one approach. In assessing the merits of different courses of action, the nurse is guided by her knowledge of the biophysical and the social sciences, her understanding of the patient's health problem and of the physician's plan of care, and

---

[4] Dorothy M. Smith: Writing Objectives as a Nursing Practice Skill. *American Journal of Nursing,* 71:319–320, February 1971.

[5] Registered Nurses Association of British Columbia: Manual of Information for the Preparation and Utilization of Nursing Care Plans. Vancouver, British Columbia.

[6] Marlene Glover Mayers, op. cit., pp. 62–65.

[7] Mayers, op. cit, p. 58.

[8] Robert F. Mager: *Preparing Instructional Objectives.* Palo Alto, Calif., Fearon Publishers, 1962.

her knowledge about the individual patient as a person.

In deciding on a course of action in relation to any one specific problem, the nurse has basically three options: she may decide (1) that no action is necessary (or possible); (2) that nursing intervention can resolve the problem; or (3) that the problem should be referred to another member of the health team.

In Mr. Jordan's case, his hunger may be the one thing the nurse can do nothing about until the order for nothing by mouth is terminated. A number of his problems do require nursing intervention. Pain is, of course, one of these. The patient's anxiety about the plan of care for him, and his prognosis, would need to be referred to the physician.

The types of nursing intervention possible should be reviewed systematically. The nurse may find it helpful here to think in terms of the various aspects of nursing discussed in Chapter 6. For example, does the problem require intervention in regard to the care aspects of nursing, the curative aspects, the protective aspects, the teaching aspects, the coordinating aspects, or the patient advocate aspects?

In Mr. Jordan's case, he requires a number of interventions in regard to care since he is unable to do many things himself. He will need help with hygiene, to list just one. In regard to the curative aspects, it is essential that he maintain the prescribed position in bed. He will require instruction (teaching aspect) in regard to maintaining the prescribed position in bed and concerning turning. The protective aspects of Mr. Jordan's care include preventing the development of pressure areas. With regard to coordinating aspects, this may involve asking the social worker to help with locating Mr. Jordan's clothes and valuables. The nurse will act as a patient advocate when she requests the physician to discuss Mr. Jordan's plan of care with him and also his prognosis. This example gives just one possible intervention for Mr. Jordan in each of the six aspects of nursing; the nurse will note others in the plan of care for him.

Nursing interventions may also be categorized on the basis of whether they are preventive in nature, palliative (as, for example, to relieve suffering), restorative, or rehabilitative. The nurse will find it helpful to review the patient's problems by including this categorization of nursing interventions in planning her care of a patient.

In assessing the relative merits of different nursing interventions, the nurse uses her judgment for deciding on the best alternative to use for this particular patient, at this particular time. For example, medications for pain are usually ordered q4h p.r.n. This is generally interpreted to mean that the medication may be repeated after an interval of four hours; it may be delayed longer than the four hours; or it may not be given at all if, in the nurse's judgment, the patient does not require it. There are several alternatives to giving medications to relieve pain. Sometimes altering the patient's position, straightening out the bedclothes and rearranging the pillows, giving a back massage, or talking with the patient may relieve his pain. (The subject of pain is discussed in Chapter 31). In Mr. Jordan's case, he is having severe pain and it is important that the medication for pain be given sufficiently early to keep him comfortable and relaxed at all times while the pain is so severe. Restlessness caused by mounting pain could cause further injury to his damaged vertebrae.

NURSING CARE PLANS

To facilitate the implementation of nursing action, many agencies have developed a system of nursing care plans. The nursing care plan is just what one would expect it to be: the plan of care for the patient. It usually includes a statement of the patient's problems, the expected outcomes that have been established and the specific nursing measures which are to be used in caring for the patient. The care plan is developed as soon after the patient's admission as sufficient data are available on which to base a plan. It is developed by the nurse who has primary responsibility for the patient's care; or, in some agencies, it is developed jointly by the nursing team responsible for caring for the patient.

TABLE 10–1.

NURSING CARE PLAN		MR. PAUL JORDAN
Patient Problems	**Expected Outcomes**	**Nursing Directions**
1. Pain due to injury, aggravated by movement	1. Quiet and comfortable at all times. Calm facial expression, decreased restlessness, statements indicating that pain is lessened or absent	1. Medication for pain q4h. Give before pain too severe
2A. Limited mobility due to pain and prescribed position	2A. (a) Maintains prescribed position at all times except when on side for care	2A. (a) Prescribed position on back/bed flat: 2 pillows under head 1 pillow supporting shoulders 1 pillow under knees Verify that pt. understands prescribed position
	(b) Keeps trunk in good alignment at all times when turning on side	(b) May turn on side for back care, linen change. Pt. can help with turning Teach "log-rolling" technique for turning; repeat p.r.n.
	(c) When allowed out of bed, maintains trunk in good alignment at all times when sitting, standing, walking	(c) Discuss long-range plans with pt.'s M.D.
2B. Potential problem of loss of strength and tone in unused muscles	2B. Prevent	2B. Same as 2A (c)
2C. Potential problem of contractures in ankle joints	2C. Prevent	2C. Apply footboard and cradle to bed
3. Sensitivity to touch in lower back area due to site of injury, bruised tissues	3. Absences of sudden involuntary movements and verbal expressions of pain or facial grimaces when given care	3. Use gentle movements, extreme care when giving back massage, assisting pt. with bath, or giving other care Avoid pressure on vertebral column, also bruised area
4. Potential deviations in vital signs because of possibility of internal injuries	4. Normal vital signs	4. Monitor v.s. q4h Report deviations from normal Observe: (a) Rate, volume, quality of pulse (b) B.P., watching for marked or sudden change (c) Rate and depth of respirations (d) Temperature (e) Color and temperature of skin
5. Difficulty in voiding, owing to possible nerve damage or internal injuries	5. Normal urinary output	5. (a) Intake and output q shift (b) Observe output: 1. Amount 2. Color 3. Blood in urine (c) Report promptly if no output >8 hr. or output under 200 cc. q shift
6. Anxiety due to uncertainty about M.D.'s plan of care, prognosis	6. Relieved by information as evidenced by verbal statements and relaxed facial expression	6. Ask M.D. to explain his plans and discuss prognosis with pt.
7. Anxiety due to loss of clothes and valuables	7. Relieved by information that belongings have been found, as evidenced by verbal statements of pt.	7. Request social worker to come in as soon as possible
8. Possible decreased mental alertness due to medication for pain (a) May fall from bed (b) May burn self when smoking or set bed on fire	8. (a) Prevent (b) Prevent	8. (a) 1. Apply siderails to bed 2. Keep siderails up at all times (b) Delegate someone to stay with pt. when smoking q shift
9A. Dry mouth due to NRO	9A. Moist lips and tongue; moist mucous membranes in oral cavity at all times	9A. Oral hygiene q4h and p.r.n. Offer chewing gum p.r.n. Check with M.D. about ice chips to suck Offer lip moisturizer q4h p.r.n.

TABLE 10–1. *(Continued)*

NURSING CARE PLAN   MR. PAUL JORDAN

Patient Problems	Expected Outcomes	Nursing Directions
9B. Potential problem of dry mucous membranes in oral cavity, lips dry and cracking (see #9A)	9B. Prevent, as evidenced by #9A	9B. As in #9A
9C. Potential problem of maintaining nutritional status due to NPO	9C. Prevent	9C. 5% D/S I.V. t.i.d. × 2 (see medication order) Check with M.D. about d/c
10. Potential pressure areas over bony prominences: sacral area, heels, elbows (due to #2)	10. Prevent, as evidenced by good condition of skin, absence of redness and abrasions	10. (a) Gentle massage of back and areas mentioned q4h Use hospital lotion Be careful when massaging back (see 1.b) Pt. can be on side for back massage (note instructions above) (b) Apply lubricant to elbows, heels
11. Potential problem of constipation due to NPO and bed rest	11. Normal bowel movement q1-2 days	11. Note B.M. record q shift Check with pt. daily in a.m. Report deviation from normal Observe stools for signs of blood (see #5)
12. (a) Inability to look after own hygiene	12. (a) Maintains good hygiene at all times	12. (a) Assist pt. with bed bath daily Pt. can clean teeth himself— needs help to hold kidney basin Comb hair daily after bath and p.r.n. Pt. can clean and cut fingernails Clean and cut toenails p.r.n.
(b) Potential problem of poor status of skin and appendages	(b) Prevent. Skin clean and in good condition at all times; hair untangled at all times; nails clean, in good condition	(b) As in #12(a)
13. Potential feelings of isolation (family far away, friends working)	13. Prevent, as evidenced by patient's verbal statements	13. Request a friend to phone family in East Encourage friends to visit when not working
14. Potential problem of anxiety over finances due to anticipated lengthy convalescence and possibility of having to change occupation	14. Prevent, as evidenced by patient's verbal statements following discussions with social worker	14. Alert social worker to potential problem (see #7)

Because the patient's problems may change from day to day when he is acutely ill, the nursing care plan for the sick person is constantly under revision. Care plans for patients in ambulatory care settings, and for those in extended care facilities, also need frequent revision but usually not as often as those for patients in acute care settings.

In some agencies, the nursing action to be taken is written in terms of nursing orders, which are prescribed and followed through in much the same way as doctors' orders. In other agencies, the term "nursing approach," "nursing actions," or "nursing directions" may be used to identify the specific nursing interventions to be used in the care of the patient.

The nursing care plan is a means of communicating in writing, to other nursing personnel and to other members of the health team, the patient's problems, the expected outcomes of nursing care, and the specific nursing action to be taken in the care of the patient. In many agencies, the care plans are incorporated into the patient's record; in some, they form part of a Kardex report. Sometimes a separate notebook is kept for nursing care plans.

A nursing care plan for Mr. Jordan is shown on pages 188–189.

Standard Care Plans

Because nurses have found that most patients with similar types of conditions have many problems in common, a number of agencies have developed standard care plans for use with patients who have a particular type of condition. There might be a standard care plan for all medical patients, for example, supplemented by a plan for all patients who have suffered a stroke. There might be another standard care plan for all surgical patients, supplemented by one for patients who are having one particular type of surgical intervention. It should be noted that space is always left on these standard care plans for unusual problems which a patient has—problems that are not anticipated and are unique to this patient.

IMPLEMENTING NURSING ACTION

Once nursing care plans have been developed, the next step is to put them into action. The nursing directions (or nursing approach or orders) must be sufficiently detailed and sufficiently specific to enable all nursing personnel to carry them out in the same manner and at the designated times.

In some agencies, the nursing care plans are supplemented by a record that lists the nursing directions (taken from the care plan) and provides spaces for the nurse to tick as each intervention is carried out. This type of record acts as a checklist for the nurse responsible for the patient's care on each shift so she may quickly see what is to be done. It is also easy to see at a glance if any intervention was omitted.

Another type of form, similar in purpose to the one described above, is the flowsheet. When one specific intervention or a group of related interventions are to be done on a regular basis (as, for example, daily, or at more frequent intervals), it is helpful to have a special form which details the intervention specifically and documents the results of that intervention. See Chapter 11 (*Recording*) for more details.

In implementing nursing action, the nurse may give direct care to a patient or engage in indirect activities which contribute to his care. She may give the patient a bath, administer his medications, or supervise others in doing these things for him. Nursing care includes a wide variety of specific nursing interventions. As the student progresses through her educational program, she will learn a good many types of interventions, and will continue to do so throughout her nursing career. Specific nursing interventions in Mr. Jordan's care have been identified in the plan of care prepared for him.

EVALUATING EFFECTIVENESS OF NURSING ACTION

Throughout her care, the nurse constantly evaluates the progress the patient has made toward reaching the pre-established objectives. Evaluation is the process of determining the extent to which objectives have been attained. It implies measurement against predetermined standards. If the expected outcome of nursing care has been carefully thought through and the standards have been clearly stated, the nurse can compare the patient's attainments with these standards. For example, in Mr. Jordan's case, one expected outcome for his problem of limited mobility has been stated as "maintains prescribed position at all times, except when necessary to turn on side for care." The physician has been very explicit in describing the prescribed position. In evaluating the patient's attainment of the expected outcome, the nurse checks through the points enumerated regarding the position. Is Mr. Jordan's bed flat? Is he on his back? Does he have two pillows under his head? Is one supporting his shoulders? Does he have a pillow under his knees? Is he maintaining this position at all times, except when it is necessary to turn on his side for a back rub or for the bed linen to be changed?

In evaluating the effectiveness of nursing action it is important to have definite

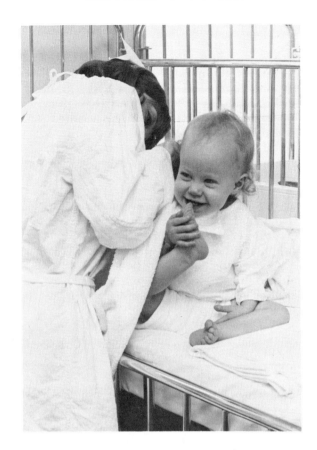

Throughout her care the nurse constantly evaluates the patient's progress toward attaining the expected outcomes of her nursing interventions.

criteria in mind. These criteria should be observable and they should be measurable. Then progress can be noted and, if a particular nursing approach does not appear to be effective, an alternative course of action can be tried. The attainment of certain objectives may mean that the patient is ready for more far-reaching ones. The patient who has learned to dress himself, for example, may be ready to learn other activities of daily living.

Stating criteria in question form helps the nurse to be objective and to look for specific indications that expected outcomes have been met. Questions are not always written down, but the beginning nurse may find it easier to develop the habit of asking herself the questions implicit in the nursing goals for the patient if she does put them onto paper.

The effectiveness of nursing care is evaluated by the nurse through her observations of the patient. Is his paralyzed arm in good anatomical position, or is the hand in a dependent position? It is also necessary to ask the patient if nursing in-tervention has been effective. Is he more comfortable? Is he free from pain?

In addition to evaluating the effectiveness of nursing action in relation to the patient's attainment of the expected outcomes, the nurse examines critically the soundness of the plan that was developed. Did she have enough information? Did she take all relevant factors into consideration in assessing the data she had? Did she omit any problems for which nursing care could have helped this patient? Were the priorities she established indeed the most important things to be taken care of? Was her plan a logical outgrowth of the problems she identified? Did she take into consideration unique factors in regard to this patient? Was her plan consistent with the physician's plan of therapy? Were the expected outcomes logical and attainable, in view of the patient's problems? Were the nursing directions clearly stated? Was the plan successful? Were there factors that interfered with its success? Factors that contributed to its success? Is the plan current and up-to-date? Have some of the problems been resolved? Have any new ones emerged?

As was stated at the beginning of Chapter 9, the nursing process is a circular one. Evaluation means a reassessment and a gathering of additional new information. On the basis of her reassessment, the nurse may identify new problems, modify her plan of care, or decide to try alternative interventions for ones that were unsuccessful.

To complete the story on Mr. Jordan: his clothes and valuables were found; they had been left in the plane and the air charter company returned them (one problem resolved). He was taken off NPO after 48 hours (another problem resolved) and progressed through a normal convalescence. His nursing care plan needed to be revised several times.

REVIEW OF THE NURSING PROCESS

The nursing process provides a methodology for a systematic approach to nursing care. The four basic steps in the process (assessment, planning, implementation, and evaluation) follow one another in logical, sequential order.

Nursing is primarily concerned with assisting an individual to cope with the daily activities of living in such a way as to promote his optimal level of health, or to cope with the exigencies of terminal illness, if such be the case. In order to help the individual, the nurse needs to know something about him as a person, his usual coping abilities, anything which is interfering with these, and his present status in relation to these abilities. She also needs to know the plans his physi-cian has for his care if the individual has a recognized health problem.

The nurse gathers the information she needs from several sources. Some of it she collects herself through the nursing history and through her observations of the patient; some comes from the individual's family, his friends, or significant others. She also utilizes data collected by other health professionals and she makes use of records, reports, and other forms of written material to extend her data base about the patient.

She analyzes the information she has gathered from all sources in order to identify problems that can be resolved by nursing actions, and to set priorities for action.

She uses relevant scientific principles gained from her studies to guide her in establishing objectives that define the expected outcomes of nursing action in terms of the patient's behavior and in developing a plan for nursing interventions that will enable the patient to attain these objectives.

Continuous reassessment takes place during the process of implementing the plan of care as new information is gathered and the patient's progress in attaining the expected outcomes is evaluated. Implicit in this reassessment is the need for constant revision of nursing care plans as new problems emerge, some are resolved, and some change. Priorities may need to be reordered, objectives modified or new ones established, and decisions made regarding appropriate nursing interventions in the light of new information, changes that have occurred in the patient's condition, and the success or failure of interventions that have been tried.

STUDY VOCABULARY	Actual problem Flowsheets Nursing intervention	Potential problem Problem	Principle Need

STUDY SITUATION: In conjunction with your instructor, select one patient:

1. Take the nursing history of this patient.
2. Do a clinical appraisal of this patient.

3. Gather other data about this patient which you feel you need in order to plan his care.
4. Identify nursing problems.
5. Develop a list of the patient's problems, in order of priority as you see them.
6. Identify principles relative to this patient's care.
7. Develop a plan of care for the patient, including:
    (a) The patient's problems.
    (b) The expected outcomes of care.
    (c) Nursing directions.
8. Explain how you would go about implementing the plan of care.
9. Describe how you would evaluate the effectiveness of the plan.

SUGGESTED READINGS

Bloch, D.: Evaluation of Nursing Care in Terms of Process and Outcome: Issues in Research and Quality Assurance. *Nursing Research, 24*:256–263, July-August 1975.

Browning, M. H., and Minehan, L. (eds.): *The Nursing Process in Practice* (Contemporary Nursing Series). New York, American Journal of Nursing Company, 1974.

Curtis, J., Rothert, M., and Christian, B.: A Practical Evaluation of Nursing Care as Part of the Nursing Process. *Nursing Digest*, p. 20, May-June 1975.

Eddy, L., et al.: Multidisciplinary Retrospective Patient Care Audit. *American Journal of Nursing, 75*:961–963, June 1975.

Ethridge, P. E., and Packard, R. W.: An Innovative Approach to Measurement of Quality Through Utilization of Nursing Care Plans. *Journal of Nursing Administration, 6*:25–31, January 1976.

Gebbie, K., et al.: Classifying Nursing Diagnoses. *American Journal of Nursing, 74*:250–253, February 1974.

Gero, S. V., and Haffke, E. D.: Two Missing Pieces: A New Formula for Solving Nursing Problems. *Nursing '73: 3*:32–35, March 1973.

Little, D. E., and Carnevali, D. L.: *Nursing Care Planning*. Philadelphia, J. B. Lippincott Company, 1969.

Marriner, A.: *The Nursing Process: A Scientific Approach to Nursing Care.* St. Louis, C. V. Mosby Company, 1975.

Mundinger, M. O'N., and Jauron, G. D.: Developing a Nursing Diagnosis. *Nursing Outlook, 23*:94–98, February 1975.

Yura, H., and Walsh, M. B.: *The Nursing Process: Assessing, Planning, Implementing, Evaluating.* 2nd edition. New York, Appleton-Century-Crofts, 1973.

11   RECORDING

The nurse should be able to:

Explain the principal purpose of the patient's record

List types of information that are kept on this record

Describe ways in which the record is used

Discuss the use of the patient's record in monitoring the quality of
    care

Describe the following parts of the traditional patient's record,
    including the type of information contained on it and nursing
    responsibilities in regard to it:
    1. Fact sheet
    2. Doctor's order sheet
    3. History sheet

Outline pertinent data that should be included in the nurse's
    notes for each of the five categories of information recorded

List information included in the data base of the POMR

Write a patient profile based on the data collected in the nursing
    history

Discuss the use of the problem list as an index to the patient's
    record

Write narrative notes using the SOAP format

Discuss the initial plans portion of the POMR as a source of
    information for the nurse

Name four guiding points to keep in mind when recording

INTRODUCTION

Recording is the communication in writing of essential facts in order to maintain a continuous history of events over a period of time. Reporting is the communication of information to another individual (or group of individuals) and may be either written or oral. A number of different records and report forms are kept by various health agencies, and the nurse will find that these vary from one agency to another. All types of health agencies maintain a patient's record or chart, however. The form of the record formerly depended on the type of agency—that is, hospitals used one type of patient record, public health agencies another, and extended care institutions yet another.

The introduction of the system called Problem-Oriented Medical Records has, however, caused a revolution in the recording practices of many agencies. Since the POMR, as it is usually abbreviated, can be utilized equally effectively in all types of agencies, it is doing much to bring about greater uniformity in health records. In fact, some authors have stated the day may be coming when each individual carries a list of his health problems and record of therapy with him and presents it to whatever health practitioner or agency he has engaged to undertake his health care.[1]

Not all agencies have yet adopted the problem-oriented system of records however, and the nurse may work in a hospital or other agency in which the traditional type of patient record is used. We will, therefore, describe briefly both systems of recording. There are, of course, some commonalities in both systems; the purpose of the patient's record remains the same, and there are some general rules for recording that are applicable in both systems.

THE PURPOSE OF THE PATIENT'S RECORD

A person's record or chart is a written record of his health history, his health problem(s), the diagnostic and therapeutic measures used to assist in the identification and treatment of his health problem(s), and his response to therapy while he is a patient in the agency. In other words, it is a record of the events that took place during the period of time he was receiving care in a particular agency.

Hospitals and other types of health agencies are required to keep records by state/provincial laws and by regulatory agencies such as those concerned with accreditation. A variety of records are kept by health agencies in addition to patient records. For example, there are financial records, records of births, details of communicable diseases, and records relevant to narcotic legislation. The nurse is concerned chiefly with the patient's health care record, which contains information regarding his nursing care as well as the care he has received from the physician and other members of the health team.

The chief purpose of the patient's record is to provide a written record of data that have been gathered about the patient; thus it serves as a means of communication among those whose professional talents are directed towards his care. This concise compilation of data serves as the basis upon which the physician plans his diagnostic and therapeutic regime for the patient and the nurse plans

---

[1]Mary Woody and Mary Mallinson: The Problem-Oriented System for Patient Care. *American Journal of Nursing*, 73:1168–1175, July 1973.

her care. Physicians other than the one primarily responsible for the patient's care (such as specialists—e.g., the radiologist, the pathologist, and other consultants called in by the attending physician) contribute information to the patient's record, as do a variety of other members of the health team. The patient's record, as we have already noted, is a valuable source of information for the nurse in the development of her plan of care for the patient.

The patient's record is a legal document and is admissible as evidence in court. Some jurisdictions, in recognition of the confidentiality of communications between the patient and his physician, have ruled that information gathered in such a setting is inadmissible in court if the patient objects. Although the record is the property of the health agency, it is generally felt nowadays that the patient has a right to the information contained on his record.[2] The current emphasis on the patient's rights has strengthened this viewpoint, although in many agencies, it is still not considered right or proper for the patient to read his own record. Some people contend, however, that, if the patient is to be considered an equal partner on the health team, it is essential not only that he have access to the information on his record, but that he also check the accuracy of it. The nurse will have to be guided by the policy of the agency in which she is working in regard to the matter of whether the patient does or does not see his chart.

With the increasing stress on the accountability of all health professionals to the people they serve, the function of the patient's record as a means of documenting the care he has received has become very important. The POMR is very helpful in this regard in that the physician, the nurse, and all other members of the health team must, in this type of recording system, not only state the care the patient has received but also give their reasons for that care. The patient's progress is systematically noted and it is easy to review

the record to make sure that all the things that should have been done for the patient have, in fact, been done. Thus, the record provides a means of checking on the quality of care that the patient has received.

Patients' records also provide material for research. Many disciplines in the health field avail themselves of this source of information in a diversity of research programs—for example, to show trends in the utilization of the services of a community health agency. The records maintained by health agencies are also a source of statistical information used by governments in the compilation of information about the health status of people and health conditions in the municipality, state/province, or country (see Chapter 4). Statistical information, such as the number of births, deaths, or hospital admissions in a health agency and the like, also serves as as basis for making plans for the future and anticipating the health needs of people in a given area. Some of the statistics are required by law; for example, the record of births must be filed with a government agency.

Another use of the patient's record is in the education of students in the health disciplines. The record provides learners with a comprehensive picture of the patient, his problems, and the care planned for him. Nursing students, medical students, interns, residents, and students in virtually all of the health disciplines utilize patient records as reference sources. The records enable them to see the application of theory in a practical situation.

Nursing Audit

The *nursing audit* consists of a review of patient records to evaluate the quality of nursing care as documented in the record. It is a retrospective audit in that it is looking back to see if the care given by the nurse has met established standards for care. The process of care, as documented in the record, is compared with criteria for good nursing care as determined by members of the nursing profession.

A nursing audit may be undertaken to evaluate either the quality of care given

---

[2]Rosemarian Berni and Helen Readey: Problem-Oriented Medical Record Implementation. St. Louis, C. V. Mosby Company, 1974, p. 17.

by individual nurses or the care provided by the entire agency. In either case, it is individual patient records that are reviewed. A nursing audit committee within the agency is responsible for determining the standards of care to be met. If the agency's quality of nursing care is being evaluated, an outside committee would be established from, for example, members of the state (provincial) nurses' association. Because these audits are done by members of the same professional group, the procedure is often referred to as *peer review*.

Criteria are established through such aspects of care as: the date base; the identification of problems; the expected outcomes of care; the selection of nursing interventions; and the degree to which the plan of care was carried out, as evidenced by the nurse's notations on the patient's record. In measuring the quality of the process of care, one asks: "Was everything done that should have been done?" In evaluating the outcomes of care, one asks: "What were the results of care in terms of changes in the patient's health status?" So far, auditing procedures for judging the quality of care have been developed to a greater extent than those for evaluating the outcomes of care.

Another mechanism for establishing quality assurance in nursing care is the development of *standards* for nursing service, which outline criteria in respect to the structure of services provided. Are the facilities, equipment, and personnel adequate to permit nurses to give good, high-quality nursing care? The ANA has developed standards with respect to both nursing care and nursing services, and the CNA is currently in the process of developing similar standards.

MEDICAL TERMINOLOGY

The nurse may find it helpful at this point to have a knowledge of some of the terminology used by physicians (and others) in their notations on the patient's record.

Pathology refers to the disease process itself; it is generally classified as either organic or functional. *Organic pathology* refers to diseases which can be identified physically—a tumor or a communicable disease, for example. *Functional pathology* refers to diseases which have no apparent physical basis; emotional disturbances frequently come under this heading. With the intensive research that is being conducted at the present time, the line between organic pathology and functional pathology has become less distinct and their frequent interrelatedness is recognized. The term *psychosomatic* illness is used to refer to the connectivity between emotional factors and organic illness as, for example, between anxiety and a peptic ulcer.

A *medical diagnosis* is the physician's opinion of the nature of the disease. *Prognosis* means the medical opinion as to the final outcome of the disease process. A prognosis can be described as negative, positive, or uncertain, and as good, poor, or fair.

A *symptom* is evidence that there is a disease process or disturbance in body function. *Subjective symptoms* are those symptoms that can be perceived only by the patient. For example, the patient is really the only person who can describe his pain. Through her observation of the patient's facial expression or his body position, the nurse may interpret that a patient has, or does not have, pain, but only the patient himself can actually describe this symptom. An *objective symptom* is one that can be observed and described by others. A flushed face, a swollen ankle, and rapid respirations can all be observed and described objectively. Subjective and objective symptoms are, in fact, the same things as the subjective and objective observations we noted in Chapter 7.

A *sign* is an objective symptom that is detected through special examination. For example, fever is detected by the clinical thermometer, an abnormal heart beat by the stethoscope.

Prefixes and suffixes commonly used in medical terms are listed in the appendix.

THE TRADITIONAL PATIENT RECORD

The traditional patient record used in a great many health agencies generally has the following components:

1. An admission sheet
2. A face sheet
3. A doctor's order sheet
4. A history sheet
5. Nurses' notes
6. Other reports and records, reports of laboratory and x-ray findings, such as preoperative anesthetic record and surgical report, and the results of other diagnostic and therapeutic measures the patient has.

The Admission Sheet

Most agencies have an admission sheet upon which are recorded basic biographical and some social data about the patient. This sheet is generally completed upon admission to an agency and then sent to the nurse or to the nursing unit to become a part of the patient's chart. Admission sheets contain accurate information which the nurse can transcribe to other records when necessary. The material on this sheet, like all the material in the chart, is confidential, to be disclosed only to professional people.

Often admission sheets record a unit number for the patient. This number serves as one means of identification and as a basis for cataloging medical records. The information on the admission sheet generally includes:

1. Patient's full name, including maiden name
2. Address
3. Classification number
4. Nursing unit or agency
5. Date and hour of admission
6. Date of birth
7. Name of physician
8. Details of financial responsibility
9. Sex and marital status
10. Nearest relative
11. Occupation and employer
12. Diagnosis
13. Previous admission or previous call
14. Religion

The Face Sheet

The face sheet is the front sheet of a chart; it has a diversity of uses. Frequently it is used to record allergies, but it is also used to record the history at discharge, in which case it is completed by the physician at the end of the patient's care.

The nurse's responsibilities are generally minimal with respect to the face sheet. Usually the headings and the notation of a patient's allergies are recorded when a patient is admitted to the agency.

The Doctors' Order Sheet

The doctors' order sheet is a written record of the orders given by the physician for the patient's treatment. The sheet may be kept with the patient's chart; however, in some hospitals it is kept in a central book on the nursing unit.

Doctors' order sheets are checked regularly by the nursing staff for new orders. Frequently a nursing unit has a method of flagging a patient's chart to indicate that a new order has been written. When the nurse has noted and put into effect an order, she indicates this in the prescribed manner on the order sheet.

In some hospitals when the physician orders a medication that is not kept on the nursing unit, he writes his order on a prescription pad as well as on the chart, so that the order can be sent to the pharmacy and a record kept on the nursing unit.

When the physician telephones an order to the nursing staff, the nurse so indicates on the order sheet. She also enters the name of the doctor, the time of the order, and her own signature. Frequently doctors are asked to countersign their telephone orders when they subsequently visit the patient.

The History Sheet

The history sheet is a record of the personal and medical history of the patient; it is filled in by the physician. Frequently the doctor also describes the therapeutic regime for the patient and makes notes on the medical progress of the patient after each visit.

The history sheet can be a valuable ref-

SPEEDISET   MOORE BUSINESS FORMS LTD.

RIVERSIDE HOSPITAL OF OTTAWA	NOV 4 77

PHYSICIAN'S ORDERS

ATTENDING PHYSICIAN _Dr. L. S. White_

ALLERGIC TO _____

SMITH   MARY   SP 1246
2321 MARKET ST OTT 234-7566 600
JONES   RICHARD   HUS
SAME
23.10.77   2PM F 23 M SURG RC

420 1

DATE	TIME	ORDERS	EXECUTED
Sept 1/77	2 pm	DAT	Noted
		Up as desired	Noted
		APC ⚬ C 30 mg tab I q4h prn for headache	T
		Seconal 100 mg qhs prn	T
		Consult to Dr. Brown regarding headaches	Notified 2:30 pm
		Hgb, Hct, WBC, Diff on admission	Done
		AC blood sugar in a.m.	Req
		Large chest x-ray in a.m.	Req
		Valium 5 mg T i.d. pc & qhs	T ordered
		Dr. White	

NURSE SHALL CLOSE OFF ORDER
SHEET IF NO PHARMACY COPY.

IMPORTANT: NURSE SHALL USE COPY BENEATH AS
PHARMACY REQUISITION.
EACH ORDER MUST BE SIGNED
PHYSICIAN'S ORDER

FORM #2 - 8208

FORM #2 - 8208   PHARMACY COPY A

A sample physician's order sheet. (Courtesy of the Riverside Hospital of Ottawa.)

erence for the nurse in making her nursing care plan for the patient. It provides information about the patient's present medical condition, previous illnesses, family history, and current medical therapy.

The Nurses' Notes

The nurses' notes in a patient's chart can serve as a record of the medical and related therapies, including nursing, and the responses of the patient to these ministrations. In some agencies only nurses record these notes, whereas in others the auxiliary nursing staff, which includes orderlies and nursing aides, also record their care and observations of patients.

Generally the nurses' notes serve to record and convey five categories of information:

1. Therapeutic measures carried out by various members of the health team
2. Measures ordered by the physician and carried out by nursing personnel
3. Nursing measures which are not ordered by the physician but which the nurse carries out to meet the specific needs of a patient
4. Behavior and other observations of the patient which are considered to be pertinent to his general health
5. Specific responses of the patient to therapy and care

In many situations the nurses' notes serve as a record of the therapeutic measures that are carried out by various members of the health team. For example, when the physician changes a dressing on a patient's wound, it is recorded by the nurse in these notes. She includes not only the name of the doctor performing the procedure but also relevant details such as the appearance of the wound, the amount and nature of any discharge, the application of a medication or dressing and the removal of sutures. In some agencies, the nurse also records visits by the doctor and other members of the health team, such as the physical therapist and dietitian. This type of charting serves chiefly as a record of care and therapy and therefore as a communication tool for all members of the health team.

Nurses also record measures that are prescribed by the physician and for which the nurse has the primary responsibility. For example, the nurse records the administration of medications ordered by the physician and the time they were given. She also notes any unusual difficulties she encountered in administering the medication or unusual reactions observed in the patient. If a patient refuses to take a medication which has been prescribed, this fact is noted, together with the patient's stated reason for refusal wherever possible.

The third type of recording comprises the nursing measures that are independent nursing functions. These are the measures not ordered by the physician, but rather those the nurse judges to be necessary for the patient's care.

The nurses' notes also serve as a record of behavior observed in the patient that the nurse considers pertinent to his health problems or which constitutes a problem in itself. Behavior in this sense includes not only body action but emotional tone, verbal communication, and autonomic physiological reactions. In this type of recording, objective observations are made and then recorded, the description being as complete and concise as possible. In describing verbal communication which reflects emotional tone, the nurse uses direct quotations rather than a paraphrase.

Often, the lack of a bodily reaction can be significant, and this information should also be recorded. For example, the lack of shortness of breath in a patient who sits in a chair after spending four weeks in bed can be significant in determining the ability of the patient to tolerate increased activity.

The fifth area of charting is the specific response of the patient to therapeutic and nursing care measures. This includes the effect of an analgesic on pain, of a sponge bath on a fever, and of the application of cold to a swollen joint. In recording such reactions, the nurse records the perceptions of the patient and objective observations, such as a reduction in temperature or in the swelling of a joint. When the patient's perceptions are recorded, this fact should be made clear in the record. Frequently, a patient perceives a situation differently from the way the nurse does, and this fact in itself could be important to his care.

When recording in the nurses' notes, the date and time that a patient receives a treatment or a medication are noted accurately. Time is often denoted by the use of A.M. or P.M., although most agencies use the 24 hour clock to avoid ambiguity. Each entry in the nurses' notes is accompanied by the legal signature of the person who does the recording.

THE PROBLEM-ORIENTED MEDICAL RECORD

The POMR is simply a method of documenting the problem-oriented approach to patient care. We have just spent two chapters discussing this approach to nursing care. The POMR system of recording reflects the increasing use of the problem-oriented approach by all members of the health team in all aspects of patient care.

The student who has understood the problem-oriented approach to nursing care and is able to apply this in the clinical situation should have no difficulty in understanding the POMRs nor in learning to record in the format prescribed. We have deliberately introduced some of the terminology that has developed in regard to the POMR in the previous two chapters in order to acquaint the student with the language used. We have also discussed some of the forms used in the POMR because they serve a dual purpose of assisting in the planning and implementation of nursing care and in the documentation of care.

Components of the POMR

The problem-oriented medical record has four components:
1. A data base
2. A problem list
3. Initial plans or orders
4. Progress notes

The Data Base. The data base contains the information that is considered necessary for the development of a comprehensive plan of care for the patient. It is a "defined" data base in that there usually are specific instructions on what information is to be gathered. Questionnaires have been developed and are used by most agencies to ensure that the needed data is gathered. What is included depends on the type of patient with whom the record is being used. For example, if the record is intended for use with patients who have one particular health problem such as hypertension, the information gathered will probably concentrate on factors particularly relevant to this condition.

The data base usually includes:
1. Information about the patient's chief complaint, or reason for admission to the health agency
2. A description of his present illness and a systems review
3. The patient's medical history
4. A patient profile
5. Findings from the initial physical examination.
6. Baseline laboratory data and x-ray findings
7. The nursing history

Most of this information is gathered by the physician and the nurse in their initial assessments of the patient. If special data have been requested to be gathered by other members of the health team, this information is also included in the data base.

The nurse who took the nursing history is usually responsible for preparing the patient profile. The profile is intended to give members of the health team working with the patient a "thumbnail sketch" of this person as an individual. The information contained in the profile varies somewhat from one agency to another. Generally, however, it includes some of the basic social data which the nurse has collected about the individual, pertinent information about his lifestyle and personal habits that may be significant in his care, any physical disabilities that he has, his ability to communicate, and the availability of family or significant others. The following patient, for example, has been referred to a rehabilitation center from an acute care hospital.

Mrs. Doe is 72 years old and was admitted to the Center on referral from _____ Hospital. She has right hemiparesis and aphasia due to left cerebral accident on 5/5/71. Historian is husband, aged 83 years, a retired civil servant on limited income. He is attentive and protective towards his wife; seems interested in learning about her care. States his goal is to assist his wife to return home and have some pleasure in life. They are proud of their four well-educated children, three sons and one daughter, all of whom live a major distance from them. Mr. and Mrs. Doe have a modern, two-bedroom, one-floor house in _____ (city) _____ (state). Mr. Doe plans to rent an apartment near the Center so he can visit his wife daily.*

The patient profile is usually affixed to the front of the patient's chart. In many agencies, the nurse also includes the profile as part of her admission notes on the chart.

The Problem List. Problems are identified from the data base of information collected about the patient. If the data base is incomplete, this becomes the first problem on the list. The patient's physician is responsible for developing the initial problem list; the nurse and other members of the health team contribute to its development.

The identified problems are listed in order of priority; each problem is dated and assigned a number. The problem list becomes an index for the rest of the patient's record and is placed at the beginning of the record. All subsequent notations made are referred to the numbered problems. Problems that are resolved are identified with the date of their resolution.

The problem list is kept current and up-to-date by the dating of resolved problems, new statements of those that have changed, and the addition of new problems that have arisen since the original list was compiled. Erasures usually are not permitted. If new information causes a change in the index, the new problem (with a different number) is added to the list, and reference is made to the previous number.

As we stated earlier, a problem has been defined as anything with which the patient requires help. The statement of the problem may be a diagnosis, a symptom, or a finding. Psychosocial, economic,

and demographic problems (such as excessive smoking or eating) are included, as well as physical ones.

An example of a numbered patient problem list is shown on page 203.

Problems are identified as either active or inactive—that is, active problems are those the patient has now and inactive ones are those he had previously. The inactive ones are usually shown in a separate column and usually are not numbered. An arrow is often placed after an active problem which requires resolution. When it is resolved, the date of resolution may be written along the line of the arrow, or in a separate column.

Potential problems—those which are suggested by findings but which have not yet developed into actual problems, such as an initial occurrence of vomiting—are not included in the problem list but are written up in the progress notes. If they do turn out to be actual active problems, they are then added to the active problem list.

Initial Plans or Orders. The initial plans for the patient's care are made relative to each problem on the active list. The plans are numbered to correspond with the number of the problem. The plan for each problem contains three parts: the diagnostic measures, therapeutic measures, and a plan for patient education. The doctors' order sheet is an extension of these plans. Orders are written, again being numbered to correspond with the number of the problem to which the order relates.

This system makes it much easier for the nurse to understand the reasoning behind the physician's diagnostic and therapeutic regimes for the patient and also the doctor's orders for medications and treatments. It also provides her with a better basis for planning nursing care. She is able to anticipate some of the patient's reactions and is guided in her observations in knowing better what to look for and what is important in her assessments of the patient. Knowing what the physician has planned in the way of patient education and what information he or she has told (or is going to tell) the patient is of considerable assistance to the nurse in planning her teaching program for the patient.

*Rosemarian Berni and Clyde Nicholson: The POR as a Tool in Rehabilitation and Patient Teaching. *Nursing Clinics of North America*, 9:267, 1974.

	PROBLEMS:	Originator's Initials	Physician	Active	Inactive
1	Left CVA	M.S.	J.B.	6/10/71	
2	Aphasia			6/10	
3	Ulcer Over Sacrum			6/10	
4	Urinary Incontinence			6/10	
5	Bowel Incontinence			6/10	6/23/71
6	Decreased Ambulation			6/10	
7	Decreased Activities of Daily Living			6/10	
8	Discharge Planning	M.S.		6/10	
9	Subluxation Rt. Shoulder		J.B.	6/11	

Problem list on patient Jane Doe. (From Rosemarian Berni and Clyde Nicholson: Nursing Clinics of North America, 9:266, 1974.)

INITIAL PLANS[3]

PATIENT: Jane Doe
(DATE, TIME)_____
#1 Lt. CVA
   a. Passive range of motion to Rt. U.E. with positioning.
   b. PROM. to Lt. L.E. to tolerance.
   c. Padded foot board.
   d. Confer with physiatrist.
   e. Teach patient and husband the exercises.
#2 *Aphasia* due to #1
   a. Record extent of language deficit.
   b. Use very short sentences or phrases.
   c. Test response to communication in pantomime only.
   d. Maintain frequent sensory input.

   e. Omit distractions when trying to communicate.
   f. Plan constant daily routine. Write schedule on patient's bulletin board for team information.
   g. Confer with speech pathologist.

Progress Notes. The progress notes provide a record of the progress made by the patient toward the resolution of his problems, as one would anticipate from the name of this component of the record. Therefore, notations made by the physician, the nurse, and other team members, laboratory and x-ray reports, the record of surgical intervention and of other diagnostic and therapeutic measures all form part of the progress notes. More strictly, however, the term "progress notes" is usually taken to refer to three parts of the overall record of progress: narrative notes, flowsheets, and the discharge summary.

NARRATIVE NOTES. These are the notations made by the physician, the nurse,

---

[3]Rosemarian Berni and Clyde Nicholson: The POR as a Tool in Rehabilitation and Patient Teaching. *Nursing Clinics of North America,* 9:267, June 1974.

and other members of the health team relative to the patient's problems. The narrative notes are numbered according to the problem to which they refer; they are dated; and the person making the notation affixes his signature and title at the bottom end of his notation. A specific format has been developed for the writing of narrative notes; it is usually referred to as the SOAP format because it contains Subjective observations, Objective observations, Assessments, and Plans.

The *Subjective notation* is the problem (or sign or symptom) as the patient perceives and expresses it. It is not the observer's interpretation of what he or she thought the patient meant. The patient's own words should be used, rather than an interpretation of what the observer thinks the person meant. If the patient is unable to communicate his thoughts or feelings, or does not do so, this section of the notation is left blank.

The *Objective notation* is what the observer sees, hears, or feels, or it includes observations made through the senses of seeing, hearing, touching and smelling, or with the aid of various tools, such as the thermometer, the stethoscope, and so forth (as described in Chapter 7). Laboratory and x-ray findings, and the findings from other diagnostic and therapeutic measures, are also included in the objective notation.

Assessments are the observer's impressions, interpretations, and conclusions drawn from the subjective and objective observations. All persons making notations are urged to state their assessments honestly, that is, at their level of skill and understanding of the situation. This is quite a change from the days not so long past when nurses were told not to write any impression or interpretations on the patient's chart, but to confine their comments to factual data.

The *Plan* communicates the specific action the observer intends to take to work toward the resolution of this particular problem. As in the initial plans, the observer is encouraged to think in terms of diagnostic, therapeutic, and teaching actions.

#5 *Bowel Incontinence* (date, time)[4]

S: Husband reports enemas given about every three days. Last accident—yesterday. Pt. "used to go to the bathroom right after breakfast."

O: Rectal sphincter tone present. Very soft stool on rectal glove. Rectum empty.

A: Loss of normal bowel function due to too many enemas.

P: 1. Evaluate bowel function for possible initiation of structured bowel program. Start daily record on flowsheet.
    2. Omit enemas.
    3. Order bedside commode and commode cushion.

Mary Smith, R.N.

FLOWSHEETS. The purpose of the flowsheet is to show in graphic form interventions or observations in respect to one particular problem. Flowsheets are usually developed for use for a designated period of time. They may cover a week or a 24 hour period. The TPR form used in most hospitals is an example of a flowsheet which is used to record vital signs for one week at a time. When it is necessary to monitor vital signs more frequently than every four hours, as is allowed for on the usual TPR form, a separate flowsheet would be used. The minute-to-minute monitoring of vital signs of patients in the intensive care unit of a hospital serves an appropriate example.

Flowsheets are helpful in ensuring continuity of care in that each nurse caring for the patient knows exactly what is to be done and when it is to be done. She can also note quickly the results of previous nursing interventions and assess the patient's progress in relation to the expected outcome. The flowsheet also serves to document the care that has been given. Notations made on it are not repeated on the narrative notes.

---

[4]Rosemarian Berni and Clyde Nicholson: The POR as a Tool in Rehabilitation and Patient Teaching. *Nursing Clinics of North America,* 9:267, June 1974.

Date	Start Related *Meal* Breakfast	Suppository Time	Toileting Time	Rectal Massage Time	B.M. Time	Description: Amount, Color, Consistency	Place
6/10/71	---	---	---	---	7 PM	Smearing, brown	Bed
6/11/71	7:15 AM	---	7:45 AM	---	10 AM	Smearing, brown	Bed
6/12/71	7:15 AM	7:45 AM	8:00 AM	8:15 AM	Noon	Smearing, brown	W.C.
6/13/71	7:15	7:45 AM	8:00	8:15 AM	8:20 AM	Small, brown, hard	Commode
6/14/71	7:15	7:45	8:00	8:15	8:30 AM	Moderate, brown, hard	Commode
6/14 PM	---	---	---	---	9:00 PM	Smearing	Bed
6/15/71	7:15	7:45	8:00	8:15	8:20 AM	Large, brown, formed	Commode
6/16/71	7:15	7:45	8:00	8:15 AM	8:20 AM	Moderate, brown, formed	Commode
6/17/71	7:15	7:45	8:00	D.C.	8:15 AM	Small, brown, formed	Commode
6/18/71	7:15	7:45	8:00	---	8:15 AM	Moderate, brown, formed	B.R.
6/19/71	7:15	7:45	8:00	---	8:20 AM	Small, brown, formed	B.R.
6/20/71	7:15	D.C.	8:00	---	8:20 AM	Moderate, brown, formed	B.R.
6/21/71	7:15	---	8:00	---	8:15 AM	Moderate, brown, formed	B.R.
6/22/71	7:15	---	8:00	---	8:20 AM	Small, brown, formed	B.R.
6/23/71	7:15	---	8:00	---	8:05 AM	Moderate, brown, formed	B.R.

Flow sheet for recording bowel program. (From Rosemarian Berni and Clyde Nicholson: Nursing Clinics of North America, 9:269, June 1974.)

An example of a flowsheet developed for a patient on a bowel retraining program is shown below. This particular flowsheet covers a 15 day period.

THE DISCHARGE SUMMARY. The physician in charge of the patient's care is usually responsible for writing the discharge summary when an individual leaves the agency. With the increasingly widespread use of the POMR system in community agencies, such as a visiting nurse agency, it may well be the nurse who prepares the discharge summary. The summary follows the format used elsewhere in the record—that is, notes are made concerning the progress attained in regard to each of the problems identified on the problem list. Again, the discharge notes are numbered by problem.

GUIDES TO CHARTING

The nurse may work in an agency in which the problem-oriented system of patient records has been implemented, or in one in which a traditional type of patient record is used. In either case, she will find that every agency has specific policies regarding charting on the patient's record.

Each nurse should be aware of the regulations for the agency for which she works. The following guides, however,

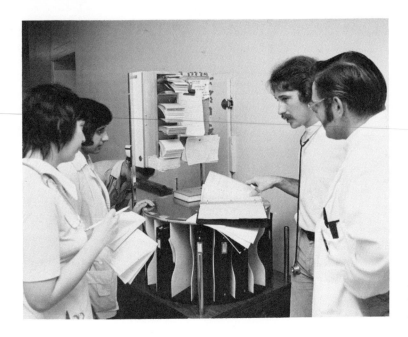

The patient's record is a valuable source of information for all members of the health team.

will help a nurse in her recording, no matter what the particular policy happens to be.

Accuracy

The nurse records all factors accurately and truthfully. The omission of a recording is as inaccurate as an incorrect recording. Time is recorded accurately in the notations the nurse makes; all treatments and medications are recorded immediately after their administration, never before. Observations are specific and accurate; for example, the pain of a patient is described in detail as to type, exact location, duration, and any precipitating factors and accompanying signs and symptoms.

Because the chart is a legal document, most agencies do not permit the use of

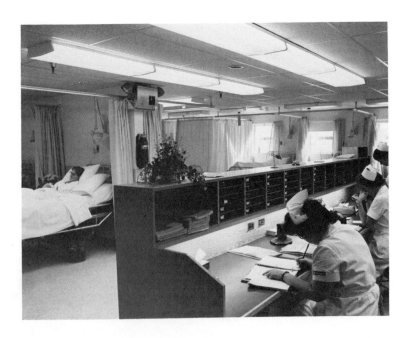

Charting is an important part of the nurse's daily responsibilities.

erasures when an error is made in recording. Each institution has its own method of correcting mistakes. It is not unusual to cross out the error with a single line and initial the error and then to insert the correct information immediately following the error.

Headings on the chart sheets are entered accurately. Many health agencies use Addressograph plates which print data about the patient directly on the sheet. An Addressograph plate usually prints the patient's name, date of admission, nursing unit (if applicable), agency unit number (some agencies have a classification system in which each patient has a number), and the name of the doctor. The Addressograph has the advantage of recording this information quickly and accurately.

Brevity

All recording is concise and complete. Vagueness is to be avoided. Extra words such as "patient" can usually be eliminated from charting because it is obvious that it is the patient about whom the nurse is recording.

Legibility

Most agencies permit either printing or script on a patient's chart, provided that the script is legible. Ink is used because pencil does not provide a permanent record.

In making entries on the patient's record, the nurse is required to sign her name following her notations. Her signature includes her first initial and full last name. In most health agencies the nurse is also required to record her status, for example, R.N.

Format

There is usually a standard format for recording, which ensures consistency and facility of communication. For example, all medications and treatments might be recorded on separate flowsheets (or in one

column of the nurse's notes if the traditional type of record is used).

Most agencies use blue or black ink for all charting, but occasionally red ink is used for night charting (2400 to 0700 hours).

COMMONLY USED TERMS AND ABBREVIATIONS

It is an important part of charting that only correct spelling and acceptable abbreviations be used. Some hospitals provide a list of abbreviations that are acceptable; others accept the commonly used abbreviations. The list below illustrates only a small portion of abbreviations in use. The student is advised to refer to medical terminology books and dictionaries that specialize in this type of material.

abd.	abdomen
A.M.	morning
amb.	ambulatory, walking
amt.	amount
approx.	approximately (about)
ax.	axillary (armpit)
B.M.	bowel movement
B.P.	blood pressure
B.R.P.	bathroom privileges
C	Celsius (Centigrade)
$\bar{c}$	with
ca	cancer
CBC	complete blood count
cc	cubic centimeters
C.D.	communicable disease
CHF	congestive heart failure
c/o	complains of pain
COPD	chronic obstructive pulmonary disease
CVA	cardiovascular accident
DC	discontinue
dist.	distilled
ECG (EKG)	electrocardiogram
E.R.	emergency room
exam	examination
F.	Fahrenheit
G.I.	gastrointestinal
G.U.	genitourinary
gr. $\bar{x}$	10 grains
gr. $\overline{iss}$.	1½ grains
h(hr.)	hour
hi-cal	high calorie
hi-vit	high vitamin

H_2O	water	p.r.n.	when necessary
h.s.	bedtime	Psych.	psychology (psychiatry)
I.M.	intramuscular	pt.	patient
invol.	involuntary	P.T.	physical therapist
irrig.	irrigate	q.	every
I and O	intake and output	r (resp.)	respirations
I.V.	intravenous	RBC	red blood cell
kg.	kilogram (weight)	R.L.E.	right lower extremity
lab.	laboratory	R.L.Q.	right lower quadrant
L.L.E.	left lower extremity	R.U.E.	right upper extremity
L.L.Q.	left lower quadrant	R.U.Q.	right upper quadrant
L.U.E.	left upper extremity	s̄.	without
L.U.Q.	left upper quadrant	S.C.	subcutaneous
mid.	middle	sp. gr.	specific gravity
min.	minute	stat	at once
no. (#)	number	staph	staphylococcus (microorganism)
noc.	night		
NPO	nothing by mouth	TL	team leader
O_2	oxygen	TPR	temperature, pulse, respiration
O.B.	obstetrics		
O.O.B.	out of bed	V.D.	venereal disease
O.R.	operating room	via	by way of
o.d.	right eye	WBC	white blood cell
o.s.	left eye	wt	weight
o.u.	each eye	×	times
p.	pulse	>	greater than
Ped(s).	pediatrics	<	less than
per	by or through	↑	increase(d)
p.o.	per os (by mouth)	↓	decrease(d)

STUDY VOCABULARY

Data base	Peer review	Psychosomatic
Medical diagnosis	POMR	Recording
Nursing audit	Problem list	Sign
Pathology	Prognosis	SOAP format
Patient profile	Progress notes	Symptom

STUDY SITUATION

Mrs. J. Rossten is a patient who has undergone abdominal surgery. She has been on the nursing unit three days postoperatively. Her orders from the physician include dressing changes once a day as necessary and Demerol, 100 mg. I. M. p.r.n., for pain.

Her dressing is soaked through with reddish brown fluid and she complains of pain. As her nurse you give her 100 mg. of Demerol and change her dressing.

The following questions should be answered for recording on:
a. A problem-oriented medical record
b. A traditional patient record.

1. Where should you check for Mrs. Rossten's orders?
2. Give a sample of the charting for the Demerol, including what should be recorded about the patient.

3. What should be included in recording the dressing change? Given an example.
4. Where are these data recorded?
5. How would a change in the physician's orders be indicated to nursing personnel?

SUGGESTED READINGS

Ansley, B.: Patient-Oriented Recording. *Nursing '75,* 5:52–53, August 1975.

Atwood, J., and S. R. Yarnall (eds.): Symposium on the Problem-Oriented Record. *Nursing Clinics of North America,* 8:2, June 1974.

Berg, H. V.: Nursing Audit and Outcome Criteria. *Nursing Clinics of North America,* 9:331–335, June 1974.

Howard, F., et al.: Problem-Oriented Charting—A Nursing Viewpoint. *Canadian Nurse,* 69:34–37, August, 1973.

Lindeman, C. A.: Measuring Quality of Nursing Care. Part 2. *Journal of Nursing Administration,* 6:16–19, September 1976.

Mitchell, P. H., and J. Atwood: Problem-Oriented Recording as a Teaching-Learning Tool. *Nursing Research,* 24:99–102, March-April 1975.

Phaneuf, M. C.: *The Nursing Audit: Profile for Excellence.* New York, Appleton-Century-Crofts, 1972.

Robinson, A. M.: Problem-Oriented Record: Uniting the Team for Total Care. *RN,* 38:23, June 1975.

Vaughn-Wrobel, W. C.: *The Problem-Oriented System in Nursing: A Workbook.* St. Louis, C. V. Mosby Co., 1976.

Weinstein, E. L.: Developing a Measure of the Quality of Nursing Care. Part I. *Journal of Nursing Administration,* 6:1–3, July-August 1976.

Woody, M., and M. Mallison: The Problem-Oriented System for Patient-Centered Care. *American Journal of Nursing,* 73:1168–1175, July 1975.

Unit III

MEETING BASIC NEEDS

12 ANXIETY

The nurse should be able to:

Discuss the importance of relieving anxiety in both the sick and the well

Discuss adaptive mechanisms that assist an individual to cope with his fears

Discuss common sources of anxiety in people with health problems

Describe physiological changes that may be observed in anxious people

Discuss some behavioral patterns that may be indicative of anxiety

Describe subjective observations by the patient which may help the nurse to identify anxiety as a problem

Discuss how the nurse can assess the level of a patient's anxiety

Name guiding principles which are helpful in determining nursing action to help the anxious person

Establish goals for nursing intervention to assist an anxious patient

Utilize specific nursing interventions to prevent anxiety or to help anxious patients

Evaluate the results of nursing interventions

INTRODUCTION

Anxiety is considered to be a modified form of fear. Both anxiety and fear are emotional responses to the threat of real or imagined danger. We used to differentiate between anxiety and fear on the basis that fear was a response to a danger that is known and identifiable, whereas the uneasiness of anxiety might have no definite basis that the individual could pinpoint. Threats of both real and imagined danger give rise to the same pattern of physiological and behavioral responses in an individual, whether he can identify the actual cause of the threat or not. The distinction would therefore seem to be an academic one, and we will not pursue it further.

Anxiety is such a universal phenomenon that almost everyone has experienced it. It affects both the sick and the well. Nurses as well as patients have anxieties. People who come to a health agency for help, whether to maintain their health, to prevent illness, or to overcome a health problem, almost always are at least a little anxious.

Those who come with health problems are under stress. Their homeostatic balance has been disturbed. They require, in most instances, technical assistance from health personnel to enable them to overcome their problems. This technical assistance forms the "curative" aspect of health care. It includes the diagnostic services and therapeutic measures that are carried out by physicians, nurses and other health workers. The curative aspect is an essential component of health care. But people also need help in maintaining their emotional equilibrium under the stress of illness. The provision of this psychological support helps the patient to maintain a motivational balance, which is conducive to recovery, and this is seen largely as a responsibility of nursing.[1] In her supportive role, the nurse is the person who "cares" for the patient. She maintains an environment that is therapeutic; she looks after the patient's physical comfort; and she helps to allay the fears and anxieties that accompany illness. That these comfort and care aspects of the nurse's role are as important to the patient's recovery as her skilled performance of nursing techniques is being increasingly recognized.

The importance of the patient's mental outlook on his health has long been recognized. Motivation is accepted as essential to recovery; it is difficult to cure the patient who does not want to get well. In the surgical field, the excessively fearful patient is generally considered to be a poor surgical risk; many surgeons refuse to operate on the patient who is convinced that he is going to die under anesthesia. It is only recently, however, that much attention has been paid to the significance of the alleviation of anxiety as a factor in preventing illness and in making the patient's recovery from illness easier and less fraught with complications.

Much of the research to date has been on the effectiveness of preoperative nursing measures in preventing or minimizing postoperative discomfort and complications. There is now much evidence that nursing action, such as that involved in preoperative teaching, and the time spent in allaying the patient's anxiety, can contribute to a smoother postoperative recovery for the patient. Anxiety, however, is

---

[1] James K. Skipper, Jr.: The Role of the Nurse: Is it Expressive or Instrumental? In *Social Interaction and Patient Care* by James K. Skipper, Jr., and Robert C. Leonard (eds.). Philadelphia, J. B. Lippincott Company, 1965, p. 41.

such a common contributing factor in illness, and its effects on the individual are so pervasive, that its alleviation is important in every field of nursing.

The nurse should know the physiological and behavioral manifestations of anxiety, and she should be able to identify these in patients. She should be aware of potential sources of anxiety and, whenever possible, take steps to prevent or minimize these. The nurse cannot, of course, anticipate all the fears and anxieties a patient may experience, but she can help to allay a good many of them.

EMOTIONAL EQUILIBRIUM

A person's emotional well-being is as important to his health as his physical or social well-being. A person who is depressed, sad, worried anxious, angry, or really frightened is not able to function at his best physically, mentally, or socially. Each component of health affects all other components, as we discussed in Chapter 2. People usually experience a variety of emotions—such as happiness, sadness, anger, fear, disgust (which are the basic ones)—in varying degrees during the course of their daily lives. It is essential, however, that a balance be maintained, or disturbances soon begin to appear in the individual's physical state, his mental functioning, and his social relationships.

Human beings have a variety of adaptation mechanisms that help them to maintain equilibrium in all areas of functioning. In the case of emotional functioning, but specifically for fear, there are mechanisms both within the body and in a person's mental processes that help him to cope with threats of real or imagined danger. In Chapter 2 we discussed the flight-fight reaction; this is the body's physiological response that prepares a person to contend with fear by either removing himself from the cause (flight), or to overcome it by standing his ground and fighting it. The defense mechanisms we discussed in Chapter 2 also help an individual to deal with real or imagined threats to his self-concept by adjusting his thinking to cope with these dangers.

When the fear extends over a long period of time, or is sufficiently intense, the normal mechanisms are unable to restore a balance, and problems arise in the individual's physical, mental, or social functioning.

SOURCES OF ANXIETY

Many anxieties which patients experience could be prevented if potential sources of fear were eliminated. Other anxieties, if not preventable, can often be minimized by nursing intervention. Some of the most common sources of anxiety are: interference with the fulfillment of basic needs, developmental crises, and other life changes.

Interference with the Fulfillment of Basic Needs

A basic source of anxiety is actual, potential, or imagined interference with a person's ability to satisfy his basic needs. Physiological needs, as we have mentioned several times, take precedence over all other needs because they are essential for survival. Hence, people who are physically ill are usually frightened; something is wrong with their physiological functioning. Among the most frequently cited causes of anxiety in this regard are fear of pain, death, or disfigurement, loss of an organ or of strength, or inability to return to a normal life. Another source of anxiety that has been found among many hospitalized patients is fear of bad reaction to medications.[2]

When people are ill, their basic body processes become a source of major worry. A healthy person takes for granted his breathing, the functioning of his heart and circulatory system, his intake of food and fluids, his elimination of wastes, and his ability to perform a multitude of activities using his motor abilities. When he is ill, the fact that something is interfering with these vital processes causes them to assume major importance. The sick person becomes very anxious and wants to know what his temperature, pulse rate,

---

[2]Betty J. Volicer: Patients' Perceptions of Stressful Events Associated with Hospitalization. *Nursing Research*, 23:235–238, May-June 1974.

and blood pressure are, the results of his physical examination, laboratory, x-ray and other tests, what they found when he was operated on and so forth. His meals, his urinary output, and his bowel movements cause him daily concern.[3]

People who are well and go to a health agency for a routine physical examination also worry about many of these things because of the threat of imagined danger (perhaps they will find something wrong). In the person who has a health problem, these anxieties are magnified because his thoughts are focused on his illness, and he knows something actually is wrong.

Fear of the unknown is one of the principal sources of anxiety for people who come to a health agency. This would seem to bear out Kalish's suggestion, as exemplified by man's curiosity, that the *need for knowledge* is the second most important of the basic needs. Health practitioners have not always been fully aware of the patient's need for information, but it has come through in a loud, clear voice in the Patients' Bills of Rights discussed earlier. The incorporation of teaching plans in the POMR initial and subsequent care plans for patients acknowledges the importance of giving the patient adequate information, and helps to ensure that he receives it.

Boredom and inactivity, or a lack of sufficient sensory stimulation in the environment, will also cause a person to be anxious. Kalish included the need for stimulation as one of the items in his discussion of basic human needs (see p. 16). The bored individual becomes restless; he wonders what to do, feels he should be doing something, and becomes anxious that he is not. If boredom or inactivity persists too long, the individual will become apathetic. This aspect of boredom is discussed more fully in Chapter 13.

Safety and security are next on the hierarchy of human needs, and threats to these constitute a very real source of anxiety for people. Imagined threats to one's physical safety, for instance, account for the anxiety a person feels walking along a dark and lonely street at night. But one's

emotional security may be threatened too. You may worry that another person, or an object, is going to make you angry, will depress you, or that the other person may explode in a temper tantrum, which will disturb your emotional equilibrium. You may also worry that you won't be able to control your emotions.

Threats may also exist with respect to a person's financial security. Particularly in illness, people worry about having sufficient money to cover health expenses. A person may fear that a health problem will interfere with his ability to earn a living. The possibility of altered family structures, or changes in social relationships caused by illness, also threaten the security a person has in knowing who he is and his place in the scheme of things.

If the individual is hospitalized, he usually experiences anxiety because of the change in his environment. When people are in unfamiliar surroundings, they become anxious. The patient will worry until he knows where to find things, how to operate the various mechanical devices attached to his bed, and why the other things in his immediate environment are there. The patient is accustomed to routines, which provide him with security in his normal existence. These are disrupted, and he must adjust to changes in his sleeping habits, meal and bath times, and other aspects of daily living. The presence of strangers, and the lack of familiar faces, will also contribute to his anxiety until he knows that he can safely trust the people who are giving him care.

A lack of fulfillment of the basic need for love and belonging was discussed in Chapter 2 as a factor contributing to illness. We mentioned especially the loneliness and feelings of depersonalization experienced by so many people in our big cities today. Among hospitalized patients, the need to feel part of a group, to feel that people like and accept them and their illness, has been cited as one of their most common concerns.[4]

Nor should we forget that threats to a person's self-esteem interfere with an-

[3]Joan Luckmann and Karen C. Sorensen: What Patients' Actions Tell You About Their Feelings, Fears and Needs. *Nursing '75*, 5:54–61, February 1975.

[4]Rosemarion Berni and Helen Readey: Problem-Oriented Medical Record Implementation. St. Louis, C. V. Mosby Company, 1974, pp. 8–9.

other of man's basic human needs. The loss, or potential loss, of independence, for example, poses a very real threat to a person with a health problem. It can cause him to lose his self-esteem and to think that other people will not respect him. It is important therefore to make sure that nothing the nurse does or says causes the patient to think that he is any less a person because of his health problem.

Potential or actual interference with achievement of self-actualization is another frequent cause of worry among people who are ill or think they have a health problem. Illness can interfere with a person's career, or with fulfillment of his need to make the best of his potentialities in any sphere. The loss or threatened loss of the ability to use one's hands, for instance, would be a major blow to a pianist or the person who uses his hand(s) in pursuing one of his principal interests in life. Similarly, the person whose hobbies are mainly outdoor ones that require motor skills, such as skiing or riding, would be very anxious about being able to continue with these activities if his health problem, actual, potential, or imagined, threatens the loss of his motor functioning abilities.

Developmental Crises

At certain times in a person's lifespan, major changes take place as he makes a transition from one developmental stage to another. Often referred to as "developmental crises," these occur as an individual reaches various stages in his physical and/or psychosocial development. Major changes occur, for example, when a child first goes to school, when he enters puberty, when he leaves the security of home or school to make his own way in the world, when he gets married, when he begins to have children and again when they leave home, when he goes through the physiological and psychological changes of the menopause (a similar state occurs in men, too), retires from active work, loses his marriage partner, and, lastly when death is near. All of these developmental crises cause anxiety, as the individual wonders if he can cope with the demands that will be made upon him in the next stage of his development.

Other Life Changes

In addition to those we have just mentioned, other changes in a person's life also cause stress and anxiety. These, too, we discussed briefly in Chapter 2. In one study assessing patients' perceptions of stressful life events, the most common situations causing stress were grouped as follows:

Changes at work
Changes in the health of self or family
Moving
Financial changes
Births (in addition to birth of the first child)
Arguments
Death (of a family member or close friend)
Involvement with law authorities
Marital situations
Changes regarding children
Changes at school
Other[5]

The results of this study indicated that the patients, all of whom were receiving care in an emergency unit, had had a greater number of life changes in the six months prior to their admission to the unit than are usually found in normally "healthy" individuals. This finding would tend to lend support to the theory that change, and the anxieties associated with it, can be a major factor contributing to illness.

IDENTIFYING THE PROBLEM OF ANXIETY

The threat of danger causes certain physiological reactions to take place within the body. These vary to a certain extent in different individuals according to their physical makeup, although many are commonly seen in the majority of anxious people. Anxiety also brings about changes in a person's behavior. The nature of these behavioral changes depends on a number of factors, such as the severity of the anxiety, the individual's basic personality structure, and the ways in which he has learned to cope with anxiety in the past. The physical condition of the

---

[5]Marcia DeCann Andersen and Jane Marie Pleticha: Emergency Unit Patients' Perceptions of Stressful Life Events. *Nursing Research*, 23:378–382, September-October 1974.

patient affects his ability to tolerate anxiety. Something which may constitute only a minor worry when one is well may create an overwhelming anxiety when the body's defenses are lowered.

Through her observations of an individual, the nurse can often tell if he is anxious. The individual's verbalizations of his feelings, and statements he makes in regard to physical or mental symptoms he is having, also help the nurse to identify anxiety as a problem this person is having.

Physiological Manifestations

The principal physiological mechanism operating in anxiety is the fundamental "alarm reaction" as the body attempts to protect itself from harm (see Chapter 2). It was originally believed that the reaction was due to the outpouring of epinephrine into the blood stream in response to strong emotion. However, this theory does not account for all the physical signs and symptoms that occur in people with anxiety. It is believed that these are the result of stimulation of the autonomic nervous system. The sympathetic portion of the system is most usually affected, although, if the stimulus is sufficiently intense, the parasympathetic portion will be affected as well. Thus, the anxious individual may show evidence of muscular tension, which is a result of sympathetic nervous system stimulation, and, at the same time, have diarrhea due to increased gastric motility resulting from overactivity of the parasympathetic system.[6]

Almost everyone has had experience with some of the physical signs and symptoms of anxiety. There are varying degrees of anxiety, ranging from a mild apprehension to overwhelming panic. In its mild form, anxiety may be beneficial in that it has the effect of putting the body into an alert state and motivating the individual to take some action to alleviate it. Few people would study or get assignments completed on time if there was not a certain amount of anxiety involved. Unresolved anxiety, however, or anxiety in more than mild degree can be harmful.

Among the most easily observable physical signs of anxiety in an individual are the *circulatory changes* which take place. The action of the heart is strengthened and accelerated. The person's blood pressure may be elevated by 10 mm. of mercury or more above normal. The nurse may find that his pulse rate may be as much as 30 per cent above normal. A person's respiratory pattern is often disturbed as well. It may be increased in rate and depth, or may become irregular. There may be a marked pallor of the skin or sometimes a flushing of the face. Often the skin surfaces are cold.

Muscular tension is almost invariably present. In some people this may be observed in a taut expression of the face or in a clenching of the fists. Some people assume a very rigid posture. At times muscular tension is revealed by a tremor of the hands; in a facial, arm, or shoulder tic; or in a generalized shivering or trembling of the body. The tightening of the abdominal muscles and the "butterflies" in the stomach which one commonly experiences with anxiety are the result of muscular tension. The tension headache is another common symptom of anxiety.

People seek relief from muscular tension in a number of ways: by biting their nails, drumming their fingers on the table, or pacing up and down, for example. Restlessness and overactivity are usually fairly reliable indications that the individual is anxious.

Many people *perspire excessively* when they are in anxiety-provoking situations. It may be the palms of the hands or the soles of the feet that are most affected. This increased perspiration combined with a coldness and pallor of the skin (due to lessened peripheral circulation) results in the typical cold and damp hand of the very anxious individual.

Changes in the patient's voice and speech patterns should also be noted as possible indications of anxiety. Some people talk very rapidly or constantly when they are anxious and sometimes the voice becomes very loud or high-pitched. The voice may quaver. In other persons there

---

[6]For a more detailed explanation of this point, the nurse is referred to the text *Function of the Human Body,* by Arthur C. Guyton. Fourth edition. Philadelphia, W. B. Saunders Company, 1974, pp. 334–337.

may be a hesitancy of speech; they may appear to be having difficulty finding the words they want to use. Stammering and stuttering are not uncommon in people with anxiety.

In anxiety, *mental activity is usually increased.* When the anxiety is mild, this may mean that the individual is simply more alert and better able to think clearly. As anxiety mounts, however, a person's perceptual awareness decreases. He becomes unaware of things in his immediate surroundings, except possibly a single thing on which his attention focuses. The anxious person often has difficulty concentrating on anything outside that one thing. His attention span is usually short and he may be unable to answer even simple questions. The very worried parents who bring a sick child into the emergency unit are sometimes so distraught that they cannot remember their own address.

With increasing anxiety, the heightened mental activity may hinder a person from getting rest, and insomnia (inability to get to sleep) frequently results. If the anxious person does manage to get to sleep, he is often troubled by nightmares.

Gastrointestinal symptoms often accompany anxiety also. The "knot" or "butterflies" in the stomach may progress to nausea and vomiting. Often people say they cannot face the thought of food when they are going to take an exam or have an important interview. Some people vomit before every exam they take. Diarrhea, as we mentioned above, is also a common symptom in anxiety. Often people have urinary frequency as well, as many a nervous traveler waiting for his plane to depart has found.

Behavioral Manifestations Of Anxiety

People react to threatening situations in a variety of ways. The behavioral manifestations of anxiety in people who are sick usually reflect the ways in which they have learned to cope with life's dangers in the past. While some people can talk easily about their fears, and openly express these to the nurse, others may be saying, "I am frightened" in less easily recognizable forms. Some people attempt to *deny* the existence of anxiety. They ask no questions and frequently make a point of keeping conversation off the subject of their illness. In our culture, many men feel that it is unmanly to say that one is afraid, particularly to a woman. Men not infrequently (and sometimes women too) cover up their feelings of anxiety with *loud assurances* that they are not frightened, and they may *joke and laugh* in their attempts to minimize the seriousness of their condition.

Some people react to the threat of danger with *anger and hostility.* They may criticize the care they are receiving and be loud and insistent in their demands for special treatment. People who react in this way often engender hostility on the part of the staff, who label them consciously or unconsciously as "difficult" patients. There is an old saying that goes, "When in danger, when in doubt, run in circles, scream and shout." It is perhaps well for the nurse to remember this when she encounters a patient who is being very "difficult." If she can accept this type of behavior as being indicative of the patient's anxiety and not take it as a personal attack on herself she will be in a better position to take positive measures to help the patient.

Crying is another way in which some people react to anxiety. Many nurses are embarrassed to find a patient in tears and find it difficult to know what they should say or do. Attempts to reassure the patient that everything is going to be all right are not usually effective in helping the patient to cope with his feelings. Crying often denotes a feeling of helplessness and inability to handle one's problems. The tears serve to relieve tension, and the nurse can perhaps be most helpful by staying with the patient and being ready to listen when the crying episode is over.

The Patient's Subjective Perceptions

As already mentioned, some people can verbalize their anxieties, others cannot. The nurse may find, however, that the patient may tell her about some symptoms he is having which, put together with her own observations, may confirm her suspicions that the individual is anxious. Pertinent observations which the patient may make relate to the physiological manifestations of anxiety described above. He may say, for example, that he has a headache which starts at the base of his neck (frequently caused by tension in the shoulder and neck muscles). He may complain that he just can't sit still, or that he can't concentrate on anything. He may describe a knot or butterflies in his stomach, or complain that he has a cramping pain, accompanied by frequent loose stools. He may tell her that he has to urinate frequently. The nurse must be careful not to jump to conclusions about these symptoms. Of course, they could very well be caused by something other than anxiety. They should, however, be reported in her observations about the patient in conjunction with her objective findings.

ESTABLISHING PRIORITIES FOR NURSING ACTION

Anxiety may be mild, moderate, severe, or it may turn into panic. In establishing priorities, the nurse assesses the level of the patient's anxiety by observing the degree of severity of the physiological and behavioral manifestations he is showing. It has been suggested that nurses sometimes project their own anxieties onto the patient, and thus may assess that the patient is experiencing more severe anxiety than he actually is. It is wise, therefore, to use objective criteria in assessment. Particular observations to note are: evidences of greatly increased muscular tension, as seen in trembling hands and frequent position changes; increased perspiration, and the presence of the cold, clammy hands; markedly decreased perceptual awareness and inability to concentrate; marked increases in pulse rate and disturbances in breathing; and disturbances in sleep patterns.[7]

Severe anxiety may become *panic*, in which the person is unable to say or do anything that is meaningful. His behavior may be completely out of context—he may laugh when he should be crying—and his thoughts and speech become incoherent. The person who has "panicked" needs someone who is calm to stay with him, to take charge of the situation, and to tell him what to do. He cannot think for himself at this point.

The nurse often encounters people in a state of panic in the emergency room unit. A calm, reassuring manner, simple directions on what to do, and, often, the familiar routine of offering a cup of tea or coffee will help to calm the person. Calming a person who is in a panic is always a matter of immediate priority. Severe anxiety is something which needs to be dealt with on a priority basis also.

In determining measures which will allay anxiety, the nurse must take into account the fact that her plan of care has to be individualized to suit each patient. No two people are alike in regard to the nature of their anxieties, their reactions to these, or the type of help they need in overcoming them. There is therefore no easy set of rules which the nurse can follow. The guiding principles given below may, however, be helpful.

PRINCIPLES RELEVANT TO THE CARE OF PERSONS WITH ANXIETY

1. It is easier to allay a known fear than anxiety from an unknown source.
2. People generally feel less anxious when they know what is going to happen to them.
3. Anxiety is lessened when people feel they have some control over their situation.
4. Loneliness aggravates anxiety.
5. A feeling of depersonalization contributes to anxiety.
6. Physical activity helps to relieve muscular tension.
7. Anxiety can often be relieved by diversional activity.

GOALS FOR NURSING ACTION

Nursing action for the individual who may develop anxiety is directed towards

---

[7]Suzanne Marek Lagina: A Computer Program to Diagnose Anxiety Levels. *Nursing Research*, 20:484–492, November-December 1971.

preventing it. For the person who is already anxious, nursing action may aim at one of three things: (1) alleviating his anxiety, (2) minimizing it, (3) assisting him to cope with it.

In order to identify actual or potential sources of anxiety, the nurse needs information about the individual's health status, information about him as a person, his stage of physical and psychosocial development, and about recent changes in his life that have caused alterations in his lifestyle.

In regard to his health status, she considers such questions as: Does this person have a recognized health problem, or does he think that he has a health problem? If so, is it one in which pain is a factor? Is death a possible consequence of the problem? Is disfigurement, or loss of an organ a possibility? Is there a possibility that the person thinks these may occur? Does he perhaps perceive his health problem (actual or imagined) as leading to a loss of strength, or interfering with his ability to pursue his normal lifestyle? Is there a possibility of surgery or might he think there is? (Surgery, even the most minor, usually brings on anxiety.)

The nurse also needs to know something about the person as an individual. What are his personality characteristics? How has he coped with anxiety in the past? Where does he stand in relation to fulfillment of his basic needs? Is he concerned with self-actualization at this point in his life, or is he struggling to make enough money to provide himself (and, if he is married, his family) with the basic essentials of food, shelter, and security? Is his career the most important thing in his life? His home? His wife? His children? His outside interests?

She considers also his age and his stage of physical and psychosocial development. Is there a possibility that he is going through a crisis time in his life? The nurse should also be aware of the individual's marital and family status. Who are the members of the family constellation? Where does this person fit into the family structure? Is he the head or a dominant member of the household? Is he in a dependent role in the family? Who are the other members of the family? If the patient does not live with his family, does he live with someone else? Who are the significant others in his life? What is this individual's occupation? His socioeconomic status? What are his hobbies and his interests? What are his immediate concerns? Another matter to consider is whether there have been any major changes in the person's life recently. If so, how many changes has he undergone? What sort of changes were they? Did they necessitate major readjustments in his life?

Some of this information will be available to the nurse from data she or other persons have gathered about the patient in the initial assessment interview and observations. Some she may learn from the physician's notations on the patient's records and his plans for diagnostic and therapeutic care, as well as other information that is on the patient's progress record. The social worker, if he or she has been called in, usually writes a lengthy social history on the patient, which is often helpful to the nurse in identifying actual or potential sources of anxiety. The nurse supplements the information she has gathered from other sources by talking with the patient. As we noted in Chapter 8, most people will talk quite freely about things that are concerning them if the nurse has established a climate in which the patient feels free to communicate, and if she takes the time to be an attentive listener. In trying to identify sources of anxiety, it is sometimes helpful to ask direct questions, such as about changes that have occurred in a patient's life, or other matters she feels are significant in relation to this particular individual.

SPECIFIC NURSING INTERVENTIONS

In deciding on specific nursing interventions to prevent anxiety, to minimize or alleviate it, or to help the person to cope with anxieties that cannot be eliminated, the nurse is guided by her assessment of the individual patient, his particular problems, and her understanding of potential or actual sources of anxiety he may have. She also considers whether she

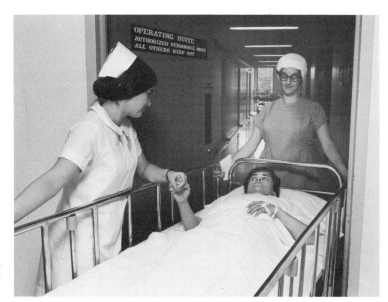

Often the comforting presence of someone who is sympathetic can help to allay some of the anxiety a patient feels in a stressful situation.

can do something to help this person herself, or whether he needs the help of another member of the health team. If we review some of the interventions the nurse may undertake in applying the principles noted above, we will find some which she might consider in the care of specific patients.

1. *It is easier to allay a known fear than anxiety from an unknown source.* We have already discussed some of the ways the nurse can gather information to help her to identify the sources of a patient's potential or actual problem of anxiety. The nurse always verifies with the patient that her interpretation of the source of his anxieties is consistent with his perceptions in this regard. The nurse may think that the patient is very worried about the treatment he is going to have tomorrow, for example, when in actual fact he is not worried about that at all; he may instead be anxious about his daughter, who has not come in to see him as she had promised.

It is important to remember, too, that talking with the patient can also be therapeutic. It gives the patient an opportunity to explore the causes of his anxieties, to discuss them with someone and perhaps to work out his own solutions to some of the things that are worrying him.

The beginning nurse, however, should not feel that she can be a skilled counselor at this stage in her career. If the nurse does not feel comfortable in dealing with a patient's anxieties, or feels he needs more highly skilled counseling than she is able to provide, she should not hesitate to call in someone else. Nor should she feel guilty in doing so. Her instructor, or the head nurse on the ward, may be able to help the patient. If a psychiatric nursing specialist is available, this person is often able to help people with their anxieties more effectively than someone without that orientation. She may also be able to provide that nurse with help in her approach to the patient. Some patients need the counseling services of a psychologist or psychiatrist, and the patient should be referred for these services.

2. *People generally feel less anxious when they know what is going to happen to them.* Providing information is important both in preventing and in allaying anxiety. If a patient knows what is going to be done during a laboratory test, he usually is less apprehensive about it. Similarly, the patient who has been told that a certain procedure may hurt a little is better able to face the pain. Teaching plans which identify information the patient needs should form a part of every nursing care plan.

3. *Anxiety is lessened when people feel they have some control over their situa-*

tion. Enlisting the patient's cooperation and having him participate in his care whenever possible help to give him this feeling. Giving the patient a voice in the scheduling of his activities, or the way some procedure should be done, is one way of helping him to feel he still has some control over events. The nurse might confer with him about the time for his bath, for example, the time he prefers to have treatments done. When would be the best time to change his dressing, for example?

4. *Loneliness aggravates anxiety.* People need someone to whom they can talk and with whom they can share their feelings. A large part of the nurse's role is providing this kind of emotional support for patients. Talking with the patient is important, but feelings can also be shared without words, and sometimes words are not necessary. It is helpful to the patient simply to have someone who is sympathetic present. Some people feel more comfortable in talking over their anxieties with non-medically oriented personnel. The nurse should not overlook the contributions that such members as the chaplain and the social worker can make in helping patients with their anxieties.

5. *A feeling of depersonalization contributes to anxiety.* When the person feels that he has lost his identity, that he is just a health agency number or an interesting "case," his confidence in the care he is receiving is diminished. It is important to help the patient to retain the feeling that he is a respected person in his own right. Referring to the patient by name, not by bed number, and taking an interest in him as an individual are among the many things a nurse can do to reassure him that he is in good hands.

6. *Physical activity helps to relieve muscular tension.* Exercise within the patient's limits of tolerance is a good way of relieving the muscular tension accompanying anxiety. Relaxation exercises also help. The assistance of the physical therapist is often helpful in teaching patients relaxing exercises or suggesting other measures to reduce muscular tension.

Two simple exercises from Yoga, which the nurse may find useful herself, are shown on pages 222 to 224.

SPONGE*

I.   *Benefits:*

The Sponge—
• promotes deep *muscular relaxation.*
• deeply *relaxes* the *nervous system.*
• restores *peace of mind.*
• results in a reduction of *anxiety* or "nerves" through the release of tension.
• is a marvellous *energy-recharger.*

II.   *Technique:*

1.   Lie on the floor, legs slightly apart, arms limply by your side. (*E.*)
2.   Point your toes away from you and hold for 5 seconds. Relax.
3.   Pull the toes up towards the body, bending at the ankle. Hold. Relax.
4.   Pull your heels up two inches on the floor and then straighten the legs, pushing the back of the knees firmly against the floor. Hold. Relax.
5.   Point the toes toward each other and pull the heels under and up, keeping the legs straight. Hold. Relax.
6.   Pinch your buttocks together. Hold. Relax.
7.   Pull your abdomen in and up as far as possible. Hold. Relax.
8.   Arch the spine back, pushing the chest out. Hold. Relax.
9.   With arms straight by your side, palms down, bend the fingers up and back toward the arm, bending at the wrist. Hold. Relax.
10. Bend the elbows and repeat step 9, bending the hands back toward the shoulders. Hold. Relax.
11. Make a tight fist of your hands, bring the arms out to the sides and move the arms up perpendicular to the floor. Move very slowly, resisting the movement all the while to make the pectoral muscles of the bust stand out.
12. Pull the shoulderblades of the back together. Hold. Relax.
13. Pull the shoulders up beside the ears. Hold. Relax.
14. Pull down the corners of the mouth. Hold. Relax.
15. Bring the tongue to the back of the roof of the mouth. Hold. Relax.

---

*Reprinted from Kareen Zebroff: *The ABC of Yoga.* Vancouver, B.C., Fforbez Enterprises, Ltd., 1971.

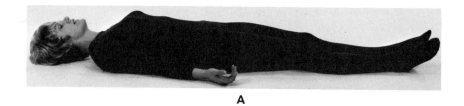

A

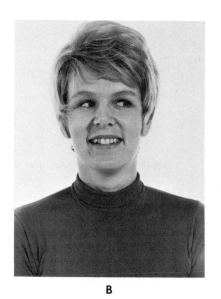

B

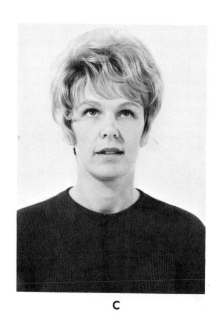

C

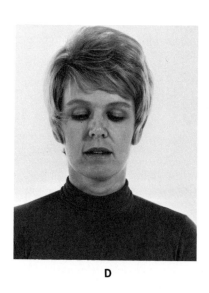

D

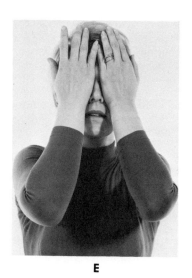

E

(From Zebroff, 1971.)

16. Purse your lips, wrinkle the nose and squeeze the eyes tightly shut. Hold. Relax.
17. Smile with the lips closed and stretch the face. Hold. Relax.
18. Yawn very slowly, resisting the movement.
19. Press the back of the head against the floor. Hold. Relax.
20. Frown, moving the scalp forward. Hold. Relax.
21. Go through the eye exercises.
22. Pull your head under and against the shoulders without moving anything else.
23. Relax, melting into the floor, for up to 10 minutes. (*E.*)

III. *Dos and Don'ts:*

DO hold each holding position for at least 5 seconds.
DO relax after each holding position, by flopping back into place after each flexing position.
DO NOT worry or think of unpleasant things as you relax at the end of the Sponge. Rather, keep your thoughts to a minimum, on pleasant things, and dispassionately watch them wander past without trying to become involved.

The Sponge is called the Dead Man's Pose or Corpse in the Sanskrit language. Really, it is a deep relaxation pose where your body has a chance to assimilate what it has learned, at its leisure. Seldom do we take the time simply to relax. We may read, watch TV or sleep. Just because we lie down does not at all mean we are relaxing our deep-seated neuromuscular tensions. The body has to relearn how to do that. After some weeks of the deliberate Sponge technique you will find that you can relax without going through all the steps.

EYE EXERCISES *

I. *Benefits:*

The Eye Exercises—
• relieve *tension*, *fatigue*, and *strain* of the eyes.
• strengthen the *eye* muscles.
• relieve *headaches*.

----

*Zebroff, op. cit.

• give eyes a clear, *shiny* look.
• give a general feeling of *relaxation*.

II. *Technique:*

1. Sit in a comfortably cross-legged position; look straight ahead.
2. Look as far to the right as is possible without moving the head. Hold 5 seconds.
3. Look to the left. Hold. (*B.*)
4. Look up under the eyebrows. Hold. (*C.*)
5. Look down past nose. Hold. (*D.*)
6. Now imagine a giant clock with the 12 just under the eyebrows and the 6 on the floor immediately in front of you.
7. Look at each digit of this clock for one second, so that your eyes are moving jerkily.
8. Repeat, moving counterclockwise.
9. Cover your eyes with the palms of both hands for 30 seconds, to rest them. (*E.*)

Variations:

1. a) Look far away out the windows. Try to look miles toward the horizon. Hold.
   b) Slowly bring your gaze back and look crosseyed at your nose. Hold.
2. Use your imagination: e.g., describe semi-circles or diagonals with your eyes.

III. *Dos and Don'ts:*

DO these exercises any time you are very tired or feel that your eyes have been strained, instead of just squeezing the eyes up in the customary fashion.
DO rest the eyes by closing them between each set of exercises.

The eyes are our most important sense and yet people neglect them greatly by taking them for granted. Eye strain and resulting headaches can be greatly reduced through exercising the eye muscles.

If exercise is not feasible or permissible, nursing interventions, such as a soothing backrub or massage, can frequently help to relieve tense muscles.

7. Anxiety can often be relieved by diversional activity. If a person has nothing to occupy his time or attention, he tends to become introspective and to brood on his troubles. Reading, watching television, and playing cards are activities which are usually available in hospitals to divert patients from a constant preoccupation with their illnesses. Women often like to knit, crochet, or do embroidery, and people of both sexes seem to like macramé; these activities should be encouraged. Frequently, the occupational therapist can make suggestions and help to interest patients in activities which divert their attention from themselves.

Tranquilizers

Drugs of the tranquilizer group frequently are ordered to help to reduce anxiety. Among those most commonly used are Valium, Stelazine, Librium, and Mellaril. These are given as directed. The nurse should be alert to the possible side-effects of tranquilizers in her patients. The most common side-effect is drowsiness, but patients may show other reactions as well, such as headache, dizziness, nausea and vomiting, constipation, or mental disturbance. Because the side-effects are usually specific for each drug, the nurse should acquaint herself with those associated with the drug ordered for her patient.

Particularly vulnerable are elderly patients, who sometimes experience a marked decrease in blood pressure after the administration of these drugs. It is not uncommon for elderly patients to develop symptoms of excitement or mental confusion when they are receiving tranquilizers.

EVALUATING THE EFFECTIVENESS OF NURSING INTERVENTION

The prevention or alleviation of anxiety is perhaps best evaluated by the absence or decrease in severity of the physical signs and symptoms and of the behaviors by which it was identified. The nurse may note, for example, that the patient's facial expression is calm and relaxed, his muscular tension is reduced, his pulse rate and breathing are normal, his perceptual awareness is improved, his voice and speech patterns are more normal, that he is not perspiring unduly, and that his sleeping patterns are normal. The patient may state that his anxiety has lessened or that he is no longer having the distressing gastrointestinal symptoms, urinary frequency, headache, or whatever his particular manifestation of anxiety was.

The nurse will also note the absence or decrease in the behavioral manifestations that were discussed as being symptomatic of anxiety in some patients. If observations in her assessment and the expected outcomes of her care have been specific, she will find that she has observable criteria on which to evaluate the patient's progress.

GUIDE TO ASSESSING ANXIETY

1. Does the patient show physical signs or symptoms of anxiety? For example, is his pulse rate above normal in the absence of a known physical cause for it? Is there evidence of muscular tension?
2. Does the patient appear to treat his illness very lightly — that is, does he laugh and joke a lot about his condition?
3. Is the patient demanding, complaining, or hostile toward the staff?
4. Is there evidence that the patient has been crying?
5. Does the patient express any fears verbally?
6. What do you know about this patient as an individual?
7. What are some of the possible sources of anxiety this patient may have?

8. Is the patient lonely?
9. Does the patient have activities to occupy his time?
10. What source people might be able to help this patient?

STUDY VOCABULARY

Alarm reaction	Curative aspects	Reassurance
Anxiety	Fear	

STUDY SITUATION

Miss Julie Allen is an attractive, 22 year old airline stewardess. She thoroughly enjoys her job and the benefits she receives through working for an airline. Although planning to be married next month, Miss Allen intends to continue working for another few years before raising a family. In a routine physical examination, Miss Allen's physician detected some evidence of tissue changes which could be indicative of early cervical cancer. He has suggested that Miss Allen be admitted to hospital for further diagnostic tests. Miss Allen appears to be very upset.

1. For what reasons would Miss Allen be upset?
2. What physical manifestations of anxiety might the nurse observe in Miss Allen?
3. When Miss Allen is admitted to the nursing unit in the afternoon before surgery, she is very restless and talks constantly. She follows the nurse around and laughs and jokes about her work as an airline stewardess. She tells the nurse she just cannot sit in her room and it is too early to go to bed. What can the nurse do to help Miss Allen?

SUGGESTED READINGS

Aiken, L. H.: Systematic relaxation to Reduce Pre-operative Stress. *Canadian Nurse*, 68:38–42, June 1972.

Bellack, J. P.: Helping A Child Cope with the Stress of Injury. *American Journal of Nursing*, 74:1491–1494, August 1974.

Bolzoni, N. J., et al.: Premature Reassurance: A Distancing Maneuver. *Nursing Outlook*, 23:49–51, January 1975.

Chaney, P.: Ordeal. *Nursing '75*, 5:27–40, June 1975.

Cohen, R. G.: Providing Emotional Support for the Seriously Ill. *RN*, 37:62–64, October 1974.

Hannan, J. F.: Talking is Treatment, Too. *American Journal of Nursing*, 74:1991–1992, November 1974.

Klopf, J. K.: Please don't go away: A crisis when nobody intervened. *Nursing Clinics of North America*, 9:77–80, March 1974.

Lederer, H. D.: How the sick view their world. *In* Skipper, J. K., Jr., and R. C. Leonard (eds.): *Social Interaction and Patient Care*. Philadelphia, J. B. Lippincott, 1965, pp. 155–167.

Ludwig, J.: Jack Wanted to Direct His Care His Way. *Nursing '75*, 5:10–11, August 1975.

Maslow, A. H.: *Motivation and Personality*. 2nd edition. New York, Harper & Row, 1970.

Murray, R. L. E.: Assessment of Psychologic Status in the Surgical ICU Patient. *Nursing Clinics of North America*, 10:69–81, March 1975.

Peterson, M. H.: Understanding Defense Mechanisms: Programmed Instruction. *American Journal of Nursing,* 72:1651–1674, September 1972.

Rickles, N. K., and B. C. Finkle: Anxiety: Yours and Your Patient's. *Nursing '74,* 3:23, March 1973.

Robinson, L.: The Demanding Patient. *Nursing '73,* 3:20–24, January 1973.

Saylor, D. E.: Understanding Presurgical Anxiety. *AORN J.,* 22:624, October 1975.

Seaver, S.: We had Misjudged Barb: Now She Was Punishing Us. *Nursing '76,* 6:18–20, August 1976.

13 SENSORY DISTURBANCES

The nurse should be able to:

Discuss sensory stimulation as a basic human need

Explain briefly and in simple terms the process of sensory perception

Explain the phenomenon of adaptation to sensory stimuli

Discuss the concept of sensory deprivation

Name and give examples of the principal causes of sensory deprivation

Discuss sensory overload as a problem in hospitalized patients

Gather appropriate data for identifying sensory disturbances in a patient

Make pertinent observations to identify sensory deprivation, sensory deficits, and sensory overload in patients

Apply principles relevant to the care of patients with sensory disturbances

Establish long-term goals for nursing actions, and short-term expected outcomes for specific nursing interventions

Evaluate the results of nursing interventions

INTRODUCTION

Sensory stimulation is a basic human need. Psychologists and educators have long been aware of the need for adequate sensory stimulation to promote the optimal growth and development of children, but only in recent years has the subject received much attention in other areas of the health field, particularly for adults.

Yet, sensory stimulation is a vital component of our lives. Our sensory abilities of sight, hearing, smell, taste, and touch are the antennae which enable us to pick up signals that give us information about our environment. Without these abilities, we would not know what is going on in the world around us; nor would we be able to communicate with other people since communication involves both visual and auditory abilities, as well as abilities to symbolize, to write, and to make sounds. In discussions of sensory functioning, the ability to communicate is usually included because of the interrelationship of sensory functioning and communication.

The receiving and accurate interpretation of sensory input from the environment is essential for survival. The person who has lost the use of one of his senses is handicapped. One of his antennae is missing, so to speak, and he must pick up more stimuli from other sources to make up for it.

The person who is blind, for example, learns to distinguish sound with much more discrimination than the person whose sense of sight is intact. He also develops the sensitivity of his fingers to allow him to read Braille. But he may still require the help of another person or of a guide dog to protect him from hazards in the environment.

Similarly, the person who is deaf learns to "listen" to other people by reading their lips; if he is both deaf and mute (unable to speak), he may learn to talk in sign language. He also develops his sense of sight more keenly to interpret the meaning of nonverbal communications. But the deaf person is still at a disadvantage; he may not hear the horn of a car warning him to get out of the way when he is crossing the street.

Inability to communicate, either in speech or in writing, lessens a person's ability to make contact with other human beings and, hence, cuts off a major area of sensory stimulation. If speech is affected, the individual must either write his messages or depend on nonverbal means of communication. If the ability to write is lost, the person is more or less at the level of a child who has not yet learned to write.

Appetite is aroused by the sight and smell of food, but it is also dependent on direct stimulation of the taste buds. Thus, if the ability to taste is lost, a person's appetite diminishes, and he may take in insufficient nourishment to meet his body's requirements. Loss of the sense of smell lessens the pleasure of a cup of coffee, since the aroma of coffee contributes a great deal to its enjoyment. The loss of the sense of smell also entails other handicaps. A person may not be able to distinguish important odors, such as fumes. He may not, for example, smell the smoke of a fire, but must depend on his senses of sight and hearing to alert him to the danger.

If a person has lost the sense of touch in a part of his body, e.g., if his left arm and leg are paralyzed as a result of stroke, he is unable to tell if tissues in the affected arm and leg are being damaged. He cannot tell if a hot water bottle is burning his left foot, for instance. Loss of the sense of touch affects the ability to

229

perceive pain, heat and cold, and pressure. It also affects a person's balance, since we use touch as a means of aligning ourselves with objects or persons in our immediate environment. We feel where we are sitting in a chair, for example, and shift ourselves around until we are comfortable. A person without the sense of touch is cut off from contact with other objects or human beings so far as the affected area is concerned. If his arm or hand is paralyzed, he is unable to feel the comfort of a soothing hand on his arm, or to feel the texture of a piece of silk in his hand.

Of course, a person can also suffer from too much sensory input. The excessive noise and constant barrage of stimuli from a variety of sources that seem to be a part of living in a large city these days can overload our sensory receiving mechanisms and result in problems in sensory functioning. One wonders, for example, about the possible damage done to the hearing abilities of people who frequent discotheques on a regular basis, since the noise emanating from them has often been measured at well above the safety limit for noise levels.

SENSORY PERCEPTION

The perception of sensory stimuli is a complex process, which has its origin in the five sense organs: the eyes, the ears, the skin, the nose, and the mouth. Receptors in the sense organs pick up stimuli from the environment and send this information along to the brain via distinct channels in the nervous system.[1] The information passes through several levels of increasing complexity in the brain, where it is modified, refined, and interpreted, this interpretation depending on a number of factors, such as the individual's state of well-being, his past experiences with stimuli of this sort, and the interrelationship of stimuli coming in from various

sources. The result of this process, which takes less than a second of time, is known as *perception.*

In order to process sensory perception, the brain (in particular, the reticular formation) depends on a constant and varied barrage of stimuli from the environment. If the receptors are not picking up enough stimuli or are getting too much of the same stimuli, *adaptation* occurs, and the brain will no longer perceive the available stimuli. To illustrate this effect, the student might try sitting in a quiet, darkened room and staring at a luminous object. Gradually the object will seem to disappear until the student can no longer see it. Extreme concentration on any object or person will produce the same effect. This phenomenon has been known to be used by some cult leaders as a demonstration of their power over their followers. A lack of environmental stimulation will likewise result in a form of sensory adaptation. It is believed that, in this case, the brain will then focus on higher thought processes and tend to disregard the small amount of external stimulation that is available. Either situation—that is, too much of one stimulus or not enough stimuli altogether—results in sensory deprivation.

SENSORY DEPRIVATION

Much research has been carried out in recent years on sensory deprivation and its effects on the human organism. In psychology departments in many universities, this subject has come under close scrutiny. Health personnel are also focusing their attention on sensory deprivation as an area of concern, as exemplified in a study reported by Dr. Florence Downs.[2] The purpose of this particular study was not to test the effects of sensory deprivation but to investigate the effects of bed rest as functions related to personality characteristics and varied auditory input. The subjects who participated in the study were healthy young adults between

---

[1] This is not so for the perception of pain. It is now believed that there is no separate and distinct channel in the nervous system which transmits information concerning painful stimuli to the higher centers of the brain. This topic is discussed further in Chapter 31.

---

[2] Florence S. Downs: Bed Rest and Sensory Disturbances. *American Journal of Nursing,* 74:434–438, March, 1974.

the ages of 18 and 35. The incidental findings of the study were astonishing. Subjects reported disturbances ranging from basic physical discomfort, space and time disorientation, sensory distortions, and difficulty in concentrating, to outright hallucinations. One woman experienced the sensation of her leg being detached from the rest of her body. Other subjects felt as though they were floating above the bed. As the subjects in this study were considered to be in an optimal state of physical and psychological well-being, one may well question what the effects of sensory deprivation might be on persons who are ill.

Sensory deprivation has been defined as "a lack or alteration of impulses conveyed from the sense organs to the reflex or higher centers of the brain. It may result from inadequate or monotonous stimuli [that is, sensory underload], poorly functioning sense receptors, or an inability to perceive environmental data."[3] When an individual is ill, his resistance to harmful stimuli and his energy level are considerably lowered; thus, the effects of sensory deprivation are bound to be more profound in the sick person. Downs states that "realistic bodily concerns probably heighten an individual's susceptibility to [indeterminate sensory experiences] by intensifying environmental disruption and encouraging introspection."[4]

CAUSES OF SENSORY DEPRIVATION

Sensory deprivation may be caused simply by a lack of stimulation from the environment. It may also result from impairment of the sensory receptors themselves or from impairment of the centers in the brain which process sensory input.

Inadequate Stimuli

People who have all of their sensory abilities intact are just as vulnerable to

sensory deprivation as are people with impairment of these abilities. The lack of stimulation may be in the physical environment, the psychosocial environment, or both. People with limited mobility, such as "shut-ins" at home, those confined to a wheelchair or a sickroom, or those whose ability to get around is limited in any way, are particularly vulnerable. Their opportunities for varying their surroundings and for meeting and talking with other people are seriously hampered. The potentialities for inadequate sensory stimulation are therefore greatly increased. People whose work or home environments are monotonous and lacking in stimulation may also suffer from sensory deprivation. The man who works on an assembly line, for example, and has few hobbies or after-work activities and the housewife who stays home day after day with the same monotonous round of housework and who has no interests outside the home are both likely to suffer from sensory deprivation.

The problem of lack of stimulation is a very common one in people who are ill, particularly in the hospital setting. Profound disturbances caused by this form of sensory deprivation have been documented in studies on patients in isolation, in intensive care units, and in coronary care units, who have minimal contact with the outside world. Whether it is in the home or in a hospital, the normal sickroom is usually lacking in environmental stimuli. Noise is kept to a minimum, lights are low, and contact with family and friends is often restricted. In the hospital setting, the walls are often bare and colors muted. All these factors were thought to act for the best interests of the patient, with the principal objective being to promote rest and comfort. Unfortunately, the reverse is often true.

Impairment of the Sense Organs

The sense organs and their accessory muscles, nerves, and blood supply must be intact for optimal sensory stimulation. Disease, injury, or a congenital defect can interfere with the receiving of adequate sensory input. The impairment may be temporary, or it may be permanent. A per-

[3]C. F. Cameron et al.: When Sensory Deprivation Occurs.... *The Canadian Nurse*, 68:32–34, November 1972.
[4]Downs, op. cit.

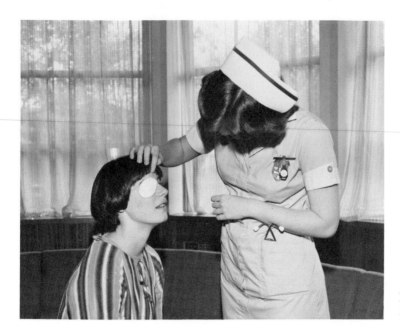

Even the temporary loss of the sense of sight is a distressing experience.

son recovering from eye surgery who has both eyes bandaged may be suffering only a temporary loss of vision, but it is a very distressing experience. While his eyes are bandaged, he must adjust to life as a blind person. The person with a permanent sensory deficit must learn to adapt by making greater use of his remaining sensory abilities and learning to live with the deficit.

The loss of the sense of sight, of hearing, or of touch may mean a complete restructuring of a person's life. The person who loses some of his hearing may be able to use a hearing aid, but not all hearing problems can be helped by this means. The person who has lost any of the three senses just mentioned or his ability to speak loses at least some of his independence and, consequently, his self-esteem suffers as he finds he has to depend on others to do things he would normally do for himself.

Sensory impairment may be either partial or total. Partial loss of any of the senses can be almost as disturbing as total impairment. A person recovering from an eye operation who has only one eye bandaged is unable to perceive depth, which depends on focusing both eyes simultaneously. The individual who is "hard of hearing" often becomes very anxious and frustrated as he tries to catch what other people are saying. His social relationships

may be impaired and he loses much in the way of sensory stimulation because of his difficulties in receiving spoken messages.

Distorted sensory perception can be equally distressing and potentially harmful to the individual. A person with distorted vision, for example, may stumble and fall as he tries to find where he should put his foot next. If you have ever walked through a "fun house" in an amusement park, you may remember how it feels to have your vision distorted in one of the convex or concave mirrors. This experience helps to give you some idea of the feelings of a person with distorted vision.

As people grow older, their sensory functioning decreases. It takes more stimulation to whet the appetite, for example, because the sense of taste is diminished. Yet older people, particularly those residing in institutions, are often given very bland meals. Of course, one has to take into consideration other factors as well, such as the person's ability to chew food, and gastrointestinal problems he may have, but the monotony of institutionalized food does not usually do much to encourage the intake of adequate nourishment by older persons.

Vision and hearing also decrease as one grows older. As a person approaches middle age, he generally finds that he needs to wear glasses, even if he did not need them before. Hearing also becomes less acute; the older person usually needs the radio or television volume to be set much higher than a younger person does. It is also often necessary to speak more loudly to him, and to enunciate words clearly and distinctly.

Impairment of the Centers for Processing Sensory Stimuli

Any factors which impair the functioning of centers in the brain which refine, modify, and interpret sensory input interfere with a person's sensory abilities. Diseases affecting mental processes, or damage to the brain itself resulting from disease processes or from injury, may cause disturbances in sensory functioning. Fever, for example, often distorts sensory perception: a very high fever may cause a person to have hallucinations. Hallucinations are something like dreams. They may be visual or auditory; the person may see persons or objects in his mind, or he may hear voices or other noises. Other senses, su :h as smell and touch, may also be involved, and sometimes several sensations may be experienced at the same time. When this occurs, the feeling that this is real, and not a dream, may be overpowering.[5]

A stroke (cerebrovascular accident) is a common cause of temporary or permanent impairment to brain tissues that interferes with sensory functioning. Paralysis often results from a stroke, and not infrequently there is interference with speech and hearing as well. Because the speech area in the brain is located in the dominant hemisphere, a stroke affecting this side of the brain may cause difficulties in speaking or aphasia (that is, a complete absence of the ability to speak). In people with heart problems, general circulation is impaired, and there may be interference with the blood supply to the brain. These people then may also experience disturbances in

sensory functioning because of the inadequate oxygenation of brain tissues.

A person's level of consciousness affects both his ability to receive sensory input and his ability to process it. His antennae are turned down low, to pick up the analogy used at the beginning of the chapter, and the complicated mechanisms in the brain that process the sensory stimuli are functioning at less than optimal efficiency when the level of a person's consciousness is decreased.

Drugs that depress the central nervous system will decrease sensory functioning, since it is this system that carries information from the sensory receptors and also handles the processing of it. Many drugs are known to cause distortions in sensory perception. The hallucinogens, such as marijuana and LSD, cause a person to have hallucinations. Other drugs commonly used in the treatment of illness may also cause disturbances in sensory functioning, such as a blurring of vision, a ringing in the ears, or a distorted taste. These are side-effects, and are specific to each drug. When caring for patients on any type of medication therapy, the nurse should be aware of potential side-effects and be alert for their appearance in the patient.

A person's emotional state can also affect his sensory abilities. A happy person sees everything in a different light than when he is worried or depressed. The flowers have more color; other people look different, perhaps more friendly. The depressed individual, on the other hand, may be unaware of things in his immediate environment—his eyes just do not see them. We have discussed the changes in perceptual awareness of the person with anxiety in Chapter 12. This is another example of emotions affecting a person's sensory abilities.

SENSORY OVERLOAD

As we mentioned at the beginning of this chapter, a person may sometimes have an overabundance of sensory stimulation. This is not an uncommon problem in the sickroom or hospital setting. Although the atmosphere of the sickroom or

---

[5]R. L. Gregory: Eye and Brain. 2nd edition. New York, McGraw-Hill Book Company, 1973, p. 131.

the hospital is traditionally quiet and conducive to rest, often this is not the case. Many humorous articles have been written by patients about the disturbances to rest in a hospital, but the situation is not always amusing. The patient may be subjected to bright lights or disruptive noises, as, for example, those produced by the machinery used to provide life-giving assistance to him, such as a respirator or a renal dialysis (artificial kidney) machine. The noise of food carts being trundled along the hall can also be disturbing. The patient's rest may be constantly interrupted by members of the health team checking his vital signs or those of a roommate. Adequate rest and sleep are important in a person's physical and psychological well-being, as well as in his sensory perception; the specific effects of sleep deprivation are discussed more fully in Chapter 18.

IDENTIFYING PROBLEMS WITH REGARD TO SENSORY FUNCTIONING

The most common sensory disturbances the nurse will encounter in patients are:
1. Sensory deprivation
2. Sensory overload
3. Sensory deficit, partial or complete

Sensory deprivation and sensory overload are relative terms. What might be sensory deprivation for one person may be peace and tranquility for another. A person who comes from a large family may enjoy a quiet time to himself. He may, on the other hand, not find noise as disturbing as one who is used to a quiet household, and in fact may miss the stimulation of an active, busy home.

In order to identify problems a patient may be having with regard to sensory functioning, the nurse will find information about the following items helpful:

The patient's usual status with regard to sensory functioning

His present status in this regard

Health problems he may have

The therapy he is receiving if he has a health problem

His personality

His usual lifestyle

His normal environment

His present environment

Sources of Information

From the nursing history and the nurse's initial clinical appraisal, the nurse can obtain information about the patient's usual and current status with regard to his sensory abilities. The report of the initial physical examination of the patient, and any tests done on specific sensory abilities, such as a hearing test, eye examination, and so forth, should be included in the patient's record, and the nurse can supplement the nursing data with this information. Similarly, information about the patient's health problems and the plan of therapy for these should also be available to the nurse from the physician's notations and doctors' orders on the record.

From these sources the nurse can usually identify long-standing sensory deficits or problems the patient has, and any which have occurred recently, and she can also obtain information about corrective devices that the patient uses, such as eyeglasses or a hearing aid. In addition, what is his mobility status? Is he confined to bed, for example? Does he use a cane? Does he need a wheelchair for getting about?

Through talking with the patient or with his family or friends (the significant others in his life), the nurse may be able to learn something about the patient's basic personality structure to supplement information from the nursing history. Is this individual normally a quiet person? Or he is usually talkative? Is he gregarious and does he like the company of other people? Or does he prefer the company of his family or of one or two close friends? What are his usual activities during the day? What is his present environment like in comparison with this usual environment?

This is by no means an exhaustive list of questions the nurse might ask herself, but it may help her to think of other questions which might be useful in relation to this particular patient.

The nurse can further extend information about the patient's sensory abilities by her observations of the patient and his subjective reporting of changes that occur. The patient is the most reliable source of information about the functioning of his senses. Much of the information about these abilities must come from him. Because it is difficult to separate the subjective observations from the objective in this particular set of problems, the two have been combined in the discussion that follows. However, in her notations on the chart, the nurse will record separately those observations the patient describes and those she observes.

Observing for Sensory Deprivation

Sensory deprivation has long been thought to be a problem requiring nursing intervention. Florence Nightingale herself was evidently concerned about this when she wrote:

It is an ever recurring wonder to see educated people who call themselves nurses, acting thus. They vary their own objects, their own employments, many times a day; and while nursing (!) some bedridden sufferer, they let him be there staring at a dead wall, without any change of object to enable him to vary his thoughts; and it never occurs to them at least to move his bed so that he can look out of the window.[6]

It is important for the nurse to be able to recognize the signs of possible sensory deprivation in her patients and to take steps to prevent this problem from occurring or to remedy the situation if it does occur. Cameron and co-workers list a continuum of behaviors manifested by the patient suffering from sensory deprivation: boredom, inactivity, slowness of thought, daydreaming, increased sleeping, thought disorganization, anxiety, panic, hallucinations.[7]

The person who is *bored* may also be *inactive*, or he may be overactive, usually with trivial or inappropriate occupations. He may annoy other patients or continually push his call button to summon staff members, usually for small requests that

are either unnecessary or which he could handle himself. Often he is irritable and tends to make mountains of molehills. If he is *inactive*, he may appear apathetic and just lie or sit in one place without seeming to respond to any form of stimulation.

A person experiencing *slowness of thought* may take considerable time to grasp even simple concepts, and there may be great lapses in his conversation as he tries to think of what he wants to say. His reaction time will be reduced and he may appear clumsy and awkward.

The *daydreaming* individual may sit for seemingly endless periods of time, happily absorbed in his thoughts and fantasies, ignoring what is going on around him. It may be difficult to rouse him from his reveries, and he may not know when he has taken a medication or that someone was talking with him. He may confuse reality with fantasy.

The person who *sleeps* for longer than usual periods of time may be bored and consider this an effective way to pass the time, or he may actually find it difficult to stay awake with no stimuli to arouse his nervous system.

The individual suffering from *thought disorganization* may find it difficult to remember what he was saying, or he may experience space and time disorientation. He may not know what time of day it is, which meal he has just eaten, or where he is. He may make inappropriate responses both in conversation and in his actions. For example, he may intend to put on his glasses, and instead removes his shoes or puts on his dressing gown. He may experience distortions in sensory perception and, for instance, think he is eating fish when in fact he is eating fruit.

The person experiencing *anxiety* may feel that he is losing all faculties one by one or that he has a terrible brain disease affecting his sensory perception. He may become frightened and resort to the use of one of the defense mechanisms, as mentioned in Chapter 2.

Panic, as discussed in Chapter 12, is a severe state of anxiety. When an individual reaches the stage of panic where sensory disturbances are concerned, he may feel that he will be permanently blind, deaf, or paralyzed, or that he is going mad.

---

[6]Florence Nightingale: *Notes on Nursing.* New York, Appleton, 1946.

[7]Cameron et al., op cit., p. 33.

Downs places *hallucinations* at the extreme of her continuum.[8] A person suffering from hallucinations has lost all contact with reality. An explanation of the reason for hallucinations appearing in people who have experienced sensory deprivation is found in the following quotation from R. L. Gregory's book, *Eye and Brain:*

It seems that the brain is always spontaneously active, and that the activity is normally under the control of sensory signals. When these are cut off [as in an isolation chamber] the brain activity can run wild and instead of perception of the world, we become dominated by hallucinations which may be terrifying and dangerous, or merely irritating and amusing.

Observing for Sensory Overload

The nurse should also be alert to factors in the patient's environment which may cause sensory overload, and she should be observant for signs of this in the patient. Ambulatory patients may suffer from an excess of sensory stimulation in their work or home environment, or in the sum of their daily activities. Everyone needs a quiet place in which to relax, to be free from the constant ringing of the telephone and from all the other noises and activities that form a part of the lifestyle of many active, busy people.

The busy mother with a houseful of noisy children may show signs and symptoms of stress, as may the harried executive whose phone is constantly ringing, and who goes immediately from one meeting to another. The noise of machines in a factory constitutes a real health hazard to employees, as does the constant noise of planes for people who work in airports. We are only beginning to realize both the physical and psychological effects of excessive sensory stimulation as stress factors contributing to illness.

People who are ill are particularly vulnerable to the effects of excessive stimulation. This, of course, has long been recognized. Rest and quiet are still considered

the best therapy for many illnesses. In many instances the body will heal itself if it is not overwhelmed with the exigencies of the usual everyday activities. Indeed, illness is frequently the body's way of telling the individual that rest is needed.

We have already mentioned some of the sources of excessive sensory stimulation in people who are ill. The nurse should be alert to the factors which have been discussed as well as to excessive noise, interruptions of the patient's rest, too many people attending to the patient, or too many visitors, particularly for the person who is acutely ill.

People usually show signs of being tired from the effects of these. They may express their weariness verbally but often it is the nurse's responsibility to note if the patient's face looks tired and drawn, if his reactions are slowing down and every movement seems an effort, or if he is lying quietly in bed, trying to ignore the noise and what he views as widespread confusion around him.

Observing for Sensory Deficits

From her other sources of information, the nurse will be aware of existing sensory deficits, but she should be alert to pick up any which have not been identified, and also any which subsequently develop. Things to watch for in relation to specific sensory areas are:

Visual: (1) Acuity, particularly lessened ability to see objects or persons. If the patient normally wears glasses, the nurse should also check to see if these are still suitable for him. Many times, people find that illness affects their sight, and the glasses they used to wear no longer help them. This may be one reason the patient is not reading.

(2) Field of vision, particularly a decreased field; the patient may be unable to see things on either side of him without turning his head as well as he could previously.

---

[8]Downs, op. cit., p. 438.

[9]R. L. Gregory: *Eye and Brain.* 2nd Edition. New York, McGraw-Hill Book Company, 1973, p. 132.

(3) Unusual sensations, such as the perception of spots in front of the eyes, or black, grey, or sometimes other colored areas obscuring part of his vision in one or both eyes; or a ring or "halo" around objects.

Auditory: (1) Ability to distinguish voices, or to locate sounds.

(2) Unusual sensations, such as ringing or humming in the ears.

Olfactory: (1) Ability to distinguish odors.

(2) Unusual sensations, such as smelling an odor when there is no stimulus for it. In this regard, it should be noted that people sometimes experience the sensation of a specific odor just prior to a seizure (convulsion).

Gustatory: (1) Ability to discriminate sweet, sour, salty, and bitter tastes.

(2) Unusual sensations, such as a bitter or metallic taste in the mouth

Tactile: (1) Ability to discriminate sharp, dull, light, and firm touch.

(2) Ability to perceive heat, cold, pain.

(3) Intactness of body image.

(4) Unusual sensations, such as prickling, a feeling of "pins and needles," and the like.

Speech: (1) The formation and perception of speech.

(2) Problems in phonation (ability to articulate words).

(3) Ability to understand and initiate speech.

PRINCIPLES RELEVANT TO THE CARE OF PATIENTS WITH SENSORY DISTURBANCES

Nursing interventions are planned for patients with sensory disturbances in accordance with their specific problem, and are based on the individual's particular needs. It is helpful, however, to keep the following principles in mind.

1. Psychosocial equilibrium requires that individuals have adequate sensory stimulation.

2. Stimuli picked up by the sense organs provide the body with information about the external environment.

3. Integrity of the sense organs is essential for sensory perception.

4. Sensory perception can be distorted in persons who are ill.

5. Damage to brain tissues caused by disease processes or by injury can interfere with sensory perception.

6. Communication provides an important means of sensory stimulation.

7. All sensory receptors adapt, either partially or totally, to their various stimuli over a period of time.

8. The brain is active even in the absence of stimuli from the external environment.

GOALS FOR NURSING ACTION

The goals of nursing action for patients with actual or potential problems of disturbed sensory functioning depend on the nature of the problem. Regardless of whether they have problems or not, two goals are common for all patients:

1. To prevent sensory deprivation

2. To prevent sensory overload

For people with sensory deprivation, the following goals would be applicable:

1. To restore adequate sensory input

2. To restore normal perception

For people with a temporary or permanent sensory deficit, the following would be applicable:

1. To assist the individual to adjust to his deficit

2. To ensure that the individual receives adequate stimulation via his remaining sense receptors.

For people with sensory overload the primary objective would be to lessen sensory input to an optimal level.

SPECIFIC NURSING INTERVENTIONS

Our sensory abilities function to provide us with information about our environment. The environment, then, is one of the principal factors to be considered in helping people with sensory disturbances. Other major factors which the nurse takes into consideration are the in-

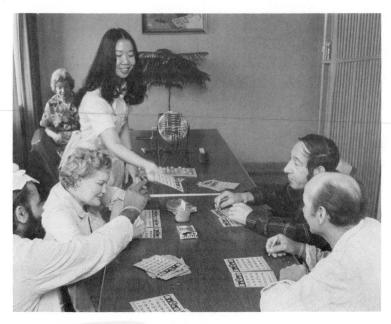

Active participation in games with other people provides a variety of sensory input that helps to keep an individual in touch with his environment.

dividual's reaction to disturbances in his sensory abilities and his needs in relation to learning to live with a deficit, if this is the problem.

Nursing interventions are considered in the light of their suitability for each individual's particular problem. The following possible approaches for nursing action are, therefore, outlined separately for each of the three common problems identified earlier in the chapter.

Sensory Deprivation

The logical approach to nursing action for the person who is suffering from sensory deprivation, or for those in whom this is a potential problem, is to ensure that the environment contains adequate stimuli to maintain or restore optimal sensory input. This implies a certain amount of environmental management on the nurse's part.

People in a home situation should be encouraged to vary both their physical and their psychosocial environment. The nurse may be able to make some suggestions in this regard, or to involve family and friends, or community organizations, to assist the individual if he is unable to do this for himself. Radio and television are great comforts to people who are un-

able to get out of their everyday environment, and they help to keep the individual in touch with the outside world. These can be supplemented with active participation in games, crafts, and other activities that keep them in contact with their environment. If the person is fond of reading, mobile libraries are available in many communities. A visit by a library staff member not only provides the person with new books and magazines to read, but also provides the stimulation of a new face and some conversation to relieve the monotony of the day.

People who deliver "Meals on Wheels" find that their clientele often look forward to the social aspects of the service as much as the actual meal. A number of service clubs, lodges, and other community groups visit shut-ins, and arrange for outings for senior citizens and handicapped persons. The nurse should be familiar with those services that are available in the community in which she works. Community centers and other organizations, such as the YWCA and YMCA, also provide a variety of activities for those who are ambulatory. Bridge clubs, arts and crafts classes, courses in a variety of subjects, academic and other subjects, such as gardening, swimming, and exercise classes, are among the many activities offered in a number of these centers.

For the person who is ill and in an institutional setting, the same types of approaches may be used. Volunteers and the resources of the community can help to provide the individual with sufficient change in both physical and psychosocial environment to ensure an adequate amount of sensory input.

Varying the patient's surroundings, even if it is just moving his bed so he can look out the window, as Florence Nightingale suggested, provides the individual with a different perspective.

For the person who must remain in an extended care facility, or one who is severely handicapped and confined at home, it is important to maintain their contact with reality. It is helpful to provide some device to enable them to do this. The use of clocks and watches, calendars, fixed time schedules for meals, arts and crafts, physiotherapy classes and so forth, regular television or radio programs, and similar means help to keep the person oriented to time and place. Newspapers and magazines provide a contact with what is going on in the world outside the agency setting.

The nurse may find brief explanations of nursing functions and treatments helpful, too, even if the activities are routine ones. They help to keep the person oriented to where he is and what is being done for and to him. The nurse should not think that just because the patient does not respond that he does not hear. It is important to maintain auditory stimuli for the person who is seriously deprived of sensory input.

Nor should the nurse forget the therapeutic effects of touch as a means of communication. A number of articles have been written recently on this topic and the nurse will find reference to some of these in the suggested reading list at the end of the chapter. The "laying on of hands" that is so much a part of nursing has been shown to have definite therapeutic healing properties, from both a physical and a psychological point of view. The nurse's presence also means the patient has someone to talk to, and the different nurses coming on for different shifts help to provide a variation in people which patients often find stimulating.

The nurse, then, functions both as a source of sensory input to the patient, and also as a resource person who can enlist the assistance of family, friends, visitors, and volunteers from community organizations to help the patient to receive adequate sensory stimulation. The nurse is frequently called upon to use her imagination to think of ways of getting people involved and providing the type of stimulation needed for a particular individual.

Sensory Overload

For the patient who is suffering from sensory overload, interventions that help to reduce the number of stimuli in the environment are indicated. In the community, the nurse may be able to help the individual to plan periods of rest in a busy day or to engage in activities that are relaxing for that individual. Physical exercise is often a good antidote for the person whose work keeps him in an office, a factory, or other enclosed surroundings. Some people need assistance in order to be able to rest and relax. Other people enjoy music or book reading or find a game of bridge relaxing. A change of stimuli is often as relaxing as a cessation of stimuli.

Some people need help in learning how to relax and clear their minds of stimuli activating them to do something. This topic will be discussed more fully in the chapter on rest, comfort, and sleep.

We have already discussed some of the ways the nurse can help to reduce environmental stimuli for the ill person, at home or in hospital. In addition, it sometimes helps to explain things in the environment, the reason for all those tubes and machines that are surrounding the patient, the purpose of treatments, and the reason why other personnel come in to see the patient. Putting a structure to the sensory input helps a person to interpret stimuli meaningfully; he is not so apt to feel disoriented, and his anxiety is reduced.

Sensory Deficit

In helping a person to cope with either temporary or permanent impairment of any one of his sensory abilities, the nurse needs to be aware of the individual's reaction to it. Loss of sensory functioning has both physical and psychosocial ramifications. We have mentioned some of the psychosocial effects in our earlier discussions. If the person has suffered a permanent and total disability of one of the senses, he feels an acute sense of loss and will grieve. If the nurse is caring for someone who has recently experienced such a loss, she may find it helpful at this point to read Chapter 32 of this book on care of the terminally ill patient. This individual goes through the same process of grieving as the person described in Chapter 32.

With a partial or a temporary loss of sensory functioning, the person will probably be anxious and worried. Will he regain total functioning? What if he becomes totally blind, or deaf, or is permanently paralyzed? What if his speech never comes back? How is he going to cope with partial impairment? These are some of the spoken and unspoken questions the person asks.

The patient needs much psychological support in coping with his anxieties, even if he does not express them (see Chapter 12). He also needs assistance with handling his physical environment in such a way that the deficit does not interfere with daily activities.

The nurse should be alert to anticipate problems in this regard, and also be aware of tools that have been developed to assist the handicapped person with maintaining, or restoring, his physical independence. The nurse should, whenever possible, provide for the patient's needs before he has to ask for help, which threatens his self-esteem. Cutting up food for the person who is having problems with vision, or for the person who has the use of only one hand; anticipating the need for help in putting on a dressing gown, or slippers; moving furniture out of the way; these and similar activities are a few examples of actions the nurse can take. It should go without saying that things on the bedside table and the light cord, the hand signal, and things the patient needs are placed within easy reach. It is amazing how often nurses, busy with treatments or medications, forget these small details.

Many new utensils and mechanical devices are now available commercially, or ordinary ones can be adapted to assist people with such activities as eating, reading, getting in and out of bed, and moving about. These items eliminate problems for people who are blind, paralyzed, or otherwise handicapped in performing necessary activities or those that provide pleasure. The physical and occupational therapists are often helpful in making suggestions for increasing an individual's independence when he has lost the use of one of his sensory abilities.

Often people with sensory handicaps need the help of specialized health professionals, or the services available in specialized agencies, to enable them to learn to live with a sensory deficit. The nurse supports the work of people such as the physical, occupational, and speech therapists by following through on activities, such as exercises, suggested by them. The patient's increased independence is ensured when all nursing personnel are aware of the goals for the patient, and are consistent in their approach to the patient.

Rehabilitation centers offer tremendous help for people who are learning to live with a sensory deficit, such as blindness, deafness, and paralysis, and those who have lost the ability to speak. The nurse should, if possible, visit one of these centers early in her career to become aware of things that are available to help these patients cope with the daily activities of living. She may encounter people who require some of these in other nursing situations, such as an acute setting where a person may be suffering a temporary loss of sensory functioning, or in a long-term care facility where she will probably meet people with multiple problems.

PLANNING AND EVALUATING THE EFFECTIVENESS OF SPECIFIC NURSING INTERVENTIONS

In planning the specific interventions to help each patient, the nurse needs to be explicit in the outcomes she expects from or hopes for in the patient. For example, for the person who remains in his room, sitting in his wheelchair most of the day, the anticipated outcome of the nurse's intervention might be to increase the number of hours he is out of his room each day, by setting definite criteria, such as two hours at first, perhaps increasing up to eight per day. Or, for the person who takes no initiative in going to arts and crafts, or other forms of activities, having him participate in these and take increasing responsibility for getting himself to arts and crafts (for example) would be worthwhile goals. For the person who is depressed or apathetic, even the patient's initiation of conversation would be a major achievement to be accomplished by nursing interventions. Having him feed himself or dress himself without help, and doing so on a regular basis, might be other goals the nurse considers important for the patient to attain. The general goals suggested earlier are helpful, but for planning specific interventions, the nurse will need to think of short-term goals that are realistic, attainable, and measurable for each patient.

If her goals have been explicitly stated, the nurse is able to evaluate the effectiveness of various interventions she has tried, and to try other alternatives if these have not been successful. It also helps the nurse to feel a sense of accomplishment when she notes the patient's progress and finds that goals are achieved, and she has been responsible in large part for their attainment. This aspect of nursing care is important for the nurse as well as the patient.

GUIDE TO ASSESSING SENSORY DISTURBANCES

1. Does the patient have long-standing deficits in regard to sensory functions, such as problems with vision, with hearing, with taste or smell, with speech communication? Is he paralyzed in any part of his body?
2. Does he normally use corrective devices for any sensory deficits he may have, such as eyeglasses, a hearing aid, a cane, walker, or wheelchair (for the paralyzed individual), or does he need the help of another person to overcome a deficit in any of the sensory abilities?
3. What is the present status of his sensory abilities?
4. Does he have any health problem that might cause, or has caused, sensory disturbances?
5. Is there sufficient stimulation in his present environment? too much? How does his present environment compare with his usual one?
6. Is he receiving enough social stimulation to maintain adequate sensory input?
7. Does the individual show physical signs or behaviors indicative of sensory deprivation? of sensory overload?
8. What are this individual's usual personality characteristics?
9. What is his usual lifestyle?

STUDY VOCABULARY

Adaptation	Hallucinogens	Sensory deprivation
Auditory	Olfactory	Sensory overload
Gustatory	Perception	Tactile
Hallucinations	Sensory deficits	

STUDY SITUATION

Mr. Jones is a 75 year old retired school principal who had a CVA with resultant hemiplegia (left-sided) nine months ago. Following the acute episode, he was admitted to a rehabilitation unit but did not progress as well as expected and was transferred to an extended care facility, where he has been ever since. His mental faculties appear unimpaired; his speech is intact; visual and auditory functioning are decreased. He has some movement in the left leg but the arm is flaccid. He is helped into a wheelchair daily and can propel himself about a little. Mr. Jones' wife died two years ago; two of his four adult children (a son and a daughter) live in town—the other two sons at a considerable distance—and both visit frequently, as do their children.

Prior to his disability, Mr. Jones was active in the local community center, played golf regularly, and liked to travel.

On the ward, he spends most of his time in his room, staring out of the window; he does not go to the TV room and has given up reading newspapers because he says he can read nothing but the headlines. He can never remember if visitors have been in or not. He has his radio on most of the time, but keeps it on low because other patients were complaining about it.

1. What can the nurse do to help Mr. Jones?

SUGGESTED READINGS

Amacher, N. J.: Touch is a Way of Caring. *American Journal of Nursing*, 73:852–854, May 1973.

Black, Sr. K.: Social Isolation and the Nursing Process. *Nursing Clinics of North America*, 8:575–586, December 1973.

Brooks, C. V. W.: Sensory Awareness. *Psychology Today*, 8:104, April 1975.

Burnett, I., et al.: Caring for Single Room Occupancy Tenants. *American Journal of Nursing*. 73:1752–1756, October 1973.

Chapanis, A.: Interactive Human Communication. *Scientific American*, 232:36–42, March 1975.

Hannan, J. F.: Talking is Treatment, Too. *American Journal of Nursing*, 74:1991–1992, November 1974.

Krieger, D.: Therapeutic Touch: The Imprimatur of Nursing. *American Journal of Nursing*, 75:784, May 1975.

Loesch, L. C., and N. A. Loesch: What Do You Say After You Say Mm--hmm? *American Journal of Nursing*, 75:807, May 1975.

Marks, L. E.: Synesthesia: The Lucky People With Mixed-Up Senses. *Psychology Today*, 9:48–49, June 1975.

McCorkle, R.: Effects of Touch on Seriously Ill Patients. *Nursing Research*, 23:125–132, March-April 1974.

Perron, D. M.: Deprived of Sound. *American Journal of Nursing*, 74:1057–1059, June 1974.

Reid, E. A., et al.: Roommates: To Have or Have Not. *American Journal of Nursing*, 73:104–107, January 1973.

Rosenthal, R., et al.: Body Talk and Tone of Voice: The Language Without Words. *Psychology Today*, September 1974.

Smith, M. J.: Changes in Judgment of Duration With Different Patterns of Auditory Information for Individuals Confined to Bed. *Nursing Research*, 24:93–98, March-April 1975.

Thompson, L. R.: Sensory Deprivation: A Personal Experience. *American Journal of Nursing*, 73:266–268, February 1973.

Wahl, P. R.: Psychosocial Implications of Disorientation in the Elderly. *Nursing Clinics of North America*, 11:145–156, March 1976.

CHAPTER 14

Spiritual Needs

14 SPIRITUAL NEEDS

The nurse should be able to:

Discuss the relationship of spiritual beliefs and illness

List criteria which are helpful in assessing the spiritual needs of the patient

Identify nursing responsibilities in the spiritual care of patients

Describe the role of the chaplain as a member of the health team

Name specific aspects of religious custom and sacraments of the Jewish, Roman Catholic, and major Protestant religions which affect the care of patients with these religious beliefs

Outline nursing responsibilities in regard to these sacraments and religious customs

Establish criteria for evaluating nursing care in relation to the patient's spiritual needs

INTRODUCTION

The need of many patients for spiritual counsel is receiving increased recognition from members of the various health and allied professions. In recent years the hospital chaplain has become a valued member of the health team and plays an important role in patient therapy.

Often the nurse is the first person to become aware of a patient's desire or need for spiritual guidance. Frequently it is up to her to inform the patient of the help available to him and to contact the hospital chaplain or the community pastor. The nurse herself may be able to help the patient in spiritual matters, for she has a supportive role as well as the role of maintaining liaison between the patient and his sources of spiritual counsel.

Most people have some type of religious philosophy. In spite of the highly publicized trend toward secularism in the twentieth century, various studies show that from two-thirds to nine-tenths of the population of the United States profess a belief in a Supreme Being. Moreover, at a time of illness many nonprofessing persons look for spiritual guidance and consolation.

To provide a person with spiritual counsel is, therefore, in keeping with treating the whole person. Just as people who are ill often require help on a physical level, so they require spiritual aid. In addition, the recent recognition of psychosomatic illness emphasizes the role of emotions in disease. Thus, to treat the whole person requires physical, emotional, and spiritual help.

The spiritual needs of patients involve answers to such questions as: Who am I? What am I like? What kind of world is this? These highly personal questions often become urgent at a time of illness, when the patient finds himself with time to think about himself and the world about him. Shut off from everyday concerns, some patients tend to question their entire system of values.

Some people look for an answer to why they are ill. They may look for moral significance to their illness and hope that religious doctrine will provide the solution. Other patients look for spiritual guidance to assist them in accepting their new role in the family. For example, the husband who normally supports his family but has become dependent upon his wife's earnings while he is ill may face a severe test. The acceptance of such changes in established roles and life patterns can be one of the most difficult adjustments a person must make.

Sometimes a person's values in life change with illness; often his horizons grow smaller, his bed becoming his domain. Spiritual beliefs can help such a patient to accept his illness and plan for the future. It can help him maintain a realistic perspective of himself and his relationship to the world about him. It can give him that inner strength which is closely interwoven with emotional health and physical well-being.

Religion is a social as well as a spiritual institution within society. Most societies have developed some form of religion, which then serves as an integrative force within the society. Traditionally, the established religions have been concerned with ethics and moral behavior. Many established religions, however, have broadened their activities to include other areas. For example, recreation centers for all age groups have become an accepted part of the facilities of the church. Such centers offer the people of the community

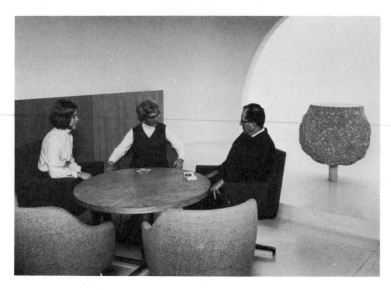

Many hospitals provide a quiet room where the patient and his family can meet with their spirtual counselor.

opportunities to find new interests and to join groups with which they can identify and in which they feel accepted.

Many churches now have special programs for youth groups designed to help adolescents and young people with their particular problems. "Drop-in centers" and other variously named gathering places are operated by a number of denominations to cater to the needs of young people.

SPIRITUAL BELIEFS AND ILLNESS

Spiritual beliefs, then, often help a patient at a time of stress. Some patients look to religious philosophy to explain illness; others look upon illness as a test of faith. Viewed in this light, illness and injury are usually accepted with forbearance and pose little threat to religious belief.

Still others interpret disease as God's punishment. "What have I done to deserve this?" they may ask. People who believe this interpretation attach a moral significance to disease, and they reason that because they have sinned they are being punished. They often believe that through prayers, promise, and penance the cause of the disease will be treated. To them the physician treats only the symptoms. When a patient who believes

this gets well, therefore, it is an indication that as a sinner he has been forgiven. On the other hand, should he die, his family either accepts his death as God's punishment or finds it to be unacceptable and unjust.

There are situations in which religious beliefs can be a hindrance to therapy and to health. Some religious groups tend to exalt faith and to disregard science. For example, many practicing Jehovah's Witnesses are by doctrine not permitted to have blood transfusions. The Church of Christ, Scientist, teaches spiritual healing; thus, when a practicing Christian Scientist seeks a physician's help, he may feel guilty because the prayers to relieve his symptoms were inadequate. He rarely blames his beliefs for the lack of cure, even when these beliefs may have caused him to delay his visit to a physician and his condition has worsened considerably during this time.

Generally speaking, religion helps people to accept illness and plan for the future. It can help a person to prepare for death, and it can also strengthen him during life. For example, the Christian belief of eternal life can help a patient face death more serenely. On the other hand, the Christian religion offers an interpretation of life that is based upon love and thus can also strengthen a person in his daily life.

A discussion of illness and religious

philosophy would not be complete without mentioning faith healing. This is an area that has received considerable publicity and research. There are religious organizations that are active in faith healing, for example, some evangelical groups. The British Medical Association appointed a committee to carry out a program of research on divine healing. The committee was able to categorize all reported instances of divine healing into six areas: mistaken diagnosis, mistaken prognosis, alleviation, remission, spontaneous cure, and combined treatment. Although the committee found no evidence to support divine healing as the sole factor in any reported cure, it did not rule out religion as an integral part of patient therapy.[1]

Generally nurses and physicians recognize the importance of spiritual counsel as a part of a patient's therapy, and pastors recognize the close relationship between spiritual, emotional, and physical needs.

IDENTIFYING THE SPIRITUAL NEEDS OF THE PATIENT

Spiritual needs, as we have noted, often become particularly apparent during a time of illness. In the hospital, it is usually the nurse who recognizes the patients who would like spiritual guidance, and it is also the nurse's responsibility to make available to the patient the sources of spiritual help.

Some patients bring articles with them which have a religious significance, and from these a nurse often can gain some idea of the importance that religious belief holds for a particular patient. For example, a Roman Catholic patient might have a rosary or a medal; an Episcopalian might have a prayer book.

Nurses should remember that there are patients who are not associated with any particular religious group. To them, spiritual need and spiritual belief are highly personal matters. Others are frankly agnostic, and for them any religious appeal would probably have a negative effect. Still others find the visits of a religious representative to be a source of discomfort rather than comfort; for example, a person might not like the particular hospital chaplain or the religious denomination that he (or she) represents. A nurse should cautiously assess the patient's attitude toward religion and his spiritual needs before she proffers suggestions or help.

Westberg has listed nine groups of people who respond best to pastoral care.[2] This list can serve as a guide to the nurse in identifying patients who might like the hospital chaplain to visit. The list should in no way be interpreted to exclude other groups, nor is it intended to replace an assessment of individual needs or to automatically include all patients to whom this classification applies.

1. *The patient who is lonely and has few visitors.* The perceptive nurse will hear a patient express loneliness in obscure ways as well as in obvious terms. The patient who continually has his signal light on to call the nurse may really be saying "I am lonely. Please stay with me." The nurse can also identify the lonely patient by making her rounds of the nursing unit during visiting hours. At this time she has an opportunity to meet patients' families and she can note those who do not have visitors. Patients whose homes are in distant communities may be lonely because their families and friends are far away.

2. *The patient who expresses fear and anxiety.* Some people will state frankly that they are afraid. Others express their fears by their questions, silence, body tension, or facial expression. The taut, pale face and the anxious eyes often express fear as emphatically as words.

3. *The patient whose illness is directly related to emotions or to religious attitudes.* Because of guilt feelings, occasionally related directly or indirectly to religious doctrine, some people might develop physical symptoms of illness. An example is the single woman who becomes pregnant and, as a result, feels that

[1]Samuel Southard: *Religion and Nursing.* Nashville, Tenn., Broadman Press, 1959, p. 63.

[2]Granger Westberg: *Nurse, Pastor and Patient.* Philadelphia, Fortress Press, 1955, p. 73.

she faces religious and social condemnation.

4. *The patient who faces surgery.* People who face operations are often afraid, and their fear is not necessarily related to the seriousness of the operation. Many people fear anesthesia, body disfigurement, pain, or even body exposure, but above all they fear death during surgery.

5. *The patient who has to change his pattern of life as a result of illness and injury.* Some people take great pride in their independence, and the prospect of any degree of dependence upon others is frightening. Some people worry about their changing roles within their families or their ability to earn a living. Illness and injury often necessitate abrupt changes in established living patterns that must be met by both the patient and his family.

6. *The patient who is preoccupied about the relationship of his religion and his health.* Such a patient may be seeking the reason for his illness in religious doctrine or may be trying to explain his illness in terms of religious philosophy.

7. *The patient who is unable to have his pastor visit or who would not normally receive pastoral care.* People who come from distant communities may not know a pastor in the immediate area. Other patients may not belong to religious groups in the community, but at a time of illness they may want spiritual counsel.

8. *The patient whose illness has social implications.* For example, the person who has had disfiguring surgery may feel that the hospital chaplain represents social acceptance or social rejection, and acceptance by the community may be important to his future plans.

9. *The patient who is dying.* Facing death, the patient may be filled with uncertainty and worry about his family. Spiritual guidance can often help him to meet death, and it can help his family accept his death and plan for the future.

THE NURSE AND SPIRITUAL GUIDANCE IN THE HOSPITAL

The nurse can play an important role in providing the patient with spiritual support. One of her most important activities is identifying people's spiritual needs. To do this effectively the nurse must take time to listen to the patient and to ascertain his emotional status. Usually a patient is not looking for answers from the nurse; he is looking for acceptance and help while he thinks out answers for himself.

Pastors appreciate referrals from nursing personnel and usually welcome the nurse's observations regarding the patient's spiritual needs. Most members of clergy prefer to look after these needs themselves, however, and nursing responsibilities are usually limited in this regard.

If the nurse feels competent and comfortable in helping to meet the patient's spiritual needs, she can assist him by helping him to read from the Bible, if he so desires. For example, if the patient is unable to read himself, the nurse can read to him. If the patient can do his own reading, the nurse can arrange privacy for him. Most hospitals provide Bibles, either at each bedside or at the nursing station or hospital library.

In addition to the Bible and prayer books, a great deal of religious literature is available. Religious tracts, for instance, are published by many groups. Since tracts are often designed to meet specific needs, particular tracts can be selected to meet particular circumstances.

Prayers are the fourth area in which the nurse can help patients. Prayer takes many forms; to many it is a means of reaching God. However, prayer does not always involve a sense of mutuality; for example, in Buddhism, Gautama is regarded as unconscious and inaccessible.

One patient may prefer to pray silently, and to him prayer is a highly personal activity. Another may like the nurse to say a prayer for him, and this becomes a source of considerable comfort. Prayers need not be long; a simple, sincerely stated prayer can be as comforting as a lengthy one.[3] A simple evening prayer that can be readily learned by the nurse is:

O Lord, support us every hour of our lives until the evening comes and our work is done. Then grant us your mercy, holy rest, and peace at last, through Jesus Christ our Lord, Amen.

[3]Ibid., p. 86.

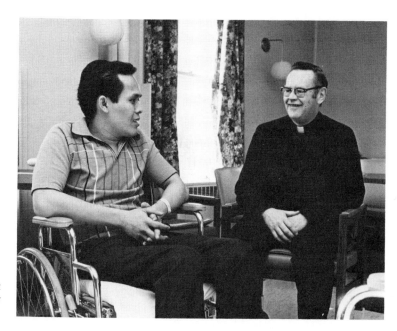

The Chaplain's visit is a source of comfort to many patients.

If the nurse does not feel comfortable praying with the patient or reading to him from the Bible, it is quite acceptable for her to suggest that someone else do this. Most clergymen are happy to assist the patient in these matters, and the nurse may refer the patient to the pastor of his faith.

Finally, the sacraments, which constitute a source of strength, are a means of providing spiritual help. Sacraments are usually administered by the designated representative of a religious group, although the nurse can administer the sacrament of baptism to a Roman Catholic patient if a priest is not available. The specific sacraments and the nurse's role in administering them are discussed later in this chapter.

THE HOSPITAL CHAPLAIN

The hospital chaplain may be a minister, priest, rabbi, or other member whose chief charges are the patients in a hospital. Large hospitals frequently have full-time chaplains representing several faiths. The Protestant faith is usually represented by ministers of various denominations, for example, Episcopalian, Methodist, Baptist and Congregationalist. The Roman Catholic faith is represented by the priest, the Jewish faith by the rabbi. Small hospitals may not have chaplains but, like their larger counterparts, they extend liberal visiting privileges to the representatives of the established religions in the community.

When the hospital chaplain or pastor comes to see a patient, he or she usually checks with the nurse to make sure the visit is convenient for the patient. At this time the nurse is afforded an opportunity to give him information which may help him in counseling the patient. She can also tell him the names of other patients who want him to visit. Hospital chaplains and community pastors are generally available day or night, and they often leave their telephone numbers with the nurse so that they can be called at any time. It could be imperative, for example, to call a priest quickly for a dying Roman Catholic patient.

Some hospitals have chapels in which religious services are held regularly for the patients and their families. The services are usually conducted by the hospital chaplain or by the pastors from the community. Patients who would like to attend these services should be assisted to do so if it is possible. They may involve rearranging nursing care activities.

The hospital chaplain is an important member of the health team. Kevin describes the Roman Catholic priest as a physician of the soul.[4] McKnight states, "The specific role of the chaplain in a psychiatric hospital is that of helping people come to a healthy relationship with God."[5] The chaplain can contribute much in the care of patients. His knowledge and his spiritual guidance are often important adjuncts to medical care. The hospital chaplain can help people clarify their anxieties and accept illness. The community pastor often maintains liaison between the hospital patient and his family and can lend his support when the patient returns home. He can also assist the physician by interpreting medical instructions for the patient and in planning the patient's future.

Many hospital chaplains are active members of the health team. As such they attend health team conferences and contribute to the plans for the patient's therapy. Their knowledge of the patient's spiritual needs and personal problems can be essential in effectively helping the whole person.

Another service provided by the chaplain is that of serving as a source of information for other members of the health team. For example, his knowledge of religious dietary preferences can be helpful to the dietitian when she plans a patient's menu. The importance of baptism in Roman Catholic doctrine is particularly relevant for nurses in the delivery room. The hospital chaplain can also provide spiritual advice to members of the hospital staff. Counsel at a time of stress can often help a nurse to be more effective in helping patients and their families.

The hospital chaplain also administers the sacraments to patients in the hospital. Through the sacraments, both the patient and his family receive spiritual strength and solace. The specific sacraments of the Roman Catholic, Hebrew, and Protestant faiths are discussed in the following section.

---

[4]Barry Kevin: The Catholic Chaplain. *Canadian Nurse*, 57:1142, December, 1961.

[5]Earle T. McKnight: A Chaplain Interprets His Work. *Canadian Nurse*, 57:1139, December, 1961.

SPECIFIC RELIGIOUS CUSTOMS

The Jewish Faith

Patients who belong to the Jewish faith probably belong to the reform, conservative, or orthodox groups. Not all Jewish people follow the same practices, so the nurse will need to be sensitive to the patient's individual wishes. Generally the Jewish patient who follows orthodox doctrine will adhere most closely to certain dietary and religious customs. The patient himself, his family, or the rabbi will assist the nurse regarding doctrinal customs.

The rabbi is the pastor of the Jewish congregation. Many Jewish patients like to have their own rabbi visit them when they are ill. He provides spiritual counsel to the patient and his family.

To the Hebrew people the act of *circumcision* is a religious rite. It marks the entrance of the male child as a potential citizen to the community. It should take place on the eighth day after birth of a male child; at the conclusion of the ceremony the child is named. Circumcision is called Brith Milah in Hebrew. The elaborateness of the ceremony depends on the preferences of the family. Ten Jewish men must always be present, including all the male members of the infant's family. Following the circumcision there may be a reception for the members of the family and their friends. The nurse will be instructed in advance by the rabbi or the mohel (one who performs the circumcision) as to what equipment will be required for the ceremony.

Upon the death of a Jewish patient, the rabbi should be notified if the family is not present. He will arrange for the patient's burial. There is no need to be concerned about baptism, since the Jewish faith does not practice this rite.

The orthodox Hebrew patient may follow certain dietary regulations. Jewish doctrine forbids the eating of certain foods, including any part of the pig. In addition, certain other foods may be eaten only when they are specially prepared. The permitted foods are called kosher. They include the meat of animals that are ruminants and have divided hoofs, such as cows and sheep. Kosher fowl are fowl that are not birds of prey, and kosher fish are fish with scales. Examples of kosher fowl are chicken and duck; salmon and sardines can be classed as kosher fish. All shellfish, such as clams, oysters, and lobster, are prohibited. Meat dishes and dishes containing milk, cream, or butter may not be eaten at the same meal.

In order for meat to be considered kosher the animals must be slaughtered and the meat prepared in a special manner. No special precautions are required for vegetables. If a hospital is not prepared to provide kosher meat, other protein foods such as vegetable protein products can be substituted. Often a patient's family will arrange to provide kosher food if the patient is anxious about this. The nurse will need to instruct the family regarding any special dietary requirements for the patient.

There are other dietary regulations that apply at the time of the Passover. At this time a Jewish patient may refrain from eating leavened food, for example, bread. The rabbi can arrange to have special Passover matzo (unleavened bread) brought to the patient. Any Hebrew patient can be excused from strict dietary customs when he is ill. If the patient is concerned about this, the nurse can notify the rabbi and he will explain this to the patient.

The Roman Catholic Faith

The Roman Catholic faith recognizes several sacraments which have particular importance for nurses. In the Roman Catholic Church, God is conceived to be a God of mercy and grace, which are mediated through the church. The sacraments are signs and seals of God's expression to his people, and through them a person attains a state of grace, which is necessary for salvation. *Baptism* is the first of the sacraments to be administered to an individual. Because it is necessary for an infant to be baptized in order to receive salvation, it is very important to see to it that an infant in danger of death is baptized. According to Roman Catholic doctrine, an infant has a soul from the minute of conception; therefore a fetus at any stage of development must be baptized if it is born.

A nurse can perform a baptism by pouring water on the head of the child and at the same time saying, "I baptize thee in the name of the Father and of the Son and of the Holy Ghost." There are forms used in hospitals to record baptism of an infant, one of which is integrated into or attached to the patient's record; the duplicate is sent to the pastor of the family.

Holy Communion is another sacrament of the Roman Catholic Church. Patients are allowed water and medications prior to communion, as well as essential medical procedures up to the time of receiving communion.

When Holy Communion is requested by the patient, the Catholic chaplain of the hospital is called, or a priest from the church which serves the hospital. In either instance, a clean towel is used as a cover on top of the bedside table, on which the nurse places a glass of water and a spoon. Hospitals usually have a communion set on each floor which is taken into the patient's room and left for the use of the chaplain or visiting priest. Privacy is to be observed for the patient and the priest during the communion service.

The *Anointing of the Sick* is a sacrament that is performed for many patients. Formerly known as Extreme Unction or last rites, it used to be given only to the person who was in danger of dying. Now, however, it is interpreted as an aid to healing and a source of strength. It may therefore be received by a patient one or more times for each illness, and may be received several times in a lifetime.

It is felt that this sacrament should be administered when the patient is conscious. It can be performed any time of the day or night. The priest anoints the eyes, ears, nostrils, lips, hands, and feet with oil, for which cotton balls should be provided. Hospitals have a form for the priest to sign after he has administered this sacrament; the form is then attached to or integrated into the patient's record.

Even if a patient of the Roman Catholic faith dies without receiving the Anointing of the Sick, a priest should be called. He can administer the sacrament immediately following death, thus providing a source of comfort to the patient's family.

With the revisions in dietary practices for Roman Catholics, meat may be eaten on Friday, except during the season of Lent. Hospitals usually have a choice of meat or fish on the Friday menu and, during Lent, on the Wednesday menu also. The patient is free to select whichever he or she wishes, unless there is a special diet prescription.

The Protestant Faith

The Protestant faith includes many denominations; Methodists, Baptists, Presbyterians, Episcopalians (Anglicans), and Congregationalists are but a few of the larger groups. Most Protestant patients prefer the chaplain of their own church, but in an emergency the chaplain of another denomination can often help.

The sacrament of *baptism* is a generally universal rite within the Protestant faith. Some denominations practice baptism in infancy; others baptize at the age of understanding, often when a child is 12 years old. For a few Protestants, baptism is a necessity before death.

Some Protestant denominations hold *Holy Communion* and for many patients this can be a strengthening spiritual food. For this sacrament the clergyman requires a table in the patient's room to be cleared and furnished with a clean white cloth. It is preferable if the patient can assume a sitting position and, of course, privacy should be provided during the service. In communion the patient partakes of wine and bread; the wine represents the blood of Christ and the bread represents the body of Christ. Some Protestants consider this rite to be a cleansing of the soul from sin.

A few Protestant churches, the Episcopal Church for example, are placing increasing emphasis upon anointing, and for this rite privacy is important.

Some Protestants have dietary customs. Some are vegetarians and some do not drink tea or coffee—for example, members of the Mormon Church. Other people do not smoke or drink alcoholic beverages because of religious doctrine. During Lent, some Protestants practice a variety of dietary restrictions. Generally speaking, however, a Protestant's eating habits are not restricted by religious doctrine.

GUIDE TO ASSESSING NURSING NEEDS

1. Is religion important in the patient's system of values?
2. Does the patient feel spiritual counsel would help his health and well-being? Or does the patient indicate that he does not want assistance with spiritual needs?
3. Is he receiving the spiritual help he wishes?
4. Does the patient have specific spiritual needs with which members of the health team can be of assistance?

GUIDE TO EVALUATING THE EFFECTIVENESS OF NURSING ACTION

1. Is the patient accorded the privacy and facilities required to fulfill his religious needs?
2. Has the chaplain, rabbi, or priest been notified if he is needed?
3. Does the patient have access to the Bible or other religious literature in accordance with his wishes?

STUDY VOCABULARY

Anointing of the sick	Kosher	Rabbi
Baptism	Pastor	Religion
Chaplain	Priest	Sacrament
Communion		

STUDY SITUATION

Mrs. J. C. D. is a 43 year old woman who has been in the hospital for 10 days. Her religion is Protestant. Mrs. D. was pregnant before she came to the hospital, but she lost her baby as a result of an automobile accident. She was scheduled to go home several days ago; however, she appeared very tired and depressed. The doctor suggested that she stay in the hospital for another week. One afternoon when the nurse walked into Mrs. D.'s room, she found the patient reading the Bible. The patient looked embarrassed and immediately put the Bible away. She said, "I am so unhappy. I lost my baby and I am sure it was a girl."

The nurse answered, "But Mrs. D., you have four wonderful sons at home now. You are really very lucky and you should think about them."

Mrs. D. said nothing more.

1. For what reasons might Mrs. D. be depressed?
2. What kinds of behavior might indicate to the nurse that this patient is worried?
3. What might the nurse have said?
4. What could the nurse do to help Mrs. D.?
5. If Mrs. D. had belonged to the Roman Catholic Church, what should the nurse consider?

SUGGESTED READINGS

Allport, G. W.: *The Individual and His Religion.* New York, The Macmillan Company, 1961.

Blum, R. H.: *The Management of the Doctor-Patient Relationship.* New York, Blakiston Division, McGraw-Hill Book Company, 1960.

Brown, E. L.: *Newer Dimensions in Patient Care. Part III. Patients as People.* New York, Russell Sage Foundation, 1964.

Daoust, J. M.: Spiritual Care of the Sick. *L'hôpital d'aujourd'hui, 16:*7:20, July, 1970.

Dickinson, Sr. C.: The Search for Spiritual Meaning. *American Journal of Nursing,* 75:1789–1793, October 1975.

Frazier, C. A. (ed.): *Healing and Religious Faith.* Philadelphia, United Church Press, 1974.

Naiman, H. L.: Nursing in Jewish Law. *The American Journal of Nursing,* 70:10:2378–2379, November, 1970.

Pederson, W. D.: The Broadening Role of the Hospital Chaplain. *Hospitals,* 42:9:58, May 1, 1968.

Recognizing Your Patients' Spiritual Needs. *Nursing Update,* 6:1, July 1975.

Spiro, D.: Jewish Patients in Hospital. *Canadian Nurse,* 57:1144, December, 1961.

Williams, D. D.: *The Minister and the Care of Souls.* New York, Harper & Brothers, 1961.

15 LEARNING NEEDS

The nurse should be able to:

Explain the importance of meeting the patient's learning needs
Describe ways of identifying the learning needs of patients
Cite factors which influence these learning needs
List principles of learning relevant to the development of an effec-
    tive teaching plan for patients
Develop realistic goals for patient learning
Name the three basic types of learning tasks
Describe methods and techniques of teaching suitable for each type
    of learning task
List factors to consider in selecting the time and place for teaching
    patients
Describe methods for the evaluation of patient learning suitable for
    different types of learning tasks

INTRODUCTION

One of the roles of the nurse identified in Chapter 6 was that of teacher. The nurse is regarded by the public as a person knowledgeable about health matters; her opinion is respected and her advice sought by people on matters that concern them about their health. By now, you have probably found that your friends, your family—and other people too—are beginning to ask you questions about health matters, even though you are just commencing your nursing program. A comment you will hear frequently throughout your lifetime is, "You should know—after all, you are a nurse." You cannot possibly expect to be able to teach everybody all that they want or need to know about their health at this stage of your career, nor even after you have completed your nursing course. But you can help them to learn what they want to learn.

The identification of learning needs and the development of plans to meet these needs are considered integral parts of the problem-oriented approach to health care (as discussed in Chapter 11).

Every individual, whatever the state of his health, has learning needs in relation to health matters. The person who is active and in good health, for example, may need to learn more about nutrition in order to control his weight, or he may want to embark on a regular exercise program to improve his physical well-being. Most people want to know how to protect their health. Parents are usually particularly anxious to learn measures they can take to protect their children from the disorders to which youngsters are particularly vulnerable, as well as steps they can take to promote each child's optimal growth and development.

Most people who become ill have learning needs relative to their new situation. They usually want knowledge about tests and examinations, about their disease process, and, if they have been hospitalized, about their environment. Some people must learn ways of planning for the future, regaining their health, or coping with physical, psychological, and sociological stresses.

Nurses and other health personnel should always keep in mind the ultimate goal of restoring the sick individual to an active, functioning role in society, insofar as this is possible. Rehabilitation should not be considered as a separate set of activities to be carried out by a specialized agency after the patient has left the hospital setting. The individual and his family must be assisted from the onset of his illness, and throughout its duration, to engage in activities that will help him achieve the highest level of well-being that is possible for him. To use an example, the person who has had a stroke needs to be encouraged to maintain independent bladder and bowel functioning and given the opportunity to do so, or, if necessary, to regain independence in this area as quickly as possible if it has been lost temporarily during a period of unconsciousness. Nurses all too often accept incontinence as an inevitable result of illness, particularly in older people—yet it need not be so. Rehabilitation is a learning process that should not be left until an episode of acute illness is over. Helping the individual to learn new skills or to relearn old ones should be a fundamental part of care throughout any illness.

Helping to meet the patient's learning needs is an integral part of the nurse's role. In order to meet these needs, the nurse must know something about the 255 learning process; be able to identify patient's learning needs; and be able to select appropriate methods and techniques to facilitate the learning process. She should also be able to evaluate the effectiveness of the patient's learning.

One of the most basic truisms of learning is that we learn what we do. Methods and techniques which encourage active participation on the part of the learner are therefore more effective than those in which the learner plays a passive role. For example, the new mother may need to learn how to bathe her infant. Telling the mother how to give the baby a bath is not a very effective way of teaching her to do this. A more appropriate way would include a demonstration of the procedure and an explanation of reasons for the various steps by the nurse, return demonstration, and subsequent practice by the mother (or patient). The effectiveness of the learning would be evaluated by the nurse by questioning the mother and observing how she bathed the baby.

THE LEARNING PROCESS

Learning is an active process which continues from birth to death. Throughout his lifetime, an individual is constantly learning as he gains information, develops skills, and applies his acquired knowledge and skills in adjusting to new life situations. Learning takes place basically in one of two ways—either informally, through the ordinary process of living, or formally, through a series of selected learning experiences designed to achieve specific goals.

People learn a great deal about health and illness through informal means. In the family environment, for example, parents usually assume responsibility for teaching children about hygiene measures, about ways to protect their health, and, often, about care during illness. The type of learning that occurs in the family is often supplemented by informal talks with people in the health field as well as by other means, such as by reading articles in the newspapers about health matters, or the health columns written by medical experts that are a feature in many of the popular magazines. People also learn informally about health and illness through programs on the radio and on television.

People who are sick and need the help of health professionals often learn much about their health problems informally through the actual life experience of being ill. However, there has been a substantial amount of evidence to indicate that many patients' learning needs are not met through informal channels. One of the most frequent complaints of patients is that they do not receive enough information. This concern has been voiced in the statements of Patients' Bills of Rights, cited in Chapter 1. Yet it has been shown that the better informed the patient is about his condition, the more effective is his therapy. The value of good patient teaching in contributing to the sick person's recovery and his rehabilitation has been well documented. Adequate preoperative instruction has been shown to be a factor in the prevention of many postoperative discomforts, such as pain and vomiting, and a contributing factor in early recovery from surgery.[1] A good teaching program for diabetic patients is accepted as an important aspect of the care of patients with this condition. Many agencies today have a diabetic teaching team whose sole responsibility is to teach patients about their disease.

The value of good instruction is by no means limited to the care of surgical and diabetic patients. One can justifiably state that all patients have learning needs, and a systematic plan for meeting these needs should be incorporated into the nursing care plan for each patient.

ASSESSING THE PATIENT'S LEARNING NEEDS

Assessing the learning needs of patients is a cooperative endeavor involving the patient, the physician, the nurse, and

---

[1] S. T. Hegyvary et al.: The Hospital Setting and Patient Care Outcomes. *Journal of Nursing Administration,* 5:29–32, March-April 1975. See also C. A. Lindeman: Nursing Intervention with the Presurgical Patient. *Nursing Research,* 21:196–209, May-June 1972.

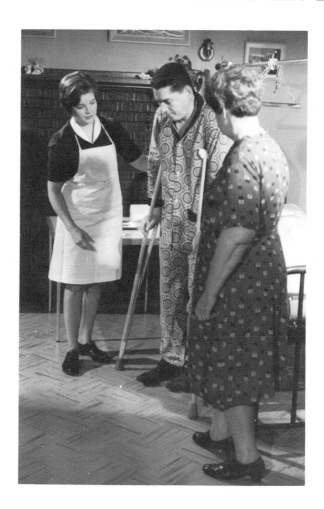

People who are ill sometimes need to re-learn skills that are commonly required in the daily activities. The regular visit of the nurse to help with exercises may be the encouragement the patient needs to start walking.

often other members of the health team. Physicians often have certain teaching regimes which they wish followed for their patients. The nurse may identify needs which are not included in a routine schedule of teaching, or routines may not have been established. The patient should be involved as an active, participating member of the health team. His perception of his learning needs is sometimes at variance with those held by the doctor and the nurse.

The patient needs to be given an opportunity to formulate and express his needs. Frequently, his anxiety about his health lessens his ability to express himself and to make known his needs and wants. Time and encouragement on the nurse's part are required. Patients are often reluctant to ask questions because nurses always seem to be so busy. Nurses usually

are busy. However, it is often a matter of establishing priorities for action. A few extra minutes spent with a patient to answer his questions or give him an opportunity to talk often minimizes the number of calls on her time later on. Providing the patient with good orientation to the health agency on admission can be extremely valuable in establishing a relationship which permits free communication between patient and nurse. Such an orientation includes welcoming the patient as an individual, describing where things are and what is going to happen to him, explaining agency policies, and answering any questions he may have. It is important also that the nurse take time to talk with the patient's family and gain their cooperation and support in the care of the patient.

The patient's learning needs will vary,

depending on the state of his health, as indicated in the introduction to this chapter. The person who is seeking to maintain or improve his health will want to learn measures to accomplish this goal. The individual who suspects that he has a health problem will want to know what tests and other diagnostic measures are going to be undertaken and why they are being done.

The sick person will want information about his condition. Is it serious? What exactly is wrong? He will also probably be concerned about the cause of his illness at this point. If he is hospitalized, he will need to learn about his new environment, including the physical layout of the hospital and of the nursing unit, and the policies and routines that will affect him, as well as something about the people who will be looking after him.

The sick person, at home or in hospital, will also want to know about the various tests that are being performed and the medical plan of therapy. As he convalesces, he begins to think of returning to his normal activities. His needs will then most likely center on the adjustment to leaving the sickroom and coping with the exigencies of daily living.

The nurse should always have the rehabilitation of the patient in mind while she is planning a teaching program for him, as mentioned earlier. Her knowledge of rehabilitative measures and understanding of preventive measures help her to identify learning needs which the patient is not always able to perceive. For example, the need for preoperative teaching in regard to coughing and deep breathing may not be apparent to the patient, but the nurse knows that these are important in preventing complications postoperatively and includes this teaching in her planning.

It is important to remember that each patient's needs are different. Teaching plans, therefore, have to be individualized for each patient. The patient's learning needs will depend on a number of factors, such as his previous experience with a health agency, prior health problems, and previous experience with his present condition. The patient who has been admitted repeatedly to a health agency because of a chronic asthmatic condition, for example, will probably have fewer learning needs than the person who has never been in hospital before. Other factors which influence the patient's learning needs and, therefore, the nurse's teaching plan, include age, sex, marital status, education, and socioeconomic background of the patient.

PRINCIPLES RELEVANT TO MEETING THE PATIENT'S LEARNING NEEDS

Several basic principles with regard to the learning process are relevant to the development of a good teaching plan for patients.
1. Learning is more effective when it is in response to a felt need of the learner.
2. Active participation on the part of the learner is essential if learning is to take place.
3. Learning is made easier when material to be learned is related to what the learner already knows.
4. Learning is facilitated when the material to be learned is meaningful to the learner.
5. Learning is retained longer when it is put into immediate use than when its application is delayed.
6. Periodic plateaus occur in learning.
7. Learning must be reinforced.
8. Learning is made easier when the learner is aware of his progress.

Using the Principles in Developing a Teaching Plan

1. *Learning is more effective when it is in response to a felt need of the learner.* It is important for the nurse to identify not only what she thinks the patient needs to know but also what the patient sees as his learning needs. Most nurses tend to view the patient's learning needs in terms of his health problem. Often, however, his needs in relation to learning about the health agency are paramount in the patient's mind. His anxiety about this problem may render ineffectual any attempts by the nurse to teach him about his condition. Some patients are not ready, when they are worried and anxious about their health, or sick and not feeling well, to learn everything they need to know, and much teaching may need to be done in follow-up home visits. For example, the hemiplegic (patient who has had paralysis of one side of his body) may need help with the activities of daily living to be able to cope with feeding and dressing himself, getting in and out of bed, and other common activities after he has gone home from hospital. Much of this follow-up teaching may be done in the specialized agencies mentioned earlier or by community health nurses who visit in the patient's home.

2. *Active participation on the part of the learner is essential if learning is to take place.* Learning takes place *in* the learner and he must be actively involved in the teaching-learning process. Telling the patient what to do or handing him a set of written instructions will not ensure that he will follow these instructions on his own. The use of discussions in which the patient takes an active part, problem-solving by the patient, and actual practice in performing procedures and handling equipment are much more effective than straight "telling," in which the activity is almost all on the nurse's part.

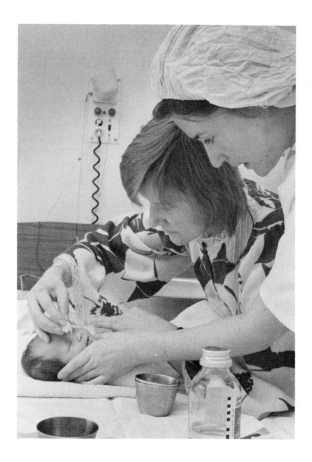

This mother is learning to bathe her new baby by doing it herself under the nurse's supervision.

3. *Learning is made easier when material to be learned is related to what the learner already knows.* It is important in this regard to find out what the patient already knows about his health status or health problems. People today are much more knowledgeable about health in general and their own health problems in particular than were patients 20 years ago. Medical information is readily available in newspapers, popular magazines, movies, television, and public school programs. Moreover, health and illness are now socially acceptable topics of conversation and have become quite popular subjects for television programs. Thus, the average layman of today knows much more about human anatomy and disease than his grandparents ever dreamed of knowing. The patient may, in fact, sometimes know more than the nurse about his particular health problem. However, the nurse should never assume that the patient, because he is well educated and perhaps even a health professional, does know everything he needs to know about tests and procedures, or as much as he wants to know about his health and health problems.

4. *Learning is facilitated when the material to be learned is meaningful to the learner.* One can of course learn nonsense syllables, and many experiments have been conducted to see how fast people can learn material which has no meaning. In nursing, however, we are more concerned with the patient's application of his knowledge than with his ability to recite facts and figures. A nurse may tell the patient that he needs so many grams each of carbohydrates, fats, and proteins in his daily diet, but unless the patient knows the foods which contain these elements and the size of a portion that constitutes so many grams, he is not likely to put the knowledge to use. It is important also to use terms which the patient can understand. The use of technical terminology should be avoided and simple words used wherever possible.

5. *Learning is retained longer when it is put into immediate use than when its application is delayed.* For this reason, the diabetic patient who has learned to test his own urine should be allowed to practice this skill immediately and, if he is hospitalized, permitted to continue to do so throughout his hospital stay.

6. *Periodic plateaus occur in learning.* The nurse should not become discouraged when the patient seems to lose interest in learning or to be unable to learn at various times. Sometimes a change in teaching method or use of a new technique will help to stimulate further learning. For example, many good audiovisual aids are now available, and these may be used in conjunction with other teaching methods. It is necessary to delay the addition of new material until the patient is ready for it.

7. *Learning must be reinforced.* Questioning the patient about material previously learned and providing for sufficient practice of skills are important ways of reinforcing learning.

8. *Learning is made easier when the learner is aware of his progress.* The patient should be given opportunity to assess his own progress. The nurse can assist the patient by giving encouragement and honest praise. The patient who is learning to walk again finds each new step a challenge, and the nurse's helpful encouragement enables this patient to take pride in his accomplishment. The nurse should be ready, too, to help the patient not to feel discouraged when he does not make as rapid progress as he would like. A recognition that no two individuals are alike and that learning does not always take place in steady progression is helpful in this regard.

DEVELOPING GOALS FOR PATIENT LEARNING

In developing a plan for teaching the patient, the first step is the identification of the patient's needs. The second step is the formulation of goals, or objectives, to be attained. Frequently, these are stated as long-range goals (or primary objectives) and short-term goals (or subobjectives). For example, one long-range goal for the patient with diabetes might be, "The patient is able to control his diabetes through medication and diet." An example of a short-term goal for the same patient could be, "The patient is able to administer his own insulin by hypodermic injection." It is always preferable to state goals in terms of what it is that the patient should be able to do rather than what the nurse is to do. Thus it is better to say, "The patient should be able to..." rather than that the goal of the teaching is "to help the patient to...." Specific goals which can be measured in terms of changes in the patient's behavior make the process of evaluating the patient's learning much easier. Thus, using the example just given, either the patient is able to administer insulin by hypodermic syringe, or he is not.

Goals should be realistic and attainable in terms of the patient's ability to reach them. To expect an elderly patient to be able to progress as quickly as a young person is unrealistic because learning occurs at a slower rate as a person gets older.

For further guidance on the development of objectives, the nurse is referred to Dorothy Smith's article, "Writing Objectives as a Nursing Practice Skill" in the February, 1971, issue of the *American Journal of Nursing*.

THE SELECTION OF METHODS AND TECHNIQUES

After the goals for learning have been established, it is necessary to decide on teaching methods and techniques to facilitate the learning process. This involves an analysis of the tasks to be learned and the selection of appropriate methods to use.

There are three basic types of learning tasks: those that involve the acquisition of information, those that involve the acquisition of skills, and those that involve the application of knowledge. Various methods of teaching are particularly suitable for each type of learning task.

The Acquisition of Information

Many of the patient's learning needs come under the heading of a need for information and knowledge. As stated earlier in the chapter, this is the need most frequently expressed by patients. Techniques for helping the patient to acquire information include the lecture or short explanatory talk, discussion, the use of programmed materials and teaching machines, and of audiovisual material such as films and film strips. The nurse may find the lecture or explanation useful in some instances, for example, when giving a talk to a group of patients, but these techniques do not involve much participation on the part of the learner. Discussion involving both patient and nurse is usually more effective for the retention of knowledge. Written material is available on a number of different health problems, and this literature may be used to supplement other instruction. It is good to vary the teaching technique, for example, by interspersing audiovisual material with talking. An individual's attention span is usually short when he is worried and concerned about his health.

The Acquisition of a Skill

Many times it is necessary for the patient to learn new skills. He may need to learn to administer a hypodermic injection (as in the example just cited); to use crutches for walking; or to change his own dressing. There are any number of instances which could be given of times when patients need to learn skills. Appropriate methods for skill-learning include the demonstration (or lecture demonstration), the return demonstration, and skill practice.

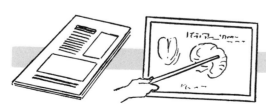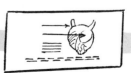

A diversity of teaching aids are available; books, posters, films and charts are all useful at times.

In demonstrating a specific nursing care measure, the type of equipment that the patient will have at home is used whenever possible. Many health agencies, for example, have standard trays of home care equipment consisting of household items. The nurse can use these to advantage in demonstrating nursing measures.

In giving a demonstration, the nurse should first of all explain to the patient what she is going to do and why it is to be done this way. She always stands so that the patient can see exactly what she is doing. For example, the patient should be able to see the numbers on a syringe when measures are explained. An overview of the procedure is given first; then the procedure is broken down into steps. Key points are stressed. The material that is being taught can often be related to something that is familar to the patient so that learning can be transferred from the familiar to the new area. The woman who is familiar with the process of preparing jars for jams and jellies can usually learn quite readily how to sterilize equipment when this procedure is shown as a similar process.

The patient should have an opportunity to perform the procedure soon after the nurse has demonstrated it. Sufficient practice sessions should also be arranged so that the patient feels competent before he is on his own.

The Application of Knowledge

Earlier in the chapter it was stated that one of the nurse's primary concerns is that the patient apply the knowledge he has learned. Giving the patient information is not enough; he must learn to apply this information in his day-to-day living. This application involves the integration of knowledge and the use of intellectual processes by the learner. The learner must be actively involved.

The problem-solving method has been suggested by educators as a very appropriate method for learning to apply knowledge. This method is useful in teaching patients. The steps in problem-solving include: (1) identification of the problem, or the perception of a felt learn-ing need by the patient (this involves gathering information and pinpointing what the problem is); (2) suggesting possible solutions; (3) selection of one solution to be tried; (4) putting the solution into action; and (5) evaluating the results of this action, reconsidering, and possibly trying other solutions.[2]

The nurse's role becomes one of supportive assistant. She helps the patient to identify his problem; to gather information and assess the relative merits of various possible solutions. She may help him to select and try one course of action, and assists him in evaluating this action.

For example, a patient may have been told by his physician that he should stay on a salt-free diet. The nutritionist, or dietitian, has talked to the patient and instructed him regarding foods that are low in salt, and the patient appears to accept the idea of salt substitutes to flavor his food. He seems worried about being able to stay on the diet at home. The nurse may help him to identify the problem by gathering information and helping to pinpoint the difficulty. The patient and his wife are elderly and they live alone. His wife does the cooking. He is afraid that it is going to give her extra work to cook his meals without salt. The nurse helps him to work through possible solutions. Has he talked to his wife about this? In this example, it would seem that the wife, who does the cooking, should be brought into the problem-solving. Together the patient and his wife might examine possible solutions. The patient's food may be cooked separately, in which case there will be two meals to prepare and two sets of pots and pans to wash. Or, food for both may be cooked together without salt, the wife adding salt to hers later. Many people find food tasteless when salt is not added during the cooking, and the wife may not like her food cooked this way. Both alternatives should be explored and a decision reached. The couple may decide to try

[2]Rosella Denison Collins: Problem Solving A Tool for Patients, Too. *The American Journal of Nursing*, 68:1483–1485, July 1968.

cooking meals for both together without salt. If this solution does not work, then they can try the alternative.

There are many examples that could be cited of situations in which problem-solving seems the logical method for helping patients to understand their disease processes and make realistic plans to care for themselves. Often the patient's family needs to be included, since many problems related to health and illness involve adjustments in family living. The family frequently provides excellent resource people to assist in developing and carrying out plans for the patient's care at home.

SELECTING THE TIME AND THE PLACE FOR TEACHING

All teaching, if it is to be worthwhile, takes time. Some of the nurse's teaching may be done informally, during the process of talking with the patient, but when specific material is to be taught, a definite plan should be developed and sufficient time should be allocated. A time that is suitable for both the patient and the nurse—when neither feels rushed and the patient is not overly tired—should be selected. The choice of time varies, depending upon the patient's activities and the nurse's schedule. In an ambulatory care setting, there may be definite times allocated when classes are scheduled for people with common concerns as, for example, the prospective parenthood classes run by some agencies, or classes for people with diabetes or other specific health problems. There may also be regularly scheduled classes in an inpatient facility to accommodate people with similar problems. Often, however, the teaching needs to be done on an individual basis. For people in inpatient facilities, the period in the morning after treatment and care have been completed, or the early afternoon, frequently can be used to advantage for teaching. For the sick, teaching periods are kept relatively short because most people, during illness, have a decreased attention span and generally do not feel well, and the nurse must be careful not to try to cover too much in any one session.

The place for teaching in a hospital is most often at the patient's bedside, although some health agencies have separate rooms for consultations with a health worker. It is important that privacy be provided in learning situations which involve personal matters.

Wherever possible, one nurse should initiate and carry through the teaching plan. Patients usually prefer to have the

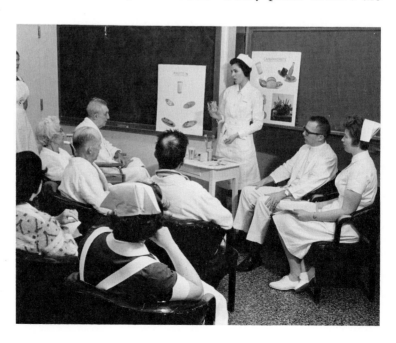

In this class, the nutritionist, the nurse, and the physician combine their efforts to teach a group of diabetic patients.

same person teaching them, and the nurse can develop a more effective relationship with the patient if she carries through the complete teaching plan. It also helps to provide for continuity in the teaching-learning situation if only one nurse is involved. If this is not feasible, however, a team approach in which each nurse is responsible for one aspect of teaching can be used quite effectively.

EVALUATING THE EFFECTIVENESS OF THE PATIENT'S LEARNING

Evaluation is the assessment of how far along the road toward attainment of the pre-established goals the learner has come. If the goals have been stated specifically in terms of what the learner is expected to be able to do at the end of the teaching program, the task of evaluating the effectiveness of his learning is relatively simple. If, for example, one goal for learning is that the patient should select foods that are low in fat content for his meals, then the extent of his learning would be evaluated through his reporting of the foods he has eaten, or the nurse's observations of the foods he selects.

Methods of evaluating effective learning will vary with each of the three types of learning task. If the task has been one of acquiring information—for example, learning the danger signals to watch for in patients with a diabetic condition—questioning the patient is a good method of finding out the extent of his knowledge. Can he list the danger signals? Does he understand their significance? Does he know what to do about them?

The acquisition of skills can be assessed by observing the patient's ability to carry out the specific procedures. Can he give himself a hypodermic injection or do his own dressing? Does he know how to prepare the equipment, handle it, and maintain good technique while doing it? Questioning the patient while he is performing the procedure helps to ascertain whether he understands the principles involved (or the "why's" of doing things a certain way).

In assessing the application of knowledge and skills, observing what the patient does in a given situation is the best way of measuring this type of learning. In the example of the patient on a fat-free diet just cited, the nurse must either rely on the patient's accurate reporting of what he has eaten or actually observe the foods he eats. Many times evaluation of the application of knowledge can be done only by observing the patient in his home situation. This emphasizes the importance of follow-up visits in the home. Indeed one of the most important responsibilities of the community health nurse is teaching the patient and helping him to apply his knowledge in day-to-day living.

SUMMARY

Meeting the patient's learning needs is a primary responsibility of nurses, yet it is one which has not received sufficient attention, particularly in the hospital field, until fairly recently. The topic deserves much more extensive coverage than it has been possible to give in this short chapter. Like the subject of communication, the nurse's role in teaching patients merits a book on its own. The nurse is therefore directed to the books and articles included in the Suggested Readings for more thorough coverage of this topic.

STUDY VOCABULARY			
Behavior	Explanation	Teaching
Demonstration	Learning	Thinking
Discussion	Practice	Visual aid

STUDY SITUATION

Jimmy Smith, who is eight years old has an infected cut on his thigh. He is at home and his physician has asked you as the community health nurse to visit his home and teach his mother how to apply hot compresses to the cut. Jimmy's mother is Spanish and speaks very little English.

1. What factors would you consider before initiating any teaching?
2. What methods would best be used for teaching in this situation?
3. What possible factors might inhibit learning?
4. What aids could you use to facilitate learning?
5. How could you evaluate the learning of the patient and his mother?

SUGGESTED READINGS

Allendorf, E. E., et al.: Teaching Patients About Nitroglycerin. *American Journal of Nursing*, 75:1168–1170, July 1975.

Cooper, I.: Group Sessions for New Mothers. *Nursing Outlook*, 22:251, April 1974.

Hartmann, K., et al.: Action-Oriented Family Therapy. *American Journal of Nursing*, 75:1184–1187, July 1975.

Merkatz, R., et al.: Preoperative Teaching for Gynecological Patients. *American Journal of Nursing*, 74:1072–1074, June 1974.

Robinson, G. C.: No One Told Me To. *Nursing Outlook*, 22:182–183, March, 1974.

Schweer, S. F., et al.: The Extended Role of Professional Nursing . . . Patient Education. *International Nursing Review*, 20:174–175, November-December 1973.

Storlie, F.: *Patient Teaching in Critical Care.* New York, Appleton-Century-Crofts, 1975.

Upcavage, A. T.: Individualized Nurse Care: How One Nurse Practitioner Succeeded Where 20 Doctors Had Failed. *Nursing '75*, 5:64–66, January 1975.

Winslow, E. H., et al.: Teaching and Rehabilitating the Cardiac Patient. *Nursing Clinics of North America*, 11:211–387, June 1976.

Wood, M. M.: 300 Valuable Booklets to Give to Patients and Their Families. A Source Guide. *Nursing '74*, 4:43–50, April 1974.

16 NUTRITIONAL NEEDS

The nurse should be able to:

Explain how food helps to satisfy basic human needs
Give examples of the role of food in the traditions, customs, super-
    stitions, and religions of different cultures
Discuss nutritional needs in health, giving examples from the na-
    tional food guide used in your country
Describe the four basic types of diet commonly used in hospital
Discuss major nutrition problems in the world
Identify factors affecting the nutritional status of specific patients
Identify observable signs of good *and* poor nutrition in patients
Identify nutritional problems requiring *prompt* intervention by
    health professionals
Apply relevant principles in the care of patients with nutritional
    problems
Establish feasible and realistic outcomes for nursing interventions
    related to nutrition
Select appropriate nursing interventions to assist specific patients
Discuss the nurse's responsibility in providing nourishment for the
    sick patient
Outline essential factors in tray service to patients
Evaluate the outcomes of nursing interventions

THE SIGNIFICANCE OF FOOD

Food and the partaking of meals have a significance in human society that goes far beyond the provision of nourishment for the body.[1] In addition to fulfilling a basic physiological need, food may also help to satisfy one or more of an individual's many other needs. It has long been recognized, for example, that food is closely related to feelings of security. This is not merely the presence or absence of food in sufficient quantity to appease hunger, but the availablity of specific foods. For many people, milk is a basic security food; for others, it may be meat, potatoes, rice, or some other familiar food which helps most to foster feelings of security.[2] When a person is ill, it is sometimes necessary to deprive him of certain foods. If any of these foods hold strong security meanings for him, it is understandable that the individual may feel threatened by its absence from his diet.

Food is often used to promote a feeling of social acceptance. Sitting down to eat with another person, even if the food that is taken is simply a cup of coffee, conveys to the other person that you consider him your equal. Offering someone a cup of tea or coffee, our "ritual of hospitality," can do much to foster an atmosphere of warmth and friendliness that is often difficult to attain in other ways. In some hospitals, obstetrical nurses use a "coffee-get-together" with the patients to provide a relaxed and informal setting in which to teach new mothers about the care of their infants.

Then, too, some foods are used for their prestige value, to enhance feelings of self-esteem. In many cultures, bread is a prestige food. For many years, steak and roast beef were considered prestige foods in North America. Now that the world has become a "global village," however, and we have been introduced to the delights of cooking from other countries, we tend to want our steak in the form of "Chateaubriand," and our fowl as "duck à l'orange" or "Tandouri" chicken. Steak or roast beef may no longer be the most expensive item on the menu. It may be flying fish imported from Barbados, or Arctic char from Alaska or Northern Canada. Food may also be used to express creativity. Many women, and a good many men also, enjoy using their creative talents to prepare gourmet meals or exotic dishes to please their families and friends.

The partaking of food in one form or another plays an important role in many religious ceremonies. One has only to think of the Christian ceremony of Communion to be aware of the significance of food in this regard. At Communion, one partakes of bread, which symbolizes the flesh of Christ, and of wine, which symbolizes His blood. In some religions, as for example, in Judaism, the preparation of food is in itself a ritual, and some hospitals maintain a kosher kitchen to cater to the needs of their orthodox Jewish patients. There are also many food taboos associated with specific doctrines of other religions. The Orthodox Muslim will not eat pork, for example, nor the Hindu, beef.

Food is, in fact, intertwined with the traditions, superstitions, and prejudices of virtually every culture. The Easter ham in our country and the Devali[3] gift of sweets in India are but two examples of the in-

---

[1] Miriam E. Lowenberg, E. Neige Tidhunter, Eva D. Wilson, Moira C. Feeney, and Jane R. Savage: *Food and Man.* New York, John Wiley & Sons, 1968, p. 109.

[2] Ibid.

---

[3] Devali, the "Festival of Lights," is a major religious festival in India.

corporation of food into traditional customs. To spill salt is considered by many people to be bad luck; this is a common example of a superstition involving food. Most of us have prejudices against certain foods; yet these foods may be eaten with great enjoyment by others. Until fairly recently, few North Americans would have eaten snails, for example, although these are considered a delicacy by most people in France.

Mealtime, in most parts of the world, is a significant aspect of family life. In many cultures, eating is considered a private affair, to be shared and enjoyed only with one's family or intimate friends. Meals often play an important role in reaffirming solidarity within the family group. In most North American homes, the mother usually likes to have all members of the family present for the evening meal. The traditional gathering of the family for Thanksgiving or Christmas dinner serves to strengthen family ties within the extended family unit. Meals, too, may provide a time when family roles are defined and clarified as when the father sits at the head of the table, a tangible symbol of his role as head of the family.[4]

In our culture, we usually like to think of mealtime as a pleasant time—a period of relaxation, when we can enjoy the company of others and engage in social conversation. Health agencies today are doing much to make mealtimes more pleasurable for patients. Trays are attractively served; there is usually a menu from which the patient may select the foods that he likes; and many hospitals now have small dining areas adjacent to the nursing units, where patients who are able may gather to eat their meals.

As well as having psychological, social, and cultural significance in our daily lives, food is vitally important to our physical being. Because all cells in the body require adequate nourishment for optimal functioning, all systems of the body may be affected by nutritional problems. The synergism between poor nutritional status and infections was discussed in the chapter on health problems (Chapter 4). The direct effect on brain tissue of malnutrition is currently receiving considerable study. The listlessness and poor concentrating ability of children who are malnourished is felt to be an important factor in lessening their ability to do well in school.

Many skin and gastrointestinal problems are directly attributable to poor dietary habits. Nutrition is certainly a factor in a person's strength and endurance, as athletes prove.

The importance of good nutrition for pregnant women and for children as well as adolescents, in promoting optimal growth and development of the fetus, the growing child, and the teenager, cannot be overstressed.

Nutrition is so vital to all aspects of health that nurses should be well versed in helping people to develop and maintain good dietary habits.

NUTRITIONAL NEEDS IN HEALTH

A person cannot exist for long without taking some form of nourishment. Food is the fuel with which we run our human bodies. It is necessary for the growth and maintenance of bones and other tissues, and for the regulation of all body processes. In order for a person to function at his optimal level, he must consume adequate amounts of foods containing the nutrients considered essential to human life. A *nutrient* is defined as any chemical substance found in foods that functions in one or more of the three ways mentioned above.[5] The amount considered adequate will, of course, vary from one individual to another, depending on age, sex, current physical status, lifestyle, physical environment, and many other factors. The essential nutrients are carbohydrates, proteins, fats, vitamins, minerals, and water.

CARBOHYDRATES. *Carbohydrates* are composed of carbon, hydrogen, and ox-

---

[4]Anne Burgess and R. F. A. Dean (eds.): *Malnutrition and Food Habits.* New York, The Free Press, 1963, pp. 63–64.

[5]L. Jean Bogert, George M. Briggs, and Doris H. Calloway: *Nutrition and Physical Fitness.* 9th edition. Philadelphia, W. B. Saunders Company, 1973, p. 8.

ygen and are used by the body primarily as a source of energy. They are the most common nutrients in the majority of diets because of their availability. Carbohydrates are found in most plants and fruit sugars, and in natural starches. The cellulose in plants is an important ingredient for digestion. Excess carbohydrates consumed are stored in the liver in the form of *glycogen* or changed into fat. For this reason, carbohydrate consumption is often restricted in weight-loss diets.

FATS. *Fats* are also composed of carbon, hydrogen, and oxygen but in different ratios than in carbohydrates. They are also primarily a source of energy to the body, and because they contain less oxygen, they release their energy more quickly and in greater quantity than do carbohydrates. Fats are found in nature in animals and in plant seeds. The most common sources of fats in our diets are butter, margarine, nuts, eggs, and oils used for cooking and in salad dressings (for example, corn, peanut, olive, soybean). It is thought that the saturated fats (eg., butter, meat fats) are a contributing factor in high blood pressure, arteriosclerosis, and other circulatory diseases.

PROTEINS. Like carbohydrates and fats, *proteins* are composed of carbon, hydrogen, and oxygen, but with the added element of nitrogen. Most proteins also contain sulfur and some contain other minerals as well. The primary functions of proteins in the human body are the release of energy and the building and repair of body tissues. For this reason, children require greater quantities of protein-rich foods than adults, since they are growing, and sick people are often prescribed high-protein diets. Protein is found in nature in animals and plants. The most common sources in our diets are dairy products, meat, fish, eggs, and legumes (such as peas and beans).

VITAMINS. *Vitamins* are a natural component of most foods. They are necessary for the growth, maintenance, and repair of body tissues and for the regulation of body processes. Since the body is unable to manufacture vitamins, they must be obtained from foods we eat. Vitamins are designated as A, B, C, D, E, and K and are classified into two main groups. The *fat-soluble vitamins* (A, D, E, and K) are transported throughout the body in fats.

Vitamin A, often considered the most important vitamin, is essential for growth and maintenance of tissues, for proper development of bones and teeth, and for good vision. It is found in yellow and green fruits and vegetables, egg yolk, butterfat, and liver.

Vitamin D promotes the growth of teeth and bones. Called the "sunshine vitamin," it is most commonly obtained through sunlight and in enriched foods. Other sources of vitamin D are fish liver oils, egg yolk, and butterfat.

Vitamin E is important for normal creatine excretion and for the prevention of blood disorders. In recent times, much attention has been given to the apparently miraculous properties of this vitamin—it is thought by some to enhance sexual powers, prevent tissue scarring, and increase sensory perception, among other things. However, these claims have yet to be clinically proved. One property has been established, though, and that is that vitamin E lowers the body's need for vitamin A. An excellent source of Vitamin E is wheat germ oil; other common dietary sources are whole grains, salad and cooking oils, liver, and fruits and vegetables.

Vitamin K is necessary to the body for blood coagulation. It can be found in liver, egg yolk, green leafy vegetables, and soybean oil.

The *water-soluble vitamins (the B complex and C)* use water as their vehicle. For this reason, foods containing these vitamins are most effective when eaten raw, since cooking tends to remove the vitamins.

The *B complex vitamins*, of which there are nine, are essential for the formation of red blood cells, for tissue growth, and for the process of digestion. They also are an important factor in nervous stability and healthy appetite. The B vitamins are found in meat, eggs, milk, green vegetables, and whole grains.

Vitamin C is essential for the building and maintenance of teeth, bones and joints, muscles, gums, and connective tissues. It also functions to protect the body from infection and promotes wound healing. Common sources of vitamin C are citrus fruits, tomatoes, and green leafy vegetables.

MINERALS. *Minerals* are necessary to the body in the building and maintenance of bones, teeth, and the various body systems. The main essential minerals are considered to be calcium, phosphorus, and magnesium. Other minerals, called trace minerals, are equally essential, but are needed in much smaller amounts. Some of the minerals required by the body are iron, copper, iodine, manganese, zinc, and fluorine.

Calcium is important for the proper formation of teeth and bones, for muscle tone and nerve transmissions, and for the coagulation of blood. The most common source of calcium in most diets is milk and other dairy products, but it is also found in dark green leafy vegetables, eggs, meat, and cereals.

Phosphorus aids in the formation and strengthening of bones. It can be obtained from dairy products, meat, fish, poultry, nuts, whole grains, and legumes.

Magnesium is an important factor in regulation of the body's temperature, nerve conduction, and muscle contractions. Common dietary sources of magnesium are green leafy vegetables, nuts, whole grains, and beans.

Water, as considered in this chapter, is the single most important nutrient in the human body. It is a component of most foods, both liquid and solid. Water is a vehicle of absorption for most nutrients in the body and is present in all body excretions and secretions. Approximately 50 to 70 per cent of the adult body is composed of water. Because water is of paramount importance in the regulation and maintenance of all body tissues and processes, it will be discussed in more detail in Chapter 29.

RECOMMENDED DAILY FOOD GUIDES

Recommended daily requirements of specific nutrients have been established in both the United States and in Canada (and in many other countries). International standards have been issued by the United Nations Food and Agriculture Organization and the World Health Organization (FAO/WHO). Food Guides have also been developed to assist people to select foods that will ensure that they have an adequate supply of essential nutrients in their daily diets.

The *Guide to Good Eating*, developed by the United States Department of Agriculture, and *Canada's Food Guide*, issued by the Department of National Health and Welfare, are shown on pages 271–272. The United States Guide shows recommended amounts for four basic food groups: milk, meat, vegetables and fruits, and bread and cereals. The Canadian Guide separates the fruits from the vegetables and adds a sixth group, of foods containing Vitamin D, for growing persons and for expectant and nursing mothers. Basically, the two guides contain the same foods, and the recommended amounts are similar, with only minor variations. The United States Guide, for example, recommends a greater number of *glasses* of milk, both for children and for adults (both guides recommend the same for adolescents), but the Canadian Guide is more specific about the number of fluid ounces in the glasses. The United States Guide suggests two servings of meat, fish, or poultry daily, whereas the Canadian one recommends only one but adds a thrice weekly serving of eggs and cheese.

The Canadian Guide recommends slightly higher amounts of fruit and vegetables, and specifies one serving of potatoes daily, which does not seem to be considered vital to the American daily intake of food.

FACTORS AFFECTING NUTRITIONAL STATUS

A person's nutritional status reflects the balance that is maintained between the body's requirements for nutrients and energy and the actual intake of food. It depends, then, on three major factors; the requirements of the individual for nutrients and energy, his intake of food, and the efficiency of his bodily processes for absorbing, storing, utilizing, and excreting nutrients.

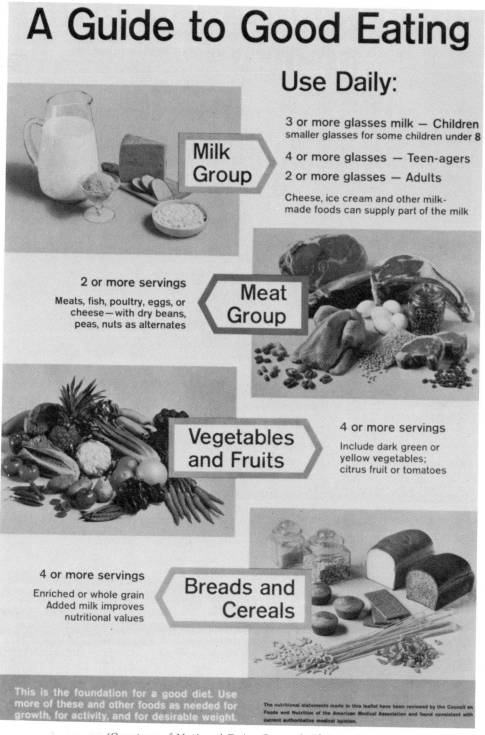

A Guide to Good Eating

Use Daily:

Milk Group

3 or more glasses milk — Children
smaller glasses for some children under 8

4 or more glasses — Teen-agers

2 or more glasses — Adults

Cheese, ice cream and other milk-made foods can supply part of the milk

Meat Group

2 or more servings

Meats, fish, poultry, eggs, or cheese—with dry beans, peas, nuts as alternates

Vegetables and Fruits

4 or more servings

Include dark green or yellow vegetables; citrus fruit or tomatoes

Breads and Cereals

4 or more servings

Enriched or whole grain Added milk improves nutritional values

This is the foundation for a good diet. Use more of these and other foods as needed for growth, for activity, and for desirable weight.

The nutritional statements made in this leaflet have been reviewed by the Council on Foods and Nutrition of the American Medical Association and found consistent with current authoritative medical opinion.

(Courtesy of National Dairy Council, Chicago.)

Keep this Food Guide handy to use in planning your grocery shopping and daily menus.

Canada's food guide

These foods are good to eat • Eat them every day for health • Have three meals each day.

Milk Children (up to about 11 years) .... 2½ cups (20 fl. oz.) Adolescents .... 4 cups (32 fl. oz.) Adults .... 1½ cups (12 fl. oz.) Expectant and nursing mothers .... 4 cups (32 fl. oz.)	Whole, 2%, skim, or powdered milk; cheese; ice cream; or soups made with milk all supply necessary calcium, riboflavin, and protein.
Fruit Two servings of fruit or juice, including a satisfactory source of vitamin C (ascorbic acid) such as oranges, tomatoes, and vitaminized apple juice.	Selections could be fresh or canned fruits (grapefruit, peaches), dried fruits (prunes, raisins), or fruit juices (tomato, orange). Most fruits are sources of vitamin C, vitamin A and iron.
Vegetables One serving of potatoes. Two servings of other vegetables, preferably yellow or green and often raw.	Raw, cooked, frozen or canned vegetables such as cabbage, broccoli, carrots, peas, turnips and potatoes provide vitamin C, vitamin A, folic acid and iron.
Bread and cereals Bread (with butter or fortified margarine). One serving of whole grain cereal.	Whole grain breads and cereals and enriched products (breads, cereals, macaroni, spaghetti) supply thiamin, riboflavin, niacin, and iron.
Meat and fish One serving of meat, fish or poultry. Eat liver occasionally. Eggs, cheese, dried beans or peas may be used in place of meat. In addition, eggs and cheese at least three times a week.	Foods such as hamburger, fish chowder, baked beans, cheese omelets, and peanut butter also contain valuable protein, iron, B vitamins and vitamin A.
Vitamin D 400 International Units, for all growing persons and expectant and nursing mothers.	Sources of vitamin D include vitamin D fortified milk and margarine, cod liver oil, or a vitamin D supplement.

(Courtesy of Health and Welfare Canada.)

Requirements

Dietary requirements are generally considered in terms of both specific nutrients and energy requirements. The body's needs for energy are usually expressed in calories (a term taken from the physical sciences), which measure heat units. A *calorie* in nutrition means the amount of heat required to raise the temperature of one gram of water by one degree Celsius.[6]

The body's requirements for nutrients and energy vary considerably from one individual to another, depending principally on age, sex, body frame, amount and kind of daily activity, and climate. The requirements of children and adolescents are greater than those of adults. During periods of rapid growth, their needs are markedly increased. One is constantly amazed at the amount of food teenage boys, especially, can consume, and, if they are active, still remain slim. Nutritional requirements are also increased during pregnancy and lactation (for cal-

[6]Bogert et al., op. cit., p. 26.

cium by 50 per cent, for most other nutrients by 20 per cent).[7] As a person passes middle age, body requirements for some nutrients are lessened.

In general, men require more food than women, because of their usually larger body frames. Women do, however, need more iron than men.[8]

The amount and kind of activity a person does in a day has a considerable influence on the caloric intake required. Strenuous activities, such as tennis, swimming, skating, exercising, or hard manual labor, burn up a large number of calories, a factor to consider if one is interested in losing weight. Nursing students are well known for always being hungry. No doubt this is due to the number of calories they use up in lifting and moving patients, making beds, and the like, which are hard physical work.

In warm and humid climates, a person usually requires less energy-giving foods and more fluid intake than in temperate zones. In cold weather, more calories are needed for energy, particularly if the body is not well insulated by sufficient clothing. People usually need more soups and nourishing hot meals in the wintertime as opposed to summer, when lighter meals and a greater intake of fluids are usually preferred.

Intake

If a person eats more food than the body requires, or, conversely, he does not eat enough to meet his energy and nutritional requirements, problems develop. A number of factors—economic, physical, and psychosocial—affect food intake.

In Chapter 4, in discussing major health problems, we mentioned affluence as being a contributing factor in the widespread prevalence of overweight or obesity in North America. We also mentioned the serious poverty that exists in many countries, and in parts of our own, that prevents people from having sufficient food to meet their nutritional needs.

Among the physical factors affecting food intake, the condition of a person's teeth, gums, and the mucous membranes of the oral cavity are important factors for nurses to consider in assessing a patient's nutritional status. A person with no teeth or with poorly fitting dentures, or one whose mouth is in poor condition, has difficulty in biting or chewing food and will limit his intake to those foods he can handle easily. Other physical factors to be considered are the person's general state of health and specific health problems he may have. (These are discussed in more detail in subsequent sections.)

A person's emotional status will also affect his intake of food. We have already mentioned this point in connection with anxiety, such as the "knots" and "butterflies" in the stomach, and the pre-examination nausea or vomiting. In one psychiatric hospital setting, the dietetic staff observed interesting correlations between food intake and the general anxiety level of both patients and staff. When they were upset by changes in their environment, such as staff changes, hospital policy changes, and holidays, the consumption of such "security foods" as bread and milk went up, as did the amount of food left on plates. When things settled down, eating patterns returned to normal.[9]

Some people use food as a source of comfort and security; they may eat excessively because of their anxieties or because of a lack of fulfillment of the basic needs of love and belonging.

Other emotions besides anxiety will also affect a person's appetite and, hence, his intake of food. The depressed patient does not want to eat; the happy individual usually does, unless he is too excited by happiness to eat. In countless poems and romantic novels, the person in love is described as someone with no appetite (among other symptoms).

The attractiveness of a meal and the en-

[7]Madelyn T. Nordmark and Anne W. Rohweder: Scientific Foundations of Nursing. 3rd edition. Philadelphia, J. B. Lippincott Company, 1975, p. 79.
[8]Ibid., p. 78.

[9]Mary Lou Chappelle: The Language of Food. American Journal of Nursing, 72:1294–1295, July 1972.

vironment in which it is served also contribute to a person's enjoyment of food, and encourage people to eat, as all restaurant managers realize.

As we noted at the beginning of this chapter, cultural, moral, and religious values play a considerable role in the food people eat. Food habits are learned, and eating habits vary considerably in different cultures and among different religious groups. They also vary from one family to the next, and from individual to individual.

Among cultural groups, food habits usually have their origins in types of food that are available in the part of the world in which the group lived. Potatoes are plentiful in many parts of Canada; hence, they are included in the National Food Guide. In many other countries, potatoes do not grow well, and rice, which may, is much more of a staple food and forms a part of the culture. When people from one culture move to another part of the world, they usually carry their food habits with them. In a country with many ethnic groups intertwined, it is important for the nurse to be aware of the cultural food heritage of her patients and of their religious backgrounds as well, since many religions have specific food rules.

In the realm of moral values, there seems to be a search for simplicity in all aspects of living, particularly among young people, and this search extends to foods too. Among the common beliefs are that it is better to eat brown bread than white (even if the white is enriched), to make your own bread if possible, and to use only naturally grown foods. Many of the diets espoused by youth are forms of vegetarianism.[10] There are varying degrees of being a vegetarian, from not eating any kind of animal product (including eggs) to the more common variety of not eating meat.

Then, too, food habits vary from one family to another, even if all other factors are constant. In some households, breakfast is a sketchy or nonexistent affair, whereas, in others it is considered one of the main meals of the day. The patterns of eating that were learned in the home have a considerable influence on the food habits children maintain later in life, and are frequently handed down from one generation to the next.

There is, however, also the matter of individual differences in taste and preference for food, as anyone from a large family knows. From the moment of birth, various factors, such as good or poor digestion, allergies and differences in taste, imagination, education, and the food habits in the home, will influence the individual's set of eating habits.[11]

A person's lifestyle affects his eating patterns. People who are busy and under pressure sometimes do not take time to eat properly. They often may skip meals or bolt their lunches in order to get on to more important business. Teenagers also are often in a hurry and want to rush off to school or afterschool activities without taking time to eat a proper meal, or they fill up on snacks and have no appetite at mealtime. Some, of course, seem to eat continuously, both meals and snacks.

Senior citizens are another group whose dietary habits do not always provide them with sufficient nutrient intake. Sometimes this is a matter of not having enough money to buy nutritious foods; sometimes it is a lack of interest in food. The Nutrition Canada survey showed that the diets of a large number of people over 65 was only "marginally adequate."

Health problems also affect a person's intake of adequate nourishment. In addition to the allergies and poor digestion mentioned above, most physical and emotional problems affect food intake in some way. We will be discussing food and the sick person in a later section of the chapter, but perhaps we should mention here two common health problems which can interfere with a person's taking sufficient nourishment to meet his requirements. These are alcoholism and drug addiction.

The alcoholic often drinks instead of eating, and his nutritional status suffers as

---

[10]Ruth P. Fleshman: Eating Rituals and Realities. *Nursing Clinics of North America*, 8:91–103, March 1973.

[11]Lowenberg et al., op. cit., p. 97.

a result. Serious nutritional problems are found in many alcoholics, and these require prompt intervention.

Drug addicts too can have serious nutritional problems. The addict may opt to buy drugs instead of food with his limited funds, or he may not feel the need for food when he is "high" on whatever drug that he is taking.

Efficiency of the Body in Processing Food

Any factor that interferes with the body's ability to absorb, store, utilize, or excrete nutrients will adversely affect a person's nutritional status. Disease processes, congenital problems, or injury to any part of the gastrointestinal system may therefore result in nutritional problems. Probably the most common type of illness affecting the gastrointestinal tract is infection, especially gastroenteritis, which is a major cause of death in many underdeveloped countries, and a very common cause of illness in both the United States and Canada. A number of other disorders, which the nurse will learn about in her courses in medical-surgical nursing, are also specific to the gastrointestinal system. Congenital problems are usually discussed thoroughly in pediatric nursing courses, so we will not go into these further at this point, except to note that there are both congenital malformations, that is, defects or abnormalities in the anatomical structures of the system, and congenital disorders affecting the physiological processes involved in the digestion and absorption of food.

Illnesses involving parts of the body other than the gastrointestinal tract may also cause disturbances in the processing of food, as well as altering the body's needs for energy and for specific nutrients. This aspect of nutrition will be discussed in the next few paragraphs.

FOOD AND THE SICK PERSON

Food as a source of nourishment is particularly important for those who are ill. Nearly all sick persons have some distur-

bances in gastrointestinal functioning.[12] They may lose their appetites or be unable to tolerate food and fluids; there may be a problem in the digestion of food or in the absorption of nutrients from the gastrointestinal tract. Whatever the problem, the sick person's nutritional needs are usually different from those of the well. Lack of exercise because of illness may decrease the body's need for energy-giving foods but, at the same time, there is a greater need for tissue-building nutrients.

The nutrients that are taken into the body, normally via the gastrointestinal tract, are digested and then absorbed into the blood stream and taken to the cells of the body. In the cells, metabolic activity takes place. Metabolism has two phases: catabolism and anabolism. In *catabolism* the glucose derived from carbohydrates, and the ketones and glycerol derived from fat, are broken down into carbon dioxide, water, and energy. Proteins are broken down into carbon dioxide, water, urea, and energy. In *anabolism* this energy is used in the synthesis of enzymes and proteins needed by the body cells. The restructuring of amino acids to form protein elements of the body is a particularly important part of anabolism.

In the well person, the processes of anabolism and catabolism are normally equal. In the sick, particularly those who are incapacitated, the catabolic activities are increased, which leads to a breakdown of cellular materials and a subsequent deficiency of protein.[13] Thus, there may be a decreased need for food to meet energy requirements but an increased need for specific nutrients in the person who is ill. Additional protein foods are important for almost all sick people. There are, of course, some conditions in which a high-protein diet is contraindicated, but the foregoing statement is a good general rule.

There are certain conditions, too, in which metabolic activity, both anabolic and catabolic, is increased, as in patients

---

[12]Edith V. Olson et al.: The Hazards of Immobility. *American Journal of Nursing*, 67:780–797, April 1967, pp. 78 –787.
[13]Ibid.

with a fever, and in these cases there is a need for additional energy-giving foods as well as proteins.

In a good many disease conditions, the patient may be unable to tolerate food or fluids, or may lose these through vomiting, diarrhea, or other means. In these cases, the replacement of lost fluids and nutrients is an important part of the patient's therapeutic care. In some disease conditions, there is interference with the absorption of food. These cases require special adaptation of the diet.

Kinds of Diet

As a part of the patient's therapeutic regimen, food is usually prescribed in the form of a diet. There are many kinds of diet. For example, the average patient is on a regular or full (normal) diet. This means that he eats any or all of the foods that he normally eats in health. Generally, fried and highly seasoned foods are not served to patients because of the difficulty many people normally have in digesting them. A modification of the full, or regular, diet is the light diet. The foods on this diet are cooked simply, with an avoidance of fried foods, rich desserts, and other fat-laden foods. Coarse gas-forming foods, such as corn, turnips, radishes, onions, cabbage, cauliflower, and cucumbers, are also usually avoided.

A third type of diet is the soft diet. This diet consists of food that requires little chewing and contains no harsh fiber or highly seasoned foods. Because soft-diet foods are easily digested, they are often indicated for people who have gastrointestinal disorders or difficulty in masticating food.

A fourth kind of diet is the liquid diet. There are usually two types of liquid diet: full liquid and clear liquid. A full liquid diet is free of irritating condiments and cellulose. Often gelatin, jelly, and junket are included in a full liquid diet, and also soft drinks and ice cream. A clear liquid diet permits water, tea with lemon, or coffee. Often a patient on a clear liquid diet is restricted in the amount of fluid he may take at one time.

Therapeutic diets are special diets which vary greatly in their composition and purpose. Many special diets are designed to eliminate substances that are irritating to the gastrointestinal tract. The amount and kind of nutrients may be varied or certain nonnutritive compounds eliminated. For example, restrictions may be placed on the flavoring or seasoning used or on the amount of cellulose to be consumed. There are also diets that restrict the amount of sodium, sugar, or protein. There are high calorie diets and low calorie diets, high protein diets and low protein diets. There are also diets which control the quantity and type of fats. Each therapeutic diet is ordered by the physician to meet the patient's specific needs. The quantity of each kind of food is calculated by the dietitian and each meal is served carefully in the prescribed amounts of specific foods.

Regardless of the kind of diet, it is important that the patient understand why he is served certain foods. The nurse and the dietitian can help gain the patient's cooperation and thereby his acceptance of the specified food as part of his prescribed therapy.

COMMON PROBLEMS RELATED TO NUTRITION

The most common problems associated with nutrition throughout the world are malnutrition, starvation, and obesity. Although malnutrition is often regarded as an affliction of only underdeveloped and poor countries, it is also of great concern to health workers in the so-called developed nations.

At least 30 per cent of the United States population shows some evidence of malnutrition in the form of inadequate intake of food and nutrients (especially iron, calcium, vitamin A, vitamin C and riboflavin), or in the form of anemias, obesity, or diseases closely associated with poor nutrition, such as the circulatory diseases (heart disease, hypertension, stroke etc.), diabetes, severe dental and periodontal disease, and alcoholism. Especially vulnerable to malnutrition are young children, adolescents, young pregnant women, families of the poor, handicapped persons, and people over 65 years of age.[14]

---

[14]Bogert et al., op. cit., p. 6.

FORM A-72A
66725 - 15M - REV. 10-73

DIET CHANGES

VANCOUVER GENERAL HOSPITAL
FOOD SERVICES DEPARTMENT

DATE	Meal B.L. or D.	STANDARD DIET SPECIFY CONSISTENCY					THERAPEUTIC DIET (Doctor Must Prescribe) SPECIFY CONSISTENCY					HOLD TRAY	NO TRAY TO O.R.	NO TRAY	Resume Tray. Specify Consistency	FORCE FLUID	NUR. INIT.	DIET. INIT.
		REG-ULAR	ADV. SOFT	REST. SOFT	FULL FLUID	CLEAR FLUID	REG-ULAR	ADV. SOFT	REST. SOFT	FULL FLUID	CLEAR FLUID							
10/11	B	✓											✓					R.S.

BED NO. R 42 A   PATIENT'S NAME MRS. ANN YOUNG

A sample diet form. (Courtesy of the Vancouver General Hospital.)

FORM A-72
66720
24M - REV. 10-73

DIET LIST

VANCOUVER GENERAL HOSPITAL
FOOD SERVICES DEPARTMENT

DATE	NUR. INIT.	DIET. INIT.	PATIENT LIKES	PATIENT DISLIKES	DIET SIGNALS
9/11	KS		BACON FOR BREAKFAST	EGGS	(PURPLE) - STANDARD DIETS
			MILK, TEA	COFFEE	YELLOW - THERAPEUTIC
			ORANGE JUICE	GRAPEFRUIT JUICE	RED - CALCULATED
					ORANGE - CHANGE (ATTN. DIETITIAN)
					BLACK - FORCE FLUIDS

NOURISHMENT (FOOD SERVICES DEPT. USE ONLY)

1000 HRS. JUICE

1400 HRS. TEA

2000 HRS. COCOA

DOCTOR R.L.S

COMMENTS:

AGE: 29 YRS.

UNIT NO.: R 4295

THIS SPACE FOR FURTHER
RESTRICTION - E.G.
ISOLATION, FEED, ETC.

BED 42A   NAME (SURNAME ONLY) YOUNG

(REG-ULAR)   ADV. SOFT   RESTR. SOFT   FLUID   CLEAR FLUID   THERAPEUTIC

A sample change of diet form. (Courtesy of the Vancouver General Hospital.)

A recent national nutrition study[15] in Canada revealed many nutritional problems in that country also. Iron deficiencies were so widespread that remedial food enrichment practices and a national nutrition education program were recommended. Protein deficits were found in a substantially large proportion of pregnant women, and protein and/or calorie deficits among a small but noteworthy group of children under the age of 5 years. Shortages of calcium and vitamin D were found to be a problem in the daily diets of many infants, children, and adolescents, and a moderate thiamine deficiency was revealed among adults. A deficiency of vitamin C was found in the Inuit (Eskimo) group, and, to a lesser extent, among the native Indian population. The survey also revealed that a large proportion of adults in the country have a problem of overweight.

There are many causes of *malnutrition*, ranging from a simple lack of food to the ready availability of convenience foods, which are deficient in the essential nutrients. Religious, social, and cultural customs, as we have mentioned, affect nutrition as well. The Buddhist, for example, may not eat meat; a person from an African tribe may have a diet consisting solely of rice and legumes; a young adult in the United States or Canada may live in a vegetarian commune. Throughout the world, people suffering from malnutrition appear to have one trait in common—that is, a diet deficient in protein. In Africa, for example, a tribe of tall, strong, and generally healthy individuals eats a diet consisting mainly of meat and dairy products, while a neighboring tribe, whose members are on the average 12 cm. (5 in.) shorter, much less strong, and generally in poor physical condition, lives mainly on a diet of rice and vegetables.[16]

In poor and underdeveloped nations, the climate and terrain may be such that those crops that do grow there are neither sufficient in quantity nor nutritionally adequate for the resident population. Overpopulation is often a concomitant factor in such cases. Most foods have to be imported and are, therefore, costly, so that only the very rich can afford to eat well. Indeed, the situation in some countries is so extreme, that many people starve to death. The United States and Canada, with other countries and international organizations (such as UNESCO, UNICEF, and WHO, for example), are participating in food distribution programs to countries in need and providing agricultural specialists to advise on food cultivation and processing.

Nutritional problems are fast becoming a major concern in the highly developed, industrialized nations as well. In such countries where food is abundant, many people suffer from inadequate nutrition, often in the form of obesity. *Obesity* may be caused by simple overeating, but more often than not it is a symptom of malnutrition. Contrary to popular belief, people do not necessarily choose naturally the foods their bodies need. In fact, most people choose their foods according to cost and preparation time. The so-called convenience foods, which are relatively expensive, are highly processed and take little or no preparation. They are also usually high in carbohydrates and low in protein, although they may be "enriched" with various vitamins and minerals. Foods rich in carbohydrates occur abundantly in nature and thus appear to be inexpensive when compared to protein-rich foods, such as meat and dairy products. With the escalating cost of living, therefore, the average person is likely to eat proportionately more rice and potatoes than meat, to use an example.

Promotion of Adequate Nutrition

The problem of inadequate nutrition affects all countries and all classes of society. As well as food distribution programs for the undeveloped nations and for the poor in the developed countries, nutritional counseling is becoming an increasingly important means of remedying the situation. Governments are becoming more conscious of the importance of proper diet for their people and are using the media to propagate information. Television and radio networks are "becoming involved," devoting time to programs em-

---

[15]Report of Nutrition Canada National Survey, 1970–1972. Ottawa, Ontario, Department of National Health and Welfare, 1975, p. 113.

[16]Bogert et al., op. cit., p. 6.

phasizing nutrition and fitness; large business enterprises are funding advertisements and programs on the subject. Community health workers are reaching out to society through classes in the schools and community centers, trying to educate the public in matters of nutrition—the roles of the various essential nutrients; food substitutions; preparation and preservation of foods.

Nurses are in a key position to assist in nutrition education. People come to them for advice and health counseling, often on an informal basis in the community in which they live, as well as in the course of their professional activities.

ASSESSING NUTRITIONAL STATUS

In order to assess the nutritional status of an individual, the nurse needs information about all the factors that affect a person's state of nutrition. These include: age, sex, height, usual weight, present weight, usual habits with regard to daily activities and current activity level, usual dietary pattern, and present status with regard to food and fluid intake. She should know whether he is on a special diet and, if so, if he is adhering to it. She should also know the person's religious affiliation, his ethnic origin, whether he subscribes to any special beliefs about food, and his attitude toward food.

She should know his socioeconomic status and something about his lifestyle. She should be aware of the person's general physical condition and his emotional status. She should also know about any health problems he may have that could cause alterations in his nutritional needs or interfere with his digestive processes. If the patient is a woman, the nurse should determine if she is pregnant or a nursing mother.

Much of this information is available to the nurse in the data gathered during the nursing history and in the initial nursing clinical appraisal. Information about the patient's current health status and health problems, special diet orders, and status relative to pregnancy or lactation should be available from the patient's record.

The nurse supplements the information she has gathered about the patient from other sources by talking with him and through her observations. She notes his general appearance. Is he fat? thin? or does he look emaciated?

The patient's current weight is compared with his usual weight. His height and weight are compared with standard weight tables, such as those shown below and on the next page.

DESIRABLE WEIGHTS FOR MEN AND WOMEN—WEIGHT IN POUNDS ACCORDING TO FRAME (IN INDOOR CLOTHING)

Men of Ages 25 and Over			
Height (With Shoes On), 1-Inch Heels Feet Inches	Small Frame	Medium Frame	Large Frame
5 2	112–120	118–129	126–141
5 3	115–123	121–133	129–144
5 4	118–126	124–136	132–148
5 5	121–129	127–139	135–152
5 6	124–133	130–143	138–156
5 7	128–137	134–147	142–161
5 8	132–141	138–152	147–166
5 9	136–145	142–156	151–170
5 10	140–150	146–160	155–174
5 11	144–154	150–165	159–179
6 0	148–158	154–170	164–184
6 1	152–162	158–175	168–189
6 2	156–167	162–180	173–194
6 3	160–171	167–185	178–199
6 4	164–175	172–190	182–204

Women of Ages 25 and Over*			
Height (With Shoes On), 2-Inch Heels Feet Inches	Small Frame	Medium Frame	Large Frame
4 10	92– 98	96–107	104–119
4 11	94–101	98–110	106–122
5 0	96–104	101–113	109–125
5 1	99–107	104–116	112–128
5 2	102–110	107–119	115–131
5 3	105–113	110–122	118–134
5 4	108–116	113–126	121–138
5 5	111–119	116–130	125–142
5 6	114–123	120–135	129–146
5 7	118–127	124–139	133–150
5 8	122–131	128–143	137–154
5 9	126–135	132–147	141–158
5 10	130–140	136–151	145–163
5 11	134–144	140–155	149–168
6 0	138–148	144–159	153–173

*For girls between ages of 18 and 25, subtract 1 pound for each year under 25.

Courtesy of Metropolitan Life Insurance Company.

ADULT WEIGHT IN KILOGRAMS
FOR WOMEN, ACCORDING TO
FRAME, IN INDOOR CLOTHING°

Height in cm (With 5-cm Heel Shoes)	Small Frame	Medium Frame	Large Frame
147 (4'10")	41.3–44.5	43.5–48.0	47.0–54.0
148	41.7–44.8	43.9–48.6	47.4–54.4
149	42.1–45.3	44.3–49.2	47.8–54.8
150	42.6–45.8	44.7–49.8	48.2–55.3
151	43.1–46.3	45.2–50.3	48.7–55.8
152	43.6–46.8	45.7–50.9	49.3–56.4
153	44.0–47.4	46.2–51.5	49.8–56.9
154	44.5–47.9	46.7–52.0	50.3–57.5
155	45.0–48.4	47.2–52.6	50.8–58.0
156	45.5–48.9	47.7–53.2	51.4–58.6
157	46.0–49.4	48.2–53.7	51.9–59.1
158	46.4–50.0	48.7–54.3	52.4–59.7
159	46.9–50.5	49.2–54.8	53.0–60.2
160	47.4–51.0	49.7–55.4	53.5–60.8
161	48.0–51.6	50.3–56.1	54.1–61.5
162	48.6–52.3	50.9–56.8	54.8–62.2
163	49.2–53.0	51.5–57.6	55.5–62.9
164	49.9–53.7	52.2–58.3	56.2–63.7
165	50.5–54.4	52.8–59.0	56.8–64.4
166	51.1–55.0	53.4–59.8	57.5–65.1
167	51.7–55.7	54.0–60.5	58.2–65.8
168	52.4–56.4	54.6–61.2	58.9–66.5
169	53.0–57.0	55.3–62.0	59.5–67.2
170	53.6–57.7	56.0–62.7	60.2–68.0
171	54.3–58.5	56.7–63.4	60.9–68.8
172	55.0–59.2	57.4–64.2	61.6–69.6
173	55.7–60.0	58.1–65.0	62.3–70.4
174	56.5–60.7	58.9–65.7	63.1–71.2
175	57.2–61.5	59.6–66.5	63.8–72.1
176	57.9–62.3	60.3–67.3	64.5–72.9
177	58.6–63.0	61.0–68.0	65.3–73.7
178	59.3–63.8	61.7–68.8	66.0–74.6
179	60.0–64.5	62.5–69.5	66.7–75.4
180	60.8–65.3	63.3–70.3	67.5–76.2
181	61.6–66.1	64.0–71.0	68.2–77.0
182	62.4–66.9	64.8–71.8	69.0–77.9
183	63.2–67.7	65.6–72.6	69.7–78.7

°E. L. Koh: Height-weight correlation in the metric system. *Canadian Medical Association Journal, 110:* 1044, 1974.

ADULT WEIGHT IN KILOGRAMS
FOR MEN, ACCORDING TO FRAME,
IN INDOOR CLOTHING°

Height in cm (With 2.5-cm Heel Shoes)	Small Frame	Medium Frame	Large Frame
157 (5'2")	50.5–54.1	53.2–58.6	56.9–63.5
158	51.0–54.6	53.7–59.1	57.4–64.2
159	51.6–55.2	54.3–59.7	58.0–64.9
160	52.2–55.8	54.9–60.3	58.6–65.6
161	52.8–56.4	55.5–60.9	59.2–66.3
162	53.3–56.9	56.0–61.5	59.7–67.0
163	53.9–57.5	56.6–62.1	60.3–67.7
164	54.5–58.1	57.1–62.7	60.9–68.4
165	55.1–58.7	57.7–63.3	61.5–69.2
166	55.7–59.4	58.3–64.0	62.1–70.0
167	56.3–60.1	58.9–64.7	62.8–70.7
168	57.0–60.8	59.5–65.4	63.5–71.4
169	57.6–61.5	60.2–66.1	64.2–72.2
170	58.2–62.2	60.8–66.8	64.9–73.0
171	58.9–62.9	61.4–67.5	65.6–73.7
172	59.6–63.6	62.0–68.2	66.3–74.5
173	60.2–64.4	62.7–69.0	67.0–75.3
174	60.9–65.2	63.4–69.8	67.7–76.1
175	61.6–66.0	64.1–70.7	68.4–77.0
176	62.3–66.8	64.9–71.5	69.2–77.8
177	63.0–67.6	65.6–72.4	70.0–78.7
178	63.8–68.4	66.4–73.2	70.7–79.5
179	64.5–69.2	67.2–74.1	71.5–80.4
180	65.3–70.0	68.0–75.0	72.2–81.2
181	66.0–70.7	68.8–75.9	73.0–82.0
182	66.7–71.5	69.6–76.8	73.8–82.9
183	67.5–72.3	70.4–77.6	74.7–83.8
184	68.2–73.1	71.2–78.5	75.5–84.7
185	69.0–73.9	72.0–79.4	76.4–85.6
186	69.7–74.7	72.8–80.3	77.2–86.5
187	70.5–75.5	73.6–81.2	78.1–87.5
188	71.2–76.4	74.4–82.1	79.0–88.4
189	72.0–77.3	75.3–83.0	79.8–89.3
190	72.7–78.2	76.1–83.9	80.6–90.3
191	73.5–79.2	77.0–84.8	81.5–91.2
192	74.2–80.2	77.9–85.8	82.4–92.2
193	75.0–81.2	78.7–86.8	83.3–93.2

°Koh, op. cit., p. 1044.

Weight tables provide a good general guide to desirable body weight, but they must be considered in terms of the individual's body frame and the amount of fatty tissue the person has in subcutaneous layers of skin. Special instruments have been developed for measuring subcutaneously fatty tissue but whether these are available for nurses to use, and whether the nurse or some other health professional takes these measurements, are matters of agency policy.

The weight tables give a good general indication of where the person stands in regard to being overweight, underweight, or in the average range for his height and age. In order to assess his state of nutrition, however, the nurse supplements her data by noting observable signs of good or poor nutrition. The table on page 281 lists characteristics of persons with good nutrition and poor nutrition, which the nurse may find helpful in her observations.

PRIORITIES FOR NURSING ACTION

Priority situations with regard to nutritional problems are those in which the in-

CHARACTERISTICS OF GOOD NUTRITION AND POOR NUTRITION°

Good Nutrition	Poor Nutrition
Well developed *body*	Body may be undersized, or show poor development or physical defects
About average *weight* for height	Usually thin (underweight 10 percent or more), but may be normal or overweight (fat and flabby)
Muscles well developed and firm	Muscles small and flabby
Skin turgid and of healthy color	Skin loose and pale, waxy, or sallow
Good layer *subcutaneous fat*	Subcutaneous fat usually lacking (or in excess)
Mucous membranes of eyelids and mouth reddish pink	Mucous membranes pale
Hair smooth and glossy	Hair often rough and without luster
Eyes clear	Dark hollows or circles under eyes or puffiness; eyes reddened
Good natured and full of life	Irritable, overactive, fatigues easily
	or
	Phlegmatic, listless, fails to concentrate
Appetite good	Appetite poor
General health excellent	Susceptible to infections
	Lacks endurance and vigor

°Bogert, Briggs, and Calloway, op. cit., p. 419.

dividual's health is being affected or jeopardized by nutritional status or is causing other health problems. The grossly overweight individual, as we have mentioned, should be referred for medical assistance, whether or not he or she is showing signs of other health problems. Malnourished individuals are also referred for medical assistance because of the possibility that malnourishment may be caused by another health problem. Severely malnourished individuals, however, require prompt intervention by health professionals. In some situations the nurse may be responsible for initiating treatment—for example, if she is working in a community where medical help is not available. However, in this situation the nurse needs additional preparation for coping with such circumstances, and this type of training is usually included in postbasic courses.

The nurse should nevertheless be alert to the signs of severe malnourishment in individuals, whether they are ill and in an inpatient facility, or in an ambulatory setting in the community. The characteristics of poor nutrition, shown in the table above, will be helpful in this regard.

People who are severely malnourished, or whose nutritional status is threatened because they are unable to take sufficient food and fluid on their own, usually require that nourishment be provided either in lieu of, or supplementary to, their oral intake by means such as intravenous feedings or gastric gavage, for example. These interventions are discussed in later chapters in this text (Chapters 29 and 26, respectively).

PRINCIPLES RELEVANT TO THE CARE OF PATIENTS WITH NUTRITIONAL PROBLEMS

1. An adequate intake of essential nutrients and energy-giving foods is required for optimal health.
2. An individual's nutritional status is determined by the adequacy of the specific nutrients and energy-giving foods taken into the body, absorbed, and utilized.
3. Nutritional needs are affected by illness.
4. Food has psychological meaning for people.
5. Foods habits are learned.
6. Food habits are related to cultural, religious, and moral beliefs.

GOALS FOR NURSING ACTION

The long-range goals for people who have actual or potential problems of nutrition are basically one or more of these three:

1. To maintain adequate nutrition of the individual
2. To promote his optimal nutrition
3. To restore the individual to a satisfactory nutritional status if his nutritional balance has been disturbed

SPECIFIC NURSING INTERVENTIONS

The nurse in the community does much nutritional counseling in the course of her work, sharing this responsibility with the nutritionist, the physician, and others. Many of the nutritional problems the nurse encounters require the specialized assistance of another health professional. The overweight person, for example, needs advice about reducing diets and exercise programs, and usually requires much support to adhere to them. Some people have found "Weight Watchers" clubs a help in this regard. Grossly overweight people frequently need medical supervision if they wish to undertake a reducing program; it can be dangerous to lose too much weight too quickly. Fatty tissue helps to support some of the body's internal structures and, if the fat is removed too quickly, there may be serious problems.

The overweight but malnourished individual needs assistance in changing his eating habits to ensure a properly balanced diet containing all the essential nutrients. Malnourished individuals need to be referred to the physician, because the malnourishment may be a symptom of some underlying health problem.

Many people, however, simply want help in planning meals to ensure that they and their families have an adequate, nutritious diet. The nurse works closely with the nutritionist and the health educator in teaching people about basic nutrition needs.

Some of the important points to stress in basic health teaching about nutrition are:

1. The need for a nutritionally balanced diet to promote optimal health (the national food guides are very helpful in this regard)
2. The special needs of children, adolescents and expectant and nursing mothers to promote their optimal growth and development
3. The need for regular mealtimes to foster the development of good eating habits
4. The need for good oral hygiene to promote an adequate intake of essential nutrients
5. The need for good standards of cleanliness in the preparation, storage, and serving of food to prevent infections

The Nurse's Role in the Provision of Nourishment for the Sick

Food for the sick person is both therapeutic and a source of pleasure and nourishment. Most patients, if they are not too ill, look forward to mealtimes; meals provide diversions in a sometimes otherwise monotonous day and a pleasant change from the necessary treatments that many people must undergo when they are ill.

Usually other personnel are employed in a health agency to prepare and, often, serve food to the patient. The nurse, however, has important responsibilities with regard to the patient's nourishment.

Illness, as we have mentioned, has a very great bearing upon a person's acceptance of food. Those who are nauseated, dyspeptic, in pain, or have a fever are less desirous of food than are healthy people. The nurse has a responsibility to modify these factors as much as possible so that the patient will accept nourishment. Small, frequent meals are often more acceptable to the sick person than larger servings at regular mealtime hours.

The sedentary patient is less likely to have a big appetite than the patient who exercises regularly. If a patient is able to perform some activity he should be encouraged to do so, for it will stimulate his appetite. It is important, however, that this activity be carried out well before meals, not directly afterward, and that the amount of exercise is not exhausting.

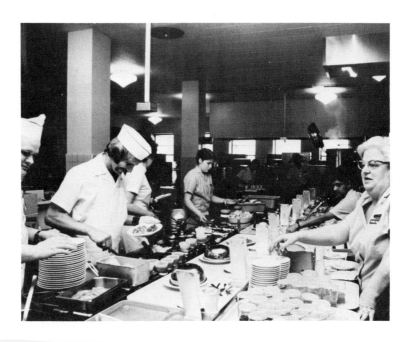

In addition to the special diets which are designed for particular illnesses, the kitchen staff must cater to a wide variety of individual preferences in preparing meals.

It is also necessary to cater to the particular tastes of the individual, to find out what he does and does not like in the way of food, in order to encourage him to take a sufficient amount of nourishment. As noted in the section on the meaning of food at the beginning of this chapter, and subsequent sections on factors affecting food intake, cultural, moral, and religious values play a considerable role in food acceptance. Many Europeans are accustomed to a small "continental" breakfast of coffee and rolls, and may reject the hearty meal which many North Americans enjoy in the morning. A large number of people from Eastern cultures are vegetarians and find it difficult to obtain a sufficient variety of nutrients from our predominantly meat-dominated menus. Beans and rice form an important part of the diet for many Spanish-Americans, but the rice may be unpalatable to them if mixed with raisins and sweetened in a pudding. With the highly diversified ethnic origins of the people of our countries, it is important that all these factors be taken into consideration in preparing meals for patients. The matter of individual differences must also be taken into account.

Then, too, anxiety may affect a patient's desire for food, as well as his ability to digest it. Sometimes anxiety is manifested in complaints about the food. The coffee is cold, the meat may be too well done. Often these complaints are a vocalization of a deeper anxiety. Understanding and acceptance on the part of the nurse can do much to help the patient to accept his illness and his diet.

The amount of food that patients eat and the amount of fluids they drink are sometimes very important therapeutically. It is the nurse who observes how much he eats and drinks and who has the responsibility for communicating this knowledge to other members of the health team. Many health agencies have a standard form (in addition to the Intake and Output chart in the patient's record) that is kept at the patient's bedside so that fluid consumption can be recorded. Often the patient can help to keep the bedside record himself. Once the record is completed, the information is transferred to the "I and O" form in the patient's record.

The nurse is also responsible for helping the patient to get ready for his meals. The patient is offered a bedpan or urinal and is provided with facilities for washing his hands prior to eating. Often a patient who has an unpleasant taste in his mouth will find his appetite improved if he brushes his teeth before eating.

Another factor which affects a person's appetite is the environment in which he eats. If a patient is served in his room, the

SPEEDISET   MOORE BUSINESS FORMS   3

FOR APPROXIMATE MEASUREMENTS ONLY

CREAMER, "TETRA PAK" _____ 20CC	★ CUP, PAPER DRINK (7 OZ) _____ 190CC
TRAYPACK CEREAL MILK OR CREAM (3 OZ) __ 90CC	POT BEVERAGE-INSULATED PLASTIC 200CC
TRAYPACK MILK (8 OZ) _____ 240CC	SOUP BOWL (4 OZ LADLE) INSULATED 120CC
★ TRAYPACK FRUIT JUICE 4 OZ _____ 120CC	★ JUG, STAINLESS STEEL (S-100) ___ 960CC
GLASSJUICE 4 OZ _____ 100CC	★ JUG, BLUE PLASTIC _____ 850CC
ONE SIP _____ 10CC	★ JUG WATER DISPOSABLE _____ 850CC
★ CUP, CROCKERY TEA _____ 150CC	CUSTARD (120 GRAMS) _____ 90CC
★ CUP, PAPER DRINK-(3 OZ) _____ 70CC	JELLO (90 GRAMS) _____ 85CC
-(5 OZ) _____ 130CC	JUNKET (100 GRAMS) _____ 80CC
★ MEASURES TAKEN ½" FROM RIM OF CONTAINER.	30CC = 1 OUNCE = 2 TBSP = 6 TSP

FORM M - 186
REV. 4 - 76
61860

December 4/77   B4
DATE   NURSING UNIT

Bed No.
206A

MRS
MR. MISS MRS.   UNIT NUMBER

DUVAL   MARIE
SURNAME   BLOCK CAPITALS

Intake Required
2500cc

DR A.S. SMITH
DOCTOR   BLOCK CAPITALS

ALL MEASUREMENTS IN CCs.

DAY			AFTERNOON			NIGHT		
HOUR	INTAKE	OUTPUT	HOUR	INTAKE	OUTPUT	HOUR	INTAKE	OUTPUT
0700		250	1500			2300		
0800	430		1600			2400		
0900			1700			0100		
1000	120	300	1800			0200		
1100			1900			0300		
1200	370		2000			0400		
1300		200	2100			0500		
1400	190		2200			0600		
Total	1000	750						

VANCOUVER GENERAL HOSPITAL
FLUID INTAKE AND OUTPUT   **DAY**

A sample bedside fluid intake and output record. (Courtesy of the Vancouver General Hospital.)

air should be fresh and free from unpleasant odors. In addition, the patient's unit should be free of unpleasant sights. Bedside treatment trays are neatly covered and any unnecessary equipment is removed.

The nurse can also see that the patient is free from pain at mealtimes and that he is not subjected to unpleasant treatments immediately before or after meals. Enemas and dressing changes should be carried out at a time when they will have little effect on the patient's appetite.

Some patients like to get out of bed to eat their meals. If this is allowed, the nurse can help the patient to get up a few minutes before his tray arrives. Patients find it very difficult to eat and to swallow when they are flat in bed. If a patient cannot be raised to a sitting position, he will be more comfortable lying on his side while he eats. A comfortable position with adequate support helps make meals more enjoyable experiences.

Some patients prefer company at mealtime. Pleasant conversation with visitors or members of the nursing staff often relaxes the patient, so that the meal is more pleasurable and his appetite and digestion are improved. If the nurse stops to talk with a patient, she is guided by the patient's wishes in regard to mealtime conversations.

Tray Service

Despite the fact that dining-room service for patients is gaining increasing popularity, the majority of patients in hospitals still receive their food on trays in their rooms. Patients are not always physically able to go to a dining room and not all hospitals have such facilities for their patients as yet.

The nurse needs to be aware of good standards for tray service and see that these are adhered to.

1. The tray should be large enough to hold the dishes and utensils needed for the patient's meal and, at the same time, be small enough to fit on the patient's overbed or bedside table.

2. Food must be served at the proper temperature; that is, hot food should not be allowed to cool and cold food should not be allowed to warm.

3. Food should always be covered when it is being carried to the patient's bedside. Covering food helps not only to maintain the proper temperature but also to prevent drying out, which affects the flavor, texture, and appearance of food.

4. Food should be served as attractively as possible, in arranged portions, with garnishes to give color appeal. Small portions are more stimulating to the appetite than large portions.

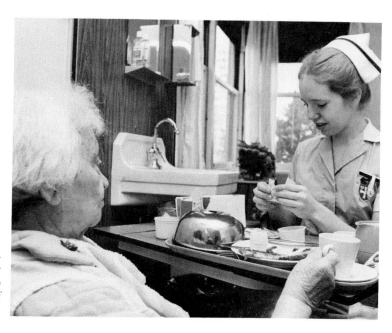

A relaxed, unhurried atmosphere and an attractively arranged tray contribute to the patient's enjoyment of a meal.

5. The napkins, dishes, utensils, and the tray itself should be spotlessly clean.

6. The arrangement on the tray should be neat and organized. Any spilled food should be replaced.

7. China and utensils should be attractive and in good condition.

8. The patient should always get the right tray with the right diet. Each tray has a card with the patient's name, bed number and type of diet. If the nurse has any doubts as to the correctness of a patient's tray, she can check the physician's orders before leaving the tray with the patient.

Feeding the Patient

If it is necessary for the nurse to feed the patient, the observance of a few simple rules will make him more comfortable:

1. Whenever possible use the utensils that are normally used for the food being served.

2. Never hurry the patient. Sit down to feed him whenever possible.

3. Offer the patient small rather than large amounts of food.

4. Offer the food in the order that the patient prefers.

5. Note whether any food or liquid is hot and if it is, warn the patient to take only small portions or sips.

6. A straw or drinking cup will often help a patient to take liquids.

7. If the patient can hold bread or toast, let him manage it himself.

8. Be careful not to spill food. Wipe the patient's mouth and chin whenever necessary. Always protect the patient with a napkin.

After the patient has finished his meal,

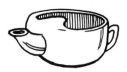

There are several types of drinking cups available commercially which can be useful to people who are ill.

the tray is removed promptly. A patient is never hurried with his meal. If his fluid intake is to be recorded, the amounts are noted on his fluid sheet. The nurse should be familiar with the amount of fluid contained in the commonly used containers. Estimated volumes of consumed fluids suffice in most situations.

Patients should be provided with facilities for washing their hands and brushing their teeth after meals. This offers a good opportunity for the nurse to teach oral hygiene and the correct method for brushing teeth.

Changing Food Habits

It is sometimes necessary for a person to change his food habits because of illness. He may be told by the physician that he can no longer use salt to flavor his food, or he may have to give up eating a favorite dish. The patient may be put on a low-fat diet, or any one of a number of special diets. In these situations, people react differently. Some accept the restrictions of a special diet fairly easily; others are less amenable to change.

One of the most common reasons for failure of a patient to adhere to a diet is lack of understanding of why it is necessary. Another underlying cause may be fear resulting from the loss of a familiar food. The person who has been used to eating pasta all his life, and for whom this represents a basic security food, will find it difficult to adjust to a diet on which this is banned. An individual may rebel against being told what to eat or may resent the loss of personal choice in the matter.

The nurse should remember that merely imparting knowledge to the patient does not ensure that dietary instructions will be followed.[17] Explaining the reasons for a specific diet is essential, but there are other factors which must be taken into consideration also. These include socioeconomic factors; the cultural, religious, and moral values of the patient; and the matter of control over the pur-

---

[17]Lowenberg et al., op. cit., pp. 115–121.

chase and preparation of food in the home.

The most influential member of a household in regard to purchasing and preparing the food that is eaten in the home is, in most instances, the mother. Younger, better-educated homemakers usually have the best nutritional knowledge and are more adaptable, but it is often necessary to work with others who are more resistant to change.

Many older people find it hard to alter the eating patterns they have been used to all their lives, yet often they are the ones on whom dietary restrictions are imposed. Then, too, in most "new American" and "new Canadian" families, it has been recognized that food habits from the homeland are retained long after language, clothing, and other aspects of daily living are altered.[18] Often, strong resistance may be encountered to suggested changes involving the removal or alteration of familiar foods.

It is usually better to work within the framework of the individual's existing food habits, and to suggest modifications wherever possible rather than complete change. The old age pensioner's protein intake may be increased, for example, by the addition of cheese to his lunch of tea and toast. Supplementing a familiar diet of beans and rice by the addition of meat and milk may be accepted more readily by the Puerto Rican family than the suggestion of a completely different way of eating.

Another important item to consider is the effect of the patient's diet on other members of the family. Can the family afford to buy the special foods that are required for the patient? What problems may develop as a result of the need for preparing a different meal for one individual? If, for example, the patient is placed on a low-salt diet, this may involve cooking meat and vegetable dishes for him separately from those for the rest of the family, an additional chore for the homemaker.

---

[18]Ibid.

In her role as teacher, the nurse must coordinate her efforts with those of the physician and the dietitian. The nurse's knowledge of the patient, his family and his home conditions can contribute much to ensuring the success of a teaching program.

PLANNING AND EVALUATING SPECIFIC NURSING INTERVENTIONS

The long-range goals for nursing action, as we have mentioned before, provide general directions for nursing care. The patient who is reluctant to eat, for example, might be expected to achieve an outcome such as "eats all of his meals each day," or the objectives might be less than that to start with and gradually increased. For people taking in a less than adequate amount of fluids, the target intake should be specific and, again, a gradual increase in daily targets may be helpful. It is essential that the patient be involved in the planning unless he is too ill to be, and, if possible, encouraged to assist in keeping track of his food and fluid intake.

Evaluation of the expected outcomes depends on targets set by the nurse, and the patient will find it helpful if these have been specifically stated. Some of the questions for the nurse to keep in mind, however, are:

1. Is the individual eating his meals?
2. Does he enjoy them?
3. Is his intake of food and fluids adequate to meet his daily requirements?
4. How do you know that it is?
5. If the patient is on a special diet, is he adhering to it?
6. If he is in hospital, does he select foods that are compatible with his prescribed diet from the diet menu?

The nurse also observes the patient to assess his nutritional status and the progress made toward achieving the long-range goals. Comparison of her observations of the patient with the characteristics of good nutrition and poor nutrition are again helpful in this regard.

GUIDE TO ASSESSING NUTRITIONAL PROBLEMS

1. What are this person's age, sex, height, usual weight, present weight?
2. What are his usual habits with regard to eating?
3. What are his usual daily activities? His current activity level? What is his present status with regard to food and fluid intake?
4. Is his intake of food and fluids adequate to meet his daily requirements for nutrients and energy-giving foods?
5. What is his general physical condition? Does he appear obese? thin? emaciated?
6. Does he show characteristics of good nutrition? of poor nutrition?
7. Does he have a health problem which may be affecting his intake of food, or his digestive abilities? What is his emotional status? His attitude toward food?
8. Does the patient have cultural, religious, or moral beliefs or values concerning food which conflict with his dietary needs?
9. Is the individual on a special diet?
10. Does he understand the purpose of it? Is he adhering to it?
11. Does the patient need extra fluids?
12. Does he need help with his meals?
13. Are there foods the patient needs to avoid or to eat?
14. Does the patient or his family need help with planning meals to provide optimal nutrition? Will altering existing patterns of dietary intake because of a special condition cause any problems? Do they need help with basic nutrition matters?

STUDY VOCABULARY

Anabolism	Fats	Minerals
Calorie	Glycogen	Nutrient
Carbohydrates	Malnutrition (malnourishment)	Proteins
Catabolism	Metabolism	Vitamins

STUDY SITUATION

Susan James, aged 20, works at a day-care center and lives on a communal farm at the edge of town with five other people. All the members of the commune are vegetarians, their staple diet consisting of rice, whole-grain cereals, and organic fruits and vegetables which they grow on the farm. Susan has not been feeling well for the past few days. She was admitted to hospital this morning suffering from severe abdominal pains and diarrhea, with a tentative diagnosis of regional enteritis. She is thin and pale. Her lab test results indicate that she is also anemic. The physician has ordered bed rest and a high calorie, high protein diet with a vitamin B_{12} supplement for Susan. He has also ordered an iron preparation to be given parenterally.

1. What are some of the factors contributing to Susan's nutritional problem?
2. What information would you need to be able to help Susan?
3. Where would you obtain this information?
4. What are some of the objective signs you might observe in Susan?

5. What subjective observations might you note?
6. What factors would you take into consideration in developing a plan of care for Susan?
7. What specific nursing interventions would you consider in Susan's care?
8. How would you evaluate the effectiveness of these interventions?

SUGGESTED READINGS

Balsley, M., et al.: Nutrition in Disease and Stress. *Nursing Digest,* 3:27–29, March-April 1975.

Birch, H. G.: Malnutrition, Learning and Intelligence. *American Journal of Public Health,* 62:773–784. June 1972.

Bozian, M. W.: Nutrition for the Aged or Aged Nutrition? *Nursing Clinics of North America,* 11:169–178, March 1976.

Dwyer, L. S., et al.: Simplified Meal Planning for Hard-to-Teach Patients. *American Journal of Nursing,* 74:664–665, April 1974.

Feingold, B. F.: Hyperkinesis and Learning Disabilities Linked to Artificial Food Flavors and Color. *American Journal of Nursing,* 75:797–803, May 1975.

Kane, L. T.: Canada Inside Out: Surveying the Nation's Nutrition. *Canadian Nurse,* 70:30–33, August 1974.

Kroog, E.: Helping People Stretch their Grocery Dollars. *American Journal of Nursing,* 75:646–648, April 1975.

LaFrance, K. H.: DX: Poor diet. *Nursing Care,* 8:16–19, February 1975.

Lambert, M. L., Jr.: Drug and Diet Interactions. *American Journal of Nursing,* 75:402–406, March 1975.

Lapointe, G.: A Nutrition Course for Nurses. *Canadian Nurse,* 71:30–31, January 1975.

Margolin, C., et al.: Vital Food Facts Every Expectant Mother Should Know. *Parents,* 50:35–37, March 1975.

Robinson, C. R.: *Normal and Therapeutic Nutrition.* 14th edition. New York, Macmillan Company, 1972.

Star, J.: Why You Choose the Foods You Do. *Today's Health,* 51:32–37, 1973.

Taif, B.: Preventing Complications of Alcoholism. *Journal of Practical Nursing,* 25:18–19, September 1975.

Walker, L.: Nutritional Concerns of Addicts in Treatment. Methadone Maintenance Treatment Program, Los Angeles, California. *Journal of Psychiatric Nursing,* 13:21–26, May-June 1976.

Wolfe, B. M.: Hypoglycemia: Some Facts About a Misunderstood Condition. *Canadian Nurse,* 69:38–40, October 1973.

17 MOVEMENT AND EXERCISE NEEDS

The nurse should be able to:

Discuss the importance of mobility in a person's life

Compare and contrast the dangers of bed rest and the benefits of exercise, relating these to the sick person and the well individual

Explain in simple terms the functions of bones, muscles, joints, nerves, and their blood supply in body movement

Discuss factors interfering with motor functioning

Assess an individual's motor abilities

Establish priorities for nursing action

Discuss relevant principles in planning an exercise program for a patient

Assist the patient in selecting and carrying out appropriate exercises

Discuss principles underlying body mechanics

Discuss how to apply good body mechanics in assisting patients to move

Evaluate the effectiveness of specific nursing interventions

INTRODUCTION

All living creatures move. The lusty cry and accompanying body movements of the newborn indicate to the doctor or midwife that the child is indeed alive. The cessation of all movement is the first observable sign of death. Movement is such a vital part of our lives that permanent loss of the ability to move any part of the body is one of the major tragedies that can occur in a person's life. Loss of mobility lessens the concept a person has of himself. His body image is affected and he thinks of himself as less a person than he was—he is less than "whole." Independence is threatened and, if the immobility affects one or more of the principal locomotor parts of the body, the threat to independence assumes major proportions. The individual's opportunities for communication are also jeopardized if he cannot move around, and sensory deprivation becomes a real possibility. Communication itself depends on motor abilities for speaking, writing, and using non-verbal "body language" to send messages to other people.

The ability to move enables the infant to explore first himself and then his surroundings. Infants deprived of sufficient opportunities for movement, for any reason, do not develop as well physically, intellectually, or psychosocially as those who are free to move. One has only to think of the ancient Chinese custom, which prevailed until comparatively recent times, of binding the feet of girl babies to keep them small—and the hobbling gait that resulted—to appreciate the importance of movement in physical growth.

Intellectual development depends to a large extent on the child's exposure to an ever-widening world. A child who has never seen an airplane and perhaps not even a bird, has difficulty understanding the concept of flying. Children whose mobility is restricted because of illness or economic reasons (whose parents cannot afford or do not bother to take them to the zoo and other cultural places) do not have the same opportunities to expand their intellectual horizons. This was one of the principal reasons behind the Head Start programs for socially disadvantaged children, who were often judged intellectually inferior to children who had had greater opportunities. Intelligence, as measured on standard IQ tests, has very often been substantially increased in children who have participated in Head Start programs.

All systems in the body function more efficiently when they are active. Disuse of the neuromuscular system quickly leads to degeneration and subsequent loss of functioning. If muscles are immobilized, the process of degeneration begins almost immediately. It has been estimated that the strength and tone of immobilized muscles may decrease by as much as 5 per cent per day in the absence of any contraction of the muscle.[1]

The process of degeneration in muscles occurs very quickly. The restoration of muscle strength and tone, on the other hand, is a very slow process that may take months or years to accomplish. In this case, then, prevention is by far the better part of cure. Nurses caring for patients during the acute stage of illnesses requir-

---

[1]Phyllis Brower and Dorothy Hicks: Maintaining Muscle Function in Patients on Bed Rest. *American Journal of Nursing*, 72:1250–1253, July 1972, p. 1250.

ing more than a few days of bed rest have a responsibility to do everything possible to prevent degeneration of unused muscles and the development of complications that will limit the person's mobility or prolong his recovery and restoration to health.

BED REST, EXERCISE, AND THEIR IMPLICATIONS

The Dangers of Bed Rest

The dangers of prolonged bed rest have been well documented in numerous study reports, books, and articles in both the nursing and medical literature over the past 30 or 40 years. The custom of early ambulation of patients following surgery, childbirth, and acute illness was introduced just after World War II. The results have been phenomenal in preventing complications and hastening patients' recovery.

Among the adverse effects of lengthy bed rest that have been noted are: a slowing down of the basal metabolic rate; a decrease in muscle strength, tone, and size; postural changes; constipation; increased vulnerability to pulmonary and urinary tract infections; circulatory problems, such as thrombosis (the development of a clot in the blood stream) and embolus (which occurs when the clot becomes detached and travels through the blood stream until it comes to a vessel too small for it to pass through, where it lodges). The degenerative process affects bone and skin tissues as well.

The pulse rate increases, as the heart works harder in an attempt to cope with the extra amount of blood "dumped" into the general circulation from the legs when the body is lying down. There is increased excretion of calcium, nitrogen, and phosphorus, and the individual may suffer severe depletion of these elements. The person usually develops feelings of anxiety and frequently hostility as a result of disturbed functioning of physical and mental activity, as well as disruption of his sleep patterns.

The Benefits of Exercise

Exercise, in comparison, increases the efficiency of functioning of all body processes. The physiological, psychological, and social benefits of exercise have been receiving increasing attention in recent years. The predominantly sedentary way of life of so many North Americans has been viewed as a major factor contributing to many of the illnesses with which we are plagued, such as coronary heart disease (the leading cause of death in North America), hypertension, diabetes, and obesity.

Many studies have been undertaken in the United States, Canada, and a number of other countries, to determine the exact physiological changes that result from a regular exercise program. Among those that have been found are: increased muscle strength, tone, and size; increased efficiency of the heart; increased work tolerance; increased pulmonary efficiency; improved digestion; better mental alertness; improved sleep patterns; increased hemoglobin levels in the blood; decreased blood pressure; decreased deposits of fatty tissue; and decreased cholesterol levels in the blood.[2] It has been demonstrated that exercise following a fatty meal will help to clear the blood of excessive cholesterol, and thus increase fat tolerance.

Implications for the Sick and the Well

The documented dangers of bed rest and benefits of exercise have implications both for the prevention of illness and for the restoration to health following illness. Physically fit people are less vulnerable to such illnesses as heart problems, hypertension, obesity, and diabetes in that the "risk factors" that predispose people to these disorders are lessened. There is evidence to support the belief that their

[2] Donald K. Mathews and Edward L. Fox: *The Physiological Basis of Physical Education and Athletics.* 2nd edition. Philadelphia, W. B. Saunders Company, 1976, pp. 271–318.

chances for survival following a heart attack are also better. They usually recover more quickly from infections than those who are physically unfit. Lest you think that it is necessary to undertake a strenuous athletic program to achieve these benefits, it has been demonstrated that a six week program of 3 one-half hour sessions per week, at such activities as swimming, jogging, cycling, or calisthenics, followed by a once or twice a week maintenance program, will significantly improve fitness in all aspects of physiological functioning enumerated in the previous section.[3]

Rest and enforced immobility are needed for recovery from many illnesses. An injured part of the body must be put to rest to prevent further injury while the tissues repair themselves. Following a heart attack, for example, it is important that the heart be relieved of as much work as possible so that the process of tissue repair can take place with no more strain on the heart than is absolutely necessary. Similarly, broken bones and torn ligaments must be immobilized to allow the bone tissues or muscle fibers to knit sufficiently to withstand the normal wear and tear they receive in the course of daily activities.

Many other illnesses also require lengthy periods of rest. Some disorders result in partial or total loss of mobility—e.g., arthritis (inflammation of the joints, which often results in limited mobility for the individual) and paralysis, which can cause total immobility of one-half or more of the body.

Any person who is on bed rest for more than a few days, or whose mobility is limited in any way, requires exercise to those parts of the body that are not immobilized of necessity. These days, even cardiac patients are being started on exercise programs at an early stage of their recovery, and gradually increasing exercise is a part of their therapy. People who have had a myocardial infarction are even receiving training in marathon running in some parts of the country. For people with most illnesses exercise is started al-

most immediately after the crisis stage is over. The new postoperative patient is out of bed and walking (with help) down the hall, within a few hours following surgery, in some cases. He may have to carry his intravenous infusion apparatus with him, or his drainage tubes and bottles, but walk he must.

People who cannot get out of bed must have their exercise in bed, in the form of active or passive range of motion exercises (and others) as tolerated. This is now an accepted nursing responsibility that is carried out on all patients unless there are contraindications. How to help patients with range of motion exercises will be discussed in a later section of this chapter.

NORMAL MOTOR FUNCTIONING

The principal systems involved in body movements are the skeletal system, the muscular system, and the nervous system. The circulatory system is also involved in that it provides nourishment to the tissues of these systems. If circulation to any part of the body is impaired, degeneration of the tissues in the area begins, since the body cells cannot live without adequate nourishment. However, it is the bones, the nerves, and the muscles that make movement possible.

The bones of the skeletal system have two functions in movement—they provide an attachment for muscles and ligaments, and they act as levers. The *proximal* end of a muscle is attached to a less movable bone, such as the scapula in the shoulder. This point of attachment is called the *origin of the muscle*. The *distal* end of the muscle is attached to a freely movable bone, such as the humerus in the upper arm. This point is called the *insertion* of the muscle.

"Lever" is a term taken from the physical sciences, meaning a rigid bar that revolves around a fixed axis called a fulcrum. The simplest example of a lever is a teeter-totter or seesaw. Two children of equal weight can balance on a teeter-totter that is resting on a fixed point or axis, if they are equidistant from the middle. If

---

[3]Ibid. See also Chapter 21.

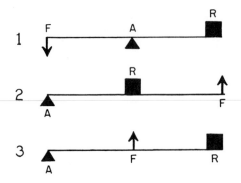

F = Force
A = Axis or fulcrum
R = Resistance or weight

Three types of levers.

one child exerts force, by pushing down, or moves his weight further backwards, his end of the board will move towards the ground, assisted by the pull of gravity. To raise his end of the board and bring down his partner, he must exert force to push upwards against the force of gravity, which is resisting his movement. Using the board as a lever, however, he is able to lift the weight of the other child off the ground—to a considerable height, if you stop to think about it—a feat he could not accomplish if he tried to do it while standing on the ground and trying to lift him in his arms.

An axis need not always be in the center of a lever. Three different types of levers are shown in the figure above.

The muscles contract to produce motion. Muscles for movement are always in pairs, one on either side of a bone or joint, and have opposing functions; as one contracts, the other extends (stretches) to cause the bone to move in a certain direction. The action is similar to that involved in the manipulation of a puppet by strings: you shorten one string and lengthen another to make the puppet move in the direction you want it to go.

Muscles also tend to work in groups rather than in single pairs. Breathing, for example, requires the coordinated activity of a number of muscles, including the intercostals, the diaphragm, and the sternocleidomastoid muscles, the scalenes, the thoracohumeral, and the thoracoscapular muscles. To move the thigh alone involves all the gluteus muscles, as well as the adductor muscles.

The spinal nerves are directly involved in trunk and limb movements. Each spinal nerve has an anterior and a posterior root in the spinal column. The anterior root conducts impulses to the muscles from the central nervous system. The posterior root conducts messages from the sensory receptors to the central nervous system.

Almost all patterns of movement can be initiated by the spinal cord alone. Balance and the progression, coordination, and purposefulness of movement, however, require participation of progressively higher levels in the brain. Motor areas located in the frontal lobes of the cerebral cortex serve as the "master control" for directing and controlling specific movement in various parts of the body.[4]

Types of Movement

The body has six large movable parts: the head, the trunk, the two arms, and the two legs. It also has smaller movable parts, such as the hand, fingers, feet, and toes, which form part of a larger part but may move independently of it. You can move a hand without moving the rest of the arm, for example, or a finger independently of any other part of the body.

These body parts are capable of various kinds of movements:

Abduction: Movement away from the central axis (midline) of the body.

Adduction: Movement toward the central axis (midline) of the body.

Flexion: The act of bending; the angle between the two moving parts is decreased.

Extension: The act of straightening; the angle between the two moving parts is increased.

Hyperextension: Extension beyond the normal range of motion—for example, in bending the head back toward the spine.

Gliding: Movement in one plane, as in sliding.

[4]Arthur C. Guyton: Basic Human Physiology: Normal Function and Mechanisms of Disease. Philadelphia, W. B. Saunders Company, 1971, Chapters 37 and 38.

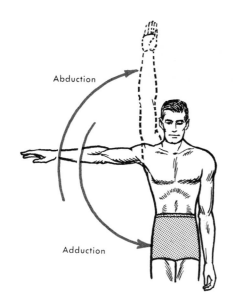

Abduction

Adduction

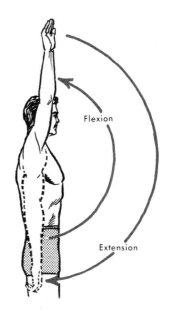

Flexion

Extension

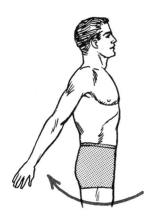

Hyperextension

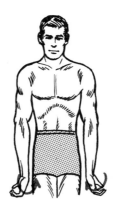

Inward rotation

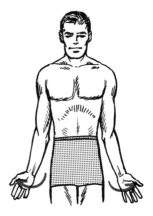

Outward rotation

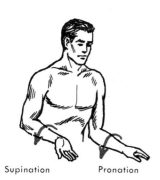

Supination   Pronation

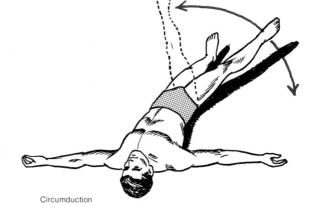

Circumduction

Rotation: Turning in a circular motion around a fixed axis.

Circumduction: Circular motion of a limb or part when the limb or part forms part of a cone, as in swinging the arm in a circular motion.

Pronation: Turning down toward the ground.

Supination: Turning upward (the opposite of pronation).

Inversion: Turning inward towards the body.

Eversion: Turning outward away from the body.

These movements are illustrated on pages 295 and 296.

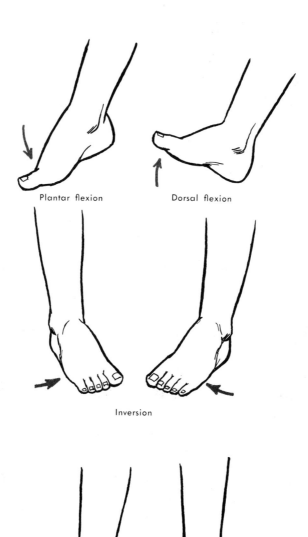

Plantar flexion   Dorsal flexion

Inversion

Eversion

Types of Joints

The various types of movements are made possible by the *joints,* which connect one bone to another. The body does have some joints that are immovable, such as those connecting the bones in the skull, but the major purpose of the joints is to serve as hinges to enable the body to move. Each movable joint is constructed to make possible a certain type of movement, and each has a circumscribed range.

The body has six types of movable joints.

Hinge. This is a uniaxial joint which permits flexion and extension. An example of a hinge joint is the knee.

Pivot. This is also a uniaxial joint. It permits rotation. An example is the atlantoaxial joint (between the first cervical vertebra and the base of the skull).

Condyloid. This is a biaxial joint. It permits flexion, extension, abduction, and adduction. A combination of these four movements is called circumduction. The wrist is a condyloid joint.

Saddle. This is another biaxial joint. It permits flexion, extension, abduction, adduction, and circumduction. An example is the thumb.

Ball and socket. This type of joint is polyaxial. Movements permitted include flexion, extension, abduction, adduction, circumduction, and rotation. The hip joint is a ball and socket joint.

Gliding. This is a *plane* joint and permits gliding movements. An example is the acromioclavicular joint of the shoulder.

Planes of the Body

Body movements are often described in relation to *planes,* another term from the physical sciences, which means that when the body is in a standing position, as shown in the figure above, the *sagittal plane* divides it into right and left sections, the *frontal plane* into dorsal and ventral sections, and the *transverse plane* into upper and lower sections.

This figure shows the body in good anatomical position—that is, the alignment of

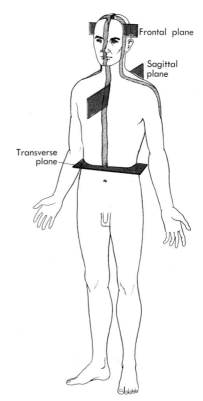

Sagittal, frontal, and transverse planes of the body.

body parts is balanced, and their weight is also balanced. In the anatomical position, the individual stands with his hands at his sides, thumbs adducted, and hands supinated. The head is erect; the spine, pelvis, legs, and feet are in good alignment with the head. The feet are slightly apart and directed forward, and the knees and fingers are slightly flexed.

Movement of the body is much easier when the body parts are in good alignment, when the weight of the body is evenly balanced, and when the feet are set a little farther apart (about one foot apart) than in the anatomical position. Setting the feet this far apart provides the body with a wider base of support for its weight than the normal standing posture does.

The center of weight (center of mass or gravity) in the body is located in the pelvis at approximately the level of the second sacral vertebra. The line of gravity is an imaginary straight line that passes from the top of an object through its

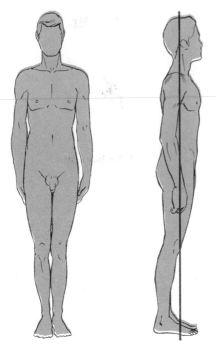

The anatomical position.

center of gravity to form a right angle with the ground.

When the body is erect, in good anatomical position, the line of gravity falls in the frontal plane downward behind the ear, through the center of gravity in the pelvis, and slightly in front of the knee and ankle joints, to the middle of the body's base of support, so that the line is perpendicular to the ground, as shown in the figure below. The body is more stable in this position because its line of gravity is in direct line with the gravitational pull of the earth.

Motor Abilities Needed for Activities of Daily Living

The ability to make parts of the body move and to control these movements enables an individual to develop the motor skills needed for the activities of daily living. A motor skill is used here to mean a series of coordinated movements. It also permits the development of more highly refined motor skills, such as playing the piano, playing tennis, dancing, and so forth.

The basic motor skills needed for the activities of daily living are those that are learned early in life:

1. Lifting the head when lying on the back
2. Grasping an object in the hand
3. Raising an object to the mouth
4. Turning over onto one side or the other from a back-lying position
5. Rolling over, from back to abdomen and the reverse
6. Sitting up from a back-lying position
7. Standing up and sitting down
8. Transferring from one place to another
9. Walking

Control over the bodily processes of elimination, which also is essential to daily living, involves control over muscular functioning. Problems in relation to these processes are discussed in Chapters 27 and 28.

FACTORS INTERFERING WITH MOTOR FUNCTIONING

The ability of the body to move its various movable parts and to control these movements so that they are performed in a coordinated fashion depends on the integrity of the muscles, the bones, the joints, the nerves innervating these structures, and the circulation nourishing them. Injury, disease, or congenital problems affecting the bones, muscles, joints, or their collateral nerve or blood supply may, then, cause impairment of motor functioning.

Even a minor injury, such as a sprained ankle, which damages muscles and ligaments in that area, will limit a person's ability to walk until the muscle fibers and ligaments have healed. Fracture of a bone limits the ability to move the part of the body in which the fracture is located. People who are injured in car accidents, severe falls, or other types of accidents may sustain injury to the spinal cord. Because the cord is essential in the transmission of nerve impulses to and from the area in the brain controlling motor function, all movements below the site of the injury may be cut off. The person may be paralyzed from the waist down (*paraplegic*), if the injury is located at that level, or from the neck down (*quadriplegic*), if the injury is in the cervical region.

A stroke is the result of a cerebrovascular accident. This problem frequently impairs the blood supply to motor areas in the frontal lobe of the brain of one hemisphere, with resultant loss of motor functioning on one side of the body (*hemiplegia*). The motor abilities needed for speech may also be impaired if the accident is in the dominant half of the brain.

Congenital abnormalities are one of the common troubles causing hospitalization in infants and small children. Many children whom the nurse will encounter on the pediatric units of hospitals are there for repair of congenital malformations that interfere with their ability to walk, as, for example, the children with "clubfoot," or a "congenital hip."

Contractures of muscles controlling movement of the joints of the body, at the wrist or ankle joints for example, will also cause limitations in mobility. These contractures frequently result from the hand or the foot not being supported in good anatomical position when the person was immobilized for another reason. It should be noted here that these contractures require intensive therapy, over a prolonged period of time, to correct. Briefly, the hand should be supported in a straight line with the lower part of the arm and the fingers slightly flexed. The foot should be at a right angle to the lower part of the leg, in walking position if the person were standing up. (These topics are discussed further in Chapter 18.)

Serious illness of any kind lessens an individual's muscular strength and tone. The individual may be completely helpless and unable to lift his head, to move himself in bed, or to turn himself onto his side. Or he may be semi-helpless, that is, requiring assistance to be able to do these activities and to sit himself up in bed. Surgical patients are usually restricted in their movements because of pain in the operative area and the need to avoid movements that could cause a freshly sutured wound to break open.

Restrictions are put on a patient's movements as soon as he is placed on bed rest for any reason in any type of illness, as we noted earlier in the chapter. The individual may have limitations placed on his mobility for therapeutic reasons, even if he is not confined to bed, as, for example, the person with a sprained ankle, or one with a "wry neck" (torticollis), which is a not uncommon occurrence in people who have been involved in automobile accidents.

A person who is isolated because of infectious precautions also has his mobility restricted (see Chapter 21).

The movements of some patients may be curtailed by the use of restraints if it is in their best interests to do so (for example, if they are confused and may hurt themselves trying to get out of bed) (see Chapter 20).

Some people may be restricted in their mobility because of other disabilities that limit their ability to get around without help, as, for example, a blind or deaf person. Others may be restricted because of their environment. People who reside in nursing homes, for example, may have limited opportunities to move about and usually they have physical mobility problems as well. The children from disadvantaged homes, whom we mentioned at the beginning of the chapter, may also be limited in mobility because of their home circumstances.

Some people, of course, limit their own mobility; probably we all know people whose only movements are from the house to their car, from the car to the office, and home again, where they sit for the rest of the evening.

COMMON PROBLEMS IN MOTOR FUNCTIONING

People whose motor abilities are impaired because of illness or injury often need help to perform the daily activities of living. Among the common problems with which they may need the nurse's help are: inability or limited ability to raise the head; to grasp objects; to move themselves in bed; to turn on their side or to turn over; to raise the buttocks when lying flat, or when sitting up (necessary for use of the bedpan); to sit up; to stand; to transfer, as from the bed to a chair, or the reverse; to walk.

The problem of maintaining the functional ability of unused muscles and preventing their degeneration is common to all patients on prolonged bed rest, and to those whose muscles are not being used for any reason. Maintaining optimal functional ability in muscles is common also to many who are otherwise well, but whose mobility is restricted either voluntarily or because of circumstances beyond their control.

Because the degenerative process affects the skin, as well as muscles and bone, in persons on bed rest and those whose motor abilities are impaired, there are problems in maintaining the skin in good condition (this is further discussed in Chapter 19). The maintenance of nutritional status is also a problem in patients on bed rest because of excessive losses of protein, calcium, and nitrogen (see Chapter 16). Maintaining psychosocial equilibrium is another problem commonly seen in patients with limited mobility. Anxiety and sensory deprivation are other potential problems, as we discussed in Chapters 12 and 13.

The patient's safety may also be of concern, because the person who is not able to move about well cannot protect himself from environmental hazards (see Chapter 20). Potential problems with regard to infections will also exist, because of the patient's possibly poor nutritional status or poor skin condition (see Chapter 21).

ASSESSING MOTOR FUNCTIONING ABILITIES

In assessing a patient's motor status when developing a plan of care for him, the nurse needs information about his usual motor abilities and his present status with regard to these abilities (see Chapter 9). She also needs information about any recent health problems he has had in addition to his current problems. If the patient has, or recently had, a health problem, she should be aware of the physician's diagnostic and therapeutic plans of care for the patient. She needs to know, for example, if other health workers, such as the physical therapist or the occupational therapist are involved in helping the patient. She needs to be aware of any restrictions that have been placed on the patient's mobility, such as bed rest or no exercise.

She should also be aware of the patient's potential prognosis. It should be noted, however, that it is often difficult to predict the patient's chances of regaining motor functioning that has been impaired by illness, such as stroke or spinal injury. Recovery is often slow, and in some cases, may take years to accomplish. One should never give up simply because a tentative prognosis is not hopeful.

Much of the information needed is available from the patient's record, the nursing history, the initial clinical appraisal form, the physician's notations on the record, and reports of assessments done by other health professionals. If a physical therapist has been called in, for example, he or she usually does a thorough assessment of the patient's motor functional abilities. When a patient has disturbances of motor functioning, specialist physicians, such as the neurologist and the physiatrist, are frequently consulted by the attending physician, and their reports should also be on the patient's record.

The patient's family are often very helpful in providing information about the patient's abilities with regard to motor functioning.

The nurse's observations and the patient's subjective observations are both important in the initial and continuous assessments of his motor status. Sensory functioning and motor functioning are usually closely interrelated, and often the patient's ability to feel pressure is the first sign of a return of functioning ability in a limb. The patient, the nurse, or a member of the patient's family may be the first to notice this in the patient. The nurse must be alert to signs of increased muscle tension, or of movement in flaccid muscles, when she is doing passive range of motion exercises for the patient, and note these on the record.

PRIORITIES FOR NURSING ACTION

In establishing priorities for nursing action for limited mobility, the nurse takes into account two sets of problems. For the individual whose mobility is curtailed, the overwhelming priority is the preventive aspect of making sure that those unused muscles whose movement is not contraindicated for therapeutic reasons receive sufficient exercise to prevent their deterioration.

When patients cannot move themselves and need the nurse's help to move, assistance in the daily activities of living ranks high on the nurse's list of priorities. The patient who cannot feed himself should not be left until his food is cold. Patients who need help in turning must be turned at scheduled times, or serious skin problems may result. The individual who needs the nurse's help to use the bedpan or a urinal needs it immediately, not half an hour from now. The person who needs assistance in getting up, getting in or out of bed, or getting in or out of the wheelchair likewise should not be left waiting for lengthy periods to be helped with these activities.

The nurse uses her judgment, then, in scheduling her activities to ensure that patients who have problems in meeting their basic physiological needs are given the needed assistance at the time they need it. The nurse must also be sufficiently flexible to interrupt other activities that can be deferred to assist patients who need immediate assistance with the basic needs. Recording, for example, can be interrupted when the nurse sees a patient's signal light go on. The ignoring of or slow response to their signals for help is one of the most common complaints patients have when they are ill in hospital.

PRINCIPLES RELEVANT TO THE CARE OF PATIENTS WITH PROBLEMS IN MOTOR FUNCTIONING

The principles relevant to the care of patients with problems in motor functioning may be divided into two categories: those relating to exercise needed to prevent muscular degeneration, or to improve muscular strength and tone; and those relating to helping people who are unable to help themselves in moving. The

specific nursing interventions that the nurse considers when developing a nursing care plan for patients with these problems may also be divided into two groups of activities. Thus, we will consider each set of principles as they relate to specific nursing interventions.

GOALS FOR NURSING ACTION

The goals of nursing action for patients who have existing or potential problems in motor functioning abilities are directed towards:

1. Maintenance of strength and tone in unused muscles whose movement is not contraindicated by the nature of health problem(s) they may have
2. Prevention of degeneration of these muscles
3. Prevention of contractures that could hinder the mobility of joints
4. Restoration, insofar as possible, of strength and tone of muscles so impaired
5. Promotion of optimal strength and tone of muscles
6. Prevention of deterioration of the patient's other functional abilities as a result of limited mobility
7. Retention or regaining of independence in the activities of daily living insofar as this is possible
Note: Goal #6 is discussed in other chapters concerned with specific functional abilities.

NURSING INTERVENTIONS FOR EXERCISE

There are very few patients for whom all exercise is contraindicated. The physician generally orders the degree of activity for patients in an inpatient health agency, that is, whether he is to be confined to bed, have bathroom privileges, and so on. The patient who has a specific need for remedial exercises—for example, the patient with a paralyzed arm—is often guided in his exercise by the physical therapist and the nurse. For many patients, exercise is part of their nursing care and most of the guidance they receive is provided by the nurse. It is an im-

PRINCIPLES RELEVANT TO PLANNING AND IMPLEMENTING EXERCISE PROGRAMS FOR PATIENTS

1. The process of degeneration starts almost immediately when muscles are unused.
2. The process of degeneration involves bone and skin tissues as well as muscle tissue.
3. All joints have a circumscribed range of motion.
4. Passive exercise of the body's movable parts through their full range of motion prevents the development of contractures that can interfere with joint mobility.
5. Active contraction of muscles is required to maintain and improve their strength and tone.
6. Active contraction of muscles on one side of the body causes the corresponding muscles on the other side of the body to contract.
7. Exercise has beneficial effects on all body systems.

portant independent nursing function to assess the patient's exercise needs and provide for suitable exercise within existing limitations and contraindications.

Patients who remain in bed for a prolonged period are prone to develop complications as a result of their inactivity, as we mentioned earlier. Exercise helps maintain and create good muscle tone and prevent atrophy. For the person in bed, this means that the strength of his muscles is maintained or developed in readiness for greater activity. Exercise also helps in the elimination of waste products from the muscles. The contraction of muscles increases circulation and the removal of wastes from the body. Increased circulation is particularly important for the person who remains in bed. Stasis of blood is a predisposing factor in the formation of clots, which can lead to serious complications.

The increased basal metabolic rate that results from exercise increases the body's need for oxygen. This in turn results in an increase in both the rate and depth of respirations, thus improving lung aeration and helping to prevent infectious processes in the lungs, which occur as a result of inactive lung areas and stagnant secretions. Improved blood circulation also increases the delivery of oxygen and nutrients to tissues, thus maintaining their health and preventing deterioration and ulcer formation.

Contracture of the muscles and stiffen-ing of the joints are other unfortunate side effects of prolonged inactivity. By putting joints through their full range of motion, these can often be avoided.

Kinds of Exercise

Basically, there are three types of exercise:

1. *Passive exercise.* In passive exercise the body part is moved by someone other than the patient. In passive exercise, the muscles do not actively contract. This type of exercise helps to prevent contractures, but it does not increase muscle strength and tone.

2. *Isometric exercise.* This is a form of active exercise in which the patient consciously increases the tension of his muscles, but there is neither joint movement nor is there change in the length of the muscle. This type of exercise, sometimes referred to as "muscle-setting exercises," can help considerably in maintaining or improving muscle strength and tone.

3. *Isotonic exercise.* This, too, is a form of active exercise. In this type, the patient supplies the energy to actively exercise his muscles and move the limb or other body part. In isotonic exercise, the muscle actively contracts or shortens, causing the limb to move. Isotonic exercises increase muscle strength and tone and help joint mobility.

Regardless of the kind of exercise the patient is to have, the nurse must see that he avoids fatigue.

Exercises are planned as a regular part of her nursing activities. During the bed bath, for example, the nurse has an excellent opportunity to move the patient's limbs through their full range of motion. The patient is encouraged to exercise actively those muscles that he is permitted to use. The nurse passively exercises those he cannot. Patients can learn to do isometric exercises on their own while they are otherwise inactive in bed, and can supplement programs of regular isotonic exercise by this means.

Regular isotonic exercise is often prescribed as part of the patient's therapy. He may go to the physiotherapy department for this, or the physical therapist may come to the nursing unit. If a program of regular exercise is not undertaken by another health worker for patients, the nurse institutes a program for all patients for whom active exercise is not contraindicated. Both individual and group exercises are used.

Group exercises are helpful from a social point of view (increasing sensory stimulation), as well as having physically therapeutic benefits. There is greater motivation to put forth more effort in a group when everyone is doing the same thing. In many agencies, group physiotherapy classes are organized by the physical therapy department, but there is no reason why a nurse cannot organize these on a nursing unit. It is frequently done on some obstetrical units to assist patients to regain lost muscle tone resulting from pregnancy and childbirth.

Occupational therapy is often used to supplement physical therapy to assist people in maintaining or regaining muscular strength and preventing loss of joint mobility.

Range of Motion. When a patient is exercising, his joints should go through their full range of motion. For example, the normal shoulder and upper arm movements are flexion, extension, hyperextension, abduction, adduction, circumduction, inward rotation, and outward rotation. The chief muscles involved in these movements are the deltoid (abducts upper arm), pectoralis major (flexes and adducts the upper arm), trapezius (raises and lowers the shoulders), latissimus dorsi (extends and adducts the upper arm), and serratus anterior (pulls the shoulder forward).

Hand and finger exercises are often a part of a patient's therapy. Flexing, abducting, extending, and adducting the hand, as well as flexing and extending the joints of the fingers, are exercises commonly carried out by patients who have some functional impairment as a result of a stroke. It is particularly important to exercise the thumb. The ability of man to bring the thumb in opposition to the tip and base of the fingers is a key factor in using the hands. It permits the individual to hold a pencil and write, and to hold a fork and eat, or to do any number of ordinary activities.

The knees and the elbows can be flexed and extended. The biceps, quadriceps, and hamstring muscles are active in these movements. The forearm can be supinated and pronated. The four principal muscles that move the forearm are the biceps brachii (flexes and supinates), brachialis (flexes and pronates), triceps brachii (extends), and pronator quadratus (pronates).

Thigh movement involves the gluteus muscles and the adductor muscles. The gluteus muscles (maximus, medius, and minimus) extend, rotate, and abduct the thigh. The adductor muscles adduct the thigh and adduct and flex the leg. Flexion, extension, abduction, adduction, and inward and outward rotation from the hip are usually possible. Circumduction of the hip involves all the movements of the hip. Most hip movements involve movement of the pelvis as well.

Movements of the feet and toes are also important. The ankle is a hinged joint that permits plantar flexion and dorsiflexion. Inversion and eversion of the feet take place in the gliding joints. The joints of the toes permit flexion, extension, abduction, and adduction.

Normally the vertebral joints permit flexion, extension, lateral flexion, and rotation of the cervical spine and trunk. The

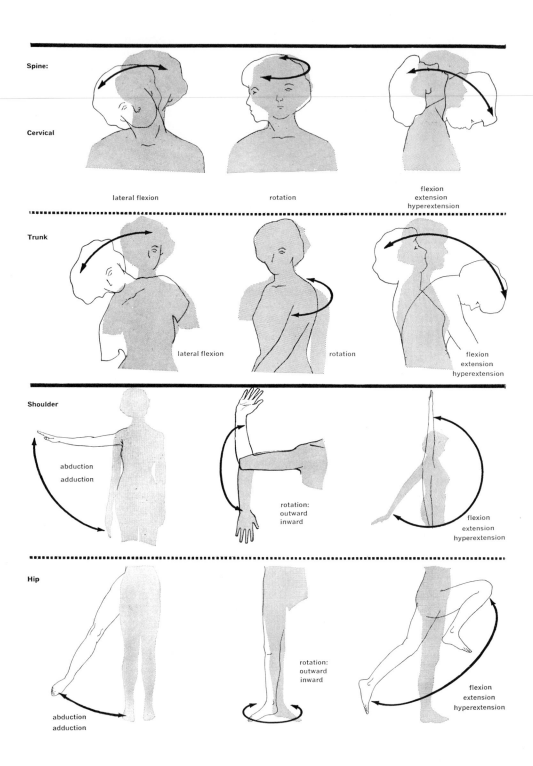

Spine:

Cervical

lateral flexion   rotation   flexion
extension
hyperextension

Trunk

lateral flexion   rotation   flexion
extension
hyperextension

Shoulder

abduction
adduction   rotation:
outward
inward   flexion
extension
hyperextension

Hip

rotation:
outward
inward   flexion
extension
hyperextension

abduction
adduction

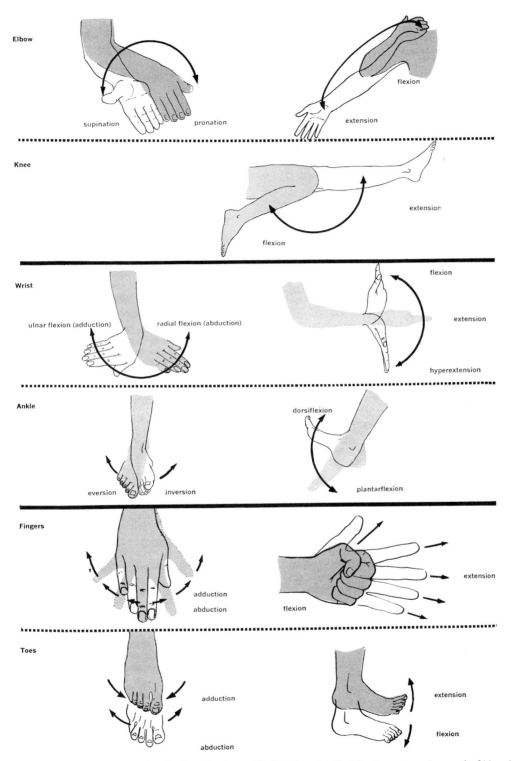

From Kelly, M. M.: Exercises for Bedfast Patients. © October, 1966, The American Journal of Nursing Company. Reproduced with permission from The American Journal of Nursing, Vol. 66, No. 10.

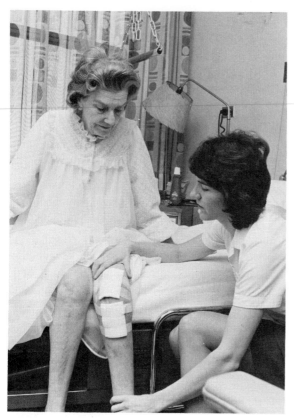

Regaining movement in an injured joint requires gradually increasing exercise.

rectus abdominus, the external and internal oblique muscles, and the sacrospinal muscle are involved in these movements.

The degree to which people can tolerate exercise varies considerably. A patient should avoid fatigue and pain while exercising. Joints need to be exercised to their full range of motion, but the nurse should not force movement when it is painful to the patient or when she meets resistance.

Exercises in Preparation for Walking. Everything should be done to help the patient to maintain strength and tone in muscles that are needed for walking, or to regain these if they have deteriorated owing to illness. Patients who may have to use a walker, crutches, or a cane need to gain additional strength in their hand, arm, and shoulder muscles because much of the weight of their body must be supported by these muscles when using such aids. All patients need their leg and abdominal muscles strengthened in preparation for

walking. If active isotonic exercises are not contraindicated, the patient should be encouraged to do these while in bed.

Active exercises for patients requiring additional strength in their arms and shoulders in preparation for crutch or walker-assisted ambulation include push-ups (lying on the abdomen with the hands under the shoulders and pushing the head and upper half of the trunk up, taking the weight on the hands), and sit-ups (pulling oneself to a sitting position from lying down). A trapeze supported from an overbed frame is often used to assist patients to pull themselves to a sitting position if they are unable to manage it themselves. Another exercise for strengthening hand, arm, and shoulder muscles is to have the patient lie flat in bed, reach his arms up to grasp the head of the bed, and pull himself up in the bed.

If isotonic exercises are not feasible, isometric exercises can be used. It is possible to develop almost as full an extent of muscular tension in muscles by exercising them isometrically as isotonically. In isometric exercises the individual alternately tenses and relaxes muscles without moving joints. The muscle does not move outwardly, and no work is performed. Hence, this type of exercise is useful for people who do not have sufficient strength to do active range of motion exercises, or it can supplement them. Isometric exercises are also useful for patients in whom active isotonic exercise is contraindicated.

For increasing muscular strength, even a one second maximal contraction done isometrically once a day is effective. Muscle strength can be increased more quickly if the maximal contractions are increased to five per day, each lasting six seconds.

[These are] particularly useful for maintaining the tone of postural muscles of the buttocks, abdomen, and thighs. The patient can set the quadriceps, gluteal, and abdominal muscles separately, or he may set all of them simultaneously by lying supine with legs extended and hands at his sides, then lifting his buttocks off the bed, bearing his weight on shoulders and heels.[5]

[5] Brower and Hicks, op. cit., p. 1252.

Exercises for the Ambulatory. All ambulatory patients should be encouraged to participate in a regular exercise program, unless there are health reasons which preclude this. Exercises are planned to suit each person's needs and his motor abilities, taking into consideration his age, sex, degree of mobility, and limitations imposed by chronic or current health problems, and his interests. The individual who starts on an exercise program should always have a complete physical examination first to make sure there are no contraindications to exercise, as well as to find out if there are any limitations on the type or amount of exercise that should be planned.

The program may planned for the patient to do either at home or outside the home. Many community organizations offer a graded series of exercise classes to assist people in maintaining or regaining optimal physical fitness. Exercises for the elderly have become a regular feature of many of these programs. Exercise programs can be found to accommodate all age groups and to cater to virtually all interests, such as hiking, swimming, and other sports, as well as simple calisthenics.

NURSING INTERVENTIONS FOR HELPING PATIENTS TO MOVE

A knowledge of the principles of body movement and skill in their application are important to both the patient and the nurse. Kinesiology is the science of human motion; its beginnings as a science date back to Aristotle, who is considered the father of kinesiology.

It is important that the nurse use her body in a way which not only avoids muscle strain but also uses energy efficiently. The practice of good body mechanics is not restricted to nursing care; it is integral to healthy living for all people. In health and in illness, good posture and efficient body movement are essential both therapeutically and aesthetically.

Once a person has a knowledge of the principles underlying body mechanics, he should put them into practice in order to establish good habit patterns of body movement. As these patterns are established, movements become smooth and place a minimum of strain upon the body muscles. The nurse will find that she can help patients to move more easily, and the patient will be more comfortable.

PRINCIPLES UNDERLYING BODY MECHANICS

1. Large muscles fatigue less quickly than small muscles.
2. Muscles are always in slight contraction.
3. The stability of an object is always greater when there is a wide base of support and a low center of gravity, and when the line of gravity is perpendicular to the ground and falls within the base of support.
4. The amount of effort required to move a body depends upon the resistance of the body as well as on the gravitational pull.
5. The force required to maintain body balance is greatest when the line of gravity is farthest from the center of the base of support.
6. Changes in activity and position help to maintain muscle tone and avoid fatigue.
7. The friction between an object and the surface on which the object is moved affects the amount of work needed to move the object.
8. Pulling or sliding an object requires less effort than lifting it, because lifting necessitates moving against the force of gravity.
9. Using one's own weight to counteract a patient's weight requires less energy in movement.

Understanding of these principles, and of their application in the correct use of the nurse's muscular energy and weight, will contribute greatly to ease of nurse-patient physical interactions and reduce the likelihood of injury to either party.

1. *Large muscles fatigue less quickly than small muscles.* Using a group of large muscles places less strain on the body than using a group of smaller muscles or a single muscle. For example, less strain results when a heavy object is raised by flexing the knees rather than by bending from the waist. The former movement utilizes the large gluteal and femoral muscles, whereas the latter utilizes the smaller muscles such as the sacrospinal muscle of the back.

2. *Muscles are always in slight contraction.* This condition is called muscle tone. If the nurse prepares her muscles for action prior to activity, she will protect her ligaments and muscles from strain and injury. For example, she will be better prepared to lift a heavy object if she first contracts the muscles of her abdomen and pelvis and the gluteal muscles of the buttocks.

3. *The stability of an object is greater when there is a wide base of support and a low center of gravity, and when the line of gravity is perpendicular to the ground and falls within the base of support.* In her motions the nurse can assume a broad stance and bend her knees rather than bend at the waist. This practice keeps the vertical line of her center of gravity within her base of support, thus providing her with greater stability. For example, in helping a patient to move, the nurse's position is more stable and she is therefore better able to maintain her balance if she stands with her feet apart and bends her body at the knees rather than at the waist.

4. *The amount of effort required to move a body depends upon the resistance of the body as well as the gravitational pull.* By utilizing the pull of gravity rather than working against it, the nurse can reduce the amount of effort required in movement. For example, it is easier to lift a patient up in bed when he is lying flat and his center of gravity has been shifted toward the foot of the bed than it is when he is n a sitting position in which

the resistance of the body to movement is much greater.

5. *The force required to maintain body balance is greatest when the line of gravity is farthest from the center of the base of support.* Therefore, the person who holds a weight close to his body uses less effort than the person who holds the weight in his extended arms. For example, when moving a patient from a bed to a stretcher, it is easier for the lifters if they hold the patient's body close to their own.

6. *Changes in activity and position help to maintain muscle tone and avoid fatigue.* If a person changes his position even slightly while he is carrying out a task, and if he changes his activity from time to time, he will maintain better muscle tone and avoid undue fatigue.

7. *The friction between an object and the surface upon which the object is moved affects the amount of work needed to move the object.* Friction is a force that opposes motion. The smoothest surfaces create the least friction; consequently less energy is needed to move objects on smooth surfaces. The nurse can apply this principle when a patient changes his position in bed by providing a smooth foundation upon which the patient can move.

8. *Pulling or sliding an object requires less effort than lifting it, because lifting necessitates moving against the force of gravity.* If, for example, the nurse lowers the head of a patient's bed before she helps him to move up in the bed, less effort is required than when the head of the bed is raised.

9. *Using one's own weight to counteract a patient's weight requires less energy in movement.* If a nurse uses her own weight to pull or push a patient, her weight increases the force applied to the movement.

Lifting the Patient and Helping Him to Move

Often the nurse is called upon to help a patient to move or to change his position. Gentle, sure motion on the nurse's part, based on her knowledge of body mechanics, not only helps patients to move easily but also gives them a sense of confidence in the nurse. Some patients, unable to move by themselves, are completely dependent upon the nurse for their changes in position and their exercise. The nurse is frequently called on to assist her patients to make the movements described in this section. It should be noted that there are various methods of performing each movement. The techniques and illustrations used here present one way of doing them.

Helping the Patient Move to the Side of the Bed. The nurse may be called upon to help a patient who is lying on his back (dorsal recumbent position) to move to the side of the bed, as when she is planning to change his surgical dressing. To lift the patient would require a great deal of effort upon the nurse's part, possibly putting unnecessary strain on her muscles as well as upon the patient. The patient can be helped to move more easily, however, if the nurse uses her own weight as a force to counteract the patient's weight and her arms to connect her with the patient so that they move as one.

1. The nurse stands facing the patient at the side of the bed toward which she wishes the patient to move.

2. She assumes a broad stance with one leg forward of the other and with her knees and hips flexed in order to bring her arms to the level of the bed.

3. The nurse places one arm under the shoulders and neck of the patient and the other arm under the small of the patient's back.

4. She shifts her body weight from her front foot to her back foot as she rocks backward to a crouched position, bringing

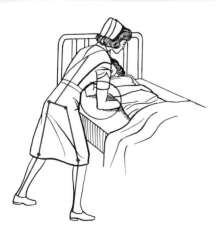

the patient toward her to the side of the bed. The nurse's hips come downward as she rocks backward. The patient should be pulled rather than lifted in this procedure.

5. The nurse then moves the middle section of the patient in the same manner by placing one arm under the small of the patient's back and one arm under the thighs. Then the patient's feet and the lower legs are moved with the same motion.

Care should be taken not to pull the patient off the side of the bed. If the patient is unable to move the arm that is nearer the nurse, it should be placed across the patient's chest so that it will not hinder movement or be injured. In moving a patient in this manner, the nurse should feel no strain across her shoulders; it is her own weight that supplies the power to move the patient.

Raising the Shoulders of the Helpless Patient. Some patients are unable to raise their shoulders, even for a short time. When the nurse finds it necessary to raise such a patient, as when changing the pillows, she should proceed as follows:

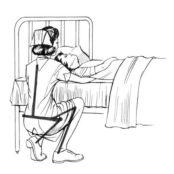

1. The nurse stands at the side of the bed and faces the patient's head. She assumes a wide stance with her foot that is next to the bed behind the other foot.

2. She passes her arm that is farther from the patient over the patient's near shoulder, and rests her hand between the patient's shoulder blades.

3. In order to raise the patient the nurse rocks backward, shifting her weight from her forward foot to her rear foot, her hips coming straight down in this motion.

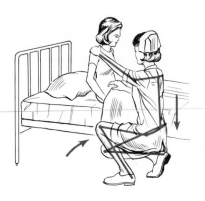

The nurse can either guide the patient with her free arm or use it for balance. Again it is the nurse's weight which counteracts the patient's weight.

Raising the Shoulders of the Semihelpless Patient. The semihelpless patient can move to some extent; however, he needs considerable support in most of his movements. In order to help the semihelpless patient raise his shoulders, the nurse uses her own arm as a lever and her elbow as the fulcrum.

1. The nurse stands at one side, facing the head of the patient's bed. Her foot next to the bed is to the rear and the other foot is forward. This position provides a wide base of support.

2. She bends her knees to bring her arm that is next to the bed down to a level with the surface of the bed.

3. With her elbow on the patient's bed the nurse grasps the posterior aspect of the patient's arm above the elbow, and the patient grasps the nurse's arm in the same manner and pushes with the other hand.

4. The nurse then rocks backward, shifting her weight from her forward foot to her rear foot and bringing her hips

downward. Her elbow remains on the bed and acts as the fulcrum of the lever.

Moving the Helpless Patient Up in Bed. Helpless patients are best assisted to move up in bed by two persons rather than one; however, one nurse can help a patient to move up in bed by moving him diagonally toward the side of the bed. By moving the patient in sections and by using her own weight to counteract the patient's weight, the nurse can safely move the helpless patient up in bed. This is most easily done if the head of the bed is lowered; then the nurse is not working directly against the force of gravity.

1. The nurse stands at the side of the patient's bed and faces the far corner of the foot of the bed. She places one foot behind the other, assuming a broad stance.

2. She flexes her knees so that her arms are level with the bed and puts her arms under the patient. One arm is placed under the patient's head and shoulders, one arm under the small of his back.

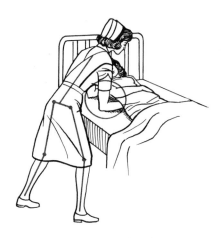

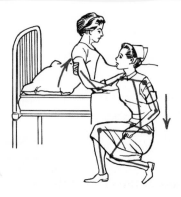

3. The nurse rocks forward, then shifts her weight from her forward foot to her rear foot, her hips coming downward. The patient will slide diagonally across the bed toward the head and side of the bed.

4. This is repeated for the trunk and legs of the patient. (See the procedure for moving the patient to the side of the bed.)

5. The nurse then goes to the other side of the bed and repeats steps 1 to 3. She continues this process until the patient is satisfactorily positioned.

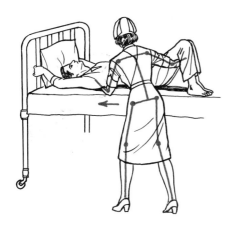

Moving the Semihelpless Patient Up in Bed. This movement is facilitated if the patient can assist by flexing his knees and pushing with his legs. In assisting the patient to make this movement, the nurse should take precautions that his head does not hit the top of the bed. Thus the nurse can lower the head of the bed and put the patient's pillow at the head of the bed, where it can act as a pad. Helping the patient move up in bed can be done by one or two nurses; in the latter instance one nurse stands at each side of the patient's bed. The procedure for one nurse is described here.

1. The patient flexes his knees, bringing his heels up toward his buttocks.

2. The nurse stands at the side of the bed, turned slightly toward the patient's head. One foot is a step in front of the other, the foot that is closer to the bed being to the rear; her feet are directed toward the head of the bed.

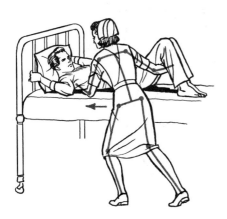

3. The nurse places one arm under the patient's shoulders and one arm under his thighs. Her knees are flexed to bring her arms to the level of the surface of the bed.

4. The patient places his chin on his chest and pushes with his feet as the nurse shifts her weight from her rear foot to her forward foot. By grasping the head of the bed with his hands, the patient can help pull his own weight.

Helping the Patient Turn on His Side. When a patient needs help in order to turn on his side, the nurse must take particular care that the patient does not fall off the bed. She can control his turning by placing her elbows on the bed as a brace to stop his roll.

1. The nurse stands on the side of the bed toward which the patient is to be turned. The patient places his far arm across his chest and his far leg over his near leg. The nurse checks that the patient's near arm is lateral to, and away from, his body so that he does not roll upon it.

2. The nurse stands opposite the patient's waist and faces the side of the bed with one foot a step in front of the other.

3. She places one hand on the patient's far shoulder and one hand on his far hip.

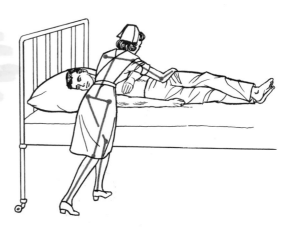

4. As the nurse shifts her weight from her forward leg to her rear leg, the patient is turned toward her. The nurse's hips come downward during this motion.

5. The patient is stopped by the nurse's elbows, which come to rest on the mattress at the edge of the bed.

Helping the Semihelpless Patient Raise the Buttocks. In this motion the nurse's arm acts as the lever, her elbow as the fulcrum.

1. The patient flexes her knees and brings her heels toward her buttocks. She is then ready to assist by pushing when the nurse tells her to do so.

2. The nurse faces the side of the bed and stands opposite the patient's buttocks. She assumes a broad stance.

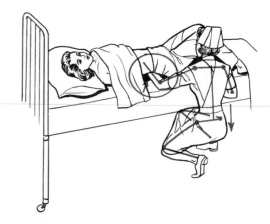

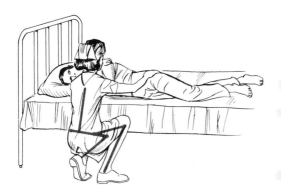

3. With her knees flexed to bring her arms to the level of the bed, the nurse places one hand under the sacral area of the patient, her elbow resting firmly on the foundation of the bed.

4. The patient is instructed to raise her hips.

5. As she does so, the nurse comes to a crouching position by bending her knees, while her arm acts as a lever to help support the patient's buttocks. The nurse's hips come straight down in this action. While the nurse supports the patient in this position she can use her free hand to place a bedpan under the patient or to massage the sacral area.

Assisting the Patient to a Sitting Position on the Side of the Bed. 1. The patient turns on her side toward the edge of the bed upon which she wishes to sit. (See the procedure for helping the patient turn on her side.)

2. After ensuring that the patient will not fall off the bed, the nurse raises the head of the bed.

3. Facing the far bottom corner of the bed, the nurse supports the shoulders of the patient with one arm, while with the other she helps the patient to extend her lower legs over the side of the bed. She assumes a broad stance, with her foot that is toward the bottom of the bed being to the rear of the other foot.

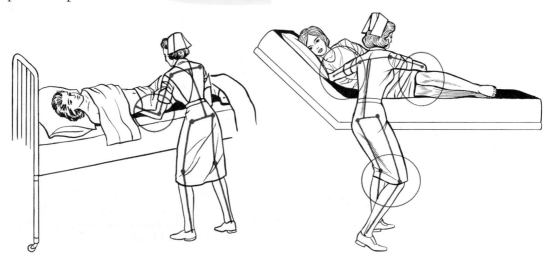

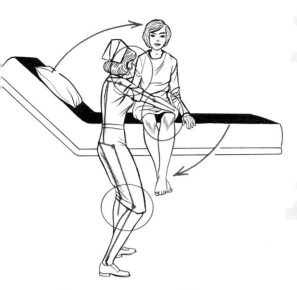

4. The patient is brought to a natural sitting position on the edge of the bed when the nurse, still supporting the patient's shoulders and legs, pivots her body in such a manner that the patient's lower legs are swung downward. The nurse's weight is shifted from her front leg to her rear leg.

Assisting the Patient to Get Out of Bed and Into a Chair. In this procedure the bed should be at a height from which the patient can step naturally to the floor. If the bed cannot be lowered sufficiently, the nurse should obtain a footstool for the patient. The footstool must be stable and have a surface upon which the patient is unlikely to slip. Also, it is advisable for the patient to wear low-heeled shoes rather than loose slippers. The shoes enable the patient to walk comfortably and provide support, but are not as likely to slip.

1. The patient assumes a sitting position on the edge of the bed and puts on shoes and dressing gown.

2. A chair is placed at the side of the bed with its back toward the foot of the bed.

3. The nurse stands facing the patient; her foot that is closer to the chair is a step in front of the other, to give her a wide base of support.

4. The patient places her hands upon the nurse's shoulders, and the nurse grasps the patient's waist.

5. The patient steps to the floor, and the nurse flexes her knees so that her forward knee is against the patient's knee. This prevents the patient's knee from bending involuntarily.

6. The nurse turns with the patient while maintaining her wide base of support. She bends her knees as the patient sits in the chair.

Lifting the Patient From a Bed to a Stretcher (Three Man Carry). To move a patient who must remain in the horizontal position from one place to another—for example, from a bed to a stretcher—three persons are usually needed. The tallest person should take the top third of the patient, because he probably has the longest reach and can most easily support the patient's head and shoulders. The second person supports the middle third of patient, usually the heaviest part. He will be helped if the first and third persons put their arms beside his. The shortest person supports the patient's legs.

Before the patient is moved, a stretcher is placed at right angles to the bed, with the head of the stretcher almost touching the foot of the bed. The stretcher wheels should be locked. To coordinate their movements, the three persons must work by counting off numbers; the person who takes the head of the patient calls the numbers.

1. The three who are to move the patient face the side of the patient's bed. Each assumes a broad stance, with his foot that is toward the stretcher being forward.

2. At the call of "one," the three bend their knees and place their arms under the patient. The first person places one arm under the neck and shoulders and the other arm under the small of the patient's back. The middle person places one arm under the small of the patient's back and the other arm under his hips. The person at the foot of the bed places one arm under the patient's hips and the other arm under the patient's legs.

3. At the call of "two" the patient is turned toward those who are lifting him. This is accomplished by rolling the patient toward the lifters. The patient's arms should not be allowed to dangle freely. The lifters hold him close to their bodies in order to avoid backstrain.

4. At the call of "three," they rise, step back (with the forward foot), and walk in unison to the stretcher.

5. At the call of "four," they bend their knees and rest their elbows on the stretcher.

6. At the call of "five," each lifter extends his arms so that the patient rolls to his back at the middle of the stretcher. Protection is needed at the far side of the stretcher to prevent the patient from rolling off.

7. At the call of "six," each lifter withdraws his arms.

In lifting the patient, the lifters should hold the patient close to their bodies. It is also important to lift and lower the patient with an easy, smooth motion in order not to jar or frighten him.

Some Devices for Assisting the Patient to Move

The Liftsheet. A liftsheet, or full sheet folded in half, placed under a helpless patient is a useful aid in moving him in many situations. The liftsheet should extend from the patient's arm level to the bottom of the buttocks.

At least two nurses are needed to move a patient by this means. One nurse stands at each side of the patient, grasps the liftsheet firmly near the patient, and moves the patient and liftsheet to the desired position—up in the bed or toward the side, for example.

To turn a patient on his side, his arms and legs are first positioned safely (see p. 311). The nurse then reaches over the patient, grasps the liftsheet on the far side, and pulls it toward her in such a way that the patient rolls on his side toward the nurse. Again the nurse should take precautions to ensure that the patient does not roll off the side of the bed.

Mechanical Devices. There are several mechanical devices available for moving a patient. One is the hydraulic lift, which can elevate a person and move him—from his bed to a stretcher, for example. Some models have heavy canvas supports which fit under the patient's buttocks and behind his back to provide support. These lifts can be used to assist a patient in and out of the bathtub and in and out of bed.

Ambulation

It is often necessary for patients to relearn to walk, often with the aid of crutches, braces, or canes. This is usually the responsibility of the physical therapy department, but there are some situations in which it is necessary for the nurse to assist the patient.

The patient may be learning to walk again following an extended period of bed rest. Preparing the patient for this task involves both psychological and physical measures. The nurse can help the patient to gain confidence in his ability to walk again. Often her encouragement and her faith in his ability can bolster his. If an appropriate exercise program has been maintained throughout his illness, the task is easier. Before attempting to stand, it is important for the patient to learn to maintain good trunk balance first in a sitting position, then in a standing position, before he attempts to walk. When he can maintain a standing position and feels confident in his balance, a few steps should be tried. Since good balance is essential and the patient must feel steady on his feet, it is important that he wear shoes with good support rather than slippers when he is standing or walking. The patient should not be allowed to become fatigued and should attempt only short distances at first. The nurse can help to promote the patient's feelings of self-confidence by helping him to set small goals for each day's activity and acknowledging his accomplishment of these goals.

Most patients who are learning to walk again following a lengthy period of bed rest require physical support when they are first starting. There are several ways the nurse can provide this support. The nurse can place the arm that is nearer the patient under his arm at the elbow and grasp his hand in hers. She synchronizes her steps with his, moving her inside foot forward at the same time as he moves his inside foot.

Another method is to grasp the patient's left hand in her left hand, and encircle his waist with her right hand. Again, the walking is synchronized to provide as wide a base of support as possible.

The patient can also be supported by being held at the waist from the rear. This can be accomplished with a towel folded lengthwise and encircling the patient's waist. There are also special belts designed for this purpose. Such support helps the patient to maintain his balance and keep his center of gravity within his base of support. If the patient requires more support than this, it is advisable for the nurse to have a second person to assist him.

In some situations, however, the nurse may have to assist a person with weakness on one side of his body to walk, with no second person to assist. A *safe* method is for the nurse to support the patient on his unaffected side. The patient puts his good arm around the nurse's shoulder and clasps her hand. The nurse puts her other arm around the patient's waist. Together, they step forward, the patient using his weak foot first and the nurse her opposite foot to provide as wide a base of support as possible.[6]

For hemiplegic gait training or ambulation training, however, the patient is encouraged to take some weight, and eventually as much weight as possible, on his affected side. During the rehabilitation phase, it is important that the nurse con-

sult with the physical therapist regarding the walking pattern being taught to the patient and the best method of assisting him.

Braces give support to a particularly weak leg. In the past braces were made of heavy material with sufficient rigidity to hold the limb in place and provide it with support. A new type of lightweight inflatable brace has been developed recently which should prove very useful for patients who need the legs supported for walking without the extra weight. There are also a variety of walkers available which provide support for a person while he is walking. When a patient uses a walker, much of his weight is borne by his hands and arms as he pushes the walker forward.

Some patients find it necessary to use crutches for a period of time. There are many kinds available: underarm, elbow extension, and Lofstrand crutches, for example. Sometimes the nurse measures a patient for crutches and helps him learn to walk with them. Several methods are used to measure a person for an underarm crutch. One method is to measure the distance from the patient's axilla to the heel of his foot while he is in bed. To this distance, 2 inches is added. A second method is to measure from the anterior

---

[6]Physiotherapy Department, Rehabilitation Unit, Royal Ottawa Hospital, 1975.

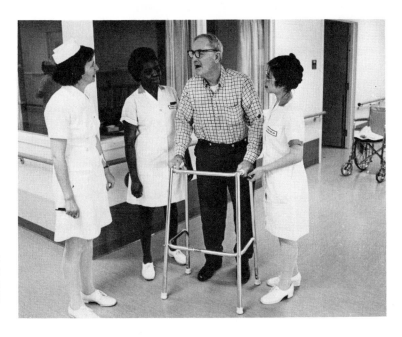

The use of a walker is part of the retraining program for many people whose mobility has been affected by illness.

fold of the axilla to a point 6 inches lateral to the heel. When crutches are of appropriate length, the hand bar permits slight flexion of the elbow, and the weight is borne by the hands and arms rather than at the axilla. The nerves in the axilla are not protected against pressure except by a layer of fat, which is compressible. If weight is borne on the axilla, then the pressure may result in nerve damage and possibly paralysis. For this reason the top of the crutch should be 2 inches below the axilla and should not be padded initially.

Gaits. There are seven basic crutch gaits:

TWO POINT CRUTCH GAIT. This gait has the following sequence: right crutch and left foot simultaneously; left crutch and right foot simultaneously.

THREE POINT CRUTCH GAIT. This gait has the following sequence: both crutches and the weaker limb; then the stronger limb.

FOUR POINT CRUTCH GAIT. This gait has the following sequence: right crutch, left foot, left crutch, right foot. This is a particularly safe gait because there are always three points of support on the floor at one time.

TRIPOD GAITS. There are two tripod gaits: in one, the patient puts the crutches forward simultaneously and then drags his body forward; in the other, he puts his crutches forward one at a time, and then drags his body forward.

SWING GAITS. There are two swing gaits: in one, the patient puts his crutches forward and then swings his body up to his crutches; in the other, he swings his body beyond them.

The advantage of possessing skill in more than one gait is twofold: the patient can use a slow or fast gait as he wishes and, since each gait requires a different combination of muscles, he can change gaits when he becomes fatigued.

Before a person uses crutches he would be wise to strengthen the muscles he will need, particularly the shoulder depressors (trapezius), triceps, and the latissimus dorsi muscles. These can be strengthened by simple exercises that the patient can carry out in bed, as mentioned earlier.

PLANNING AND EVALUATING SPECIFIC NURSING INTERVENTIONS

Nursing interventions are planned to suit each individual patient, his problems, and his needs. It is again helpful to set specific targets to be accomplished by nursing action and then to decide on the appropriate interventions to accomplish these objectives. The patient and his family should be involved in the establishment of expected outcomes and in the selection of the interventions to be used, and should participate in the implementation of exercise programs as much as possible. The nurse works closely with the physical therapist and the occupational therapist in planning appropriate exercises that are consistent with the physician's plan of care for the patient. The prevention of muscle deterioration and the maintenance and improvement of muscle strength and tone in patients whose mobility is limited require the intensive effort of all concerned.

The process of recovery for people who have lost partially or completely one or more of their motor abilities is often a long one. Short-term goals are therefore very important. The achievement of each small step of progress is something to work toward and provides the nurse, the patient, and his family with motivation to work towards further goals. The outcomes of nursing interventions, such as range of motion exercises, might include, for example, that the patient be able to put his arm or leg (or a smaller appendage, such as a hand or a foot) through a more complete range of motion and that he accomplish this feat daily (or twice a day). Specifics should be included as to what his range of motion was at the start and what the expected outcome will be at the end of a given period. The expected outcomes of passive exercises done by the nurse would be the prevention of contractures that could hinder joint mobility, such as in the wrist, the ankle, the shoulder, the knee, and so forth.

For the patient who needs help in moving, the expected outcomes would be related to the various activities and functional abilities. For example, helping the patient to turn might be related to maintaining the status of his skin, his respiratory functioning, or his circulatory status, and to the prevention of complications with regard to these abilities. Assisting the patient to use the bedpan or urinal would be related to the maintenance of adequate elimination.

For the patient who needs help in sitting up, or in learning to move from bed to chair and the reverse, or in learning to walk again, the nursing interventions are directly related to motor functioning and increasing the patient's independence in carrying out the activities of daily living. Again, outcomes should be established on a short-term basis, with explicit details as to what is to be accomplished in a given period of time. An example could be the patient's being able to pull himself up to a sitting position using a trapeze in bed, and doing it so many times a day. Or, the patient is able to sit or maintain himself in an upright position while sitting for gradually increasing specific periods of time.

It should be noted that the road to recovery is not always a smooth one. Patients need encouragement and support when temporary setbacks occur in their progress. A major nursing responsibility is providing the support the patient needs, both physically and psychologically.

If the expected outcomes of her nursing interventions have been sufficiently explicit, the process of evaluating the effectiveness of these becomes relatively simple. Have the expected outcomes been achieved? Is the patient's range of motion extended? Can he do more of the exercises himself? Does he carry out isometric exercises on his own the prescribed number of times as stated in the goals? Is he able to sustain the contraction for one second, or for the number of seconds specified as his target goal?

The nurse also keeps in mind the long-range goals of nursing action. Have unused muscles whose movement is not contraindicated been maintained in strength and tone? Has the process of degeneration been prevented in these muscles? Have contractures that could interfere with joint mobility been prevented? Has joint mobility been maintained? Have muscular strength and tone been improved? Has the patient regained independence in carrying out activities of daily living? Or is he making progress towards this? What progress has he made towards this goal? If the patient requires help in moving to carry out these activities, has he received this help when he needed it and in such a way as to enable him to maintain his other functional abilities? Is there optimal functioning of his other abilities?

GUIDE TO ASSESSING MOTOR FUNCTIONING ABILITIES	1. Is the patient able to walk normally? Or does he need aids for mobility, such as a cane, crutches, a walker, a wheelchair, another person, or a stretcher?
	2. Does he have limitations in mobility due to chronic health problems, as, for example, paralysis, weakness, difficulty of movement in one or more limbs and/or other parts of the body? Has he had an amputation?
	3. How does his present motor status compare with his usual status?
	4. Does he have any current health problems which may be interfering, or could interfere, with his motor functioning abilities? Or, has he had any recently?
	5. What is the patient's response to activity?
	6. Does the patient need help with raising his head and shoulders? With moving in bed? With turning? With sitting up? With using the bedpan or urinal? With standing? With transferring from the bed to a chair and the reverse? With walking?

7. What are the physician's diagnostic and therapeutic plans of care for this patient?
8. Have reports been received on diagnostic tests or examinations done on this patient? If so, how do these affect the planning of nursing care for this individual?
9. Have restrictions been placed on the patient's mobility? On exercises he can perform?
10. Is the physical therapist involved in helping this patient? The occupational therapist? What are their plans for the patient? How can you help with these plans?
11. Can the patient do these exercises himself?
12. Can the patient's family help the patient in carrying out exercise activities?

STUDY VOCABULARY

Abduction
Active exercise
Adduction
Basal metabolic rate
Circumduction
Embolus
Eversion
Extension
Flexion
Friction

Frontal plane
Gliding
Gravity
Hemiplegic
Hyperextension
Insertion (muscle)
Isometric exercise
Isotonic exercise
Kinesiology
Origin (muscle)

Paraplegic
Passive exercise
Quadriplegic
Pronation
Rotation
Sagittal plane
Supination
Thrombosis
Transverse plane
Transversion

STUDY SITUATION

Mr. George Ellis, age 28, had his leg crushed in a logging accident three days ago. He works as a scaler for a large forest products company. Following surgery to repair the damaged tissues, the physician has applied an over-the-knee cast and put the leg in traction. He has ordered that Mr. Ellis remain in bed for an unspecified period of time. He has told Mr. Ellis that when he is allowed up, he must learn to walk with crutches or use a wheelchair to get around in. Mr. Ellis is a healthy, active individual, and objects strongly to being confined to bed. He says he is not going to use a wheelchair if he can help it. He wants to know if there is anything he can do while in bed which will help him when he is allowed up from bed.

1. What information would you need to help you in planning Mr. Ellis's care?
2. What sources would you use to obtain this information?
3. What problems might Mr. Ellis have in addition to his mobility?
4. What other health professionals might be involved in Mr. Ellis's care?
5. What factors would you take into consideration in planning Mr. Ellis's care?
6. What exercises might Mr. Ellis do on his own to prevent the deterioration of muscular strength and tone? To prepare himself for using crutches?
7. What other help would Mr. Ellis require in carrying out daily living activities?

SUGGESTED READINGS

Beck, R.: Helping to Make His Last Dream a Reality. *Journal of Gerontological Nursing, 1*:10–12, May/June 1975.

Ciuca, R., et al.: Range of Motion Exercises, Active and Passive: A Handbook. *Nursing '73, 3*:25–37, December 1973.

Cluclasure, D. F.: Medical Benefits From Space Research. *American Journal of Nursing, 74*:275–278, February 1974.

Foss, G.: Body Mechanics: Use Your Head and Save Your Back. *Nursing '73, 3*:25–32, May 1973.

Germain, C. P.: Exercise Makes the Heart Grow Stronger. *American Journal of Nursing, 72*:2169–2173, December 1972.

Griffin, W., et al.: Group Exercise for Patients With Limited Motion. *American Journal of Nursing, 71*:1742–1743, September 1971.

How to Negotiate the Ups and Downs, Ins and Outs of Body Alignment. *Nursing '74, 4*:46–51, October 1974.

Jordan, H. S., and M. A. Kavchak: Transfer Techniques. *Nursing '73, 3*:19, March 1973.

Kamenetz, H. L.: Exercises for the Elderly. *American Journal of Nursing, 72*:1401, August 1972.

Kern, F. C., et al.: Transfer Techniques. *Nursing '72, 2*:25–28, July 1972.

Krafchik, H.: Fitness for 39¢. *Canadian Nurse, 71*:45, August 1975.

Ranalls, J.: Crutches and Walkers. *Nursing '72, 2*:21–24, December 1972.

Wilson, R. L.: An Introduction to Yoga. *American Journal of Nursing, 76*:261–263, February 1976.

Works, R. F.: Hints on Lifting and Pulling. *American Journal of Nursing, 72*:260–261, February 1972.

Young, Sr. C.: Exercise: How to Use It to Decrease Complications in Immobilized Patients. *Nursing '75, 5*:81–82, March 1975.

18 COMFORT, REST, AND SLEEP NEEDS

The nurse should be able to:

Define the terms "comfort," "rest," and "sleep"

Discuss the importance of comfort, rest, and sleep to the health and well-being of the individual

Describe the characteristics of the five stages of sleep

Discuss normal patterns of rest and sleep

Explain the relationship between illness and sleep disturbances

Identify factors interfering with a patient's comfort, rest, and sleep

Identify signs of sleep deprivation in an individual

Identify common sleep problems

Determine priorities for nursing actions related to the patient's comfort, rest, and sleep

Apply relevant principles in selecting and implementing appropriate interventions to help patients with comfort, rest, or sleep problems

Evaluate the effectiveness of nursing interventions to promote the patient's comfort, rest, and sleep

320

COMFORT, REST, AND SLEEP NEEDS 18

INTRODUCTION

Comfort has been defined as "a state of ease or well-being."[1] When a person is comfortable, he is at ease with himself and with his environment. Rest is synonymous with repose or relaxation and implies freedom from emotional tension as well as physical discomfort. Sleep is a period of decreased mental alertness and lessened physical activity which is a part of the rhythmical daily pattern of all living creatures.

Discomfort can result from stimuli of both psychosocial and physical origin. A person who is afraid or worried is uncomfortable, as is one who is cold or in pain.

There are innumerable causes of emotional discomfort; many have been mentioned earlier in this text. For example, the newly admitted hospital patient is subjected to the stresses that accompany going into any strange environment. The ill person often fears pain, death, and disability, and he worries about his ability to cope with forthcoming stresses. Neglect by the nursing staff or care by an unyielding, unconcerned nurse also contributes to a patient's discomfort. The patient looks to the nurse for understanding and support in order to attain some degree of psychological comfort.

Physical discomforts can cause mental distress and interfere with a person's psychosocial equilibrium. Pain, nausea, heat, and even an untidy environment are stimuli which the patient finds uncomfortable and sometimes unbearable. By the selection of appropriate interventions, the nurse can prevent the development of many situations which could be a source of discomfort. Many discomforts can be alleviated if they do occur. The nurse should, therefore, be alert to the earliest signs of discomfort in a patient and aware of interventions that can be used to relieve discomfort or prevent it from increasing.

The nurse has many resources at her disposal to relieve a patient's discomfort, but it is only through a systematic approach to the problem that the effective measure or measures can be selected. It is important that the nurse record her observations of the results of her nursing interventions in order that other members of the health team may be made aware of her findings and can avail themselves of this knowledge for the patient's benefit. For example, some people like the head of the bed elevated to a certain degree; others like it flat. If there are no therapeutic reasons to the contrary, the bed should be maintained at the elevation the patient finds most comfortable.

Interventions vary in their effect from one person to another. Consequently the nurse should find the measure or combination of measures which is most effective for a specific patient.

Rest does not necessarily mean inactivity. People often find a change of activity as relaxing as sitting or lying down to rest. The person who has a sedentary job, for example, may find that physical activity in the form of a leisurely walk, skating, or swimming is relaxing and restful for him. The person who has been physically active all day may obtain his rest in watching television, reading, playing cards, or just sitting down and talking with his family or friends. People who are ill also find

---

[1] The American Heritage Dictionary of the English Language. New College Edition. Boston, Houghton Mifflin Company, 1976.

these same activities sometimes more restful than lying in bed with nothing to do.

Freedom from anxiety is important in rest, as it is in comfort. This subject was discussed in Chapter 12, so we will not go into it further here.

Sleep is an essential part of our lives and takes up approximately one-third of our time. All body cells need a period of inactivity to refresh and renew themselves. It has been found, too, that sleep is essential for growth and the repair of body tissue. The secretion of the human growth hormone is increased during sleep, as is that of some other hormones (for example, testosterone in early puberty).[2]

Whether everyone needs the full recommended eight hours of sleep a night is currently under debate. A recent survey by Hartmann and others at the Sleep and Dream Laboratory in the United States would seem to cast some doubt on this. These investigators found that people who usually sleep less than six hours a night appeared better able to cope with their daily activities than those who slept for long periods. The "short-sleepers" were generally efficient, energetic people who worked hard, felt good in the morning, and were socially adept, decisive people who were happy with their lives and their work. "Long sleepers," that is, those who slept nine hours or more tended to be worriers. They also had many aches and pains, discomforts, and concerns, and were not very sure of themselves, their careers, or their lifestyles.[3]

NORMAL FUNCTIONING IN REGARD TO SLEEP AND REST

Human bodily functions follow a pattern over the course of a 24 hour period that has been called a "circadian rhythm," a term derived from two Latin words: *circa*, meaning "about," and *dies*, meaning "day." It is as if the human body had been constructed with a biological time clock that regulates its activities. Body temperature, pulse rate, and blood pressure all fluctuate during the course of a day, usually being lowest during the early morning hours. The circadian rhythm varies in different individuals. Some people awaken bright and alert in the morning; others do not begin to function at their best until 9 or 10 o'clock. It is believed that this is due to temporal differences in the low point of an individual's temperature. People whose lowest body temperature occurs late in their sleep period find it difficult to get up in the morning and take longer to "get going." These are the ones who are irritable and cross, or uncommunicative, until after their legendary first cup of coffee. In general reaction time for most people, however, is slower in the early morning than later in the day. Efficiency peaks about 11 A.M. when body temperature is usually approaching its highest.

Our sleep and wakefulness periods occur in a regular cyclical fashion. The average healthy adult sleeps about seven hours a night. The amount of sleep needed decreases with age. Newborn infants usually sleep about 20 of the 24 hours. This is gradually decreased until the individual reaches adulthood, when it levels off and remains fairly steady until old age. Teenagers seem to require longer periods of sleep, which is possibly related to their growth needs. People over the age of 65 years generally sleep less than younger adults, and they usually have frequent periods of wakefulness during the night.[4]

The human "biological clock" is made up of hours of approximately 90 minutes in length. Infants are believed to have a biological hour of 60 minutes. Elephants, if you are interested, are said to have a biological hour of 120 minutes.

Stages of Sleep

Sleep occurs in 90 minute cycles in the human being. There are usually four to six 90 minute cycles in a person's normal

---

[2]Sleep (Editorial). *Lancet*, 1:963, April 26, 1975.
[3]James Quig: Morning Becomes Who? *The Canadian*, Dec. 20, 1975.

[4]Frederick H. Lowy: Recent Sleep and Dream Research: Clinical Implications. *Canadian Medical Association Journal*, 102:1069–1077, May 1970.

sleep time. In addition, there are believed to be five stages in each 90 minute sleep cycle. These stages have been identified from readings on an electroencephalogram (EEG), which provides a graphic representation of the electrical waves emanating from the brain.

As an individual is dropping off to sleep, he begins to feel relaxed and drowsy. His vital signs, such as heart and pulse rate, become slower, and his body temperature becomes lower. Alpha waves begin to form on the EEG. As he enters the first stage of sleep, the individual may experience a sudden jerk.

In *Stage 1 sleep*, the vital signs become even slower and the muscles more relaxed. The EEG reading becomes very flat. At this point, however, the individual is easily aroused.

He becomes a little harder to waken as he enters *Stage 2 sleep*. Some activity appears on the EEG and the individual can still be aroused fairly easily, although he is in a more completely relaxed state.

A person in *Stage 3 sleep* is difficult to rouse. His blood pressure and body temperature have dropped and the EEG waves appear larger and slower.

As the individual enters *Stage 4 sleep*, delta waves begin to appear on the EEG. The person is completely relaxed and may not move. It is extremely difficult to awaken a person in this stage of sleep. It is believed that it is during this stage that the increase in release of the hormone regulating growth and promoting tissue healing occurs. Bedwetting and sleepwalking are most likely to occur during this stage.

After the individual has completed Stage 4, it is thought that he retraces the cycle back to Stage 2 and then enters REM sleep, that is, *Stage 5*. REM sleep is a light sleep; this is the time when dreaming occurs. Vital signs fluctuate and the eyes move rapidly back and forth, which is the reason for the name given to this stage (rapid eye movement or REM for short). There is, however, increased muscular relaxation, particularly in the face and neck. The EEG reading is similar to that of a person in a waking state in deep concentration. During this stage adrenal hormones are released into the blood stream in spurts; these affect vitality, fa-

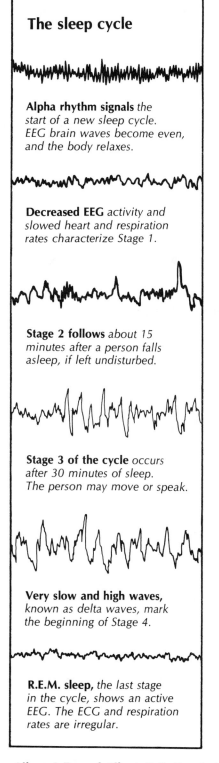

The sleep cycle

Alpha rhythm signals *the start of a new sleep cycle. EEG brain waves become even, and the body relaxes.*

Decreased EEG *activity and slowed heart and respiration rates characterize Stage 1.*

Stage 2 follows *about 15 minutes after a person falls asleep, if left undisturbed.*

Stage 3 of the cycle *occurs after 30 minutes of sleep. The person may move or speak.*

Very slow and high waves, *known as delta waves, mark the beginning of Stage 4.*

R.E.M. sleep, *the last stage in the cycle, shows an active EEG. The ECG and respiration rates are irregular.*

From Albert, I. B., and Albert, S. E.: Penetrating the mysteries of Sleep and Sleep Disorders. RN, 37:36–39, August, 1974, p. 37.

tigue, metabolism, and the ability to resist infection. They also influence the transmission of nerve impulses. Dreams, which occur during this stage, are believed to promote the psychological integration of daily activities.

With the completion of the REM stage, approximately 90 minutes after falling asleep, the individual recommences the cycle at Stage 2, follows the sequence to Stage 4, returns to Stage 2, and experiences the REM stage. In the final cycle, the individual continues beyond REM to Stage 1, and the individual wakens.

During the first few hours of sleep, the individual will spend more time in Stage 4 than in later cycles, and the length of the REM stage increases toward morning. Hormonal activity also increases toward morning.

Sleep Deprivation

Sleep deprivation has profound effects on an individual's functioning abilities, whether he is in good or ill health. A person deprived of sleep is likely to appear irritable, nervous, or anxious, or he may be apathetic. His thought processes may be impaired, and often he will not respond appropriately to stimuli. Minor troubles may become major problems. His sensory perception may be distorted and he may experience delusions or even hallucinations. It is believed that "after 48 hours of sleep loss, the body produces a stress chemical belonging to the indole group and related in structure to lysergic acid diethylamide—LSD-25. This may account for the behavioral changes."[5]

Deprivation of REM sleep can be especially disturbing for the individual. The adrenal hormones enter the blood stream but not at the proper biological time, causing the person to feel depressed and fatigued, and to have poor powers of concentration. It has been shown that when a person experiences gross deprivation of REM sleep, his body will try to catch up and he may enter the REM stage almost

immediately after falling asleep instead of following the stages as they normally occur.

Deprivation of Stage 4 sleep results in a decrease of the growth hormone in the blood stream and will cause the individual to feel tired, depressed, and generally unwell. As this hormone promotes tissue healing, deprivation of Stage 4 sleep can be particularly harmful to persons recovering from illness or injury.

In some instances, it is thought beneficial to depress REM sleep, as in the case of persons suffering from certain heart conditions or peptic ulcers, since most nocturnal attacks occur during the REM stage of sleep.

FACTORS AFFECTING COMFORT, REST, AND SLEEP

Age, as we have discussed, is a major factor to consider in assessing the adequacy of an individual's sleep and rest. Growing persons require more sleep than others. Expectant mothers usually find that they are drowsy and require a great deal of sleep, particularly during the first and last trimesters of pregnancy. During the last few weeks, however, the enlargement of the abdomen often makes it difficult for them to find a comfortable position in which to rest.

Most people have a bedtime ritual which forms part of their sleep habits. It has been reported that a substantial proportion of adult Canadians sit up to watch the 11 P.M. (11:30 in Newfoundland) national news on television and this is one of their nightly rituals. Many people enjoy a light snack before going to bed. Some like a cup of coffee or tea and find that, for them, it does not interfere with getting to sleep. For many people, a warm bath or shower is part of their nightly ritual. Each person has his own habits in regard to going to bed and getting ready for sleep. Most people also have a particular position they find most comfortable for sleeping. Some like to curl up in a ball; some are "tummy" sleepers; still others prefer a back-lying position.

Interference with these bedtime habits is likely to cause a disturbance in sleep

---

[5]Barbara Long: Sleep. *American Journal of Nursing,* 69:1896, September 1969.

patterns. People who are in a strange environment often find it hard to get to sleep the first night or so. A major change in habit patterns can disturb all body functions, as we mentioned in Chapter 2 in connection with the stress of change. Nurses in the course of their work frequently have to work evening or night shifts, and this disturbs their normal circadian rhythm. It usually takes a few days to accustom oneself to sleeping in the daytime and having one's first meal late in the day. Other people who work shifts also have the same problems.

Excessive stimulation, that is, more excitement than one is usually accustomed to, will make it harder to get to sleep for most people, unless they are exhausted by the stimulation. A lack of sufficient exercise may be another reason some people find it difficult to sleep; the muscles are not tired enough. A person who is hungry often cannot rest. On the other hand, an excessive intake of food, particularly highly seasoned food that may cause problems in digestion, may also interfere with sleep. A larger than usual amount of fluid intake before retiring usually means that an individual has to get up during the night to relieve a distended bladder.

Noise and other disturbances when a person is asleep may arouse him and disturb the cyclical pattern of his sleep. If he is suddenly awakened from deep sleep, he is likely to be confused and disoriented, a condition that has been described in the literature as "sleep drunkenness." It appears to be most pronounced in children and in people with sleep disorders.[6]

Many of the sources of excessive sensory stimulation mentioned in Chapter 13 are things hospitalized patients have described as disturbing to their comfort, rest, and sleep. In addition to these , environmental factors can be a problem, such as the warm temperatures of most hospital rooms, the hardness of most hospital pillows, the lights that are turned on, or forgotten to be turned off, the noise of nurses at the nursing station, and the sudden stillness after patients have been awakened by some noise.[7]

Other things that often disturb rest are medications that must be taken at night, and the early morning awakening that is still part of the routine in many hospitals, often followed by a long delay before breakfast is served.

Discomfort of any kind interferes with a person's ability to rest and to sleep. A number of causes of discomfort were discussed in the introduction to this chapter. Pain is, of course, always a deterrent to rest and sleep. Often, however, it is the minor irritations and discomforts that are most troublesome to patients. Discomfort may be physical or psychological. *Anxiety,* about big or little things, is probably the most common cause of inability to rest. A person lies awake and worries, and the worries magnify as sleep eludes him.

Illness and sleep problems go hand in hand. Illness disturbs the normal rhythm of sleep and wakefulness. People who are ill require more sleep because of their need for increased growth hormone to promote tissue repair, but as just stated, their normal sleep pattern is usually disturbed. Sleep deprivation, as we mentioned, can itself be a cause of illness. It is interesting to note that people who have been deprived of sufficient REM sleep usually spend more time in this stage when they are catching up on lost sleep. Apparently dreaming is a very necessary part of our lives.

Drugs will also distort sleep patterns. The reticular formation in the brain is belived to control sleep. Cerebral depressant drugs which induce sleep work in one or more of several ways:

1. They may depress the reticular formation so it no longer responds to stimuli

2. They may depress the response of the cerebral cortex to stimuli from the reticular formation

3. They may cause a specific reduction in the response to stimuli producing wakefulness (for example, anxiety, depression, or pain). Alcohol, for instance, has this

---

[6]Lowy, op. cit.

[7]Donna Allan Grant and Cynthia Klell: For Goodness' Sake, Let Your Patients Sleep. *Nursing '74,* 4:54–57, November 1974.

effect, as do many of the tranquilizing drugs.

Barbiturates are the most widely used drugs for people with sleep problems because they depress REM sleep in particular. A person who is taken off these drugs after having taken them for several days, or fails to take them, usually has a considerable increase in dream activity, and he may be convinced that he never slept at all. Barbiturates also depress parts of the brain that are responsible for inhibitory activity. Hence, they not infrequently have an excitatory effect, somewhat like alcohol. Older people are particularly susceptible to this reaction and may become confused and excited instead of going to sleep when they are given barbiturate sedatives.[8]

COMMON PROBLEMS

The most common sleep problems are insomnia (inability to get to sleep, or excessive wakefulness), hypersomnia (excessive sleeping), narcolepsy (sudden, irresistible sleep attacks), somnambulism (sleepwalking), enuresis (bedwetting), and night terrors.

Most people have problems in getting to sleep at some time or another, usually during periods of stress and anxiety; for many people this is a serious problem. *Insomnia* may be symptomatic of illness, or may be caused by anxiety, nervous tension, habitual lifestyle patterns, or any one of a number of causes. People for whom bedtime was not a pleasant experience when they were children—going to bed may have been used as a form of punishment—may become insomniacs later in life. Insomnia is by far the most common of all sleep disturbances.

It is felt that people who have a tendency to *sleep excessively* may be using this as a defense mechanism to escape from anxieties or frustrations in the fulfillment of their basic needs. This, of course, is not always the case; a person who seems to require more than the average amount of sleep should always be referred to a physician for a complete medi-

cal examination to see if there are other reasons for the excessive sleeping.

Narcolepsy is a problem which affects a small but significant number of people. The irresistible sleep attack may last from 10 to 20 minutes. The person often has vivid dreams and may often be unable to move on awakening. Accidents are more common among narcoleptics than among the general population, as one might expect. People with this problem are usually prohibited from working with machinery or at occupations where their problem could be a safety hazard. They should also be under medical supervision.[9]

Sleepwalking is more common among men than women. It usually occurs during Stages 3 and 4 of the sleep cycle; hence people who are sleepwalking are usually confused and disoriented. Their safety needs to be protected (see Chapter 20).

Enuresis, or bedwetting, is a common problem in children and may occur in some adults. It is generally found more frequently in males and in emotionally disturbed children. Some reports indicate that enuresis is more prevalent among children in low socioeconomic groups than in higher ones. It is believed to be caused in many cases by immaturity of the bladder, and many children just "grow out of it." Enuresis should, however, always receive medical attention because it may not be just a developmental problem, but could be a sign of other health problems.[10]

ASSESSING COMFORT, REST, AND SLEEP STATUS

Making sure that patients are comfortable, that they receive sufficient rest, and that they are able to sleep are among the nurse's most important responsibilities. In order to assess the individual's status with regard to comfort, rest, and sleep, the nurse needs information about his usual sleep and rest patterns, specific sleep problems he may have, and the nature of

---

[8]Stephen E. Smith: Drugs and Sleep. *Nursing Times*, 67:1248–1249, October 7, 1971.

[9]Ira B. Albert and Sharon E. Albert: Penetrating the mysteries of sleep and sleep disorders. *RN*, 37:36–39, August 1974.

[10]Lowy, op. cit.

any health problems that may be causing alterations in his sleep patterns.

She also needs to be aware of any restrictions that have been placed on his mobility. Is he confined to bed, for example? Or is he restricted to a certain position in bed for therapeutic reasons or because of the nature of his illness? People with heart conditions and those with respiratory problems are usually most comfortable when sitting up in bed or in a semi-sitting position. This then would be best for them therapeutically. The person with a fracture may have to be flat on his back, as Mr. Jordan (Chapters 9–10) was, or he may have to have the injured appendage maintained in a specific position. The nature of the surgical intervention a patient has had often determines the position he must take in bed. Even an intravenous infusion limits the patient's position in bed.

The nurse also needs to know the physician's plan of care for the patient. She must be aware of the medications the patient is receiving, and the nature of the diagnostic and therapeutic measures planned for the patient. Anxiety is such a common cause of sleep and rest problems that the nurse needs to know if there are any particular worries he has in connection with his health, real or imagined health problems, and whether he has reasons for worry about these. It is helpful also to know of any other stresses which may be causing the patient anxiety (see Chapter 12).

Information about usual sleep patterns, chronic disorders, and the present comfort, rest, and sleep status of the patient are available to the nurse from the nursing history and the initial nursing clinical appraisal. The patient's record provides information about the nature of his current health problems, and the physician's plan of care. Reports of diagnostic tests will also be found there, as well as requests for consultation by specialists and their reports. Medication the patient is receiving will be listed on the doctor's order sheet; the nurse needs to be aware also of medications the patient may have been taking at home, since drugs may distort sleep patterns, as we discussed above.

The nurse supplements this information by talking with the patient and through her objective observations. Many people are aware of the sources of their discomfort, and, when given the opportunity, will make them known. The nurse who communicates her understanding of the patient's problems and who takes the time to listen to him can frequently identify specific sources of worry and discomfort. Then she can take steps to relieve them.

There are other avenues of expression besides the verbal ones, of course. The patient who is uncomfortable may appear restless, pale, or tense; he may perspire profusely or lie rigidly in bed. All in all, there are a multitude of ways of expressing discomfort, and the nurse needs to be aware of them and alert to their possible meanings.

The person who is unable to sleep may communicate this verbally to the nurse, but she must also watch for the signs of sleep deprivation in the patient, as previously described. Nurses make frequent rounds of patients when they are on the night tours of duty and they note patients who are having difficulty getting to sleep or are wakeful during the night. Nurses on the day staff always check the night nurse's report to see if their patients had disturbed sleep during the night. The nurse also observes patients during the day and evening shift to see if they are getting sufficient rest and the extra sleep needed in illness.

PRIORITIES FOR NURSING ACTION

All aspects of promoting comfort, rest, and sleep are priority items insofar as nursing action is concerned. Particularly with ill patients, in whom rest and sleep are essential components of their therapy, the nurse must do everything possible to ensure that factors causing the patient discomfort or interfering with his rest and sleep are eliminated, or minimized if they cannot be eliminated entirely. Factors which will increase comfort, and promote rest and sleep, should be well known to the nurse so that she can assess the relative merits of specific actions to help each particular patient. This aspect of nursing care is considered so important that, in some agencies, the nurses have developed "sleep care plans" for patients.[11] This would seem to be a good way of ensuring that a definite series of nursing activities are planned to help each patient obtain adequate sleep. Interventions that nurses have found helpful for a particular patient are communicated to others so that there is consistency in the approach used by all nursing personnel.

GOALS FOR NURSING ACTION

The principal goals of nursing action with regard to the patient's comfort, rest, and sleep status are:
1. To promote comfort
2. To prevent discomfort
3. To alleviate discomfort
4. To ensure that the patient has rest
5. To assist the patient to obtain an adequate amount of sleep to meet his requirements

NURSING INTERVENTIONS TO PROMOTE COMFORT, REST, AND SLEEP

There are innumerable nursing interventions which nurses have found helpful

[11] Grant and Klell, op. cit., pp. 54–57.

in making patients comfortable and promoting their rest and sleep. Every experienced nurse has a repertoire of interventions which she has tried with patients and can tell you those which she has found to be successful. The beginning nurse must learn these, and she will find older, more experienced nurses very good sources of information about comfort measures and aids to promoting rest and sleep for patients.

Some general considerations might prove helpful to the student; these will be given first, and then we will discuss specific nursing interventions.

General Considerations

People usually get to sleep more quickly and sleep better when their lifestyle permits regular habits for mealtimes, work or school hours, periods of relaxation, and bedtime hours. Adequate nutrition and adequate exercise are important in promoting restful sleep. People should be encouraged to pursue restful and relaxing activities prior to preparing themselves for sleep. Many people have found specific relaxing techniques helpful, as, for example, the relaxing exercises described in Chapter 12. Tea and coffee are

---

PRINCIPLES RELEVANT TO COMFORT, REST, AND SLEEP

In developing a plan of care for patients to ensure that they are comfortable and have sufficient rest and sleep, the nurse may find the following principles helpful:
1. Definite periods of sleep are an essential component of the circadian rhythm in human beings.
2. Adequate amounts of sleep are needed for optimal physical and psychosocial functioning of the individual.
3. Individual needs for sleep vary with age, growth patterns, health status, and individual differences.
4. Lack of sufficient sleep impairs a person's physical functioning, his mental alertness, and his social relationships.
5. Individual habits vary with regard to bedtime rituals.
6. Sleep patterns may be disturbed by changes in a person's normal daily living patterns, by social and emotional problems, by physical problems, and by minor irritations or discomforts, as well as by pain.
7. Sleep patterns are almost invariably disturbed by illness.

both stimulants and most people find it best to avoid these prior to bedtime. Almost everyone has an occasional sleepless night. If the sleeplessness continues, however, for more than one or two nights, one should consult a physician for a thorough investigation of the problem and assistance in resolving it.

The sick person finds his normal patterns of daily living disrupted. It is helpful to provide diversional activities during the day, if these are compatible with his health problem, so that he does not sleep too much in the daytime and find himself unable to sleep at night. Morning naps are considered to be more beneficial than afternoon ones, because they are a continuation of the light REM sleep, whereas if a person sleeps in the afternoon, it is often a heavy sleep from which he wakens feeling groggy.

If some of the usual bedtime rituals can be maintained for the patient, he will feel more secure and better able to rest. The dietary department should be alerted to his usual bedtime snack and, if he is used to having a bath or shower before retiring, he should be given opportunity to continue this practice if his condition permits.

Patients should be offered a bedpan or a urinal if they are unable to go to the bathroom themselves, or should be assisted to the bathroom, so that they can wash their hands and face and clean their teeth, which are part of most people's bedtime rituals at home.

Some people are very fond of their own pillow, and may find hospital pillows hard. There would seem to be no reason why the patient could not have his own pillow if he so desired. A familiar object or routine helps to promote security; he may like the pillows arranged in a certain way; the head of the bed elevated to a certain angle; his position just so; his clock turned so he can see it during the night. It is small things like these that contribute so much to a person's comfort.

The nurse will find that it is worthwhile to spend a few extra minutes "settling" patients and attending to all the small details that are important to them. They will rest better and they are not so apt to need additional help later on in the evening or during the night.

Most people find a back massage soothing and an aid to sleep. For some, relaxing techniques are helpful. Besides the relaxing exercises, a number of techniques for learning to control tension in the muscles and bring relaxation have been developed. The nurse will find reference to some of these in articles listed in the suggested readings at the end of the chapter.

If hypnotic (sleep-inducing) drugs have been ordered, they should be given a few minutes before the lights are turned out. Analgesics to relieve pain should be administered sufficiently early for them to take effect before the hypnotic is given. This enhances the effects of the hypnotic.[12]

When the patient is "settled," and all details attended to, the lights should be dimmed. Noise should be kept to a minimum, and the patient not disturbed unless absolutely necessary.

The Bed of the Ill Person

The bed is especially important to most people who are ill. To the patient in the hospital, the bed may be the one thing that he feels is entirely his. Moreover, much of a patient's comfort is dependent upon the condition of his bed, particularly if he is in it for long periods of time. When a patient appears to be unduly particular about his bed, the nurse should remember that he may spend 24 hours of his day in it. To him a neat, clean, and wrinkle-free bed is necessary for comfort. Other patients who are exacting in regard to their beds and bed units may be clinging to a position from which they can control some aspect of their environment at a time when they believe that many decisions and activities are beyond their control. The ill patient's horizons often narrow, and matters about which he normally would have no concern become important.

Traditionally, the hospital bed is made in the morning after the patient's bath. When the bed is made, soiled linen is changed and the entire bed is aired and

[12]Grant and Klell, ibid.

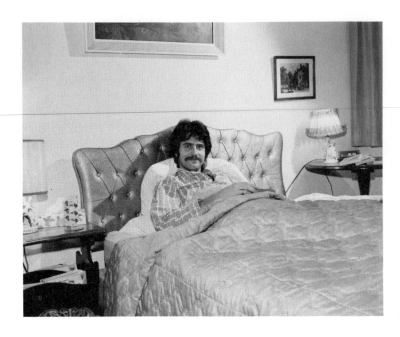

For the person who is ill at home or in the hospital, much of his comfort depends on the condition of his bed.

remade. It is equally important that linen be changed whenever it becomes damp or soiled. Soiled or wet linen predisposes a patient to skin breakdown and to infections.

Types of Beds According to Purpose. There are several ways of making a bed and each has its purpose. The *closed bed,* which is defined as an empty bed, is made after its occupant is discharged from the hospital. In a closed bed the spread extends over the bedclothes to the top of the mattress and the pillows are placed on top of the spread. In some hospitals the spread covers the pillows as well as the entire mattress.

The *open bed* refers to a bed that has been assigned to a patient. It may be prepared for a new patient, or may be made for any patient who is out of bed. The spread is folded back with the blankets, and the top sheet is turned back on the spread. One side of the top bedclothes is sometimes turned back so that the patient can get into the bed easily.

The *occupied bed,* as its name implies, refers to a bed which is occupied by a patient. Generally in this situation the person must remain in bed continuously, even while the nurse is making the bed. It is important for the nurse to learn to change linen and make a bed smoothly and quickly while the patient remains in it. Often the patient in an occupied bed is seriously ill and a great deal of activity is contraindicated.

The *anesthetic bed* or *recovery bed,* a variation of the basic hospital bed, is used for the patient immediately after surgery. Its purpose is to provide a clean area into which a patient can be easily moved. It is also important that the bed linen can be easily changed, with a minimum of disturbance to the patient. Frequently this type of bed is made in such a way that a part of it can be changed without remaking the entire bed; for example, a separate short sheet might be placed under the patient's head in such a manner that it can be removed when it is soiled without disturbing the rest of the bedclothes.

The *diagonal toe bed* is designed to expose the leg or foot of the patient and at the same time to provide warmth and adequate covering. A variation of the open bed, it is often used to air wet casts and for the patient whose leg is in traction. In the latter situation, ropes and pulleys extend from the patient's leg over the end of the bed, thus making it impossible to completely tuck the covers under the mattress at the foot of the bed.

Linen for the Hospital Bed. The linen required for the basic hospital bed comprises two sheets, two pillowcases, one plastic or rubber drawsheet (optional), one cotton drawsheet (optional), one or two blankets, and one spread. (Blankets are also optional.)

Cotton and rubber drawsheets have been traditionally used on the sick person's bed for two reasons: They are easier to change than the bottom sheet, and they protect the mattress. With the availability of plastic-covered mattresses, however, and increasing use of cotton mattress pads, (similar to the ones that are commonly used in the home), the routine use of drawsheets, both rubber (or plastic) and cotton, is disappearing. In many agencies the use of drawsheets is now reserved for the beds of patients who need them; they are no longer put on every bed.

When a plastic or rubber drawsheet is used, it is placed under a cotton drawsheet since the rubber (or plastic) retains heat and is uncomfortable. The drawsheet usually extends from above the patient's waist to his midthigh. Thus it can serve to absorb secretions in cases of urinary or fecal incontinence.

The cotton that is used for sheets, pillowcases, and drawsheets must be of a heavy weight that wears well in spite of strong pulling and frequent washing. Moreover, because linen is often washed in disinfectant solutions in order to kill microorganisms, a heavy weight is necessary to withstand the laundering.

The blankets that are used in hospitals and most other health agencies are frequently made of a loose cotton weave or a mixture of flannel and cotton. The blankets should be able to withstand frequent washings without damage or shrinkage. In many hospitals, the temperature of patients' rooms is such that no blankets are needed. However, blankets are sometimes necessary for warmth. Usually one or two blankets suffice. An extra blanket is sometimes used as a throw blanket over the spread. Blankets should never be used by more than one patient because of the danger of transferring microorganisms from one patient to another. The extra blanket can be rolled and stored at the foot of the bed, fanfolded down to the bottom of the bed, or put in the patient's closet until he wishes to use it. Elderly patients are often more sensitive to the cold than younger patients and require more covers for warmth.

Changing the Hospital Bed.   There are two basic procedures in changing a hospital bed: stripping the bed and making the bed. When the nurse is changing a bed, she should remember that microorganisms are present in the environment and be aware of the methods by which they are spread. The following principles should be kept in mind.

1. Microorganisms are present on the skin and in the general environment.

2. Some microorganisms are opportunists; that is, they can cause infections when conditions are favorable. For example, a break in the skin or mucous membrane of the patient may become a site of infection.

3. Patients are often less resistant to infections than healthy people because of the stress resulting from an existent disease process.

4. Microorganisms can be transferred from one person to another or from one place to another by air, by fomites, or by direct contact among people. A *fomite* is an inanimate object other than food which can harbor microorganisms. The nurse should therefore avoid holding soiled linen against her uniform, should never shake linen, and should wash her hands before going to another patient.

The use of good body mechanics is also important in making a bed. The principles that underlie body movements in helping the patient to move are equally applicable in bedmaking (see Chapter 17). Some guides based on these principles are useful here:

1. *Maintain good body alignment.* For example, the nurse stands facing the direction in which she is working and works in such a way that she does not twist her body.

2. *Use the large muscles of the body rather than the small muscles.* For example, flexing the knees in order to bring the body to a comfortable working level is preferable to bending at the waist. The former uses the large abdominal and gluteus muscles, whereas the latter puts strain upon the back muscles and shifts the center of gravity outside the base of support.

3. *Working smoothly and rhythmically is less fatiguing* because the muscles are alternately contracted and relaxed.

4. *Pushing or pulling requires less effort than lifting.*

5. *Using one's own weight to counteract the weight of an object decreases the effort and strain.* For example, if the nurse shifts her weight when she is pulling a mattress, it requires less effort than if she pulls the mattress with her arms. In addition, she places little strain upon her back and arm muscles.

The method of stripping and making a bed differs from place to place. Basically, however, every health agency wants the end product to be neat, clean, comfortable, and durable, and the bed changing process to be economical in use of time, equipment, and the patient's and nurse's energies. The following methods are suggested as guides to the student.

STRIPPING THE BED. Stripping a bed necessitates removing the linen and detachable equipment from the bed.

1. *Obtain the necessary equipment.* Generally all that is needed to strip a bed is a receptacle for soiled linen. Some hospitals provide a small hamper cart which the nurse takes to the door of the patient's room and into which she places the soiled linen. Care must be taken that microorganisms are not transferred by means of the hamper cart from one patient to another. Ideally, a linen hamper is provided for each patient.

If hampers are not provided, the nurse can tie the bedspread by its corners to the post at the foot of the bed to serve as a receptacle for soiled linen. Placing soiled linen on the floor facilitates the spread of microorganisms.

The nurse can avoid extra trips by taking several bundles of linen out to the linen hamper at one time. The nurse would also be wise to bring all her clean linen and clean equipment at one time in order to save time and effort. (See the procedures for making the open bed.)

2. *Remove the equipment from the bed.* First the nurse places the patient's bedside chair beside his bed. The back of the chair is in line with the foot of the bed and the front faces the head of the bed. Sufficient room is left between the chair and the bed for the nurse to pass in order to save her steps when she goes around the foot of the bed. If a chair is not available, a movable table may be used. The patient's call light, refuse bag, and so on are detached from the bed and placed on the bedside table. The patient's pillows are placed on the seat of the bedside chair; soiled pillowcases are put in the linen hamper.

3. *Remove the linen from the bed.* Starting at the head of the bed, the nurse loosens the top and bottom bedding from the mattress as she walks around the bed. When she returns to the first side of the bed, she grasps the spread at the center and near side and folds it to the bottom of the bed. She then picks up the spread at the center and lays it folded in quarters across the back of the bedside chair. This step is repeated for the blankets and the sheets, if they are to be reused. None of the linen should touch the floor.

If drawsheets are used they are folded with as little contact as possible and then picked up in the center and placed over the back of the chair. The reason for folding linen in such a manner is that it is ready to be placed back on the bed with a minimum of movement. Conservation of energy and movement is important to a nurse's efficiency and to the quality of her care. The remaining linen that is not to be reused is rolled into itself and discarded into the laundry hamper or linen bag.

4. *Turning the mattress.* After the linen has been removed from the bed, the mattress may be turned from side to side, if the nurse feels this is needed, and pulled to the head of the bed. By grasping the lugs at the side of the mattress and by using good body mechanics, the nurse can turn a mattress with little effort.

5. The nurse washes her hands when she has finished stripping the bed and before putting on the clean linen. The used linen and the mattress harbor microorganisms that should not be transferred to clean linen.

MAKING THE OPEN BED. Frequently patients who are in bed much of the day are able to get up while the nurse makes the bed. However, the decision regarding the patient's activity is usually the physician's, and the nurse should not help a patient out of bed unless there is a written order. Because a patient states that he feels well enough to get up is not

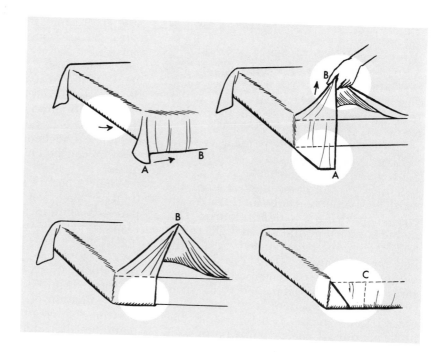

Mitering a corner.

sufficient reason for him to do so. On the other hand, even though the patient has permission to get up, his condition may change and the nurse may suggest that he stay in bed. In order to meet the needs of her patient, the nurse must continually use her judgment and her knowledge.

1. *Obtain the necessary equipment.* The nurse brings all the linen and equipment that she needs for making the bed in as few trips as possible. A few minutes' thought beforehand can often save time later. Clean linen for the bed and equipment for patient hygiene can often be collected at the same time. The linen is placed on the bedside chair in the order in which it is to be used.

2. *Make the bed.* The bottom sheet is placed on the bottom half of the mattress in such a way that the open edge is away from the center and the sheet just hangs over the bottom edge of the mattress. The sheet is then opened to the head of the bed and centered over the mattress. The sheet is tucked under the mattress at the head of the bed and the corner is mitered or squared on one side. The sheet is then tucked in smoothly along the sides. To miter the corner of a sheet the following steps are performed.

a. Tuck the sheet in securely under the mattress at the head of the bed.

b. Lift the sheet at A (see illustration above), and bring it along the side of the mattress.

c. Grasp the sheet at B and bring this point directly up, releasing the sheet at A.

d. Tuck in the part of the sheet that hangs below the mattress.

e. Bring B down firmly and tuck under the mattress. The underfold of the corner (C) should be even with the edge of the mattress.

To square a corner means to tuck in the end of the sheet and then to fold the side under so that the fold runs parallel to the corner and gives a boxed appearance to the corner.

After the bottom sheet has been tucked in on one side of the bed, the drawsheets are placed on the bed if they are indicated. They are tucked in on the near side.

The top sheet is then placed across the foundation near the foot and opened so that the bottom half of the bed is covered. It is then carried to the head of the bed until the edge of the sheet is even with the edge of the mattress. The blankets and bedspread are applied in the same manner but are brought to within approximately 23 cm. (9 inches) of the edge of the mattress.

When the bed has been made completely on one side, the other side is made up in the same manner. The foundation is pulled tightly so that it is free of wrinkles. Wrinkles are uncomfortable and can be irritating to the skin. Many agencies now use contour (fitted) sheets which make it easier to provide a firm wrinkle-free foundation for the bed.

The head of the bed is completed by folding back the top covers. The pillows are replaced on the bed.

3. *Replace the equipment.* Before the nurse leaves the bedside she replaces any equipment that the patient requires. This includes attaching the signal light to the bed, placing the bedside chair beside the bed and arranging the bedside table within the patient's reach. All unnecessary equipment is removed, and small articles that the patient is not using are placed safely in his bedside table. The nurse should ask the patient's permission before discarding any of his belongings, including flowers.

MAKING THE CLOSED BED. This procedure is usually carried out nowadays by staff of the Housekeeping Department. In some situations, however, it may be a nursing responsibility. To make a closed bed the nurse follows the same method as for an open bed except that the spread is brought to the head of the bed so that it is even with the top sheet, and the top sheet and blanket are not folded back. There are many variations of this pattern in hospitals.

MAKING THE OCCUPIED BED. Making an occupied bed is similar to making an open bed except that the nurse is concerned with maintaining the patient's body alignment, safety, and comfort. It is preferable to make the bed while the bed is level; however, some patients are unable to assume the supine position because of their condition—for example, because of difficulty in breathing. In such cases, the nurse is challenged to make a comfortable, neat bed while the head of the bed is elevated. Although the physician usually orders the position in which the patient is to be maintained, it is often the nurse's decision whether the patient's position can be changed while the bed is made.

When a bed is stripped while the patient remains in it, a pillow is left for the patient's comfort. After the spread and blankets have been removed, a bath blanket is placed over the top sheet, which is then removed by drawing it down from under the bath blanket. If the patient is to be washed, it is done at this time, before the foundation of the bed is changed, to prevent the clean sheet from becoming damp or soiled during the bath.

It is easier to change the foundation of the bed if the patient is moved to the far side of the bed. The foundation on the near side is loosened and if the linen is to be removed, it is folded to the center of the bed. Clean linen is placed on the near side of the bed and tucked in. The patient then rolls over the folded linen to the near side of the bed. The soiled linen is removed, and the clean linen is pulled tightly across the bed and tucked in.

The patient is assisted to the center of the bed and the second pillow is replaced. The top covers are replaced as for an open bed. The nurse must remember to withdraw the bath blanket after she has put on the top sheet. For some patients, as for example, orthopedic patients in traction, the bed may be made from top to bottom rather than from side to side.

When the nurse replaces the top covers,

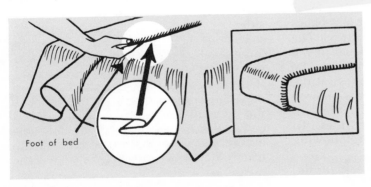

Foot of bed

A vertical toe pleat is made while the nurse is standing at the foot of the bed.

she should allow sufficient room for the patient to move his feet. Toe pleats in the top covers will provide this extra space for the patient. To make a vertical toe pleat, the upper sheet and the blankets are raised and a 5 cm. (2 inch) fold is made in the sheet and blankets parallel to the foot of the bed. The linen is then tucked in. As an alternative, the nurse can loosen the top covers at the foot of the bed, or the patient can cross his feet before the corners are mitered in order to ensure sufficient foot room.

After the nurse completes the bed she tidies the unit. This involves putting away personal utensils that the patient is not using and placing articles such as his water glass and radio within easy reach. The hospital patient's signal cord is attached to the bed so that it is always within easy reach. It gives the patient a feeling of security to know that the nurse may be easily and quickly summoned.

Today, hospitals often employ a housekeeping staff which is responsible for cleaning the patient's unit. It is the staff's responsibility to clean the bed-unit tables, change the patient's drinking water, and look after his flowers. Floor washers are assigned to clean the hospital floors regularly. In a hospital where a specialized staff is not employed for these purposes, these duties may very likely become the nurse's responsibility. In any case, the nurse is often responsible for checking that the patient's environment is clean and comfortable. It is a good idea for the nurse to stand back and check that everything is neat and tidy and that the patient is comfortable.

MAKING THE ANESTHETIC BED (RECOVERY BED). The anesthetic bed is an adaptation of the basic hospital bed. It is customarily made directly after the patient goes to surgery. If the patient is to go to the recovery room (postanesthetic room or P.A.R.) after surgery, the bed is usually taken there so that the patient is transferred to his own bed immediately after the operation is over.

The purpose of the anesthetic bed is to provide a safe, comfortable, and convenient bed for the postsurgical patient. Usually the foundation for an open bed is completed, and then one or two rubber

(plastic) and cotton drawsheets are placed over it to protect the bottom sheet. This is done because a short drawsheet is more easily changed than an entire bottom sheet; therefore the patient will be disturbed less if it is necessary to change any part of the foundation of the bed.

The top covers on the anesthetic bed are generally folded back in order to make it easier for the patient to be transferred into the bed. One method of arranging the top covers is to fold the bedclothes up on both sides and both ends. Then all the covers can be quickly folded to one side or the other when the patient is transferred to the bed.

The anesthetic bed is always made with clean linen, as free from microorganisms as possible. A clean bed lessens the danger of infection and is generally more comfortable. If a pillow is needed for the postoperative patient, it should have a plastic covering to protect it from any vomitus and drainage. In many agencies today, all pillows are plastic covered for easy cleaning.

The bed unit for the postoperative patient is arranged for efficiency of care. The patient's personal belongings are put safely away, and the bedside table is left clear. Tissues should be immediately available and a kidney basin should be nearby so that it can be obtained quickly if it is needed. Siderails should be attached to the bed. An intravenous standard should be either attached to the bed or available in the patient's room. Blood pressure equipment is needed also. Since oxygen or suction equipment is often required at the bedside the nurse must check that a space is set aside for this equipment and that the equipment is ready for the patient when he returns from the operating room.

The Mattress. There are many different kinds of mattresses available for both therapeutic and comfort purposes. The regular mattress for the hospital bed is firm and often covered with a plasticized material. Patients who are allergic to these mattresses require mattresses made of foam rubber. This type offers the patient support but molds somewhat to his body. The foam rubber mattress also has an advantage in that it places less pressure upon the patient's bony prominences. Because of this it is often used in the prevention and treatment of decubitus ulcers in patients who must remain in bed for long periods of time.

Also available are split foam rubber mattresses. These mattresses are divided horizontally into three sections. The sections at the head and foot of the bed are approximately ¾ meter (2½ feet) in length and the middle section ½ meter (1½ feet) in length. The middle section is in turn divided lengthwise into two parts, one of which can be pulled out in order to insert a bedpan without moving the patient. The split foam rubber mattress is generally used for debilitated patients and for those who are unable to move.

A third type of mattress is the alternating pressure mattress, which is run by a small motor. This mattress can be filled with either air or water. Areas of the mattress are alternately deflated and inflated with the result that there is a continual change in the pressure upon the various parts of the patient's body. These alterations of pressure stimulate circulation to the skin, thus facilitating the nourishment of tissues and the removal of waste products. Before a patient is placed on an alternating pressure mattress he requires an explanation of the use of the mattress and reassurance about his safety. Some patients feel nauseated initially because of the motion, but this usually disappears within several hours. The nurse must also warn the patient and staff to be careful not to prick the mattress with safety pins or sharp instruments. This bed is more effective with only a single layer of linen between the mattress and the patient. Care must be taken not to pinch or shut off the tubing to the motor when the bed is being made.

Another type of bed, the air-fluidized bed, uses the flotation principle to provide uniform support to all parts of the body. The mattress portion of the bed is made of very fine medical-grade optical glass spheres. Air is blown through these spheres to keep them constantly moving, and the patient experiences a comfortable sensation of floating without feeling unstable.[13]

Sawdust mattresses are also used by some agencies for patients whose movement is limited, to provide more equal distribution of pressure. Gel flotation and Silastic flotation pads are frequently used when the patient is transferred to a normal bed. These pads are often used in home care.

It should be noted that the use of any of these special mattresses or pads is *not* a substitute for nursing care. Patients still need frequent turning, good skin care, and proper positioning, topics we will discuss shortly.

The Overbed Cradle

The overbed cradle is a device that attaches to the mattress of the bed and extends over the top of the bed. It is used to keep the top bed covers off the patient. Some overbed cradles are hoop arrangements which extend from one side of the bed to the other; others extend only to the midline of the bed. Overbed cradles are usually made of metal or plastic.

The primary purpose of the overbed cradle is to keep the weight of the top bedclothes off the patient. Patients who have burns, uncovered wounds, or wet casts often need to keep the top bedclothes away from the injured area. When the nurse is applying a cradle to the patient's bed, she should ensure that it is securely fastened to, or under, the mattress. The cradle is carefully positioned so that the area of the patient's body that is to be free from the weight of the top bed covers is directly under the cradle. The top bedclothes must be pulled up higher than normally so that they cover the shoulders of the patient.

---

[13]J. Shand Harvin and Thomas S. Hargest: The Air-Fluidized Bed: A New Concept in the Treatment of Decubitus Ulcers. *Nursing Clinics of North America*, 5:181–186, March 1970.

The Footboard

The footboard is a device that is placed toward the foot of the patient's bed to serve as a support for his feet. Some footboards fit onto the bed frame across the foot of the bed; others attach to the sides of the bed frame and thus may rest on the mattress at any point along the bed. Footboards are usually made of wood, plastic, or heavy canvas.

Footboards are also used to keep the weight of the top bedding off the patient's feet as well as to support the patient in maintaining his feet in a neutral position. Normally the feet of the patient who is lying in the dorsal position will be bent into plantar flexion (see p. 296). In time, if his feet are not exercised or supported, they may become fixed in plantar flexion. This condition, known as footdrop, is the result of contractures of the gastrocnemius and soleus muscles. With this complication, the patient is unable to stand with his heels on the floor. Footdrop is usually treated by physiotherapy, but sometimes it can be modified only by surgery.

When the nurse applies a footboard to the bed, it is placed so that the patient can rest the soles of his feet against it while the rest of his body is in good alignment. The top bedclothes need to be brought higher up on the bed so that they cover the patient's shoulders. The footboard is securely fastened to the frame of the bed; it usually has to be removed when the foundation of the bed is stripped.

A *footblock* is a block of wood or a box that is placed at the foot of the bed. Its purpose is the same as that of the footboard. The footblock has a disadvantage: it is not adjustable to the height of a patient. On the other hand it is easily obtainable for the patient who is confined in bed at home.

The Fracture Board

The fracture board (bed board) is a support that is placed under the patient's mattress to give added rigidity to the mattress. It is usually made of wood or of wood and canvas and is constructed to fit the standard hospital bed. One type of fracture board has hinges so that the head and knee gatches of the bed can be used with the board in position. Another type is made of slats, which provide for flexibility so that the head and knee gatches of the bed can be raised or lowered if desired.

The fracture board is used in situations in which the patient needs additional support for his back. Patients who have spinal injuries often have fracture boards ordered by the physician.

The fracture board is easily applied to an unoccupied bed. Usually an orderly can slide the fracture board from a stretcher to the bed, making sure that the hinged joints of the board correspond to the gatches of the bed. The nurse should explain to the patient that the purpose of the board is to provide firmness and thus should not be modified by the extensive use of pillows.

The Balkan Frame

The Balkan frame is a frame made of wood or metal which extends lengthwise above the bed and is supported at either end by a pole. A trapeze may be attached to the frame just above the patient's head as an aid to the patient in lifting himself up in bed. Often the Balkan frame serves as an attachment for the pulleys and weights of traction equipment, which is used for pa-

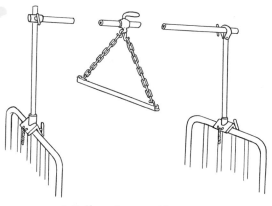

A Balkan frame with trapeze.

tients who have fractures of the lower limbs, particularly the femur.

Often the sole purpose of the Balkan frame is to provide a trapeze. Some frames use only one pole when it is necessary to support only a trapeze. The nurse can show the patient how to use this as an exercise device or as an aid in moving.

The Bradford Frame

The Bradford frame is a canvas, stretcher-like device that is supported by blocks on the foundation of the bed. It is often used to immobilize patients who have injured spines. The canvas is divided into three parts so that the small center portion can be removed to insert a bedpan. In many fracture beds the canvas covering of the frame is in strips to facilitate care of the patient.

One of the nurse's responsibilities is to reassure the patient that he is not likely to fall off the frame and that he should lie quietly. Bradford frames have been replaced in many instances by Stryker frames and Foster beds.

A number of other beds have been devised for patients who will be helpless for long periods of time and for those with specific health problems, as, for example, the Circ Olectric bed, the HighLow Tilt bed, the Rocking bed, and the Chair bed. These are usually discussed in Medical-Surgical Nursing courses and the student is directed to texts in this field for additional information.

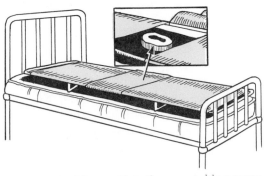

The Bradford frame. Note the removable canvas strip in the center to allow the insertion of a bedpan.

Positioning the Patient

Generally patients assume the positions which are most comfortable for them. For the patient who can move easily and freely in bed without therapeutic considerations, the nurse's chief responsibility in regard to his position is his comfort. The astute use of pillows and the provision of a firm foundation will help him remain comfortable.

Patients assume positions for therapeutic reasons as well as for comfort. There are many possible reasons for positioning a patient therapeutically: to maintain good body alignment, to prevent contractures, to promote drainage, to facilitate breathing, and to prevent the development of skin breakdown over bony prominences are but a few.

The physician often prescribes the appropriate therapeutic position for a patient. There are many situations, however, in which the nurse uses her judgment as to which position is best. Intelligent assessment of a patient's problems and a knowledge of anatomy and physiology are important bases for such judgments. Also, the nurse needs to be aware of the variety of positions that it is possible for the patient to assume and the supportive measures which promote his comfort in these positions.

The following are guides with which the nurse should be familiar in assisting patients to assume different positions:

1. Positions as close as possible to the basic anatomical position provide good body alignment, which is, of course, desirable.

2. Joints should be maintained in a slightly flexed position. Prolonged extension creates undue muscle tension and strain.

3. Positions should be changed frequently, at least every two hours. Prolonged pressure on one area of the skin may cause the skin to break down, with resultant pressure sores (decubitus ulcers). The tolerance of the skin of individual patients is not generally known.

4. All patients require daily exercise unless it is medically contraindicated.

5. When a patient changes his position, his joints should go through the full range

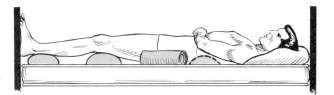

Supine (dorsal recumbent) position with padding for support and to prevent pressure on bony prominences.

of motion unless this too is medically contraindicated.

Anatomical Position. The anatomical position was discussed in Chapter 17 (p. 298). In positioning patients in bed, the principles of the anatomical position are maintained—that is:

   a. Good alignment of all body parts
   b. Equal weight distribution of body parts
   c. Maximal space in body cavities for internal organs
   d. Joints in functional position (for walking, grasping objects, etc.)

Certain positions which do not follow the therapeutically anatomical position fully may be best for some patients. The basic principles should be kept in mind and applied insofar as is possible, however.

Supine (Dorsal Recumbent) Position. In the supine (dorsal recumbent) position the patient lies on his back with his head and shoulders slightly elevated. Usually one pillow suffices for this purpose. The lumbar curvature of the back is best supported by a small pillow or a folded towel if necessary.

If the patient does not have support for his thighs, they will tend to rotate outward. Two rolled towels or a rolled bath blanket tucked in at the lateral aspects of the thighs under the trochanter of the femur will maintain the patient's legs in alignment. His legs should be slightly flexed for maximal comfort. This is attained by placing a small pad under his thighs just superior to the popliteal space. Direct pressure should be avoided upon the popliteal area because of possible interference with circulation to the extremities and injury to the popliteal nerve. The *trochanter roll* (or hip roll) is often used for this purpose; it is made from a bath towel. The towel is folded lengthwise once and then rolled to within 6 inches of one end. The roll is secured by two safety pins that are fastened between the body of the roll and the tail of the roll. To support the thigh of the patient so as to prevent external rotation, the tail of the roll is placed under the patient's thigh, with the safety pins away from the patient. The roll is then firmly secured along the patient's leg. Trochanter rolls may also be used to raise a patient's heels off the foundation of the bed.

In the supine position, the patient's feet will normally assume a plantar flexion position. Prolonged positioning in plantar flexion, however, can result in footdrop, a condition in which the gastrocnemius and the soleus muscles remain involuntarily contracted. Preventive measures for this complication include the use of the footboard, which helps the patient to maintain his feet in dorsal flexion and removes the weight of the bedclothes from his toes. Flexion, extension, and circumduction of the patient's ankles help maintain muscle tone and ankle joint mobility.

When the patient is lying in the supine position (and in all positions described

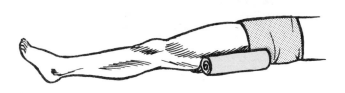

A trochanter roll can be used to prevent external rotation of the hip. The safety pins used to secure the roll initially are placed so that they face away from the patient.

subsequently), care should be taken to maintain the fingers in a functioning position, that is, fingers flexed and thumb in opposition. A small hand roll may be placed in the palm of the hand and the fingers curved around it. This is particularly important for unconscious patients and for those who have difficulty of movement in one or both hands. Wristdrop must also be prevented. The hand should never be left in a dependent position. It should be supported so that it is in a straight line with the lower arm.

Sponge rubber pads, sheepskin pads, and *small pillows* also serve as supportive devices. Placed under bony prominences, they relieve pressure; placed in the lumbar curve or under a limb they support or elevate an injured part. A small sponge rubber pad placed in the patient's hand can be used as an exercise implement. It can also be used to prevent severe flexion of the hand and to separate skin surfaces in conditions of spastic contraction. The size of the pad allows slight flexion of the hand and fingers, with the thumb comfortably placed in normal anatomical position.

Sandbags also serve as a means of providing support to the patient. They are firmer than trochanter rolls and, because of their weight, are less easily moved. For this reason, sandbags are desirable when body alignment must be maintained—for example, in fractures. Sandbags should be pliable so that they can be shaped to the contours of the body.

In some cases, the patient's head and shoulders are not elevated by pillows and rolls. The patient lies on his back with his head and shoulders on the flat surface. Supports similar to those just described are used when indicated.

This position is frequently prescribed for patients who have had spinal anesthetics.

Prone Position. The prone position is a position in which the patient lies on the abdomen with the head turned to one

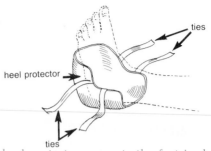

The heel protector supports the foot in dorsal flexion and protects the heel simultaneously. (From Lucile A. Wood and Beverly J. Rambo: Nursing Skills for Allied Health Services. Vol. 1, 2nd Ed. Philadelphia, W. B. Saunders Co., 1977.)

side. Many people are relaxed and sleep well in this position; some find it most comfortable to flex their arms over their heads.

Supportive measures for the patient in this position include a small pillow or pad, as needed, under the abdomen at the level of the diaphragm in order to give support to the lumbar curvature and, in the case of the female patient, to take weight off the breasts. A small pillow or towel roll under each shoulder helps to maintain the anatomical position. In addition, a pillow under the lower legs elevates the patient's toes off the bed and permits slight flexion of the knees. Alternatively, the patient can extend the toes over the end of the mattress to take the weight off the tips. Plantar flexion is minimized if the patient's lower legs are also supported. When the patient is in a prone position, there is pressure on the knees. A small pad under the thighs can be used to relieve this pressure. Sheepskin or sponge rubber pads may also be used under the knees.

The patient may prefer a pillow for his head. Unless the physician wishes the patient's head on a flat surface, in order to promote drainage of mucus, for example, a small pillow is often more comfortable;

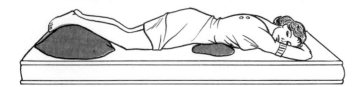

Prone position with padding for support and to prevent pressure on bony prominences. Note that the head is turned to the side and no pillow is provided.

Lateral position. Notice the pillow supporting the patient's upper arm in order to allow for chest expansion.

however, it should not be so thick as to hyperextend the patient's head.

Lateral (Side-Lying) Position. In the lateral position, the patient lies on his side with both arms forward and his knees and hips flexed. The upper leg is flexed more than the lower leg. Weight is borne by the lateral aspects of the patient's ilium and by his scapula.

The upper knee and hip should be at the same level; the upper elbow and wrist should be at the same level as the upper shoulder to prevent the limbs from being in a dependent position. The patient's heels and ankles may be protected by using small pads (for example, of sheepskin or sponge rubber) to keep them from rubbing on the bedclothes.

If the patient's upper arm falls across his chest, his lung capacity may be restricted; a pillow to support the patient's arm permits greater chest expansion and enables the nurse to readily observe the character and rate of his respirations.

The person who lies laterally will probably prefer a pillow for his head. A pillow of proper depth should prevent lateral flexion of the head. Frequently the patient will also require the support of a pillow placed lengthwise behind his back.

The lateral position is prescribed in order to take weight off the sacrum of the patient; in addition, the patient can eat more easily in this position than in the supine position. It also facilitates some kinds of drainage. Finally, many people find it a relaxing position.

Fowler's Position.[14] Fowler's position is probably one of the most frequently as-

sumed positions. It is a sitting position in which the head gatch of the patient's bed is raised to at least a 45 degree angle.

In Fowler's position the patient is usually comfortable with at least two pillows for the back and head. The first pillow is best placed far enough down the patient's back to provide support for the lumbar curvature. A second pillow supports the head and shoulders. An emaciated patient will probably need three pillows. For patients who are very weak, pillows placed laterally will support the arms and help to maintain good body alignment.

Small pillows or a pad under the patient's thighs permits slight flexion of the knees, and a footboard permits dorsal flexion and prevents the patient from sliding toward the foot of the bed. Occasionally the knee gatch of the bed is used to support flexion of the knee. If the knee gatch is used, it should not be flexed too much because of the danger of putting pressure on the popliteal nerve and major blood vessels which are close to the skin surface in the popliteal area. Prolonged pressure can cause serious interference with both nerve supply and circulation to the lower limbs. Hence, the knee gatch is seldom used for patients now.

In Fowler's position the main weight-bearing areas of the patient are the heels, sacrum, and posterior aspects of the ilium. The nurse should pay particular attention to these areas when she gives skin care.

Fowler's position is indicated for patients who suffer either cardiac or respiratory distress, since it permits maximal chest expansion.

Two variations of Fowler's position are the *semi-Fowler* and *high Fowler* positions. The semi-Fowler position refers to an elevation of the head of approximately 30 degrees. This is a comfortable position

---

[14]In some agencies, Fowler's position refers to the elevation of the upper part of the body without flexion at the hips; any elevation with hip flexion is referred to as the semi-Fowler position.

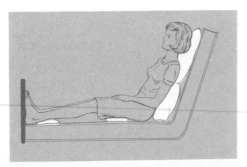

Fowler's position. Pillows can be provided for the patient's arms if such support is required.

for the patient who must remain with his head and chest slightly elevated. The high Fowler position refers to the full sitting position, that is, with the head of the bed elevated to a 90 degree angle. The head gatches of most hospital beds can be elevated to this height. A position somewhat similar to the high Fowler is the sitting position in which the patient leans over an overbed table upon which several pillows have been placed for comfort. Some patients with respiratory problems find this position makes breathing easier for them. Patients who have difficulty exhaling tend to lean forward to compress the chest for additional expiratory force.[15] The pillows on the overbed table provide support for the arms and help to maintain the individual in as erect a position as possible to increase his total lung capacity.

Sims's Position (Semiprone or ¾ Prone Position). The Sims position is similar to the lateral position except that the patient's weight is on the anterior aspects of the patient's shoulder girdle and hip. The patient's lower arm is behind him, and his upper arm is flexed at the shoulder and elbow. The upper leg is acutely flexed at the hip and knee, and the lower leg is slightly flexed at the hip and knee.

A rolled pillow placed laterally and in front of the patient's abdomen will support the patient in this position. Pillows for the patient's upper arm and upper leg will prevent adduction of these limbs, and

a small pillow for the patient's head will prevent lateral flexion. If, however, the patient is unconscious and the nurse wants to promote mucus drainage from the mouth, a pillow under his head is contraindicated.

In the Sims position the patient's feet naturally assume the plantar flexion position. If the patient is to maintain the Sims position for some time, supports should be provided in order that his feet assume the dorsal flexion position. A footboard or sandbag can be used for this purpose.

The Sims position can be established on both the left side and the right side. The patient's position should be changed frequently; if he is unable to move himself, the nurse can help him turn every two hours, or oftener as needed. When turning the patient who is unconscious, the nurse should be sure that the patient's eyelids are closed to prevent the possibility of the cornea's being scratched by the bedclothes. Good skin care, particularly to the anterior aspects of the patient's ilium and shoulder girdle, is also indicated.

This position is prescribed for patients who are either unconscious or unable to swallow. It permits the free drainage of mucus. The Sims position also allows maximal relaxation and is therefore a comfortable sleeping position for many people.

Trendelenburg Position. This position is used for some kinds of surgery and occasionally in situations involving shock and hemorrhage. In the modified Trendelenburg position shown (page 343), the patient lies on her back. The foot of the bed is elevated at a 45 degree angle so that the patient's hips and legs are higher than her shoulders.

This adaptation of the Trendelenburg position is sometimes used for a patient who requires vaginal irrigation. In this procedure it is important that the patient's hips be higher than her chest in order that the irrigating fluid will reach the posterior fornix of the vagina. Draping for this position is similar to that used in the lithotomy position. (See Chapter 23.)

In a regular Trendelenburg position the foot of the bed is elevated but the patient is not flexed at the waist. This position is also used in some situations when the patient is in shock.

[15]Jane Secor: *Patient Care in Respiratory Programs.* Saunders Monographs in Clinical Nursing, Vol. 1. Philadelphia, W. B. Saunders Company, 1969, p. 75.

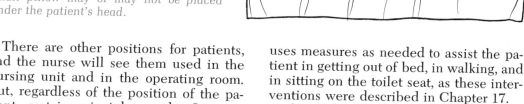

Sims's position (semiprone position). A small pillow may or may not be placed under the patient's head.

There are other positions for patients, and the nurse will see them used in the nursing unit and in the operating room. But, regardless of the position of the patient, certain principles apply: In positioning the patient in bed, it is most important that the nurse drape the patient adequately. In many situations it is equally important that she change the patient's position frequently. Adequate exercise, good skin care, and supportive measures for maintaining good body alignment should also be carried out.

Helping the Patient With a Bedpan or Urinal

People are uncomfortable when their bladder is distended or when they need to defecate. Elimination is a very basic physiological need that is essential for optimal functioning of all body systems. People who are ambulatory can take care of their elimination needs by using bathroom facilities. Often sick patients need the nurse's help to get to the bathroom and to use the facilities. Many hospitals and other inpatient facilities are equipped with specially constructed toilets, washbasins, and supportive bars to help patients who find the use of ordinary bathroom equipment difficult. The nurse uses measures as needed to assist the patient in getting out of bed, in walking, and in sitting on the toilet seat, as these interventions were described in Chapter 17.

The ill person, however, is often confined to bed and must use the bedpan or the urinal for elimination purposes. Women patients use the bedpan for both urination and for defecation. Male patients need the bedpan for defecation and the urinal for voiding. Having to use these articles for such a basic need is embarrassing for most people, and the nurse does everything possible to assure the patient's privacy, to avoid unnecessary exposure of bodily parts that are considered by most people to be very private, and to make the procedure as safe and as comfortable as possible for the patient, both physically and psychologically.

To ensure privacy, the curtains are drawn around the patient's bed, or the door of a private room closed. If the patient can use the bedpan or urinal himself, the nurse may wait outside the curtain or door if she feels the patient might need assistance. Otherwise, she places the patient's call signal within easy reach for him.

Unnecessary exposure can be avoided by folding back one corner of the bedcovers for easy insertion of the pan or urinal.

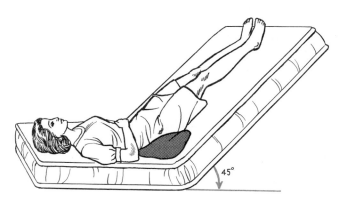

The modified Trendelenburg position.

The procedure can be made as comfortable as possible for the patient by using the proper equipment and handling it competently. Assistance is given to the patient as needed, e.g., cleansing the perineal and rectal area. Male patients, however, do not usually need cleansing after using the urinal since the urine does not normally dribble onto the skin. The nurse provides the patient with the means for washing his hands after he has finished. The entire procedure should be handled in a matter-of-fact manner. Since the bedpan is extremely uncomfortable to use, the patient should never be left on it any longer than necessary. Thus, the call signal must be answered promptly.

Excretory products from the gastrointestinal tract contain a very large number of microorganisms. In the sick person, urine may also contain harmful microorganisms. To prevent cross-infection, a separate bedpan and urinal are kept for each patient's use in almost all agencies today. They are stored in the patient's bedside locker, in an adjoining bathroom, or, in some agencies, in a separate room on the nursing unit.

Metal bedpans and urinals usually become cold when they are stored, so they need to be warmed before using them. Rinsing them with warm water helps to eliminate this problem and lessens the patient's discomfort. The nurse's hands should also be warmed if they are coming in contact with the patient's skin. Recently, more agencies are using disposable equipment that is used for one patient only, and then discarded. If this is not the case, or if there is multiple usage, the equipment must be sterilized after every use.

The nurse helps to prevent infection in the patient, herself, and other patients and workers by washing her hands before and after assisting patients. The patient should always be provided with the opportunity to wash his hands after using these articles (as he would at home after voiding or defecating). After use of the bedpan, the perineal and rectal areas are cleansed with toilet paper and/or washed with soap and water if the patient has had a bowel movement.

The nurse protects the patient's safety at all times when helping the patient with a bedpan or urinal. In addition to being uncomfortable, bedpans are also awkward to use. The patient should be helped to a secure position on the pan and supported to ensure that his balance is not going to be upset. The toilet paper should be within easy reach if the patient can use it himself. The patient may need something to hold onto to support himself if he is going to get off the pan himself; the siderails may be helpful in this regard.

It is more comfortable for the patient to be in a sitting position for using the bedpan. The head of the bed is elevated unless this is contraindicated. The bedpan can be used in the supine position if necessary; measures to assist the helpless or semi-helpless patient onto the bedpan were discussed in Chapter 17 in connection with helping the patient to raise his buttocks.

An alternative measure, which may be used with some patients, is to have the bed flat, with the siderail up on the far side of the bed to the nurse. The patient is instructed or assisted to roll onto his side and grasp the siderail. The bedpan is placed in position under the patient's buttocks, and the patient is then returned to the back-lying position. The head of the bed should then be elevated, if permissible, to bring the patient into a sitting position. The position of the bedpan may need some slight adjusting for the patient's comfort and to prevent spillage.

A fracture (or slipper) pan, which is smaller, both in diameter and height, than the standard bedpan, may be used when patients are unable to use the regular sized one. It is slipped under the patient's buttocks from the front of the body. It is easier to use if the patient is in a squatting position with the legs wide enough apart to permit the pan to be placed between

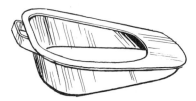

A fracture (slipper) pan. (From Lucile A. Wood and Beverly J. Rambo, eds.: Nursing Skills for Allied Health Services. Vol. 1, 2nd Ed. Philadelphia, W. B. Saunders Co., 1977.)

them and then slipped under the buttocks. Care must be taken not to injure the patient's skin in using this fracture pan; this is important with all bedpans, but particularly important to keep in mind when the fracture pan is used, because it is very narrow at the base that is slipped under the patient and could easily tear tissues.

The male urinal was designed to fit over the patient's penis so that urine could be excreted without spillage. It has a handle for convenience (specially designed urinals are available for patients who have the use of only one hand) and it is usually flat on either one side or the bottom so that it can be set down on a flat surface after use without the contents spilling.

The patient can use the urinal when in the supine position, the lateral position (either side), or Fowler's position, or when standing at the side of the bed. If at all possible, patients prefer to use the urinal without help, particularly if the nurse or other attendant is female. He sometimes needs the nurse's help, however, and this should be given without embarrassment and treated as any other procedure with which the patient needs help.

The patient should be exposed only as much as necessary. The patient's legs are separated sufficiently to allow the urinal to be placed between them. Holding the urinal with one hand, the nurse gently inserts the penis into the urinal sufficiently far to prevent urine from leaking out onto the bedclothes or the patient's skin. The nurse holds the urinal in place if the patient cannot do so.

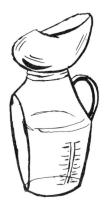

A female urinal. (From Wood and Rambo, 1977.)

A female urinal may be used for some patients. It is similar in design to the male urinal, but has a long, wide top, shaped like a spout. The patient may stand at the side of the bed to use this article, sit on the edge of the bed, or sit in bed. If necessary, it may be used when the patient is in a side-lying position. Because of its shape, the spout must be in contact with the patient's skin or urine will leak out. The spout end should point towards the rectum and the handle should be on top so that it can be easily grasped.

If the patient is on measured intake and output, the contents of the bedpan or urinal are examined and urine measured before they are disposed of in the toilet (in rooms with adjoining bathrooms) or in the hopper, if this system is used in the agency.

The Back Massage (Back Rub)

In helping the patient relax in preparation for sleeping, after his bath and at other times as indicated, the patient's back is rubbed with an emollient lotion or cream. Although alcohol was for many years the traditional solution for rubbing the backs of patients in hospital, and is still used in some agencies, it is no longer recommended as a back rub. Alcohol dries and hardens the skin, leaving it more susceptible to cracking.[6] This is a particular hazard in the elderly, whose skin tends to be dry and thin, and in patients whose nutritional status or hydra-

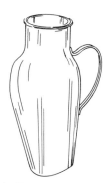

A male urinal. (From Wood and Rambo, 1977.)

[6] Edith V. Olson et al.: The Hazards of Immobility. *American Journal of Nursing* 67:780–797, 1967.

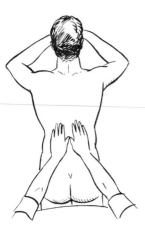

Long, smooth, and circular motions increase the blood circulation to the skin.

tion is poor. Emollient creams and lotions are considered preferable. Most agencies have their own preference as to the type of cream or lotion used for back care.

When the nurse gives the patient a back rub, the best position for the patient is the prone position. The side-lying position is the next most preferable. These positions permit the nurse to use long, firm strokes, which are both soothing to the patient and stimulating to the blood circulation. A circular motion over the bony prominences of the shoulder blades and at the base of the spine helps to keep the skin in good condition.

When giving a back rub, the nurse should warn the patient that the solution may feel cold. It is more comfortable for the patient if the nurse warms the solution in her hands before she applies it to the patient's back. The nurse starts at the shoulder area and, using her fingertips, rubs the patient's neck with circular motions extending to the hairline. This helps to relax the shoulder and neck muscles which so often are tensed in anxious people. She then moves her hands to the sacral area and repeats the circular motions with the fingertips. Then, starting at the sacrum, she rubs up the center of the back to the hairline, using long smooth strokes, then over to the shoulders, where she proceeds down the sides of the back, using broad circular motions. The circular motions are made to increase circulation to these bony prominences. The pressure

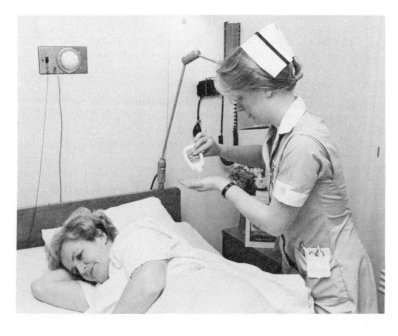

A soothing back rub helps to relax the patient and promotes comfort and rest.

of the nurse's motions should be sufficiently firm to stimulate the muscle tissue. However, if the patient is very thin or the skin is in poor condition, the nurse should be careful not to use undue pressure in rubbing or massaging. After the circular motions over the shoulders, the nurse brings her hands down to the lower edge of the patient's buttocks and to the patient's sacrum, continuing with the broad circular motions. This process is continued until the circulation to the skin has been stimulated and all lotion is rubbed in well. The nurse also rubs the patient's knees, elbows, heels, and any other reddened areas on bony prominences. Care should be taken, however, not to massage reddened areas on the patient's thighs or lower legs. Sometimes, when circulation is poor, a person may develop a clot in one of the blood vessels supplying the limbs. Surface areas in the vicinity of the clot often become reddened, warm to the touch, and tender. Massage may loosen the clot and cause it to circulate in the blood stream. This can be dangerous because the clot may subsequently block another vessel (for example, in the heart), where it can cause much damage. The nurse should always report the presence of reddened areas on the patient's skin and particularly those which may be indicative of clot formation in the blood vessels below the surface.

PLANNING AND EVALUATING NURSING ACTION

Interventions to promote comfort, rest, and sleep are an integral part of nursing care for all patients. A specific "sleep plan," or a sleep and rest plan, is helpful in focusing attention on these important aspects of patient care and in facilitating communication about each individual's needs, preferences, and problems with regard to comfort, rest, and sleep. Expected outcomes for specific interventions are related to each of these three needs. The expected outcomes of comfort measures might be that the patient is comfortable at all times, as evidenced by facial expression, by absence of restlessness and of other outward signs indicative of discomfort, and by verbal expressions that communicate to the nurse that he is comfortable. A decrease in frequency of requests for analgesics (or requests for other things) also helps to indicate to the nurse that the patient is comfortable.

Expected outcomes of interventions to promote rest and sleep relate to the amount of rest and undisturbed sleep the patient has, and to the ease with which he is able to get to sleep. The outcomes then might be expressed in terms of the amount of additional rest considered desirable for the patient, the time taken to get to sleep, the number of hours slept, and the number of times his sleep is interrupted by wakeful periods. A decrease in the last-named might be a criterion for measuring the effectiveness of the nursing interventions taken.

As with nursing interventions used with other problems, the setting down in writing of the expected outcomes in sufficient detail that they can be used as criteria for evaluation by all nursing personnel helps to direct observations used in both assessing and evaluating the patient's comfort, rest, and sleep status.

GUIDES TO ASSESSING COMFORT, REST, AND SLEEP STATUS

1. What are the patient's usual habits in regard to sleep and rest (e.g., usual hours for sleeping, taking naps, snacks at bedtime, hygiene practices before retiring, placement and number of pillows, sleeping position, other aids for sleeping)?
2. Does he have any long-standing problems with resting and sleeping? Has he any problems now?
3. Does he have a health problem(s)? If so, what is the nature of the problem or problems? What are the diagnostic and therapeutic plans of care for him? If diagnostic reports

have been received, what do they indicate about this patient's problem(s)?

4. Have hypnotic drugs been ordered for the patient? Analgesics? Was the patient using any medications before admission to this agency? If so, what drugs were they?

5. Are there any restrictions on the patient's mobility? Has a therapeutic position been prescribed?

6. What potential or existing sources of anxiety does this patient have? (See Chapter 12 for further questions in this regard.)

7. What position is best for this patient? Does the patient need assistance to maintain a position of good body alignment?

8. Does he need help with meeting his needs for elimination? If so, what kind of help does he need?

9. Does he say that he is uncomfortable, unable to rest or to sleep? If so, what things are causing him discomfort? Is he in pain? Is his bed comfortable? Does his dressing need changing? Can he reach everything he needs?

10. Do you observe any signs of discomfort in the patient (e.g., is he restless? pale? tense? perspiring profusely? lying rigidly in bed? Are his bed and his unit neat and tidy? Is the foundation of the bed firm and free of soiled or damp linen? Does he look uncomfortable?)?

11. Does he have difficulty getting to sleep at night? Is he wakeful during the night?

12. Is he getting sufficient rest and sleep?

13. Is the environment conducive to sleeping and resting?

STUDY VOCABULARY

Anatomical position	Enuresis	Narcolepsy
Anesthetic bed	Fomite	Open bed
Balkan frame	Footboard	Overbed cradle
Biological clock	Fowler's position	Prone position
Bradford frame	Fracture board	REM sleep
Circadian rhythm	Fracture (slipper) pan	Sims's position
Closed bed	Hypersomnia	Somnambulism
Comfort	Hypnotic drug	Supine (dorsal recumbent) position
Cradle	Insomnia	
Decubitus ulcer	Lateral (side-lying) position	Trendelenburg position
Diagonal toe bed	Miter	
Emaciated		

STUDY SITUATION

Mrs. R. Rogers is a 56 year old woman who was admitted to the hospital with acute rheumatoid arthritis involving her back, her knees, and her feet. Mrs. Rogers is an obese woman and she finds it difficult to breathe when the head of her bed is flat. She complains of pain in her joints continually. Mrs. Rogers has a limited income and lives by herself in a small apartment. Her husband died four years ago, and her one daughter lives out of town and finds it difficult to visit her mother frequently.

The physician has ordered that Mrs. Rogers be maintained in good body alignment at all times. Her position is to be changed every four hours. She is on a low calorie diet. Her medications include acetylsalicylic acid (0.6 gm. four times a day) and Seconal (50 mg. at bedtime).

1. Would you expect Mrs. Rogers to be uncomfortable? in pain? to have problems with sleeping?
2. What factors might cause Mrs. Rogers to have problems with regard to comfort, rest, and sleep?
3. How would you assess Mrs. Rogers' present comfort, rest, and sleep status?
4. What objective signs would indicate to you that Mrs. Rogers is uncomfortable, is not resting, or is not sleeping well?
5. What subjective observations by Mrs. Rogers might you note?
6. What other members of the health team are, or might be, involved in helping Mrs. Rogers? For what purpose?
7. What positions do you think might be most comfortable for Mrs. Rogers?
8. What supportive devices might make Mrs. Rogers more comfortable? How should you use them?
9. Outline a nursing care plan for Mrs. Rogers.

SUGGESTED READINGS

Feinberg, I.: Changes in Sleep Cycle Patterns With Age. *Journal of Psychological Research,* 10:283–306, October 1974.

Felton, G.: Body Rhythm Effects on Rotating Work Shifts. *Nursing Digest,* 4:29–32, January–February 1976.

Fowler, M. J., et al.: Sleep and Memory. *Science,* 179:908–910, March 2, 1973.

Guilleminault, C.: Insomnia With Sleep Apnea: A New Syndrome. *Science, 181:* 856–858, August 31, 1973.

Lowthian, P. T.: Portable Urinals for Women. *Nursing Times,* 71:1739–1741, October 30, 1975.

Martin, I. C. A.: Some Therapeutic Concepts of Sleep. *Nursing Times,* 71:1611–1614, October 9, 1975.

Tom, C., and D. Lanuza (Guest Editors): Symposium on Biological Rhythms. *Nursing Clinics of North America, 11:4,* December 1976.

19 HYGIENE NEEDS

The nurse should be able to:

Discuss the importance of good personal hygiene to optimal health

Briefly explain the basic anatomy and physiology of the skin, its appendages, the teeth, and other structures in the mouth

Identify factors which may be contributing to impaired status of an individual's skin, its appendages, his teeth, and his mouth

Identify common potential or existing problems people have in regard to the status of these structures

Identify problems with regard to an individual's ability to maintain good hygiene

Identify and take action in situations requiring immediate nursing intervention

Select, plan, and implement appropriate nursing interventions to maintain or restore the optimal status of an individual's skin, its appendages, his teeth, and his mouth

Evaluate the effectiveness of nursing interventions

INTRODUCTION

Hygiene is the science of health and its preservation; it also refers to practices that are conducive to good health. Good personal hygiene is important to a person's general health.

Good personal hygiene usually means those measures a person takes to keep his skin and its appendages (his hair, fingernails, and toenails), and his teeth and mouth, clean and in good condition. The healthy unbroken skin is the body's first line of defense against infection and against injury to underlying tissues. The skin is also important to the regulation of body temperature. In addition, it serves as one means for the excretion of body wastes. Healthy teeth and gums are essential for maintaining nutritional status. Decayed teeth and poor condition of the oral cavity are potential sources of infection as well as sources of discomfort and pain for the individual.

Bathing and personal grooming are important rituals in every culture. In our cleanliness-conscious North American society, most children are taught to wash their hands before meals, after voiding or having a bowel movement, and at other times when their hands are dirty. Washing the hands and face, and cleaning the teeth, the first thing in the morning and again before retiring, are habits many people acquire at an early age. With the increased emphasis on dental health these days, many people also brush their teeth after every meal.

Looking after one's personal hygiene and grooming are important independent functions both for children (once they have learned to do this themselves) and for adults. When an individual is ill, he must often depend on others to help him with personal hygiene that he is no longer able to take care of himself. This, of course, threatens a person's self-esteem. Having someone else wash your hands and face and look after the very personal aspects of hygiene is demeaning and most people find it embarrassing. They often hesitate to ask for help and their mental distress in having to ask adds to their physical discomfort.

It also puts the nurse somewhat in the role of substitute mother, a situation that is sometimes difficult for young students. If they can anticipate the patient's needs and provide help in a competent, matter-of-fact manner, before it is requested, acknowledging the patient's feelings and not treating him like a child, this will help both the nurse and the patient to feel more comfortable.

The person who is ill usually has a lowered resistance to infection; consequently the presence of pathogenic bacteria in his environment poses a constant threat of infection. Helping the patient to keep clean, by removing dirt, excretory products, and secretions, eliminates many substances in which these bacteria flourish. In addition, hygienic measures help the patients to be comfortable and relaxed. Most people feel better when they are fresh and clean, and many who have been unable to rest will sleep soundly after a relaxing bath.

People who are ill are frequently concerned about unpleasant odors. Excessive perspiration and the presence of bacteria in the mouth and on the skin are common causes of such odors. Bad breath (halitosis) is most frequently caused by bacteria and old food particles in the mouth. Good oral hygiene usually eliminates this source of unpleasantness.

Another reason that good personal hygiene is desirable for the sick person is that a clean, refreshed feeling helps his morale. Generally, a well-groomed appearance is indicative of good mental health. The nurse often observes that a patient who is very ill does not care about grooming; once he begins to feel better, he often suggests to the nurse that he shave or, in the case of a female patient, asks for her cosmetics. Such requests are usually signs that a person is feeling better, and that he is more aware of his immediate environment.

ANATOMY AND PHYSIOLOGY WITH RESPECT TO HYGIENE

The skin is composed of two main layers, the outer, thinner layer or epidermis, and the inner, thicker layer or dermis. Underlying these layers is subcutaneous tissue and adipose tissue. The epidermis itself has four layers on most areas of the body except the palms of the hands and the soles of the feet, where there are five. The outermost, horny layer of epidermis continually flakes off. This horny layer is particularly thick on elderly people.

The nails of the fingers and toes are composed of epidermal cells that have been converted to keratin. Epithelial cells lie under the crescent of each nail, and it is from these cells that the epidermal cells of the nails grow. The mucous membrane, which is also composed of epithelial tissue, lines the body cavities and passageways. For example, mucous membrane lines the digestive tract, the respiratory passages, and the genitourinary tract.

Hair is the term applied to the threadlike appendages of the skin which are in particular abundance on the scalp, pubic, and axillary areas of the body. The term is also frequently used to refer to the aggregate of hair in the scalp. Each hair is composed of a long, cylindrical shaft and a root that is embedded in a depression, called a hair follicle, which penetrates the epidermis to the subcutaneous tissues.

The hair receives its nourishment from the blood supplying the skin tissues through the root.[1] *Dandruff* is the term used for the dry, scaly material that is normally shed from the skin of the scalp.[2]

There are three kinds of skin glands in the body. The sebaceous glands secrete oil and are present wherever there is hair. The oil (sebum) keeps the hair supple and pliable. A second type of gland is the sweat gland. These are most numerous in the axilla, on the palms of the hands and the soles of the feet, and on the forehead. Their function is to help maintain body temperature and to excrete waste products. Sweat from these glands has a distinctive odor, which is distasteful to some people of Western culture. The ceruminous glands, located in the external ear canal, secrete cerumen (wax). Some people accumulate a large amount of cerumen in their ears, and this can impair hearing. In such cases, the excessive wax can be removed by cleansing with a syringe, a technique that many nurses are learning to do in more senior courses these days.

The *mouth* is the anterior opening of the alimentary canal. It is lined with mucous membrane and contains three important anatomical structures, the tongue, the teeth, and the gums. The tongue is a movable muscular organ which is an important sensory receptor. It also assists in the acts of chewing (*mastication*), swallowing, and sound articulation. The teeth are small, hard structures set in the jaw, which are essential for the chewing of food. Each tooth has a crown and a root or roots. The tooth is solid except for the inner soft pulp cavity. The crown is covered with a hard inorganic substance called *enamel,* which protects the soft structures beneath it. The root is protected by *cementum,* which is true bone. The teeth protrude up through the gums *(gingivae),* which are made up of mucous membrane with supporting fibrous tissue. The hard portion of the gum is firm, dense, normally pink in color, stippled,

---

[1]*Dorland's Illustrated Medical Dictionary.* 25th edition. Philadelphia, W. B. Saunders Company, 1974, p. 677.
[2]Ibid, p. 408.

and tightly attached to the teeth, the periosteum, and the bone of the jaws. A soft portion of the gums protrudes upward in the spaces between teeth.[3]

FACTORS AFFECTING THE SKIN, ITS APPENDAGES, THE TEETH, AND THE MOUTH

Each person's skin is different. Just as each individual is unique in other aspects of his biological being, so, too, his skin is unique. There are individual differences in texture, pigmentation, thickness of the skin tissues, the amount of subcutaneous fat, susceptibility to bruising, and ability to tolerate heat, cold, and exposure to the sun's rays. There are also variations in hair texture, color, and thickness, whether the hair curls or not, and the rapidity with which it grows. Variations also occur, of course, in the teeth, the mucous membranes, and the nails. Each person has inherited a different set of genetic factors which determine the nature of these parts of his anatomy, and these have been influenced by his environment, his lifestyle, and the health care he has received.

The skin changes throughout life. An infant's skin is less resistant to injury and infection than an adult's skin; therefore, his skin should be handled particularly carefully in order to prevent injury. Often infants need special soaps and lotions which are mild and nonirritating.

The adolescent's skin is often a source of embarrassment to him. Acne is a common problem in many teenagers. Hormonal changes occurring at this stage in the life cycle, blockage of the excretion of the sebaceous glands onto the skin surface, and possible bacterial infection are thought to be factors in teenage acne.[4] Cleanliness and a good diet are of the utmost importance during this period in order to prevent secondary infections from acne. Severe acne requires medical attention.

As the adult advances in age, two kinds of skin change take place. First, there is wrinkling, sagging, and increased pigmentation due to exposure to sunlight. Secondly, there is a general thinning of the skin accompanied by increased dryness and inelasticity. This aging takes place in the epidermis and dermis and in the subcutaneous fat. The epidermis is generally thinned and flattened, and sometimes there is an increased growth of the outer layer of the epidermis. A decrease in oil secretions leads to increased dryness and scaliness, and as a result, older people tolerate soap less well than younger adults. If the elderly person bathes too frequently, his skin will become very dry. Oily liquids and skin creams are often better for the elderly patient than too much soap and water or alcohol rubs.[5]

The aging process also takes its toll on the hair, the nails, the teeth, and other structures in the mouth. Hair often becomes thin and loses its texture (this does not always occur of course—one comes across many older persons whose hair has retained its color, thickness, and vitality). The mucous membranes lining the mouth become thinner and more fragile with age; many of the taste buds atrophy as a person get older, too[6] (this is one reason why it often takes more stimulation to whet the appetite). The fingernails and toenails become tougher and more difficult to cut. A very large proportion of older people in North America have lost all or most of their teeth. It is hoped that with better dental care for children, and throughout life, this situation will improve in the future.

The skin is nourished by nutrients delivered by the blood. Since the skin itself has limited absorbent ability, the nutrient creams that are so widely advertised on television and in magazines have only a limited value in promoting skin health. If food and fluid intake is interfered with, the skin will very likely show some ill effects. If fluid intake is insufficient, the patient becomes dehydrated, and his skin appears dry and loose, a condition called

[3] Marie Reitz and Wilma Pope: Mouth Care. *American Journal of Nursing*, 73:1728–1730, October 1973.

[4] Joan Luckmann and Karen Sorensen: *Medical-Surgical Nursing: A Pathophysiological Approach.* Philadelphia, W. B. Saunders Company, 1974, pp. 1258–1259.

[5] Robert G. Carney: The Aging Skin. *American Journal of Nursing*, 63:112, June 1963.

[6] Reitz and Pope, op cit., p. 1729.

poor tissue turgor. The skin of a patient who has suffered prolonged nutrient insufficiency heals very slowly after injury.

Exercise, as we mentioned in Chapter 17, also affects the health of the skin and its appendages. Exercise improves circulation in general and helps to bring a nourishing supply of blood to the surface tissues; it also aids in the elimination of waste products, both through the skin and through other excretory routes.

The weather also affects the skin. In cold weather, the skin often becomes dry and chapped, and, if the internal environment is dry also (as in many homes and apartment buildings with central heating), this contributes to the drying out of the skin tissues. You have no doubt found that it is necessary to use skin creams and hand lotions more frequently in cold weather. Very warm weather can also be hard on the skin. A person perspires much more than usual in hot weather and frequent bathing is needed to rid the skin surface of bodily wastes excreted through this route. Sunshine is an important factor in the health of the skin, but overexposure to the hot sun has a "weathering" effect on the skin, and can be as harmful as too little sun.

The health of the skin and its appendages is also affected by a person's hygiene habits.

Hygienic practices vary widely among individuals. These differences are accounted for by cultural patterns and home education, as well as by individual idiosyncrasies. Some people, for example, are accustomed to bathing daily, others once a week. Not every patient needs a bath every day, and indeed for some patients a complete bath daily may be harmful. This is particularly true of the elderly, whose skin tends to be thinner, drier, and less elastic than the young person's.

Then, too, some people are not aware of the beneficial effects of keeping the skin clean to prevent infection, and to rid the body of the waste products excreted through this route, nor of the importance to their health of maintaining their teeth and mouth in good condition. One also encounters people in whose value system these things simply are not important. We sometimes forget, too, that hygiene is more difficult when the facilities for maintaining good practices of cleanliness are not available or are difficult to obtain. People who live in poor, crowded, or unsanitary conditions often do not have the opportunity to practice good personal hygiene even if they would like to do so. The person who has to cut a hole in the ice to obtain water in the winter-time, or the one who has to share a bathroom with a dozen other people (or more sometimes) may not make a practice of bathing regularly. Teeth are frequently neglected because the individual cannot afford to go to the dentist, and sometimes diet is also poor and contributes to dental caries.

A person's general health status is also very important, both in relation to the person's ability to maintain his own hygiene and with respect to the effect of health problems on the skin and its appendages. Poor health, for whatever reason, is usually reflected in the condition of the skin. The ill person is more susceptible to infection, and illness renders a person more vulnerable to malnourishment, to gastrointestinal problems, and to other disturbances of body functioning that can affect the condition of the skin. There are also many types of disorders specifically affecting the skin, in addition to the common acne that plagues so many teenagers. The student will learn about a number of these skin problems in her courses on medical-surgical nursing.

One particular skin problem to which nurses should be alert from the beginning of their course, however, is the allergic skin reaction, which may occur as a result of a reaction to certain drugs. Penicillin is perhaps the most outstanding culprit for causing allergic reactions, but many other drugs do too. The nurse should watch for skin eruptions, lesions, reddened or weeping areas on the skin, or sloughing of the skin tissues and report these promptly, so that they can be investigated and treatment initiated early. Allergies may be due to a number of causes other than drugs, such as specific foods, dust, and many other things, but the possibility of a drug reaction must always be kept in mind. This again underscores the need for the nurse to be aware of the possible side-effects of drugs she is administering to the patient.

Other forms of therapy may also cause reactions in a person's skin and its appendages. Radiation therapy, which is used extensively in treating patients with cancer, is one example of a form of therapy which may affect the skin. Because the irradiation must penetrate the skin to reach and destroy cells in the part being treated, the skin and its underlying tissues may also suffer damage. The nurse should be alert to redness, sloughing of the skin, and spider-like spots under the skin (these result from damage to the small capillaries underlying the skin surface) in patients on any form of radiation therapy.[7]

Perhaps of most concern to the beginning student, who will be looking after ill people in a hospital or other institutional setting, are the people who need help to maintain the integrity of the skin and to carry out their personal hygiene. This is affected by the individual's motor abilities and the degree to which he is rendered helpless by his illness, as well as the nature of his illness. Fever, for example, usually causes increased perspiration which is uncomfortable for the individual. Irritating drainage seeping onto the skin from surgical or other wounds can cause problems in the surrounding skin area. Incontinence of urine or feces is a major factor in skin breakdown in the vulnerable sacral area. This area is already predisposed to tissue breakdown in the ill person because the sacrum bears most of the weight of patients who are in bed. It is also subject to a considerable amount of friction from rubbing on the bed linen. We mentioned in Chapter 17 that friction is caused by the rubbing together of two irregular surfaces—in this case, the body surface rubbing against the bedsheets. Wrinkled sheets, crumbs in the bed, and the like, increase the irregularity of the sheet surface and hence increase the friction. A smooth, firm foundation on the bed helps to lessen this friction and thus is an aid in preventing tissue breakdown.

The skin also needs to be kept dry.

---

[7]Luckmann and Sorensen, op. cit., p. 378.

Wetness of the bed linen also contributes to the possibilities for tissue breakdown.

COMMON PROBLEMS WITH REGARD TO THE STATUS OF THE SKIN, ITS APPENDAGES, THE TEETH, AND THE MOUTH

Probably the most common problem the nurse encounters in looking after ill people is the inability to maintain their own hygiene. The patient may be completely dependent on other people to bathe him, to clean his teeth, to comb his hair, and to cut his fingernails and toenails, or he may need assistance with some (or all) aspects of only one or a few of these. The nurse must put herself in his place and think of the things that need to be done to ensure that his hygiene is maintained the way he would wish and in a manner that is conducive to good health.

Problems resulting from the patient's inability to maintain his own hygiene are numerous. The skin, the hair, and the teeth may become dirty, and offensive odors from his own body may cause him discomfort, both physical and mental. Ingrown nails frequently result from uncut toenails, and may even interfere with the person's ability to walk. If skin care is neglected, or carried out inadequately, pressure areas are likely to develop and the skin may break down, causing the patient considerable discomfort and pain, rendering him more vulnerable to infection, and causing the nursing staff untold hours and effort to restore the skin to a healthy condition.

If the patient has been unable to look after his own oral hygiene and has not been assisted with it, the teeth and the mucous membranes lining the mouth soon show evidence of this. The nurse will probably see many patients in whom the poor condition of the mouth has become an existing rather than a potential problem, not necessarily because of poor nursing care, but because these patients did not get help in time. A common problem nurses may encounter in the mouths of patients is gingivitis, that is, inflammation of the gums. When orgal hygiene is not carried out adequately, a film of mucus and bacteria (plaque) and calculus (tartar) accumulate on the surface of the teeth and particles of food gather around the teeth and in the crevices of the gums. Normally, these substances are removed by brushing the teeth and rinsing the mouth. When this is not done, the substances accumulate and become a source of mechanical irritation. The tissues of the gums become swollen and inflamed and may separate from the teeth.

Gingivitis not only is uncomfortable for the patient, it also leads to poor nutrition and is a potential source of infection—e.g., in the parotid glands and the gastrointestinal and respiratory tracts. When oral hygiene is neglected the teeth and the tongue also suffer. Decay of the teeth (caries) may result; this problem requires the assistance of dental health professions. The tongue becomes coated with a thick, furry substance that is often referred to as *sordes*. This adds to the patient's discomfort and diminishes the ability of the taste buds to receive stimuli, contributing to the potential problem of malnourishment.[8]

One of the common problems affecting the hair is excessive dandruff. Small flakes of the outer layer of the skin are continuously being sloughed off from all skin surfaces. Excessive dryness of the scalp results in excessive dandruff. Normally, dandruff is removed by combing, brushing, and washing the hair. These procedures also help to remove the accumulation of excess sebum, the oily secretion of the sebaceous glands which keeps the hair supple and pliable. People who have oily hair due to the excessive secretions of sebum need to shampoo their hair frequently to remove the oil. If there are breaks in the skin surface, infection may develop. Thus, people who have irritation of the scalp should be referred to the physician for investigation into their problem.

The nurse may encounter patients whose hair and body are infested with lice or some other vermin. This problem is not as uncommon as one would like to think, particularly in persons who, for one reason or another, have neglected their personal hygiene.

Some patients may need help in acquiring good hygiene habits. The nurse serves as a role model as well as teacher in this regard. If she is careful to wash her hands before and after caring for the patient, maintains good personal standards herself regarding cleanliness and good grooming, and is meticulous in adhering to techniques that have been developed to prevent infection, she presents an excellent role model for the patient. Patients notice all of these things, and their opinions of the care they receive are often based on such criteria as these.

ASSESSING THE STATUS OF SKIN, ITS APPENDAGES, THE TEETH, AND THE MOUTH

The nurse's assessment of the status of the patient's skin, hair, nails, teeth, and mouth is based principally on her objective observations. She *looks* at the condition of the skin and the hair; she *examines* the fingernails and toenails; she opens the patient's mouth, or has him open it, and *observes* the condition of the teeth, the gums, and the soft tissues in the oral cavity (see Chapter 9).

She also takes into consideration the patient's motor abilities; is he able to carry out his own hygiene? Does he need help with this? She assesses his nutritional status and considers the possibility that other health problems may be affecting the condition of his skin. She also considers the effect of age on the individual's skin, hair, nails, and the condition of his teeth and mouth. She notes the therapeutic care plans for the individual. Is he going to have to remain in bed for a long period? Are there restrictions on his position in bed? Is he receiving medications that may be causing problems with his skin condition? Are there necessary treatments that could potentially cause skin irritation or damage to skin tissues? Is the patient incontinent? Is he perspiring profusely? These are some of the questions the nurse asks herself.

The nurse also needs information about the individual's usual hygiene habits (see

---

[8]Reitz and Pope, op cit.

Chapter 9), and his attitude towards cleanliness and grooming. Are these important to him?

The nurse can obtain much information about the patient's usual hygiene practices from the nursing history, and about the current status of his skin, hair, nails, teeth, and mouth from the initial clinical appraisal. Information about the patient's motor and nutritional status should also be available from these sources. None of this information, however, substitutes for the nurse's own observations.

Information about the patient's past and current health problems, and the therapeutic plan of care for him, will be found on the patient's record. From this source the nurse can obtain data on medications prescribed for the patient and restrictions on his mobility, as well as on the nature of his illness and treatments prescribed for him.

The nurse often contacts nursing personnel about the status of the patient's skin and appendages, such as other nurses, nursing orderlies, or attendants. Observations made by the nurse herself in her assessment, and those made by other members of the nursing team, should always be communicated both orally and in writing to all other nursing personnel caring for the patient. The first sign of redness over bony prominences or of breaks in the skin should be reported promptly so that adequate steps can be taken to prevent deterioration of the skin tissues.

The patient is also, of course, a good source of information about the condition of his skin, provided that he is able to communicate. Pain is one of the body's warning signs that tissues are being damaged. Discomfort (which may increase to actual pain), heat (which the patient may describe as a warm feeling or a burning sensation), and redness (as noted above) in any area of the body are all early warning signs of potential tissue breakdown. The patient may be the first one to notice some of these signs.

The nurse also learns from the patient the details of his particular preferences and habits with respect to hygiene and personal grooming. Each person has his own idiosyncrasies about the way he likes to take his bath, the times to clean his teeth, the kind of soap to use, the way to comb his hair, and many other small details of bathing and grooming. Attention to these small details can contribute immeasurably to the patient's feelings of comfort and well-being.

The patient's family (or significant others in his life) can often help the nurse to learn about the patient's usual habits and preferences in regard to hygiene and grooming. They are also usually very observant of the condition of the patient's skin (they worry about him) and are also often very helpful in assisting patients with many details of personal hygiene and grooming. They may like to take care of helping the male patient with shaving, for example, or fixing the hair of the female patient. This gives family members a feeling that they, too, are doing something for the patient, which helps to assuage some of the helplessness they often feel as visitors, and possibly some guilt feelings they may have about having to turn over the care of their loved one to someone else.

Older people, however, are sometimes reluctant to have their children do things for them; it is a reversal of roles that is sometimes very difficult to accept.

PRIORITIES FOR NURSING ACTION

Patients who need help in carrying out hygiene measures are the nurse's most important priority. Serious problems can develop if basic skin care and oral hygiene are not attended to on a regular, planned schedule. As with problems in mobility, *prevention* is the priority. Deterioration of the condition of the patient's skin and the condition of his mouth can develop very rapidly, sometimes with little forewarning. Repair of the damage is a slow process that entails much discomfort and suffering on the patient's part and much work on the nurses' part—work that could have been avoided if simple precautionary measures had been taken.

PRINCIPLES RELEVANT TO HYGIENE

The nurse may find the following principles helpful in guiding her selection and implementation of appropriate interventions in the care of patients who need help with personal hygiene.

1. The intact skin is the body's first line of defense against infection and against injury.
2. Individual differences exist in the nature of the skin and its appendages.
3. Changes occur throughout the life span in the skin, the mucous membranes, the hair, the nails, and the teeth.
4. The health of the skin and mucous membranes is highly dependent on adequate nourishment, fluid intake, and exercise.
5. A person's general health affects both the status of his skin and appendages, teeth, and mouth, and his ability to look after his own hygiene.
6. Hygiene practices are learned.
7. Hygienic practices vary with cultural norms, personal idiosyncrasies and values, and the ability to maintain good habits of cleanliness and grooming.
8. The ability to look after one's own hygiene is an important independent function in older children and adults.
9. The skin and its appendages may be affected by drugs and other forms of therapeutic treatment.

GOALS FOR NURSING ACTION

The goals of nursing action with regard to the patient's hygiene are basically four:
1. To maintain good hygiene in respect to bathing, mouth care, and the care of nails and hair
2. To maintain the integrity of the skin
3. To maintain the skin tissues in good condition
4. To maintain the teeth and soft tissues in the oral cavity in good condition

SPECIFIC NURSING INTERVENTIONS

A regular schedule of basic hygiene measures for all patients is established on most nursing units in inpatient health agencies. These usually include morning and evening care, and a daily bath. For patients requiring additional skin and mouth care, interventions are planned on an individual basis as part of their total nursing care plan.

General Morning Care

Before breakfast is served, patients are usually awakened. They are offered a bedpan or urinal, or assisted to the bathroom if they can get up. Each patient who must remain in bed is provided with the necessary materials for washing his hands and face and for mouth care, and assisted with these activities if he requires help. The patient is then helped to prepare for his meal—that is, his bed is straightened, he is assisted to the most comfortable position for eating, and a place is prepared for his tray.

General Evening Care

The evening care routine is somewhat similar in that the patient is offered a bedpan or urinal (or assisted to the bathroom), and is given the opportunity to wash his hands and face and clean his teeth. In many agencies, the bed patient's back is washed and a back massage is given as

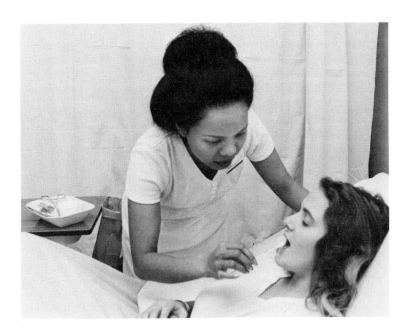

Good oral hygiene is essential for the patient's comfort.

part of the evening routine. As we mentioned in the last chapter, a back massage is beneficial for all patients prior to bedtime, not just those who are confined to bed. The nurse makes sure that the foundation of the patient's bed is clean and free from wrinkles, crumbs, and so forth. The bottom sheet and drawsheet (if one is used) are tightened, and top bedclothes straightened and tucked in. If the patient needs an extra blanket, this is put in place. The patient's bed is placed in the position the patient finds most comfortable for sleeping (unless otherwise specified), he is assisted to his most comfortable position and his pillows fluffed and arranged to his preference. Siderails, if they are needed, are put up on *both* sides of the bed. The call signal is put within easy reach, and any other items the patient feels he wants near at hand, such as a clock, his jug of water, and a glass, are placed within easy reach on his bedside table.

Mouth Care

Oral care includes regular care by dental professionals as well as adequate cleansing of the teeth. Brushing the teeth removes food particles that provide a likely medium for bacterial growth. Brushing also massages the gums and stimulates circulation. It helps to keep the tongue, mucous membranes lining the mouth, and the lips moist as well as clean. A clean, fresh taste in the mouth is important in the desire for and the enjoyment of food. Thus, good oral hygiene helps to promote good nutritional status.

Most people brush their teeth at least twice a day, in the morning and before going to bed. Many dentists advocate brushing the teeth after every meal or at least rinsing the mouth after food is taken. These measures help to prevent the accumulation of food particles on and between the teeth, which predisposes to dental caries. Patients usually bring their own toothbrushes and their own dentifrice with them to hospital. If they do not, they should be provided with a brush and toothpaste or other substance to use. A mixture of salt and sodium bicarbonate flavored with peppermint has been recommended as an inexpensive and effective substitute for toothpaste.[9] Many agencies now are using disposable toothbrushes for patient use.

---

[9] Reitz and Pope, op. cit., p. 1730.

If a patient cannot brush his teeth himself the nurse assists him. When brushing teeth, it has been recommended that the brush should be moved from the gum to the crown of the tooth. This motion is carried out on both the inner and outer aspects of the teeth. The procedure is easier if the lips are pulled back with one hand and the brush is held in the other.[10] This is just one method. Currently, there is much debate over how the teeth should be brushed.

Mouth care is also essential for patients with artificial dentures. Usually the patient with dentures prefers to take them out and clean them himself with a dentifrice and water, then to rinse his mouth before reinserting the dentures. A mouthwash is often refreshing to these patients. If a person cannot remove his own dentures, the nurse can remove and clean them for him. Care should be taken in removing dentures, in handling them while cleaning, and in storing them. Dentures are expensive articles; their replacement takes time; and the person who wears them is uncomfortable without them. He cannot eat anything that has to be chewed, he finds speech difficult, and he often is embarrassed to be seen without a full complement of teeth.

In removing dentures, it is usually easier to remove the upper plate first, grasping it between thumb and forefinger and wiggling it slightly to break the vacuum that holds it to the roof of the mouth. It is placed in a container and the lower plate is then removed. This plate usually slides out easily but may be difficult to remove if the person uses a dental adherent substance. If it does not come out easily it can be loosened by lifting upon the lower edge and gently wriggling it. For washing, it is safer to put the plates in a basin full of water than to wash them under the tap. The plates are often slippery and hard to hold. They can easily fall from the nurse's hands while being washed. Sinks are made of hard substances which can damage the dentures if they slip out of the nurse's hands. The teeth should be brushed with a dentifrice and rinsed with cold water. Care should

be taken not to use water that is too hot on dentures; they may crack or become misshapen. Since many people remove them at night, a container should be provided for the safe storage of dentures when they are not in use. Agencies often have a special container for this purpose; it should be labeled with the patient's name, hospital, and bed number. Dentures are one of the most frequently lost articles in a hospital, and precautions should be taken for safeguarding them.

Patients whose food and fluid intake is restricted, either because of NPO orders, or because they are unable to eat and drink sufficiently (as, for example very weak patients and those who are unconscious), require mouth care at frequent intervals (q4h and as indicated is usually recommended) to keep the tongue, teeth, gums, and mucous membranes lining the oral cavity clean, moist, and in good condition, and the lips from drying out and cracking. If the patient is able to use it, chewing gum is helpful in stimulating the secretion of the salivary glands and keeping the mouth moist. Rinsing the mouth is another means of providing moisture without violating imposed restrictions. Sometimes the patient is permitted to suck ice chips, but permission for the patient to do so must be obtained from the physician.

If ordinary oral hygiene is not feasible, the mouth and teeth must be cleaned by other means. Although cotton-tipped applicators soaked in a glycerine and lemon solution have traditionally been used for this purpose, it is now held by some authorities that the teeth *must be brushed* for the cleansing to be adequate and for gingivitis to be prevented. Rinsing of the mouth before brushing helps to remove food particles that have accumulated; rinsing after brushing is essential. If the patient is unable to do this himself, an Asepto syringe may be used. If the person cannot spit out the material, it must be removed by suction, so that it is not aspirated into the respiratory tract.

In some agencies, gauze sponges may be wrapped around a tongue depressor and used for cleaning the mouth. Both the cotton-tipped applicators and the tongue depressors are hazardous when used with

---

[10] Ibid.

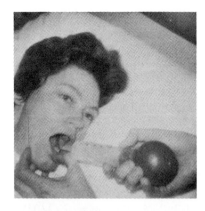

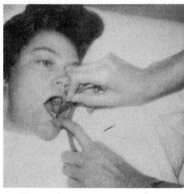

For the patient who cannot rinse her mouth, an Asepto syringe can be used to help remove food debris. And for the person who cannot expectorate, suction is used. (From Marie Reitz and Wilma Pope: Mouth Care. © October, 1973. The American Journal of Nursing Company. Reproduced with permission from The American Journal of Nursing, Vol. 73, No. 10.)

patients who may chew on them or bite off the end that is in the mouth. There is also the danger of injuring the delicate mucous membranes if hard objects are used for cleansing inside the mouth. Sometimes gauze is wrapped around the fingers to clean the mouth and this lessens the danger of injuring tissues. Great care must always be taken in cleansing the mouth of a patient to avoid injuring the mucous membranes.

Petrolatum substances sold commercially for chapped or dry lips can be used to lubricate the lips.

The Patient's Bath

Bathing has several purposes: It cleanses and it promotes comfort. Bathing

also stimulates blood circulation and affords an opportunity to exercise. When a nurse assists a patient to bathe she has an opportunity to incorporate the teaching of desirable hygienic measures and other health teaching as needed. In addition, she has an opportunity to assess the status of his skin and appendages, his motor status, and his nutritional, circulatory, and respiratory status; she may also observe his status in relation to comfort, rest, and sleep. For example, during the bath is a good time to observe the condition of the patient's skin, nails, and hair and to note such factors as the presence of edema, the quality of respirations, and any difficulty or pain the patient has on moving.

It is also a good time to assess the patient's mental and emotional status. Many patients find it much easier to talk to the nurse when she is assisting them with their bath than at other times. Davis suggests that the reason for this is that the act of giving physical care is perceived by many patients as caring about them.[11] Thus, the bath provides an excellent opportunity for the nurse to establish rapport with the patient and facilitate communication between patient and nurse.[12]

The hospital patient may have a bed bath, a tub bath, or a shower. The type of bath that a person can have is often prescribed. The decision is based not only on the amount of activity involved but also on the specific problems of the individual. For example, a patient who has had a recent abdominal operation will probably not have a tub bath or shower until his incision is healed, because of the danger of getting it wet and contaminated. (To contaminate is to soil or make unclean.) Both the tub bath and the shower require more activity on the part of the patient than a bath in bed.

In the bed bath, the nurse may give the entire bath to the patient, or the patient may participate within the limits of his physical condition. Patients usually prefer to help themselves as much as possible and should be encouraged to do so. This

[11]Ellen D. Davis: Giving a Bath? *American Journal of Nursing*, 70:2366–2367, November 1970.
[12]Ibid. See also Virginia Henderson: *Basic Principles of Nursing Care*. New York, S. Karger, 1969, pp. 33–35.

provides an opportunity to exercise muscles and stimulate blood circulation, and gives the patient a feeling of accomplishment and increasing independence.

It is believed by many, however, that the nurse should be careful to retain some aspects of assisting the patient with personal hygiene. If she does not, she loses a valuable time for free and spontaneous talk with the patient, for which other opportunities must be found.[13]

Not all patients require a bath every day while they are in hospital; nor is it necessary for all patients to receive a bath in the morning. For the patient who tires very easily or who is very ill, the bath may be contraindicated. The older person's skin will often become overly dry if he bathes too frequently. For these people as well as for other patients who do not require complete bed baths, a partial bath is indicated. This includes washing the patient's hands and back, axilla and perineal area, as well as providing for oral hygiene and massaging bony prominences. The nurse makes these judgments based upon the needs of the patient and her assessment of the situation.

The Bed Bath. The equipment required for the bed bath includes bath towels, wash cloths, a water basin, and soap. A bath blanket is also required to cover the patient so as to avoid embarrassing exposure and to keep him warm. The kind of soap used will depend largely on the individual needs of the patient and on the policy of the health agency. Some institutions permit patients to use their own soap; others prefer that the patient use the soap provided by the agency. Many agencies have their own particular procedure for giving a patient a bed bath. One suggestion is as follows:

1. Offer the patient a bedpan or urinal
2. Provide for oral hygiene
3. Remove the upper bedclothes
4. Cover the patient with a bath blanket
5. Bathe the patient
6. Cut fingernails and toenails if needed
7. Remake the bed

Guiding Principles for the Bed Bath
Heat is conveyed from the body by the *convection of air currents.* Care should be taken not to expose the body surface unduly. Drafts are to be avoided and the patient should be kept warm during his bath. The nurse can close the windows of the patient's room if it is cool outside or if there is any danger of a draft. The bed unit is screened for privacy, the patient's spread and blanket are removed, and a bath blanket is placed over the patient. The top sheet is then slipped out from under the bath blanket to prevent exposing the patient unnecessarily. The patient then removes his gown. Dirty linen should be placed in a container (dirty linen hamper) as soon after it is removed from the bed as possible. Agency procedures vary in this regard, but it is generally accepted that bed linen is a potential source of infection and suitable precautions are taken in handling it.

People differ in their tolerance of heat. Most patients require bath water between 43.3° C. to 46.1° C. (110° F. and 115° F.). Water at this temperature is comfortable to most patients and it does not injure skin or mucous membranes. Water at 50° C. (120° F.) in the basin will cool to the safe temperature range by the time it comes in contact with the patient's skin. The nurse collects the equipment and takes it to the patient's bedside before she gets the water so that the water does not cool too much before it is used. It may be necessary to add additional hot water during the procedure, or to change the water. Patients who are particularly sensitive to heat may require cooler water.

The skin is sometimes irritated by the chemical composition of certain soaps. Soap can be irritating to a patient's skin and particularly to his eyes. Therefore patients are often advised not to use soap on their faces.

Long smooth strokes on the arms and legs that are directed from the distal to the proximal increase the rate of venous flow. Distal means farther from the point of attachment; proximal means closer to the point of attachment. For example, the hand is distal to the elbow.

Moving the body joints through their full range of motion helps to prevent loss of muscle tone and improves circulation. The nurse can use the bed bath as an op-

---

[13]Davis, ibid.

portunity to help the patient to put his joints through their full range of motion (see Chapter 17).

The following order is suggested for bathing the patient

1. Eyes—inner to outer canthus (no soap)
2. Face
3. Arms, hands, and axilla
4. Chest and breasts
5. Abdomen
6. Legs
7. Back and buttocks
8. Perineal area
9. Rectal area

When bathing the patient, the nurse folds the wash cloth in such a way that the corners are folded on the palm of the hand to form a pad.

Only the area being washed should be exposed. This lessens the patient's embarrassment and helps him keep warm. Each area of the skin is dried immediately after it has been washed and rinsed and before the next area of the body is exposed.

If the patient soaks his hands and feet in the basin of water he will feel more refreshed. This practice also serves to soften the patient's nails so that they can be easily cut and cleaned. The pan of water should not be too full or the water may spill when the hands or feet are immersed. Washing the patient's back is best done with the patient lying on his abdomen. If this is impossible the patient can turn to one side while the nurse washes the other side of his back and then can reverse his position. A back massage is given after the back is washed and dried.

The nurse should take special care to wash, rinse, and dry well the creases in the patient's skin and to massage bony prominences. These areas are particularly prone to irritation. The body skin creases become excoriated if they remain moist; the bony prominences are irritated by constant friction and pressure against the bedclothes. Excoriation is the superficial loss of skin substance. Also, the areas that bear the weight of the patient while he is in bed are prone to irritation.

The patient's skin is then dried well. Skin that remains wet over a long period is uncomfortable and becomes irritated.

Usually patients prefer to wash the genital areas themselves, if they are able to do so. If, however, they are not able, the nurse does this for them. In some agencies, when the patient is male and the nurse female, the nursing orderly is asked to assist the patient. In some situations, however, the nurse may have to undertake this part of the bath for the male patient. In doing so, the nurse uses a washcloth or towel to hold the genitals while she washes between the folds of the body with another washcloth. The genitals are washed as with other parts of the body, rinsed, and dried.

The Tub Bath. Tub baths are taken for hygienic and therapeutic reasons. The physician may order a therapeutic bath for some patients as, for example, hip baths for the patient who has had rectal surgery. Patients with skin diseases often have oatmeal or medicated baths. Various types of therapeutic baths are discussed in Chapter 25. Aside from these therapeutic measures, a tub bath is most often a hygienic measure enjoyed by most people.

Bathtubs in hospitals frequently have rails, or the adjacent wall is equipped with handles to help the patient climb in and out of the tub. Most tubs also now have safety strips on the bottom which help to prevent slipping. No sick person should lock himself into the bathroom unattended; he may require help. The nurse or attendant should know when a patient is bathing, and often it is wise to check that he is all right. If a patient is out of bed for the first time after even a few days of bed rest, it is generally unwise to leave him alone in the bath; an attendant can stay just outside the curtains if the patient prefers privacy.

The bathtub is filled one-third full of water. Unless otherwise ordered, the water is drawn at 40 to 41° C. (105° F.), a comfortable and safe temperature for most people. The length of time that a person bathes depends upon his endurance and strength. If the bath is too lengthy, it may fatigue him unnecessarily. A very hot bath will cause the blood to be diverted away from the vital centers of the brain to the surface areas of the body; as a result he may feel faint and lose consciousness.

A

B

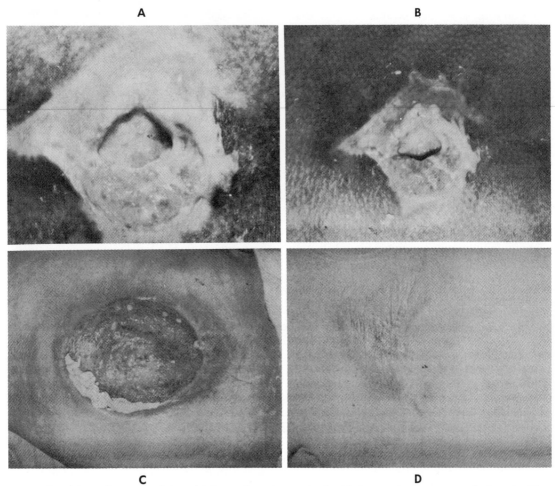

C

D

A, A decubitus ulcer, on a hip, which needs to be packed with benzoyl, 20 per cent lotion. B, The same decubitus ulcer as in A, after 4 weeks of treatment with benzoyl lotion. C, Severe decubitus ulcer on buttocks area. Note packing in lower left area of the ulcer. D, Same decubitus ulcer as in C. This ulcer completely healed after treatment. (Reprinted with permission from The Canadian Nurse, Vol. 69, No. 10, October 1973.)

Getting into and out of the bathtub is often a difficult maneuver, and the patient may need assistance from the nurse. Usually it is easier if the patient first sits on the edge of the tub with his feet inside the tub, then reaches over to grasp the rail on the other side and gradually eases himself down. In helping the patient out of the tub, it is a good practice to let the water out before the patient attempts to stand up. There are many mechanical devices available today for assisting with the tub bath procedures. A mechanical lift (or hoist), for example, can be used in either hospital or home situations. The use of a shower stool, so that the patient can sit while having a shower, is another solution to the bath problem.

Decubitus Ulcers

Decubitus ulcers (bedsores, pressure sores) are areas from which the skin has sloughed. These sores may develop in persons who are ill in bed for a long period of time, especially if the patient is unable to move about freely, or they may occur in people who sit in wheelchairs for several hours at a time. They occur as a result of prolonged pressure on one part of the body with resultant loss of circulation to the area and subsequent tissue destruction. Although decubitus ulcers may occur in any patient, if there is sufficient pressure on one area to cause ischemia, they are seen most frequently in individuals with poor nutritional status, especially if there is a negative nitrogen balance. They are most often seen on the bony prominences of the body. If decubitus ulcers are not treated, they quickly increase in size and become very painful. Secondary infection often complicates the picture.

The conditions that predispose to decubitus ulcers include continuous pressure on one area, dampness, a break in the skin surface, poor nutrition, dehydration, poor blood circulation, thinness (bony prominences unprotected by adipose tissue), and the presence of pathogenic bacteria. Early signs of a decubitus ulcer include redness and tenderness of an area. The patient usually complains of a burning sensation. Other early warning signs include coldness of an area and the presence of edema. Unless special measures are taken at this time to relieve pressure and increase local tissue nourishment, a break in the patient's skin usually follows. The sore then increases in depth and the tissue gradually sloughs off. Decubitus ulcers are difficult to cure; some require surgical intervention. Consequently, preventive measures are always indicated.

There are many nursing care measures that can be employed in order to prevent decubitus ulcers. Frequent changes in position to rotate the weight-bearing areas relieve pressure on any single group of bony prominences. The normal healthy individual shifts his body position every few minutes. For the patient who is unable to do this himself, it is the nurse's responsibility to see that his position is changed. A regular schedule should be set up for turning the patient as often as necessary to keep the skin in good condition. Usual recommendations are every 2 hours and as needed.

Massage and exercise stimulate circulation and thus improve the nourishment to the cells of the skin. Keeping the skin dry and clean inhibits the growth of disease-producing bacteria and prevents skin from becoming excoriated; body secretions and excreta are particularly irritating to a patient's skin. The nurse should take particular care that a patient's linen and dressings are dry and clean. In areas where secretions cannot be prevented, protective ointments, such as zinc oxide or petrolatum, can be used to prevent excessive irritation.

Another preventive measure for decubitus ulcers is the use of devices to relieve pressure on specific areas of the patient's body. An overbed cradle will keep bedclothes off the patient, and other aids such as alternating pressure mattresses, oscillating beds, and fluidized air or water mattresses may also be used. Many hospitals use a special bed frame, which permits the patient to be turned easily. Another measure which has been found helpful in the prevention of decubitus ulcers is the use of sheepskin under pressure areas. It is considered preferable to use the whole skin, but small pads have been found effective in protecting areas such as the heels or elbows of the patient.[14] These woolskins are being used extensively in many hospitals and nursing homes. They are particularly helpful in home situations where expensive mechanical devices may not be available.

Attention to the patient's nutritional status is essential. Since decubitus ulcers occur most frequently in patients with a negative nitrogen balance, the protein intake should be increased. Foods which contain complete proteins, such as eggs, milk, and meat, are recommended. The proteins are needed for the regeneration of body tissue. Usually, supplementary amounts of vitamin C are prescribed also because of the role of this vitamin in the healing process. Care must be taken also that an adequate fluid intake is maintained. Dehydration results in poor tissue turgor, which is another predisposing factor in the development of decubitus ulcers.

When a decubitus ulcer develops, the nurse faces a challenge in curative nursing care. The outside area of the decubitus ulcer is often less extensive than the inside area. The preventive measures just mentioned can be employed therapeutically and, in addition, the application of dry heat, such as that from an infrared lamp, increases circulation to the area and

---

[14]Miriam A. Brownlowe, Florence R. Cohen, and William E. Happich: New Washable Woolskins. *American Journal of Nursing*, 70:2368–2370, November 1970.

dries secretions. The latter measure is generally ordered by the physician. Decubitus ulcers are prone to infection by bacteria; the moist, poorly nourished tissue provides a good medium for the growth of pathogenic bacteria. The use of aseptic technique in the care of an infected ulcer prevents secondary infection and the transfer of bacteria to other areas of the body and to other patients.

A therapeutic regimen for the care of the patient who has a decubitus ulcer is planned. Antiseptic solutions, soap and water, and antibiotic creams have all been advocated at one time or another. Sometimes it is necessary to graft skin over a decubitus ulcer. Ulcers are very difficult to cure; the best nursing care is prevention.

Hair Care

Care of the patient's hair is important to both his grooming and his sense of well-being. As part of the daily toilet each patient's hair needs to be brushed and combed. Thorough brushing stimulates circulation to the scalp and improves the nourishment of the epithelium. Most patients can attend to this themselves, but the nurse may have to assume the responsibility for the aged or very ill patient.

The nurse, by seeing to daily care of the hair, can ensure that the patient's hair does not become matted. Often, long hair is braided so that it will stay neatly in place and make the patient feel more comfortable. Patients who are in the hospital for some length of time may want a shampoo. Permission for this may have to be obtained from the physician in some agencies. For the patient who is out of bed a shampoo is no problem. The sink in his room or the shower bath affords facilities for hair washing.

If a patient must remain in a supine position, however, the shampoo is given while he is in bed or on a stretcher. If a stretcher is used, it is best to move the patient to a sink and support his head on the edge of the sink. If it is necessary for the patient to remain in bed, then the nurse can use a folded plastic sheet or a specially constructed waterproof pad to direct the water from the patient's hair into a pail. The nurse uses pitchers of water, taking precautions to keep the patient's bed dry. The patient's hair needs to be dried quickly after the shampoo in order to avoid chilling. Most hospitals have hair dryers for this purpose. Many brands of dry shampoo are now available, and these may be used for patients whose condition contraindicates a regular shampoo.

Today many large hospitals have hair dressing and barber services for patients. Often the patient will request the services of the barber or the hairdresser, and the nurse then makes arrangements. The nurse is usually responsible for telling the patient what services are available and what charges are made for them.

Shaving the Male Patient. Male patients usually feel better when they are shaved. If the male patient cannot shave himself the nurse may be asked to do this for him. If the patient has an electric razor this is no problem, but a safety razor requires more skill. Very warm water is needed to give an adequate shave. After the skin has been lathered with shaving soap, the skin is held tautly and the razor is drawn over the skin in short strokes. The nurse will find that the safest way to shave the patient is to stretch the skin over the bone in a particular area and then to shave in the direction in which the hair is growing. Areas around the mouth and nose are particularly sensitive; in these areas the nurse's motions need to be firm but gentle. After the patient has been shaved he will likely prefer a shaving lotion for his skin. Most shaving lotions are refreshing and have a slightly antiseptic effect.

After a shave, the male patient will not only look better but he will also in all probability feel better. Relatives are often reassured when the male patient is well groomed, chiefly because this is the way they are accustomed to seeing him.

Many women are accustomed to shaving the hair in the axilla and to removing superfluous hair from their faces and legs. Opportunity should be provided for them to maintain these practices while they are ill if they so desire. Women are usually particularly sensitive about unwanted hairs on the chin and upper lip. A number of good depilatory creams are available. These preparations should be used with caution, however, because they are irritating to the skin and many people cannot tolerate them. Tweezers may be used instead to remove facial hairs.

Nail Care

Care of the nails is another area of grooming that most patients can attend to themselves. For the very ill patient or the patient who has difficulty in moving, however, nail care may be the nurse's responsibility. Often nail polish is not advised for a patient because the physician or the nurse may want to check the color of the tissue underneath the nails. This is particularly true for patients who are to undergo surgery. Most hospitals prohibit the use of colored nail polish for these patients.

The responsibility for cleaning and trimming the nails of patients who are unable to do this themselves usually falls to the nurse. Toenails are cut straight across, fingernails in an oval shape. Many people prefer that their fingernails be filed rather than cut so that they can be shaped attractively. For patients who are particularly prone to infection—for example, patients with diabetes mellitus or circulatory problems—it is advisable that the nurse not cut the toenails herself for fear of injuring the skin or cuticle around the nail.

To prevent hangnails, it is best to keep the cuticle of the nail pushed well back and lubricated with oil. Some patients have very hard fingernails and horny toenails. If the patient soaks his feet for 10 to 15 minutes in warm water, the nails will soften sufficiently so that they can be cut with nail cutters. Special nail clippers are available which are particularly helpful in cutting thick toenails. If the nails are too thick and difficult to cut, the services of a podiatrist (foot specialist) should be obtained.

Eye Care

Nursing care also involves the care of the eyes. On occasion the nurse will be called on to help a patient to care for his eyes when they have become irritated or infected. The physician usually orders a special solution to cleanse the eyes. Tap water or normal saline is also used. With absorbent cotton dipped in the solution, the eye is wiped from the inner canthus to the outer canthus. The nurse uses a clean piece of cotton each time she wipes the eye. Water or normal saline will soften crusts so they are easily removed. The motion from the inner to the outer canthus washes the discharge away from the nasal lacrimal duct, which is located on the inner aspect of the orbit of the eye.

Unconscious patients require special attention to protect their eyes from damage. The upper and lower lids should be kept clean and free from discharge. The lids should be closed when the patient is being turned to prevent scratching of the cornea.

Patients' glasses, contact lenses, and other prostheses should be looked after carefully and the patient assisted with their care if he is unable to care for them.

Care of Patients with Pediculosis

Occasionally a patient will be found to have pediculosis (infestation with lice). His care involves killing and removing all the pediculi (lice) and their eggs (nits) that have infested the skin, hair, and clothing. There are three main types of pediculosis: pediculosis capitis or infestation of the scalp with lice, pediculosis corporis or infestation with body lice, and pediculosis pubis or infestation of the pubic hair with lice. There are several methods of ridding patients of pediculi. For body lice, the patient's clothing is removed for washing or cleaning and the patient is usually given a cleansing bath. Then drugs, such as gamma benzene hexachloride, are applied. The treatment is repeated after 12 hours and again on the next two days. Usually three days of treatment are sufficient to overcome this infestation. In the case of head lice, or if the body lice have infected the scalp, Kwell shampoo is often used for treatment.[15] Infested pa-

---

[15]Mary W. Falconer et al.: *The Drug, the Nurse, the Patient.* 5th edition. Philadelphia, W. B. Saunders Company, 1974, p. 390–391.

tients are often separated from other patients for 24 hours after treatment has been initiated to avoid spreading the pediculi. The treatment is repeated until pediculi cannot be found on the patient.

Pediculi are spread by direct contact and through vehicles such as clothing, eating utensils, and combs. Pediculi are usually found in environments where poor hygienic measures are practiced.

PLANNING AND EVALUATING SPECIFIC NURSING INTERVENTIONS

Nursing interventions to ensure that the patient's skin and its appendages, hair, fingernails and toenails, and teeth and mouth are kept clean and in good condition are planned as an essential part of the nursing care of every patient. Basic hygiene measures are normally a part of the nursing care plans for all patients on the nursing units of inpatient agencies. If the patient requires help in carrying out these measures, or if these need to be modified in any way, this is drawn to the attention of all nursing personnel through notations on the patient's nursing care plan. A regular schedule outlining specific instructions is developed for those patients requiring additional skin or mouth care. A flow sheet may be helpful in this regard, in addition to incorporating the directions on the care plan. When writing the schedule out, space should be left for the initialing of each intervention as it is done, to ensure that the required care is carried out as planned. The nurse notes her observations in the progress notes of the patient's record.

For patients who need help in acquiring good hygiene habits, a teaching plan is incorporated into the nursing care plan. Much of the teaching may be done while carrying out specific nursing interventions, such as in the bed bath. Because personal hygiene is a very personal matter, tact is needed in this teaching, and care taken that the patient's self-esteem is protected in the process. Putting the teaching in terms of promoting optimal health and including an explanation of the reasons for the development and maintenance of good hygiene practices help to put the teaching on a more objective, less personal basis.

The expected outcomes of nursing interventions are often expressed in terms of prevention of potential problems, and specific criteria are given concerning the state of the skin and its appendages, or the oral cavity, that is to be maintained or restored. An expected outcome for the potential problem of poor mouth condition might be that the patient's lips and tongue are moist and normal tissue turgor of the mucous membranes is maintained at all times.

Successful nursing interventions are evidenced in the healthy state of the patient's skin, hair, nails, and mouth. Continuous reassessment of the status of all of these is required. The poor condition of any is a sad reflection on the nursing care the patient has received.

GUIDE TO ASSESSING STATUS OF THE SKIN, ITS APPENDAGES, THE TEETH, AND THE MOUTH	1. What is the condition of the patient's skin, hair, teeth, and nails? Is the skin clear, intact, warm to the touch? Did you notice any abnormalities with regard to color, blemishes, temperature, breaks in the integrity of the skin, poor tissue turgor? Is the hair clean, well-groomed, and in good condition? Are the nails clean and in good condition?
	2. What did you observe about the patient's lips, tongue, gums, and teeth? Did you notice any abnormalities such as dryness or cracking of the lips? a furry coating on the tongue? a film on the teeth, or tartar? food particles and mucus in the mouth or around the teeth? Are the mucous membranes pink, or are they red and inflamed? Are the gums swollen and inflamed? receding from the teeth? Is

there any bleeding in the mouth? Are the teeth in good condition? Are there missing teeth? caries? Does the patient wear dentures?

3. What are patient's usual habits with regard to hygiene practices?
4. Does the patient need help in maintaining his hygiene? What is his motor status in this regard? Is he weak, helpless, or unconscious?
5. Does he have a health problem(s) that may be affecting the status of his skin and appendages? that interferes with his ability to maintain his own hygiene?
6. Is he receiving medications or other therapy that may affect the status of the skin or its appendages?
7. Does he require additional skin or mouth care over and above the usual hygiene measures?
8. How old is the patient?
9. Are there any signs of body or head lice?

STUDY VOCABULARY

Calculus (tartar)	Enamel	Mucous membrane
Cerumen	Epidermis	Pediculosis
Cementum	Excoriation	Perspiration
Ceruminous	Gingival	Plaque
Contaminate	Halitosis	Sebaceous
Dandruff	Hygiene	Sebum
Dermis	Keratin	Sordes
Distal	Mastication	

STUDY SITUATION

Mr. Charles Rose, who was admitted to hospital yesterday for investigative procedures, has been assigned to your care. He is a 32 year old bachelor and has been working on a trapline in the north woods for the past two years. He lives alone in a remote cabin, coming into town only occasionally to replenish his supplies, which consist mainly of canned and dried foods. The cabin does not have electricity or running water; it is heated by a wood stove and Mr. Rose has to fetch his water from a stream a quarter of a mile away.

He spends several days at a time out in the woods inspecting his lines, with only his dog for company. He tells you he hit his head two or three weeks ago on a fallen tree trunk when he was straightening up after looking at a trap one day. He hasn't been feeling too well since, and has had headaches of increasing severity, so he went to the doctor in town, who admitted him to hospital. You notice that Mr. Rose is thin, his skin is dry, and he has some lesions on his arms and legs; his long hair is matted, his nails are dirty and chipped, and his teeth and fingers are stained with nicotine. The physician has ordered bed rest for Mr. Rose.

1. What problems can you identify relative to Mr. Rose's hygiene? to the status of his skin, its appendages, and the teeth?
2. What factors do you think contributed to these problems?
3. What principles would assist you in planning hygiene measures for Mr. Rose?
4. What specific nursing interventions would you plan?
5. What would be the expected outcomes of these interventions?

Mr. Rose's condition deteriorates over the next few days; he appears to be very weak and drowsy. The physician and a neurosurgeon who has been called in are contemplating surgery.

6. What additional nursing interventions would you plan for Mr. Rose with regard to hygiene?
7. How would you evaluate the effectiveness of your interventions?

SUGGESTED READINGS

Barrett, D., Jr., et al.: Collagenase Debridement. *American Journal of Nursing,* 73:849–851, May 1973.

Berecek, K. H.: Etiology of Decubitus Ulcers. *Nursing Clinics of North America,* 10:157–210, March 1975.

Brown, M. S., and M. M. Alexander: Physical Examination, Part 3: Examining the Skin. *Nursing, '73,* 3:39–43, 1973.

Carbary, L. J.: Foot Problems. *Nursing Care,* 8:10–14, June 1975.

DeWalt, E. M.: Effect of Timed Hygienic Measures on Oral Mucosa in a Group of Elderly Subjects. *Nursing Research,* 24:104–108, March-April 1975.

Don't Lose Your Head Over Hair Care. *Family Health,* 8:43–44, April 1976.

Greene, R.: Ostomy Skin Barriers for Decubitus Ulcers. *Canadian Nurse,* 71:34–35, February 1975.

Greenleaf, J., et al.: Portable Shower for Bed Patients. *American Journal of Nursing,* 74:2021, November 1974.

Lang, C., et al.: Gelfoam for Decubitus Ulcers. *American Journal of Nursing,* 74:460–461, March 1974.

Roach, L. B.: Assessing Skin Changes: The Subtle and the Obvious. *Nursing '74,* 4:64–67, 1974.

Shiery, S.: Insight Into the Delicate Art of Eye Care. *Nursing '75,* 5:50–56, June 1975.

Torelli, M.: Topical Hyperbaric Oxygen for Decubitus Ulcers. *American Journal of Nursing,* 73:494–496, March 1973.

Wallace, G., et al.: Karaya for Chronic Skin Ulcers. *American Journal of Nursing,* 74:1094–1098, June 1974.

Wilson, R.: The MUD Bed and Its Implications for Nursing Care. *Nursing Clinics of North America,* 11:725–730, December 1976.

Yentzer, M., et al.: Conquering Those Obstinate Decubiti. Foam Leg Supports . . . the Screen Box. *Nursing '75,* 5:24–25, March 1975.

CHAPTER 20

Safety Needs

20 SAFETY NEEDS

The nurse should be able to:

Discuss the nurse's role in protecting against environmental
    hazards
Identify factors affecting a person's ability to protect himself from
    environmental hazards
Identify existing and potential environmental hazards for ill
    people
Apply relevant principles in selecting planning and implementing
    safety precautions for ill persons
Take appropriate action in emergency situations to protect the
    safety of ill persons
Evaluate the effectiveness of nursing interventions

INTRODUCTION

As with so many other aspects of her role today, the nurse's responsibilities with regard to environmental safety are rapidly expanding. Time was when the nurse thought only in terms of protecting the sick person from hazards in his immediate environment. Today, however, nurses, as informed and knowledgeable health professionals, are concerned with health hazards in the communities in which they live and work. They are taking action and making their voices heard, both individually and collectively, through their professional associations, to make the environment more conducive to healthy living. Local, state (provincial), and national nursing associations are expressing their concerns about air pollution, the pollution of our rivers, lakes, and coastal waters, highway safety, the safety of our water, milk, and food supplies, the safety of drugs and cosmetics, and the presence of disease-carrying animals, insects, and other potential sources of infection that are adversely affecting health. They are issuing statements and petitioning municipal, state, and provincial authorities to take action to eliminate environmental hazards to health, as well as actively participating in community action themselves to detect, minimize, or eliminate these hazards.

Our international nursing association has strongly urged nurses to participate in actions to safeguard the human environment. The following statement[1] is pertinent for all nurses:

---

[1] Reprinted from the Registered Nurses Association of Ontario, *RNAO News*, 32:19, January/February 1976.

The Council of National Representatives (CNR) of the International Council of Nurses, meeting in August 1975, adopted a policy statement which outlines the role that nurses can play in protecting and improving the environment and thereby contribute to better health for all people. The ICN Policy Statement reads as follows:

"The preservation and improvement of the human environment has become a major goal of man's action for his survival and well-being. The vastness and urgency of the task places on every individual and every professional group the responsibility to participate in the efforts to safeguard man's environment, to conserve the world's resources, to study how their use affects man and how adverse effects can be avoided.

"The nurse's role is to:—help detect ill-effects of the environment on the health of man, and vice-versa;

—be informed and apply knowledge in daily work with individuals, families and/or community groups as to the data available on potentially harmful chemicals, radioactive waste problems, latest health hazards and ways to prevent and/or reduce them;

—be informed and teach preventive measures about health hazards due to environmental factors as well as about conservation of environmental resources to the individual, families and/or community groups;

—work with health authorities in pointing out health care aspects and health hazards in existing human settlements and in the planning of new ones;

—assist communities in their action on environmental health problems;

—participate in research providing data for early warning and prevention of deleterious affects of the various environemtnal agents to which man is increasingly exposed; and research conducive to discover ways and means of improving living and working conditions."

In courses in community health nursing, which are being incorporated into virtually all nursing education programs today, the student will increase her knowledge of environmental hazards in the community at large and will develop skills in identifying and taking appropriate nursing action concerning these. We will, therefore, concentrate in the next two chapters on the nurse's responsibilities with regard to protecting the safety of persons who are handicapped in their abilities to protect themselves because of illness or infirmity.

Since the safety aspects of prevention and control of infection are discussed in Chapter 21, this chapter will deal with safety with regard to other environmental hazards.

FACTORS AFFECTING A PERSON'S ABILITY TO PROTECT HIMSELF

In Chapter 13, we discussed the fact that our sensory receptors provide us with

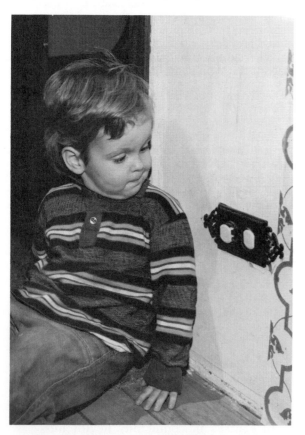

The use of safety covers on electrical outlets is one way to protect the young child from harm since he has no sense of danger.

information about the surrounding environment. It is through our abilities to see with our eyes, hear with our ears, smell with our noses, taste with the taste buds in our mouths, and feel through touching that we are alerted to dangers in our environment. Impairment of any of the sensory receptors, of the neural pathways carrying sensory impulses to and through the central nervous system, or of the ability to interpret these impulses results in lessened ability to sense harmful, or potentially harmful, factors in the environment.

The person with limited vision may not see the footstool that he is about to trip over. The person who is hard of hearing may not hear the warning call to watch his step. Someone who has lost his sense of smell may not be aware of the odor of escaping gas from the kitchen stove. Loss of the ability to taste prevents one from detecting the slightly "off" flavor of food that has been improperly preserved. A person who cannot feel does not receive the warning signal that he should remove himself from a seat too close to the fire.

As a person gets older his sensory abilities diminish: His vision is not as good as it used to be; his hearing, too, is not quite as sharp and sometimes may be considerably decreased; the sensory receptors for smell in the nose are not infrequently damaged in accidents when people have suffered any type of head injury and are, in any case, usually diminished with age. Atrophy of some of the taste buds is one of the unfortunate aspects of growing older, and even the receptors for touch lose some of their acuteness with the changes that occur in the aging skin.

The young child, on the other hand, may be able to perceive objects in the environment which can cause his harm, but his experience may not be sufficient for him to be able to interpret the stimuli as dangerous. He plays with matches and is fascinated by the flame. Until he burns himself, or mother is sufficiently impressive in her admonishments, he does not, however, perceive matches as dangerous objects. Similarly, he cannot read the warning label that tells him that the cleaning fluid is poison. The very young child has no sense of danger; it is only as his experiential world enlarges that he is able to interpret the meaning of the potentially harmful stimuli that he perceives.

It is through education and trial and error that individuals learn to identify harmful and potentially harmful situations. Children often encounter situations about which they have not yet learned and which could prove harmful were it not for suitable guidance. Likewise, an adult in a strange environment encounters situations for which he has no frame of reference, and as a result he may make judgments which could be harmful to him. A good orientation for patients, which includes showing them where bathrooms, showers, and other facilities are located, helps to familiarize them with their surroundings. It also helps to minimize some of the anxiety of being in a new situation.

If a person's mental faculties are clouded, or impaired for any reason, his sensory perception is diminished, as is his ability to interpret stimuli. The perceptual abilities of the person suffering from sleep deprivation are usually diminished, or his perception may be distorted (see Chapter 18). A person who is merely drowsy is a hazard when he is driving on the highway, because his sensory abilities are dulled; he may not see the car approaching on his side of the road. His own car may veer suddenly because his sense of touch is impaired; he does not perceive the infinitesimal shift in the steering wheel that tells him that he is not on his proper course (in addition to not being able to see as well where he is going). It may also take him longer than usual to realize that he is dangerously close to the edge of the road or in the wrong lane. Alcohol and drugs, which are central nervous system depressants, have the same effect of dulling the senses.

In fact, any alteration in state of consciousness will affect a person's ability to perceive sensory stimuli, to interpret them, and to react appropriately. The confused or disoriented individual may mistake the door leading to the stairs for the door to the bathroom. Thinking that he is at home, he may also try to get out of a hospital bed to go to the bathroom, and climb over the bedrails to do so. The person who is roused out of a sound sleep, as

we mentioned earlier (Chapter 18), is often confused and disoriented. Older people may become excited and confused by medications given to help them get to sleep (Chapter 18).

Anxiety and other emotional states may also affect a person's perception of harmful stimuli in the environment, his interpretation of these, and his ability to react to them. We discussed the perceptual changes accompanying anxiety in Chapter 12 (mild anxiety increases perceptual awareness, increased levels of anxiety progressively decrease it). A person can only attend to so many stimuli at one time, and if other stimuli are of more importance, a person may not be alert to potential dangers in his environment. The person whose thoughts are turned inward or fixed on one object, or who is lost in reverie, may bump into objects because he does not see them, step off the curb without looking, or do any one of a number of things that endanger life and limb. The stereotypes of the absent-minded professor and the person in love exemplify this problem.

Then, too, there is the phenomenon of adaptation to sensory stimuli, which can also provide hazards (Chapter 13). The smell of leaking gas may be so insidious that a person becomes accustomed to it or is never even consciously aware of it. The sense of smell is one that adapts very quickly, it seems. The nurse should keep this in mind in relation to offensive orders on the nursing unit. It is sometimes helpful to breathe fresh air for a change; then one's nose will be able to pick up the stimulus again.

Distorted sensory perception can also cause problems in relation to safety, as discussed in Chapter 13.

The individual's ability to respond to stimuli must also be considered. The brain must be functioning sufficiently well to make decisions and to initiate appropriate action in response to sensory stimuli. Some of our actions are reflexes that are initiated in the spinal cord; for example, the withdrawal of the hand from a hot stove becomes an almost instinctive reaction that is a learned cord reflex. A cord reflex can be developed in the bladder of a paralyzed patient to enable him to control his voiding when neural pathways to and from the brain itself have been sufficiently impaired to cut off voluntary control by the cerebral cortex.

Most actions, however, are initiated and controlled by higher centers of the brain (see Chapter 17); an example is the ability of a person to move himself out of the way of approaching danger. If the ability to initiate, coordinate, and carry out motor actions is impaired for whatever reason, the person's ability to protect himself from environmental hazards is decreased. The sleepy driver we mentioned may not be sufficiently alert to turn his steering wheel fast enough to get himself back on course before he goes over the edge of the road or runs into an approaching car. His reaction time is slowed. Alcohol is well known for its effect of slowing a person's reactions, thus making the person who has been drinking a potential hazard both to himself and to others. The relationship between alcohol consumption and a substantial proportion of motor vehicle accidents, fires, and other types of accidents was mentioned in Chapter 4. This life style factor is a definite health hazard.

Injury or illness affecting the specific areas of the brain initiating and controlling movement, or the neural pathways transmitting motor impulses will also limit a person's safeguarding abilities. People who have lessened mental faculties because of congenital problems, such as the mentally retarded or those with cerebral palsy (a motor disorder from nonprogressive brain damage) are hampered in their abilities to protect themselves.

Anyone with lessened motor abilities of any kind, or who has had restrictions placed on his mobility, is at a disadvantage when it comes to protecting himself from environmental hazards. The person in a wheelchair, for example, is severely handicapped. He cannot move as quickly as a person on two feet, and he is hampered by having to maneuver the chair around obstacles or out of the way of dangerous objects. One who cannot grasp objects or move his arm or leg with normal agility and speed is disadvantaged insofar as his protective abilities are concerned.

The sick person is particularly prone to accidents and injury by virtue of the nature of illness itself. He is often physically weak and impaired in his ability to carry out normal daily activities. As a result, he may fall while walking or easily lose his balance on an uneven surface. The protective senses of the sick person (as, for example, his sight) may be so impaired that he cannot perceive dangers to himself. Moreover, the anxiety that goes along with illness may interfere with his perceptual abilities and his capacity to concentrate, as well as his ability to make judgments, and thus expose him to injury. Many people who are ill suffer temporary or prolonged periods in which there is altered state of consciousness. The preoperative patient who is under sedation, the postoperative patient recovering from anesthesia, the person with a severe head injury, and the unconscious patient all have their sensory perceptual abilities decreased, as well as their abilities to respond to environmental stimuli and to make decisions based on good judgment.

In many illnesses, a person is rendered helpless or semihelpless by the nature of his illness (as we discussed in Chapter 20). He must then depend on other people to protect him fron environmental hazards. In some instances, it is necessary to restrain a person in his movements to protect him from his own actions, which may cause him injury. Restraining a confused or disoriented person, however, often distresses him and he may fight against the restraints, creating additional safety problems.

Sometimes the therapy that is prescribed makes the person more vulnerable to accidents or injury, or has inherent hazards in itself. Medication therapy carries with it many potential hazards, such as adverse reactions or the possibility that the wrong patient will get the medication. Radiation therapy also has its hazards, as discussed briefly in Chapter 19. The very act of penetrating the skin surfaces for surgery renders a person more vulnerable to infection and causes physiological stress, which makes the individual more susceptible to other disturbances of body functioning, such fluid and electrolyte imbalance—to mention only one.

Then, too, it is generally recognized that some people are accident-prone; that is, they are more likely to have accidents than the average person. For example, some children always seem to have more bruises and scrapes than their brothers and sisters. Some people may drive a car for 20 years without an accident, while others have one accident right after another. It is believed that emotional disturbances underlie accident proneness. Tension of any kind is more likely to make an individual susceptible to accidents by impairing his critical functions and exhausting his defenses.

A person who has a history of being accident-prone will need extra safety precautions when he is ill. The nurse's alert observation of potential hazards is an important measure in preventing accidents, as is provision of adequate support to the patient—when he needs help with walking, for example. Efforts to minimize anxiety should also be made. Sometimes accident-prone people need psychiatric assistance to learn to cope with their problems.

COMMON SAFETY PROBLEMS

An accident has been defined as "anything that occurs unexpectedly and unintentionally" or "an unexpected and undesirable event: a mishap."[2] Almost all accidents that occur could have been prevented if the person or persons involved had thought more carefully about their actions, used protective equipment, taken recognized safety precautions, or thought about their own safety and that of others.

The most common types of accidents occurring at home, at work, in school in hospitals, and elsewhere, are those due to:

1. Falls and other injuries caused by mechanical objects in the environment
2. Fire and other types of thermal injuries
3. Chemical injuries

A hospital is generally thought of as a place where the sick and injured come for care; it is seldom thought of as a place where people are injured. Yet, the number of accidental happenings in hospitals is extraordinarily high compared with those in most industries.

The problems of safety in health agencies concerned with caring for the sick and the injured are multiple. There are three groups of people to consider: the patients, who require additional protection because they are ill; the staff, who because of the nature of their work are vulnerable to many types of accidental injury (such as backstrain, from lifting heavy patients incorrectly, and infections); and the visitors, who are usually anxious and worried about the person they have come to see.

A hospital is a busy place, and is usually fraught with tension and stress. It must function as a hotel, and the staff members have all the responsibilities of an innkeeper for the safety of the guests. There is usually a large mechanical plant with heavy equipment that keeps the establishment running. Food service is part of the daily activities, and safety in good preparation, handling and serving must be considered. Diagnostic procedures for patients are often hazardous from the point of view of possible chemical and mechanical injuries to patients and staff, as well as being potential sources of infection. In addition, there is the ever-present threat of fire, the hospital administrator's nightmare, which could be a major catastrophe since the majority of the resident population are weakened by illness or otherwise limited in mobility. Thus, the hospital atmosphere itself is a contributing factor in likelihood of accidents occurring.

ASSESSING PROBLEMS WITH REGARD TO ENVIRONMENTAL SAFETY

The nurse's assessment of problems in protecting patients, visitors, and staff from environmental hazards involves two sets of activities:

1. Assessment of factors interfering with the patient's ability to take adequate precautions to protect himself

[2]*The American Heritage Dictionary of the English Language.* New College Edition. Boston, Houghton Mifflin Company, 1976, p. 8.

2. Assessment of potential hazards in the environment which could be harmful to patients, visitors, or staff

We will discuss the second aspect of the assessment when we cover specific nursing interventions to assist in preventing mechanical, chemical, and thermal injuries, and will concentrate here on assessing the patient's ability to protect himself.

In her assessment, the nurse needs to be aware of both the patient's age, and the integrity of his sensory abilities. She should be alert to any sensory deficits he has, such as impairment or loss of sight, hearing, smell, taste, or touch. She also needs information about his mobility status and any restrictions that have been put on his mobility, such as bed rest, position restrictions, or immobilization of a part (as with a cast or traction apparatus). She should be aware of any aids he requires for mobility (a cane, a walker, or a wheelchair, for example).

She also needs information about his general state of health, the nature of any health problems he has, and the physician's plan of diagnostic and therapeutic care. She should know if the patient is helpless, or semihelpless, or whether the nature of his illness may cause loss of strength, impairment of sensory or motor functioning, or short or prolonged periods of altered state of consciousness. Is he to have surgery, for example, with its attendant preoperative and postoperative periods when the patient's mental faculties may be lessened by sedation or anesthesia? She should be aware of diagnostic procedures being performed that may involve the use of potentially hazardous equipment, potentially harmful reactions, and the possibility of infection. She also needs information about medications the patient is receiving and the nature of other treatments planned for the patient. Is he receiving medications that may diminish his ability to perceive and respond to harmful stimuli, such as analgesics for pain? May his medications cause him to be confused? Is he having treatments, such as oxygen therapy, which require extra safety precautions?

We have said that all patients are anxious, and the nurse should be particularly watchful for evidence of this in the patient, and to the level of anxiety the patient is showing. The emotionally upset person (patient, visitor, or staff member) may rush blindly into danger. A person who is worried, preoccupied, or emotionally distressed is often less able to make judgments that are in the best interests of his physical or mental health. These patients require extra vigilance from nursing staff. The nurse also needs to know if the patient is an accident-prone individual.

The nurse can obtain much of the information she needs from the nursing history and clinical appraisal concerning the patient's usual status and current status at the time of admission with regard to sensory and motor abilities, state of comfort, rest, and sleep, and emotional and mental state. The patient's status changes constantly, however, and the nurse must rely on her own observations and her own judgment regarding safety precautions that need to be taken.

The patient's record is, of course, the most reliable source about diagnostic procedures, medications, and other therapeutic measures in the patient's overall plan of care. The nurse supplements this information by increasing her own knowledge about medications, tests and examinations, and treatments by asking knowledgeable people, such as the physician, her nursing instructor, the nursing team leader, or the head nurse, and by reading up on these matters in her texts and in the library.

The patient's subjective observations are also very helpful to the nurse. He may say that he cannot reach the things on his bedside table, for example, or that he is weak or feels dizzy when sitting up, or standing, or trying to walk. He can alert the nurse to things that are causing him pain or discomfort so that she can take appropriate action to remove the cause. For example, his arm may be in the wrong position under him. The astute observant nurse should be aware of this, but patients can be very helpful in assisting the nurse to adjust his position to the most comfortable and safe one for him. The patient is often aware when his mental faculties are impaired—he may say that he just cannot think clearly, or that everything seems to be fuzzy.

The patient's family or significant others often alert the nurse to dangerous situations for the patient. Many agencies permit family members to stay with confused or sedated patients, if they wish to do so, and this can be of great assistance to the nurse. She must be careful, however, that the family member knows what to do in helping the patient or will call the nurse if he needs additional help; the nurse does not neglect her responsibilities in watching over the patient's safety because a family member is with him.

Again, nothing substitutes for the nurse's own observations. She must be alert to all factors interfering with the patient's protective abilities and to all factors in the environment that have the potentiality for causing him harm.

PRIORITIES FOR PATIENT SAFETY

Safety and security needs were designated by Maslow as the second most important in his hierarchy of human needs, and assigned to third place by Kalish in his modification of the Maslow hierarchy (see Chapter 2). Regardless of whether one considers them second or third on a priority listing, however, safety needs are among the most basic of all human needs. Safety is important for all people, but especially to those who are ill. The protective aspects of the nurse's role are among the most important of all her functions and the nurse incorporates the patient's safety as the number one priority in all aspects of patient care.

One situation which takes precedence over all others is patient safety in the event of fire. The nurse must know the procedure used in the event of fire in the agency in which she is working, she must understand how to use the equipment for controlling fire, and know her responsibilities with regard to patient safety. She must be ever alert to potential fire hazards and take action to see that the danger is eliminated, if possible, or minimized if it can't be eliminated.

GOALS FOR NURSING ACTION

The goal of nursing action in regard to patient safety is the prevention of accident or injury to the patient.

PRINCIPLES RELEVANT TO PATIENT SAFETY

Basic to safe nursing practices and accident prevention are the following concepts, which can guide the nurse in many of her actions to ensure the safety of her patients:

1. Normally functioning body senses inform the individual about his environment.

2. A person's age affects his ability to perceive and interpret sensory stimuli from the environment.

3. Familiarity with the environment makes it less hazardous.

4. A person's ability to protect himself is affected by his sensory status, his mental status, his emotional status, his mobility status, and his status of comfort, rest, and sleep.

5. Illness renders a person more vulnerable to accidents and injury.

6. Diagnostic and therapeutic measures have inherent potential for causing a patient harm in addition to aiding in the resolution of his health problems.

SPECIFIC NURSING INTERVENTIONS

In nursing, a knowledge of safe nursing practices is essential. This involves not only a sound knowledge of the nursing and allied sciences, but also a knowledge of preventive nursing measures. To recognize circumstances which could result in an accident and to intervene effectively are essential. The nurse therefore needs to be alert to any activity which could cause injury and to any evidence of potential accident. Her observations should encompass the patient's total environment, in which she can look for such hazards as dangling electric cords, misplaced footstools, and slippery floors — in short, any situation that could result in an accident.

General considerations of environmental factors include arranging everything for the patient's maximal comfort and convenience, as well as that of his family, other visitors, and the staff. The equipment used in hospitals is generally portable, so that it can be moved easily to a more convenient position or location. Hospitals try to obtain equipment that is also quiet, durable, simple to operate, and easily repaired. More and more facilities are being built into the patient's unit so that they are easier to use and always conveniently at hand, and as a result there are fewer hazardous objects in and around the patient's bed.

The patient's unit and the nursing unit itself should be kept as free of clutter as possible. When giving care to a patient, the nurse always makes sure that she has a clear space in which to work, that she can see what she is doing, and that she is able to practice good body mechanics in any lifting and moving that is involved. It is awkward to work over siderails, for example, or to have to reach around objects to get at things she needs.

All accidents — that is, all events that have resulted or could have resulted in injury to a patient, a visitor or a staff member are reported so that remedial measures may be instituted. For example, if a patient receives an incorrect medication, notifying the nursing supervisor or the physician permits the initiation of measures to prevent a recurrence of this error or to remedy the effects of the incorrect medication.

Another purpose of reporting accidents is to guide the safety committee of an agency in its preventive program. The findings of these committees can be used as the bases for changes in medical and nursing practices and as indications of the need for the education of patients and personnel.

The Prevention of Mechanical Trauma

Among the most frequently occurring types of *mechanical* accidents are falls. Falling from beds, from chairs, or while walking is not an uncommon occurrence, but it is often preventable. A person who is weakened by illness can lose his balance and fall while simply leaning toward a table that is out of reach. Nurses can prevent many accidents of this kind by being alert to potentially dangerous situations and remedying them. For example, beds that can be raised or lowered can be left in the low position when the nurse is not present. At this level the patient will be able to get in and out of bed more safely. Also, patients who have been in bed for several days or who are weakened by illness can be helped to recognize their need for assistance in getting about.

Slippery floors can be dangerous to people in any situation not only to patients. To minimize this danger non-slippery materials are used on the floor surfaces of hospitals. Also, since any material spilled on a floor is likely to make it slippery, it should be mopped up before someone slips on it. Floors should be washed and polished at a time when there is little traffic upon them, and signs should be prominently placed to notify people that the floor is wet and slippery.

Untidiness can also contribute to accidents. People can trip over electric cords, footstools, bed gatches, and equipment that is left on the floor. Walkways, such as areas from patients' beds to bathrooms, can be particularly hazardous when they are not kept clear. Patients have fallen from their beds while reaching for articles on their bedside tables or while looking

NOV 4 77

RIVERSIDE HOSPITAL OF OTTAWA
CASUALITY OR COMPLAINT REPORT
DETAILS OF CASUALTY OR COMPLAINT
casualty complaint

```
BLACK    GRACE        SP 1242
451  TOLL RD    OTT  234-7566-600
BLACK    GEORGE    HUS
SAME
8.30.77  1PM  F 36 M  SURG    RC
     420    1
```

Date of Casualty
or complaint ___Sept 2/77___

Time of Casualty ___7³⁰___ (A.M.) P.M.
or Complaint

Examined by Doctor(name) ___White___

Date of Examination ___Sept 2/77___ Time ___8¹⁵___ (A.M.) P.M.

Attending Doctor Notified   Yes [✓] No. [ ]

On entering Mrs Black's room (212) I found her sitting on the floor between her bed and an armchair. She stated she had wanted to go to the bathroom and felt dizzy on getting oob. She didn't want to fall so she sat on the floor and grabbed the foot of the bed with her left hand. She is complaining of left wrist being sore — no signs of swelling or bruising. Patient is allowed up and about as desired. She received an oblation at a since bedtime fall-bed attached to pillow & bed lowered to floor. Supervisor & doctor notified.

Ward __4N__ Date __Sept 2nd__ 19__77__   Signature __W Stratton, Reg N.__

REPORT OF INVESTIGATION

No evidence of Nursing neglect — patient allowed to be up and about without assistance

Date __Sept 2__ 19__77__ Signature of Investigator __E Able__ Position __Supervisor__

NOTE: SEND THIS FORM, WHEN COMPLETED, TO NURSING
       OFFICE IMMEDIATELY

2-8750

(Courtesy of Riverside Hospital of Ottawa.)

RIVERSIDE HOSPITAL OF OTTAWA

DOCTORS CASUALITY REPORT

NOV 4 77

BLACK   GRACE   SP 1242
451 TOLL RD   OTT 234-7566-600
BLACK   GEORGE   HUS
SAME
8.30. 77 1PM F 36 M SURG   RC
   420   1

Date of Casualty *Sept 2/77* TIME *7³⁰* A M

Date of Examination *Sept 2/77* TIME *8¹⁵* A M

NATURE OF CASUALITY:

Patient apparently tried to go to the washroom and felt dizzy when she got up – slipped to the floor.

PHYSICAL FINDINGS ON EXAMINATION OF PATIENT

– No signs of swelling a discoloration
– Complaining of left wrist being sore

DATE OF X-RAY EXAMINATION   *Sept 2/77*   TIME *10²⁵* (A.M.)
                                             P.M.

X-RAY FINDINGS: *NIL*

Ward *4N*   Date *Sept 2/77*   *G. White*   M.D.

(To be filled out by the Doctor and forwarded to the Office of the Administrator of the Department of Nursing, immediately on completion.

To be filled on patient's chart on discharge.

(Courtesy of Riverside Hospital of Ottawa.)

for a misplaced call light. The nurse can help the patient to arrange these items so that they are within easy reach.

Other possible causes of falls are movable wheelchairs or stretchers. So often, just as a patient is about to sit in a wheelchair, it moves out of place. Most movable equipment is furnished with locks for the wheels. These locks should be set when the equipment is to be used and released only after the patient is secure.

When a patient first becomes ambulatory after a period of time in bed, he often requires some physical support (see Chapter 19). Many hospitals and other health agencies have rails in the halls to guide and support patients while they are walking. These, as well as rubber treads on stairs, can prevent many falls.

A procedure that poses a threat chiefly to people working within the hospital is the discarding of broken glass and sharp instruments. Most institutions have special containers for glass, razor blades, and the like in order that they can be disposed of separately from other materials. In this way there is less danger of injuring hospital personnel. It is the policy of many hospitals that an employee who is injured at work should report to the employees' health clinic or to a physician for care. In addition, a written report is usually required.

Safety Devices. In her concern for her patient's safety, the nurse may employ specific safety devices. Many of these devices can be deathtraps, however, and should not be used unless absolutely necessary. In most institutions devices are used either upon the request of the attending physician, or when, in the judgment of the nurse, they become necessary. Policies vary from place to place, however, and the nurse should be familiar with the practice in the institution in which she works. The student should always check with the team leader or with her teacher before using safety devices for patients.

SIDERAILS. Siderails on beds can stop the patient from rolling off the bed. They do not deter the patient from climbing out; rather, they serve merely as reminders to the patient that he is in bed and should exercise care. Most hospitals have policies regarding the use of siderails; it is not uncommon to require them on the beds of patients who are blind, unconscious, or sedated, or who have muscular disabilities or seizures. Some hospitals require that the beds of all patients over the age of 70 years have siderails. A number of hospitals have adopted a policy of using siderails on the beds of all patients, particularly at night.

It is important when siderails are in use that both rails be up. For example, even when the patient's bed is against the wall both rails should be used; the wall does not serve as a good replacement for the rail. When caring for the patient whose bed has siderails, the nurse normally takes down the siderail on the side at which she is working. She should go no further than an arm's length from that side of the bed without returning the siderail to its "up" position. Many patients dislike the use of siderails; they may find them an embarrassing reminder of their childhood crib. Some people are fearful of them, while to others siderails signify a loss of independence and control over their situation. An explanation of the purpose for using siderails often helps such patients to accept them. Generally side-

rails will not keep a patient in bed against his will; if a patient needs restraining, a safety jacket should be used.

SAFETY JACKET AND POSEY BELT. Patients who are confused sometimes try to climb over the siderails of the bed. They are frequently unaware of their surroundings; they just want to leave the bed. These patients can often be restrained comfortably in bed by means of a safety jacket or Posey belt. The jacket is an inconspicuous sleeveless garment which has long crossover ties in front or in back that can be attached to the frame on either side of the bed. The ties are secured to the frame out of the reach of the patient. The Posey belt performs the same function as the jacket. It is secured around the patient's body, and ties are attached to the bed frame. Both the safety jacket and the Posey belt allow the patient to move relatively freely in bed, yet restrain him from climbing over the siderails and possibly falling to the floor.

ARM AND LEG RESTRAINTS. Occasionally it is necessary to apply arm or leg restraints to patients in bed. Generally this is an undesirable nursing care measure because it limits a patient's movements, and this in turn often causes anxiety, increasing restlessness and subsequent fatigue. It is a particularly dangerous practice to restrain only one side of the body (as, for example, the right arm and leg). This practice tends to increase the patient's restlessness, and he may injure himself as he tries to move the arm and leg that are restrained. If only two limbs are restrained, they should be opposite limbs. Few patients like to be tied down, regardless of how irrational they are. Their reaction is usually to struggle against whatever is hampering their movement and they may become quite agitated. Injury to the tissues of the wrists and ankles may result from the friction engendered by rubbing against the restraints. Occasionally, leather restraints may be used. Many agencies will not permit their use except on a doctor's order. There is a greater possibility of both adverse patient reaction to leather restraints and injury to the patient from them.

An arm restraint may be prescribed during an intravenous infusion. Its chief purpose in this instance is to remind the patient to keep his arm immobilized during the treatment.

Arms and legs should not be restrained any longer than is absolutely necessary, and at least every four hours the restraints are loosened and the limbs are exercised. There is a danger that a patient's circulation may be restricted if a restraint is tight or if a limb is restrained in an abnormal position. In some agencies a washcloth or other soft cloth may be used to pad the skin under the restraint. A knot over the pad serves to keep the restraint from being too tight. Absorbent cotton should never be used because it has a tendency to flatten out and form into lumps. At any sign of blueness, pallor, cold or complaints of tingling sensations in the extremity, the restraint is loosened and circulation restored by exercise and massage. A limb is best restrained in a slightly flexed position.

MITTENS. Mittens are indicated for patients who are confused or semiconscious and may pull at their dressings and tubes. The mittens are often used, for example, for a patient with a head injury or for a patient who is confused following a stroke. They have the advantage of not permitting the patient to grasp such objects as dressings, tubing, or bedrails, but they do not limit movement. A mitten is like a soft boxing glove which pads the patient's hand. Commercial mittens are available, or mittens may be made using dressing pads, gauze bandage, and adhesive tape. One method of making mittens is as follows.

Before applying a mitten the patient's hand is placed in a naturally flexed position. This allows unrestricted circulation and places little strain upon muscles. A soft rolled dressing is grasped by the patient so that his thumb approximates his fingers. The soft pad permits the patient to flex his hand while the mitten is in place. All skin surfaces are separated to avoid irritation. The patient's wrist is padded with a dressing to avoid rubbing bony prominences.

Two dressings are then placed over the patient's hand; one medial to lateral, one dorsal to ventral. Large 20 by 25 cm. (8 by 16 inch) dressings are suggested. These are secured by a gauze bandage applied in figure eight patterns (Chapter 22).

To secure the dressings a stockinette is fitted over the hand and secured by adhesive tape just beyond the wrist pad. A double fold of stockinette open at one end suffices.

Mittens need to be removed at least once every 24 hours. At this time the patient washes his hands and exercises them, or the nurse may do this for him. Mittens should not be so tight as to impede circulation, but they must be secure and pad the patient's hands well.

The Prevention of Chemical Trauma

Accidents involving *chemicals* generally result from the incorrect use of pharmaceutical preparations. Physicians and nurses are well aware of the dangers incurred through errors in the administration of medications. Many institutions have special policies and rules that are designed to prevent errors of this nature. Thus, medicines are generally kept in locked cupboards in special areas away from patients and busy nursing-unit offices. Medicines for topical use are separated from medicines administered orally or parenterally. Drugs that are poisonous are well marked. Usually narcotics such as codeine and morphine are kept in a separate double-locked cupboard, and they are counted at the end of each nursing shift and the tally recorded in a special book. Medicines that are provided for use at home are labeled with complete instructions as to dosage and frequency of administration. It is becoming fairly common practice for the name of the drug to be included on the label of medications for home use so that the patient will not inadvertently take the wrong drug or one to which they are allergic.

It is common practice for medications which a patient brings in with him from home to be picked up by the nurse who admits him to the nursing unit. The nurse should ascertain the nature of the drugs contained in these medications. She should also notify the attending physician of any medications the patient is using that were prescribed by another doctor. For example, the patient may be under the care of a surgeon while in hospital and yet have an eye condition for which his ophthalmologist has prescribed twice daily eye drops. The attending physician (in this case, the surgeon) should be alerted to the medication the patient is receiving for his eye condition.

In addition to these generally accepted practices, many agencies require that the nurse have her computations of doses checked by another nurse before the drug is actually prepared. In this way any errors in arithmetic are found before a patient can be harmed. Most hospital pharmacies try to provide nurses with the exact dosage ordered by the physician in order that arithmetical calculations and the division of prepared medicines can be avoided.

Many hospitals now use drugs which are packaged in individual dosages. This practice makes the administration of medications both easier and safer; there is less chance of error. In an increasing number of agencies, medications are delivered from the pharmacy directly to the patient's room, where they are administered by the nurse. This practice helps to reduce the possibility of giving a medication to the wrong patient, another potential hazard in the administration of medications.

Specific orders by the physician help to avoid errors due to ambiguity and misinterpretation. This does not mean that a nurse does not require a thorough knowledge of the pharmaceutical preparation that she is administering. She needs this knowledge in order to protect the patient from harm, to make intelligent observations, and to give intelligent nursing care.

If an error is made in the administration of a medicine, it should be reported immediately to the nursing supervisor and to the patient's physician. In this way steps can be taken to protect the patient from injury. Hospitals usually require that a written account of the error be submitted subsequently. The nurse's responsibilities in the administration of medications are further discussed in Chapter 24.

The Prevention of Thermal Trauma

Thermal accidents involve the presence of harmful levels of heat or cold. The most common sources of thermal injuries are fire, hot appliances, or any electrical circuit which is improperly functioning. It is generally a hospital policy that electrical appliances be regularly checked and adequately maintained in order to prevent injury. As an added precaution, patients are often required to have their radios, electric razors, and other appliances checked by the hospital maintenance staff before they use them in hospital. Hot water bottles, heating pads and infrared lamps are also possible sources of thermal injury. Heat that is applied to a patient is generally regulated well within the safety limits for that patient.

Fire is a constant threat in institutions. Even though modern construction materials have lessened the danger of the actual building catching fire, there are many materials within a hospital that are highly combustible. For example, oxygen supports combustion and substances such as ether are highly inflammable.

For a fire to start there must be three elements present: a combustible material, heat, oxygen. A *combustible* material is anything that will burn. Among the most common materials involved in hospital fires are: paper, as in wastebasket or garbage chute fires; textiles, such as patient's bedding or oily rags; flammable liquids, such as ether or other liquid gases (for example, those used as anesthetic agents); and electrical equipment. Heat sufficient to ignite the combustible material may come from such sources as a lighted match, a live cigarette, a spark, or friction. There is usually enough oxygen in the atmosphere to support combustion if the other two elements are present. Fire prevention is usually directed, therefore, toward controlling the first two elements, that is, the combustible materials and heat; fire extinguishing measures toward the reduction of heat (as by water cooling) and the exclusion of oxygen.

Fire Prevention. Most hospitals have active programs in fire prevention. Education of the patients, the personnel and the public in safe practices is an essential part of such programs. Some of the areas that are included in the fire control programs of hospitals are discussed in the following paragraphs. One of the most common causes of fire is carelessness with cigarette smoking. In some agencies smoking is prohibited except when authorized by the patient's physician.

SMOKING REGULATIONS. Usually smoking is prohibited in certain areas of the hospital, and these areas are well marked. The no smoking rule is enforced within 12 feet of equipment for administering oxygen, in operating rooms where combustible gases are used, and in places where combustible materials are stored.

Patients who do smoke require ashtrays which do not easily tip and which are so constructed that if a cigarette is left burning it will fall into the ashtray. Some patients—for instance, those who are confused or under the influence of a sedative or hypnotic drug—should not smoke unattended. It may be necessary to keep matches and cigarettes locked in a cupboard if the patient is confused.

SCRUPULOUS HOUSEKEEPING. Thorough housekeeping and adequate maintenance of equipment lessen the likelihood of fires. For example, oily rags, paints, and solvents are stored carefully in a special area so as to prevent spontaneous combustion.

ADEQUATE STORAGE AND DISTRIBUTION OF VOLATILE LIQUIDS AND GASES. Generally large quantities of ether should not be kept in patient areas because of the danger of fire. *Volatile* (easily turned into vapor) gases and liquids are distributed to the various areas of the agency under strict control and all the necessary fire precautions are observed.

FIRE PREVENTION AND FIRE EXTINGUISHING. In an active fire prevention program all employees must be educated in fire prevention and fire extinguishing.

Types of Fires and Fire Extinguishers. There are basically three classes of hospital fires. Class A fires involve paper, wood and similar solid combustible materials. Class B fires involve flammable liquids, for example, anesthetics. Class C fires involve electrical equipment.

Many kinds of fire extinguishers are available and the nurse needs to know how to operate the ones used at the agency in which she works. Five widely used extinguishers are:

SODA AND ACID EXTINGUISHER. This extinguisher, which supplies water under pressure, can be used to put out rubbish or mattress fires (Class A). It is not used for electrical fires, because water conducts electricity. To operate the extinguisher it is turned upside down. The sulfuric acid mixes with the bicarbonate to produce carbon dioxide which in turn releases the water under pressure. To stop the flow, the extinguisher is turned right side up.

WATER PUMP CAN. This extinguisher also provides water under pressure, and it also can be used for nonelectrical fires (Classes A and B). To operate this extinguisher the nurse merely has to pump the handle up and down, directing the stream of water with the nozzle.

CARBON DIOXIDE EXTINGUISHER. This extinguisher is used for compressed-gas fires and electrical fires, as well as fires involving grease (Classes B and C). In order to operate the extinguisher the nurse presses the trigger, directing the horn toward the root of the fire so as to exclude the oxygen from the source of the fire.

WATER OR ANTIFREEZE EXTINGUISHER. This extinguisher stores water under pressure. It has a pressure gauge which indicates its readiness for use. To operate the extinguisher the nurse pulls the pin and squeezes the handle. It is used for class A and class B fires.

DRY CHEMICAL EXTINGUISHER. This extinguisher contains bicarbonate of soda, dry chemicals, and carbon dioxide gas. It contains no water and operates on the principle of blanketing the burning substance to exclude air. It is used on electrical fires (Class C) and is also effective on Class A fires. To operate the extinguisher, the nurse pulls the pin and opens the valve (or presses the lever) and squeezes the nozzle valve.

Fire extinguishers must be accessible to personnel. Generally they are kept in obvious places in all patient and service areas. The kind of extinguisher that is placed in a specific area depends upon the type of fire most likely to occur there. Part of a safety program is the regular inspection and maintenance of fire extinguishers.

In addition to having fire extinguishers, nursing units and other departments of a hospital are usually equipped with fire hoses, and personnel are instructed in their use. In the event of a small fire, it may be easier and quicker to use material near at hand, for example, to smother the fire with a blanket or mattress pad, or to pour a pitcher of cold water over it.

The Nurse's Responsibilities in the Event of Fire. If a fire does occur in a nursing unit the nurse should make sure that the following steps are carried out.

1. Remove patients from the immediate danger area

2. Notify the local fire department

3. Shut off the fire area and decrease the ventilation to the area

4. Employ available extinguishing equipment.

In some health agencies it is accepted practice to telephone the fire department, directly reporting the exact location of the fire. Other agencies have a fire alarm system which when set off causes an alarm to ring in the fire station. A third method of reporting a fire is to telephone the operator at the central hospital exchange, who then notifies the fire department. When reporting a fire, it is important that the nurse give the exact location of the fire clearly.

THE REMOVAL OF PATIENTS. When a fire occurs, the nurse in charge of the nursing unit assumes the responsibility for directing the activities of the hospital personnel until the firemen arrive. All fire doors should be closed. Patients in immediate danger must be moved to safety quickly. Generally, ambulatory patients are assisted in walking to safety. In moving immobilized patients, the entire bed is wheeled to a safe area. When it is not feasible to move the entire bed, a portable stretcher can be employed to move immobilized patients. The nurse may occasionally find it necessary to carry a patient in order to remove him from danger. Four basic carries are:

Pack Strap Carry. With the patient in a sitting position in bed, the nurse faces the patient and grasps the patient's wrists, the right wrist in the left and the left wrist in the right hand. The nurse then pivots and slips under the patient's arm so that the patient's chest is against her shoulders and the patient's arms are

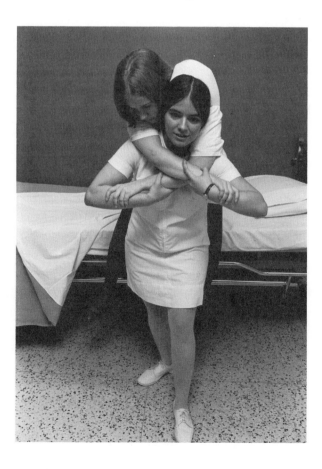

Position for the pack strap carry.

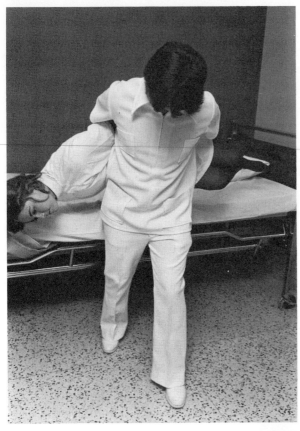

Position for the hip carry.

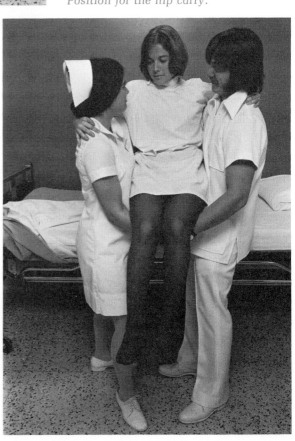

Position for the swing carry.

crossed on the nurse's chest. With one leg forward for balance the nurse then rolls the patient off the bed and on to her back.

Hip Carry. The patient lies on her side near the edge of the bed. The nurse faces the head of the bed and puts her arm that is nearest the patient around the patient's back and under the armpit. She then turns so that her hips are against the patient's abdomen and puts her other arm around the patient's thighs and under her knees. The patient is then drawn up on the nurse's hip and the nurse carries her from the bedside.

Swing Carry by Two Nurses. One nurse stands on each side of the patient. The patient's arms are extended around the nurses' shoulders and each nurse grasps one of the patient's wrists with the arm that is farthest from the patient. Each nurse then reaches behind the patient's back with her free arm (nearest the patient) and grasps the other nurse's shoulder. The patient's wrists are then released. Each nurse reaches under the patient's knees and grasps the other's wrist. The patient is then in a sitting position between the nurses.

Three Man Carry (see Chapter 17).

As part of any fire prevention and fire extinguishment program all agency personnel require information about specific policy and practice. Demonstrations in the use of fire equipment, practice in moving patients, and a knowledge of the established practice to be followed upon the discovery of a fire are important. It is only through a continuous in-service educational program in fire prevention and extinguishing methods that the safety of all is safeguarded.

Safety Programs

A safety program is an endeavor to control the physical environment in such a manner that accidents can be prevented. In order to be effective, a program must involve all the people who are concerned with the agency. Many hospitals have safety committees whose job it is to plan a safety program for the institution. Nurses are frequently members of these committees.

The committee's function is to conduct a continual analysis of the kind of accidents that occur in the hospital and their causes. On the basis of this analysis an active program is developed. Continual assessment of hospital practices and continual education of employees are important. Another part of a safety program is the regular inspection of agency facilities; for example, fire extinguishers are checked as often as recommended by the manufacturer. To be effective, a safety program must motivate all employees to accomplish the purpose of the program, for it is only through the active cooperation of all the people in an agency that accidents can be prevented.

PLANNING AND EVALUATING SAFETY MEASURES

Adequate precautions for the patient's safety are an integral component of all nursing measures and of all nursing care planning. Additional safety precautions are needed when the patient is very young or very old, when his perceptual abilities are lessened for any reason, or his ability to react to harmful stimuli is decreased, when potentially harmful equipment is being used in his care, and when he is an accident-prone individual.

All patients have learning needs in relation to protecting their own safety while in the agency and these are included in the nursing care plan. A good orientation to the physical layout of the nursing unit and the equipment in his immediate surroundings is essential. He also needs to know how to call for assistance if he needs it (and his call bell must be placed within easy reach). He needs to know how to use the various pieces of equipment that are in and around his bed, and be alerted in regard to safety precautions in their use. An explanation of all safety measures is important to ensure his cooperation, as, for example, an explanation of why the siderails are put up on the bed at night, or, when he is sedated, why it is important not to smoke when oxygen equipment is in use. Each nursing measure, each diagnostic test or examination done, and each therapeutic measure undertaken has important safety precautions that the patient needs to be aware of to protect him from harm. When the patient is unable to protect himself, it is the nurse's responsibility to do it for him.

The expected outcomes of nursing interventions with regard to patient safety are usually expressed in terms of prevention of the undesirable event. Usually the potential problem, such as "the patient may fall from the bed," is stated and expected outcome is written simply as "prevent."

Potential safety problems almost always result from another problem the patient has, or from the nature of the diagnostic or therapeutic plans of care for him. The patient's safety may be jeopardized, for example, when he is under sedation for pain relief. The basic problem is pain; that the patient may fall from the bed when sedated is a potential problem resulting from the nature of his therapy. Evaluation of the effectiveness of nursing interventions is the absence of accidents. If the potential problems are stated explicitly, the nurse can evaluate the success of her interventions, in this case by the fact that the patient did not "fall from the bed," or did not "burn himself or set the bed on fire," if he is a smoker and these are potential problems.

The patient's condition is subject to constant change. It is therefore necessary for the nurse to continuously reassess his abilities to protect himself from environmental hazards and modify her nursing care plans in accordance with his changed status. She must also be constantly alert to new dangers in the environment that could harm the patient, herself, visitors, or other staff.

GUIDE TO ASSESSING SAFETY NEEDS	1. Is the patient alert, conscious and in full command of his mental faculties?

1. Is the patient alert, conscious and in full command of his mental faculties?
2. Does he require additional safety precautions because of his age, his physical condition, or his mental state?
3. Is the patient receiving medications that impair his senses?
4. Does the patient require restraints of any sort?
5. Does he smoke?
6. Is electrical equipment in use in the patient's room? Does the patient have electrical appliances at his bedside?
7. Is heat used as a therapeutic agent in the care of this patient?
8. Is the patient on oxygen therapy?
9. Are there any information or safety practices which can help the patient to avoid injury or accident?
10. Is the patient comfortable?
11. Can he reach everything he needs?
12. Is his call signal within easy reach?
13. Is he safe from mechanical injury, such as that resulting from falls?
14. Is he being protected from burns, as for example from a heating pad of a hot water bottle?
15. What precautions are taken to ensure that medications are given safely?

STUDY VOCABULARY   Combustible   Thermal trauma   Volatile

STUDY SITUATION — Mrs. R. Ross, who is 73 years old, is in the hospital because she has a fractured femur. The physician has ordered that she sit in a chair for 15 minutes twice a day. Mrs. Ross walks with considerable difficulty and requires support.

1. What factors should the nurse be aware of in providing a safe environment for Mrs. Ross?
2. Give six specific measures that the nurse should take to prevent mechanical injury to Mrs. Ross.
3. If there is a fire in this patient's room, what should the nurse do? How should this patient be moved?[5]
4. By what criteria can the safety of Mrs. Ross's environment be evaluated?

SUGGESTED READINGS

Feyock, M. W.: A do-it-yourself restraint that works. *Nursing '75*, 5:18, January 1975.

Hefferin, E. A., et al.: Analyzing nursing's work-related injuries. Veterans Administration Wadsworth Hospital Center, Los Angeles, California. *American Journal of Nursing*, 76:924–927, June 1976.

Hillman, Harold: The optimum human environment. *Nursing Times*, 69:692–695, 1973.

Kukuk, H. M.: Safe precautions: Protecting your patients and yourself. *Nursing '76*, Part I, 6:45–51, May 1976; Part II, 6:49, June 1976; Part III, 6:45–49, July 1976.

Mylrea, K. C. et al.: Electricity and electrical safety in the hospital. *Nursing '76*, 6:52–59, January 1976.

Phegley, D., et al.: Improving fire safety with posted procedures. *Nursing '76*, 6:18, July 1976.

Reid, J. A.: Controlling the fight/flight patient. *Canadian Nurse*, 69:30–34, October 1973.

Roberts, M.: Hypothermia. An aid for the elderly. *Nursing Times*, 70:1926–1927, December 12, 1974.

Roth, H. et al.: *Electrical Safety in Health Care Facilities.* New York, Academic Press, 1975.

Swartz, E. M.: Preventing Burn Injuries. *Journal of Nursing Administration*, 3:9–10, February 1973.

Trought, E. A.: Equipment Hazards. *American Journal of Nursing*, 73:858–862, May 1973.

21 THE PREVENTION AND CONTROL OF INFECTION

The nurse should be able to:

Explain the importance to health of preventing and controlling
    infection

Briefly explain the infectious process, including common pathogens
    infecting man, the cycle of infection, and the body's reactions
    to infection

Discuss common sources of infection in health agencies and ways
    infection is spread in these agencies

Identify people who are particularly at risk to infection

Identify potential or actual problems of infection in patients

Apply relevant principles in planning and implementing nursing
    interventions to prevent and control infection

Evaluate the effectiveness of nursing interventions to prevent and
    control infection

INTRODUCTION

In Chapter 4, when we discussed health problems, we pointed out that the control of infectious diseases has been one of the principal reasons for the dramatic reduction in infant and child mortality, and the consequent lengthening of the life span in the developed countries of the world. Four major factors have contributed to this achievement: the development and widespread use of specific immunizations against many of the common communicable diseases; the discovery and widespread use of antimicrobial agents (such as the antibiotics); the application of basic sanitary measures to protect the safety of water, milk, and food supplies, along with the disposal of garbage and sewage; and the overall raising of standards of living, with its resultant improvement in the general health of people (from better nutrition, better housing, and the like).

The infectious diseases are certainly a much greater health problem in developing countries than in developed ones, but we have by no means eliminated all illnesses caused by infections in the Western world. The respiratory infections continue to be an important cause of death and of acute illness throughout the life span of the peoples of North America. Gastrointestinal infections are one of the most common causes of short-term illness. The venereal diseases have attained epidemic proportions in the past few years, and such diseases as chickenpox and hepatitis are still prevalent. Institution-acquired infections (called nosocomial infections) continue to plague hospitals throughout the United States and Canada.

The prevention and control of infection is one of the principal concerns of all health personnel, whether they work in ambulatory care settings in the community or in inpatient facilities for the care of the sick. The most common causes of infection are microorganisms. Wherever there are sick people, microorganisms that are capable of producing infection pose a constant and serious threat, since the average patient is highly susceptible to infection as a result of his generalized debility. Moreover, since some patients have particularly serious infections, their close proximity to other patients produces situations conducive to the transfer of microorganisms.

Microorganisms capable of producing infection are found in the air, on the floors, on equipment and furniture, and on articles that have come in contact with a person who has an infection, as well as on the skin and mucous membranes, and in the expired air, secretions, and excretions of the person himself. They can be spread through the air and by such things as linen, dishes, and even a nurse's hands. Health personnel sometimes unknowingly act as a carriers of microorganisms. When handwashing techniques break down, for example, microorganisms are passed on to others. In spite of stringent cleaning practices, health agency personnel are continually working in an environment which harbors many varieties of organisms. Every once in a while a particularly virulent organism is introduced, and a worker with an open cut or lowered body resistance becomes infected. An unbalanced diet, fatigue, scratches, cuts, or other wounds all predispose any person to infection.

In order to understand the rationale behind nursing measures taken to protect 393 patients and staff from infections, it is important to keep in mind the sources, methods of transfer, and modes of spread of microogranisms. In her courses in microbiology and anatomy and physiology, the student will have gained a good knowledge-base about the infectious process and the body's reactions to it. In subsequent courses in medical-surgical nursing, she will increase her knowledge of specific communicable diseases. We will, therefore, confine ourselves here to a brief review of the infectious process and the body's reactions to it, in order to provide a framework for discussion of the care of patients with existing or potential problems of infection.

THE INFECTIOUS PROCESS

Infection is a process in which a pathogen (infectious agent) gains entrance to the body and grows and multiplies.[1]

Common Pathogens

Common agents causing infections in man are the pathogenic bacteria, some protozoa, fungi, viruses, and helminths.

The *pathogenic bacteria* include those that are true pathogens—that is, they are virulent microorganisms capable of invading healthy tissue, as, for example, some species of Salmonella, which can cause an acute form of gastroenteritis; the parasitic bacteria, which are opportunists—that is, they do not usually invade body tissue but will do so if given the opportunity, as, for example, some of the streptococci and staphylococci, which can cause wound infections; and those bacteria which do not invade body tissue but produce toxins capable of producing disease, such as *Clostridium tetani,* which is the causative agent of tetanus.

Protozoa are single-celled animals; some varieties cause disease in man; an example is *Entamoeba histolytica,* which causes the intestinal infection of amebiasis.

Fungus infections include those caused by yeasts and molds, such as ring worm and athlete's foot, which are caused by cutaneous mycoses.

Many of the common communicable diseases are *virus infections;* measles, mumps, chickenpox infectious hepatitis, and smallpox are all viral infections.

The *helminths* are worms; some are common parasites in humans, as for example, the pinworms often found in children.[2]

The Cycle of Infection

The *cycle of infection* is best visualized as a circle. There must first of all be an *infectious agent,* such as one of those organisms we have mentioned above. The agent must have a place (*reservoir*) in which it grows and multiplies. It leaves the reservoir by an *exit route,* and utilizes means to travel, or a *vehicle of transmission.* By using this vehicle, it gains entrance through a *portal of entry* to the body of a *susceptible human being,* who then becomes its *host* and constitutes a potential reservoir to start the cycle again.

Common *reservoirs* for infectious agents causing disease in man are: human beings, animals, plants, the soil, and arthropods, such as mosquitoes, fleas, ticks, and lice.

Exit routes whereby the infectious agent leaves its reservoir are usually the respiratory tract, the gastrointestinal tract, the skin or mucous membranes, the blood, or the secretions or excretions of the individual. No portal of exit is required for organisms harboring in the soil.

Vehicles of transmission for infectious agents include:

1. *Air.* For example, *Mycobacterium tuberculosis* frequently adheres to dust or other small particles and is subsequently carried by air currents.

2. *Water.* For example, *Vibrio comma,* which causes cholera, may be carried in fecally contaminated water.

3. *Food.* For example, some strains of Staphylococcus, which is the causative

---

[1]Madelyn T. Nordmark and Anne W. Rohweder: *Scientific Foundations of Nursing.* 2nd edition. Philadelphia, J. B. Lippencott, 1967, p. 321.

[2]Ibid., pp. 311–320

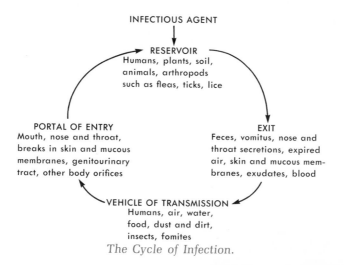

INFECTIOUS AGENT

RESERVOIR
Humans, plants, soil,
animals, arthropods
such as fleas, ticks, lice

PORTAL OF ENTRY
Mouth, nose and throat,
breaks in skin and mucous
membranes, genitourinary
tract, other body orifices

EXIT
Feces, vomitus, nose and
throat secretions, expired
air, skin and mucous mem-
branes, exudates, blood

VEHICLE OF TRANSMISSION
Humans, air, water,
food, dust and dirt,
insects, fomites

The Cycle of Infection.

agent of gastroenteritis, may be transmitted by improperly refrigerated food.

4. *Dust and dirt.* For example, *Clostridium tetani*, which causes tetanus, may be carried by soil, dust, and human or animal feces.

5. *Insects.* For example, flies pick up pathogens from open garbage and sewage and carry them to food and drink.

6. *Inanimate objects* (called *fomites*). For example, the spirochete *Borrelia vincenti*, which causes Vincent's angina or "trench mouth," may be transmitted via poorly washed dishes (it often harbors in cracks of cups and dishes).

Endogenous contact is a mode of transmission of infection from one area of the body to another in the same person, as from an infected wound to a scratch on the skin.

Person to person contact is a common mode of transmitting infection. It may be direct, as by kissing or sexual contact, or through touching infected parts of the body or discharges such as exudates from an infected wound. People may also infect one another through *droplet infection*, that is, the spray of droplets from the nose and mouth onto the skin or mucous membranes of another (as, for example, in the common cold) . Person to person contact may also be indirect; for example, organisms may be transferred from one patient to another via the nurse's hands if she does not wash them adequately before and after giving patient care.

Portals of entry whereby infectious agents gain access to the body of a suscep-

tible human being are, in many instances, the same as those by which the agents left the host reservoir, that is: the *gastrointestinal tract*, usually via the mouth in food or drink; the *respiratory tract*, in inspired air; the *skin and mucous membranes*, usually through breaks in these tissues; and the *genitourinary tract*, usually through the external openings, whence the infection travels up the tract via its mucous membrane lining.

The portals of entry to the human body and exit routes from the body used by different infectious agents vary, as do their capacities to live outside their original reservoirs. The method of transfer for each infectious agent depends on the specific portal of entry, exit route, and ability to live outside its reservoir.[3] In order to plan adequate precautionary measures to prevent and control infection, then, it is important that the specific causative agent of the infection be identified.

The Body's Reaction to Infectious Agents

The human organism is equipped with various mechanisms that help to prevent the invasion of body tissues by infectious agents and to control their growth and multiplication in the body if they do get past the first lines of defense.

Innate Immunity. The body has an *innate immunity*—that is, built-in mech-

---

[3]Nordmark and Rohweder, op. cit., p. 310.

anisms to ward off diseases through such factors as

1. The skin's resistance to microbial invasion

2. The ability of the acid digestive juices and digestive enzymes to destroy ingested bacteria and other organisms

3. The ability of the white blood cells and the reticuloendothelial system to destroy microorganisms and toxins

4. The ability of certain chemical compounds in the blood to attach themselves to infectious agents or their toxins and destroy them

Adaptive Immunity.[4] The body also has an *adaptive immunity,* which permits it to develop specific resistance to various infectious agents or their toxins. In response to an infectious agent that has penetrated the first lines of defense, the lymph tissues develop *specific antibodies,* which are specialized protein molecules, and *sensitized leukocytes;* both of these are capable of attacking and destroying the antigen (any substance capable of producing antibody formation; this reaction is believed to be a response to large protin molecules or polysaccharides in the infectious agent or its toxin) in its host.

---

[4]Arthur C. Guyton: *Function of the Human Body.* 4th edition. Philadelphia, W. B. Saunders Company, 1974, pp. 70–79.

Active immunity may be acquired by a person in response to actual invasion by an infectious agent; if a person has measles in childhood, for example, he is usually immune to it for the rest of his life. Active immunity may also be acquired artificially by the injection into the body of (1) attenuated organisms—that is, live organisms that have been processed so they will no longer cause the disease but still carry the specific antigen (smallpox vaccination is an example); (2) dead organisms which still have their chemical antigens (as in typhoid fever inoculations); or (3) treated toxins whose toxic nature has been destroyed but which still retain their antigenic properties (as, for example, tetanus inoculation).

Passive immunity may be conferred by the administration of preformed antibodies or specifically sensitized leukocyte cells in the form of immune serum globulins, antitoxins, or antiserums.

Other Responses of the Body to Infection. As we discussed briefly in Chapter 2, the body has both a generalized reaction to stress (the General Adaptation Syndrome or G.A.S.) and a localized reaction that occurs at the site of stress (the Local Adaptation Syndrome). The early *general reaction* of the body to the stress of invasion by infectious agents is the same as the "just feeling sick" phenome-

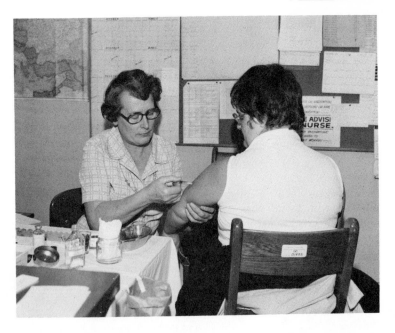

Immunization programs have helped to lessen the number of deaths from infectious diseases.

non described by Selye. This usually includes headache, malaise, a feeling of tiredness, slight elevation in temperature, and loss of appetite (sometimes followed by nausea and vomiting). In response to infectious agents there is usually a swelling of the lymph nodes as well.

It is in the second stage of the syndrome that the signs and symptoms of the specific infectious disease usually appear; an example of this is the typical vesicular rash seen in chickenpox.

The *localized reaction* that occurs at the site of injury or invasion represents the body's attempt to wall off the invader and destroy it before it can travel further to other parts of the body.

Inflammation is the localized protective response that is the body's reaction to injury or destruction of tissues, whether caused by the invasion of infectious agents, or by chemical, thermal, or physical means.[5]

When body tissues are damaged, an increased supply of blood is always diverted to the area and certain substances are released by the injured cells to promote the repair and regeneration of the tissues. Among these substances are *leukotaxine* and *histamine*. Leukotaxine draws white blood cells to the area, where they help to destroy and remove foreign substances such as bacteria and decaying tissue cells. Histamine, along with other substances increases permeability of the capillary walls, which allows the fluids, proteins, and white blood cells to move into the area. The clotting mechanism is also activated, so that the fluids clot and serve to "wall off" the injured areas.

Typically, there are five observable results from the inflammatory process: heat, redness, pain, swelling, and limitation of function. The redness is due to the local dilation of blood vessels and consequent increase in the supply of blood to the part. The warmth of the area is also the result of the increased blood supply. The swelling results from the exudative process, in which serum and leukocytes leave the blood stream to invade the area. The pain is believed to result from the stimulation of pain receptors in the area by certain substances released by the damaged cells and possibly also by the pressure of accumulated fluid (see Chapter 31). Limitation of function is usually due to the swelling and the pain.

Factors Affecting an Individual's Susceptibility to Infection

A person's resistance to infection is much better when he is in good general health. As we have mentioned in previous chapters, good nutrition, adequate exercise, a sufficient amount of rest and sleep, and good hygiene practices all contribute to increasing the body's ability to fight off infections. To supplement this general type of resistance, immunization is an effective method of preventing many communicable diseases, such as whooping cough, smallpox, measles, tetanus, typhoid fever, poliomyelitis, and many other formerly common infectious diseases.[*]

Infants and small children are particularly vulnerable to infections, as are the very old. So, too, are sick people, as we mentioned earlier, because of their general debility. People with cuts or lesions in the skin (such as the surgical patient, or anyone with a wound of any kind) have an obvious portal of entry for infectious agents. Individuals who have been exposed to infectious diseases and have not been adequately immunized are also on the list of those "at risk" to infections.

If any of these individuals are malnourished, do not have optimal strength and tone in their muscles, are tired, or have not maintained good hygiene practices, their vulnerability to infection is increased.

COMMON SOURCES OF INFECTION AND TRANSMISSION MODES IN HEALTH AGENCIES

In the introduction to this chapter, we mentioned that institution-acquired infec-

---

[5]Ibid., p. 71.

[*]For additional information on this topic, the student is directed to Dorothy Marlow, *Textbook of Pediatric Nursing*, 4th edition. Philadelphia, W. B. Saunders Company, 1973.

tions continue to be a problem in hospitals in the United States and Canada (and in many other countries, too). The nurse should be aware, then, of common sources of infection and some of the ways infection is spread in health agencies.

The most important reservoir of organisms within a health agency is probably the patients themselves. Usually, every patient who comes into a hospital or other inpatient facility is observed for any sign of infection: any boils, fever, septic wounds and the like are reported for further investigation. In most hospitals, the charge nurse has the authority to order precautionary techniques for a patient if she suspects that he harbors pathogenic organisms which could be spread to other patients and the staff.

A routine measure for most newly admitted patients in a clinic, nursing home, or hospital is the chest x-ray. The intent of the x-ray is to detect pulmonary tuberculosis. This is considered particularly important diagnostically for elderly patients. Serological tests for syphilis are done also on all newly admitted patients in many agencies. With the alarming increase of venereal disease among the population in recent years, this is another important diagnostic measure.

As mentioned earlier, people working in a health agency can also be reservoirs of infection. Any person with a fever, diarrhea, nausea, and most certainly, a cold, may be spreading infectious organisms. This is particularly serious in the operating room, the nursery, and the intensive care and coronary units, where infection seriously threatens the safety of patients and where the transmission rate is high.

Patients' visitors can also transmit infections, although normally the length of their period of contact is minimal in comparison with that of personnel. Food, vermin, and dirt also transmit disease, but they are an unlikely source in a modern institution. Hospital dust is probably heavily laden with pathogenic organisms; however, dryness inhibits their growth, and most hospitals have housekeeping policies which eliminate unnecessary moisture and maintain a high standard of cleanliness.

Among the common sources of infection in hospitals and other inpatient facilities for the care of the sick are:

1. Nose and throat secretions and the expired air of people with respiratory infections.

2. Vomitus and feces (feces more than vomitus, since microorganisms do not flourish well in the stomach)

3. Urine from patients with genitourinary tract infections

4. Discharges from body orifices

5. Exudates from infected wounds or skin lesions

6. Equipment used in the care of patients with infections

7. Bed linen and personal linen used by patients with infections

Common Vehicles for the Transmission of Infection in Health Agencies

The most common means by which infection is spread in health agencies are:

1. *Personal contact.* One child with measles, for example, may give measles to a whole ward of children. A nurse with a cold may give the cold to all her patients.

2. *Aerial routes. Staphylococcus aureus*, which has been the cause of so many hospital infections, is air-borne. The organisms are often transferred by droplet infection from the nose and throat passages of carriers; they may also travel quickly from one place to another by attaching themselves to dust particles in the air. *Staphylococcus aureus* organisms in large quantity have frequently been found on patient's bedding. The nurse must take particular care, therefore, when changing the bed linen, not to shake sheets and blankets. Used linen should be put into a hamper (preferably a closed one) as soon as possible after removal from the patient's bed.

3. *Animals and insects.* Rats and mice may be a concern in some agencies. They spread *Salmonella* and *Shigella* organisms, among others. Flies also are well-known carriers of microorganisms. Windows in a health agency should always be screened. This is not usually a problem in modern hospitals but may be in a neigh-

borhood health center or a remote nursing station.

4. *Fomites*. Inanimate objects, such as needles and syringes, are possible sources of infection in health agencies. A number of cases of infectious hepatitis, for example, have been traced directly to contaminated needles or intravenous equipment which has been inadequately cleaned and sterilized. The use of disposable equipment has reduced this hazard, but in agencies where needles, syringes, and infusion or drainage sets are reused, cleaning and sterilizing standards must be scrupulously enforced.

5. *Food and drink.* Impure water and contaminated food are known to cause outbreaks of such diseases as cholera, typhoid fever, and infectious hepatitis. Although regulations to safeguard the water supply are stringent in most parts of the United States and Canada, there are still remote areas where this is a problem. Contamination of food by workers who are carriers of disease (as, for example, the well-known cases of typhoid carriers), is another concern of all institutions, hotels, restaurants, and other eating places.

6. *Endogenous spread.* Spreading of organisms from one area of a person's body to another, as from the skin to an open wound, is also common. The maintenance of strict aseptic technique, while doing dressings, for example, is important to prevent the endogenous spread of organisms.

ASSESSING THE PATIENT FOR EXISTING AND POTENTIAL PROBLEMS OF INFECTION

Every patient in a health agency has a potential problem of infection, as does every health worker. The nurse must be alert to watch for infections in those who are particularly "at risk": (1) the very young; (2) the very old; (3) people who are generally debilitated, e.g., malnourished, tired, or weak; (4) those who have not maintained good hygiene practices; and (5) those who have been exposed to infectious disease.

From the nursing history and the initial clinical appraisal, the nurse can obtain information about the general health status of the patient, i.e., current state of functional abilities and state of health at the time of admission to the agency. This information is supplemented by data about the patient's past and current health problems, and the physician's diagnostic and therapeutic plans of care, as found in the patient's record. Laboratory tests and x-ray reports are also very helpful, if they have been done.

Frequently, all new patients undergo chest x-rays and serologic tests for syphilis. Other laboratory tests may be ordered to identify the specific agent causing an infection. The nurse must be alert for medical orders that place the patient on infection precautionary status or that require special handling of urine, feces, or other bodily secretions, of excretions, or of wounds.

Ultimately, the nurse's observations of the patient are of prime importance in identifying infections. She watches for signs and symptoms of the body's general and local responses to invasion. The vital signs—temperature, pulse, and respirations—are particularly helpful observations in early detection of infection in the patient. His complaints of tiredness, headache, or loss of appetite, or that he generally is not feeling well, are also among the early warning signs the nurse should watch for as possible indications of a generalized reaction to infection. If a patient complains of any of these it is always wise to check his temperature, pulse, and respirations to see if they are elevated. The patient's subjective observations and the nurse's objective findings are both reported promptly.

The patient may be able to tell the nurse about localized symptoms, too, such as pain, warmth in the area, and loss of function. Combined with her observations of redness and swelling (she may also observe the patient's reactions indicating pain, feel the warmth of the area, and observe limitation of movement), these would certainly lead her to suspect a localized infection.

She should also be alert to secretions from the nose and throat, coughing, sneezing, or the expectoration of sputum by a patient. Exudates from wounds or other breaks in the skin, or from any of the body orifices, should also warn her of the possibility of infection, as would any vomiting or diarrhea.

The patient and his immunization record are usually the best sources of information about prior exposure to infectious diseases. In some agencies, this information is included in the data gathered during the nursing history. If the patient is a child, a very ill adult, or unable to communicate, the family would be the best source of information on this point.

COMMON PROBLEMS

Potential or actual infections are the basic problems in this instance. A known or suspected infection brings with it additional problems, such as control of the spread of infection to other patients, to visitors, and to staff. The patient who is placed on special precautionary measures because he has, or is suspected to have, an infection, will have increased anxiety, as well as potential problems of sensory deprivation and feelings of isolation. He will no doubt be worried about the cause of the infection, about spreading it to other people, about the seriousness of the infection, and about what it means. He is usually set apart from others physically, as, for example, by being placed in a private room, or by having his unit demarcated by signs that advise staff, visitors,

and other patients that he is "infected." He also has to learn how to prevent the spread of his infection to others. The patient's family and other visitors also need to learn the reason for the precautionary measures and the various other measures they need to take to protect themselves and others.

PRIORITIES FOR NURSING ACTION

If a patient is suspected of having an infection—that is, if the nurse observes signs of localized or general infection in the patient, she reports these promptly to the physician so that appropriate diagnosis and therapy can be initiated and precautionary measures started. In many agencies, as mentioned earlier, the head nurse has authority to institute these measures based on her own judgment, to safeguard other patients, visitors, and staff from acquiring the infection. Some organisms are particularly virulent, and even their suspected presence constitutes an emergency situation. The variola virus, which causes smallpox, for example, is very virulent. A person suspected of having smallpox is isolated immediately and the room in which he was examined is thoroughly disinfected before being used again.

PRINCIPLES RELEVANT TO THE PREVENTION AND CONTROL OF INFECTION

1. Of the many varieties of microorganisms, only a few are true pathogens.
2. Many microorganisms normally present in the environment and in the body are opportunists and will become infectious agents if given the chance to do so.
3. The integrity of the skin and mucous membranes is the body's first line of defense against invasion by infectious agents.
4. A person's resistance to infection is lessened when he is very young or very old, when his health status is poor, when hygiene is neglected, and when he has not been adequately immunized against infectious diseases.
5. Infectious agents may be transported by a number of different routes to a susceptible human being.
6. The modes of transfer of infectious agents vary depending on their usual portal of entry, exit route, and ability to live outside their reservoir.
7. Some individuals carry infectious agents but do not themselves show clinical signs and symptoms of the infection.
8. Infectious agents may be destroyed by sufficient heat, by chemical agents, and by other known means.

GOALS FOR NURSING ACTION

The basic goals of nursing action in regard to infection are threefold:

1. To prevent infection
2. To control infection
3. To ensure the patient's comfort, safety, and psychosocial well-being when he is placed on precautionary measures for infection

SPECIFIC NURSING INTERVENTIONS

Cleaning Methods, Disinfection, and Sterilization Techniques

Clean equipment is essential to safe patient care. Many hospitals have a central supply department where all equipment is cleaned and prepared for use. The availability of disposable equipment has contributed greatly to patient safety and has also lessened the amount of time spent by nurses in cleaning and steriliz-ing equipment. In spite of the increasing use of disposables and the current practice of employing other personnel to clean and prepare equipment and supplies, the nurse is nonetheless well advised to be familiar with standard cleaning methods and disinfection and sterilization techniques to ensure the safety of her patients.

Cleaning Methods. Articles are referred to as *clean* when they are free from disease-producing organisms (pathogens). Dirty or contaminated materials harbor pathogens. An article is said to be *sterile* when it is free of all microorganisms, and unsterile when there are any living organisms on it.

Most utility rooms have a "clean" area and a "dirty" area. The clean area is used for the storage of sterile and clean supplies and the preparation of treatment trays. The dirty area is used for washing and cleaning trays and equipment and for storing used equipment prior to its return to the central supply (or other) department.

A basic cleaning procedure which is

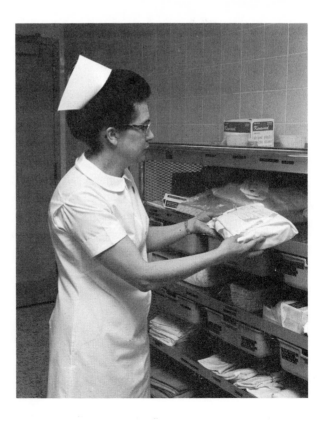

Many health agencies have separate departments in which supplies and equipment are prepared for use. The nurse selects a sterile dressing tray from the central supply cart which has been brought to the service room of a nursing unit.

applicable to most equipment is the following:

1. Rinse the article in cold water in order to remove any organic material. Heat coagulates protein and thus tends to make blood and pus stick to equipment.

2. Wash the article in soap and hot water. The emulsifying power of the soap, as well as its surface action, facilitates the removal of dirt. The water helps wash the dirt away.

3. Cleanse with an abrasive when necessary.

4. Rinse well with hot water and then dry.

5. Sterilize or disinfect as necessary.

A stiff brush helps in cleaning many types of equipment; it makes it easier to reach crevices and corners. There are specially constructed brushes for cleaning the lumina of test tubes, tubing, and the like.

Disinfection and Antisepsis. Disinfection and antisepsis are processes by which disease-inducing organisms are killed or their growth is prevented. A *disinfectant* is an agent, usually chemical, which kills many forms of pathogenic microorganisms but not necessarily the more resistant forms, such as spores. An *antiseptic* prevents the growth and activity of microorganisms but does not necessarily destroy them. Disinfectants are commonly used to destroy pathogens on inanimate objects such as scalpels, whereas antiseptics are used on people's wounds or skin. A substance is also spoken of as *bactericidal* if it kills bacteria and *bacteriostatic* if it merely prevents their growth.

Many disinfectants and antiseptics are available commercially. When choosing a disinfectant, five factors are considered:

1. The disinfectant should kill the pathogens within a reasonable time

2. The disinfectant should not be readily neutralized by proteins, soaps, or detergents

3. The disinfectant should not be harmful to the material on which it is to be used

4. The disinfectant should not be harmful to the human skin

5. The disinfectant should be stable in solution

The choice of the disinfectant for a specific purpose is best made after tests have been made of their conformity to these criteria.

Sterilization. Sterilization refers to the killing of all forms of bacteria, spores, fungi, and viruses. It can be accomplished by heat or chemicals. The autoclave is considered to be the most effective method of sterilizing hospital supplies. Generally, it is thought that steam at a pressure 15 to 17 pounds per square inch and at a temperature of 121° to 123° C. (250° to 254° F.) for 30 minutes is effective in sterilizing supplies. Prior to autoclaving, the equipment to be sterilized is washed and wrapped in such a way that it will remain protected after it is removed from the autoclave. A piece of autoclave tape which indicates when the sterilization is completed is often put on a package before it is sterilized. One type of tape has white lines which turn dark during the process to indicate that the equipment has been sterilized. Glass indicators are also available for this purpose. A chemical inside the glass changes color upon autoclaving.

When the nurse loads the autoclave for sterilization certain guides are best followed:

1. Place equipment in the autoclave in such a manner that steam circulates freely around each item

2. Turn bowls and other vessels on their sides so that water will not collect in them

3. Separate rubber surfaces so that they will not stick together as a result of the extreme heat

4. Check to be sure that the autoclave is set to sterilize the specific equipment

Boiling is another method of rendering articles free of microorganisms. It is believed that boiling for 10 to 20 minutes will destroy all pathogens with the exception of spores and the virus of infectious hepatitis. The article to be sterilized must be completely submerged in water during the entire time, the boiling time being counted after the water comes to a full boil.

Dry heat is sometimes used to sterilize supplies. Heating most objects for two hours at 170° C. (340° F.) has been found to be effective for sterilization, but petrolatum and oils require a higher temperature or more prolonged exposure to heat. In the home, an oven can be used to sterilize materials.

Chemical sterilization necessitates the submerging of the object in a sterilizing solution for a specified period of time. Many pharmaceutical preparations are available for this purpose; the choice depends upon the article to be sterilized and the kind of microorganism present. The object is soaked for the specified time before it is considered sterile.

Gas sterilization with ethylene oxide has also been found satisfactory in many situations. According to research reports, all microorganisms subjected to a temperature above 43.3° C. (110° F.), a relatively high humidity, and a concentration of ethylene oxide of 440 mg. per liter have been destroyed. Ethylene oxide sterilization has been suggested for plastics, rubber, and fabrics. Its effectiveness, however, is reduced in the presence of biological products such as blood.[6]

Exposure of articles to direct sunlight for a period of 6 to 8 hours is also considered an effective method of disinfection. It may be used in some areas for articles that are difficult to disinfect by other means—as, for example, rubber drawsheets.

Asepsis

The term *asepsis* refers to the absence of all disease-producing organisms. Both medical and surgical asepsis are practiced in patient care. *Medical asepsis* comprises those practices which are carried out in order to keep microorganisms within a given area. For example, if a patient has active tuberculosis, the patient and any articles with which he has had contact are considered to be contaminated with *Mycobacterium tuberculosis* and are therefore able to pass on the infection. In medical aseptic practices microorganisms are kept within a well-defined area, and any articles or materials removed from this area are immediately rendered free of

bacteria so that they cannot transfer the infection.

Surgical asepsis refers to practices carried out in order to keep an area free of organisms. It is just the opposite of medical asepsis in that surgical aseptic practices are designed to keep organisms *out of* a defined area. Thus, an operative wound is kept surgically aseptic.

Handwashing

Handwashing is an important measure in preventing the spread of microorganisms. Good aseptic technique involves limiting the transfer of organisms from one person to another. By washing her hands after contact with a patient, the nurse can limit the spread of microorganisms to other people, particularly other patients. In handwashing, both mechanical and chemical means are used to remove and destroy organisms. The running water mechanically washes away organisms, while soaps emulsify foreign matter and lower surface tension, thus facilitating the removal of oils, greases, and dirt.

For cleansing after contact with a person or an object such as a sputum cup, which harbors pathogenic organisms, it is recommended that a two minute wash be done with an alkaline detergent or a bar of ordinary soap. In surgical asepsis, handwashing is indicated prior to working with sterile equipment in order to render the hands as free as possible from bacteria. In either medical or surgical asepsis it is advantageous to wash one's hands at a deep sink where the water can be regulated by a foot or leg control. One procedure for the handwash is as follows:

1. Roll up sleeves above elbows and remove watch.

2. Clean the fingernails as necessary. Disposable sticks are often provided for this purpose.

3. Wash hands and arms to the elbow thoroughly with soap and warm water. Wash in continuously running water, using a rotary motion and taking care to clean the interdigital spaces.

   a. In surgical asepsis, always hold the hands higher than the elbows so that water will flow from the cleanest to

---

[6]James J. Shull: Ethylene Oxide Sterilization. *Canadian Nurse,* 58:603–607, July 1962.

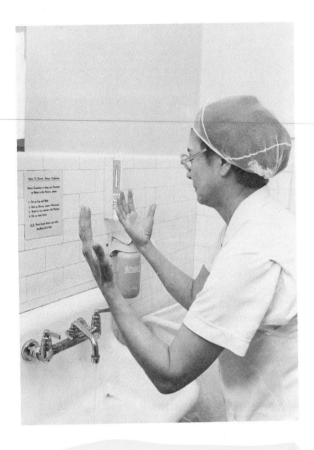

The hands are held higher than the elbows during a surgical asepsis handwash so that the water will flow from the hands to the elbows, i.e., from the cleanest to the dirtiest areas.

the dirtiest area. A surgical scrub brush is sometimes used, although the danger of creating abrasions on the skin needs to be considered.

 b. In medical asepsis hold the hands lower than the elbows while washing in order to prevent microorganisms from contaminating the arms.

 4. Rinse hands and arms, allowing water to flow freely.

 5. Repeat steps 3 and 4.

 6. Dry hands thoroughly with paper towels or a fresh clean towel. Many agencies now use hot air hand driers, which eliminates the use of paper or cloth towels. During the drying process the hands and arms are held higher than the elbows whichever method of drying is used.

When washing her hands, the nurse should take precautions to protect her uniform from getting wet. She should stand so that her uniform does not touch the wash basin and should hold her hands and arms away from her body when she is drying them. When turning off water at a

sink that does not have foot or leg controls, a dry towel is used to handle the taps; they are considered grossly contaminated. The basin is considered contaminated also. If a break in technique occurs—for example, if the nurse accidently touches the side of the basin during or after the handwash—the wash should be repeated from the beginning. It is important that the nurse keep the skin on her hands in good condition. Hand lotions or creams should be used frequently.

In caring for patients with some infections, it is often advisable to wear rubber gloves in handling excreta or in giving direct care. The topic of putting on sterile gloves is discussed in Chapter 22.

Masking

Masks are used in a variety of situations. Their general purpose is to limit the spread of microorganisms. Putting a mask over one's mouth and nose serves to filter both inspired and expired air. In some sit-

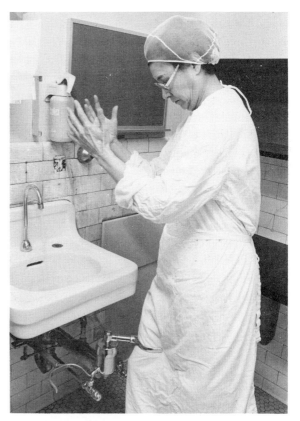

The taps are considered grossly contaminated, therefore, most sinks in health agencies are equipped with foot or leg controls to turn off the water after the handwash.

uations visitors and patients wear masks—for example, to protect an open wound.

Masks may be made of cotton, gauze, or glass fiber, although disposable paper masks are increasingly being used. Generally a mask should be worn only once, then discarded. It is a violation of technique to hang a mask around one's neck when it is not in use. Masks are changed when they become wet, since moisture fa-

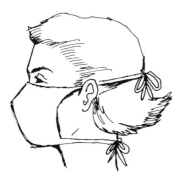

Masks are worn to filter both inspired and expired air. (From Lucile A. Wood and Beverly J. Rambo, eds.: Nursing Skills for Allied Health Services. Vol. 2, 2nd Ed. Philadelphia, W. B. Saunders Co., 1977.)

cilitates the passage of bacteria through the mask.

In surgical asepsis, masks are generally worn by personnel to keep equipment sterile or a wound free from microorganisms. It is inadvisable to cough or to sneeze while masked, and one talks only when necessary. Although the mask acts as a barrier, bacteria can escape around the sides of the mask and through the material itself, particularly during forceful respirations. Masks should be changed frequently. Although the length of time a mask is effective has not been precisely determined, LeMaitre and Finnegan suggest that a mask should be worn no longer than two to three hours in the operating room even for the same patient.[7]

When doing dressings or other treatments for a number of patients, it is good practice for the nurse to don a new mask for each patient.

Policies on the use of masks in medical asepsis vary from place to place. It is

---

[7]George LeMaitre and Janet Finnegan: *The Patient in Surgery.* 3rd edition. Philadelphia, W. B. Saunders Company 1975, p. 103.

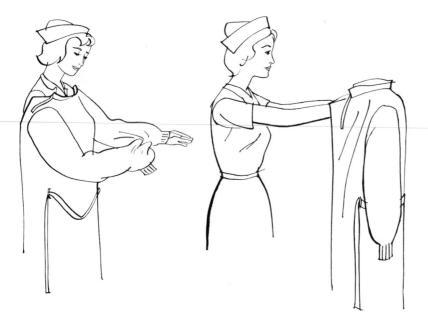

When taking off a contaminated gown that is to be discarded, the nurse keeps her "dirty" hands and the contaminated side of the gown away from her.

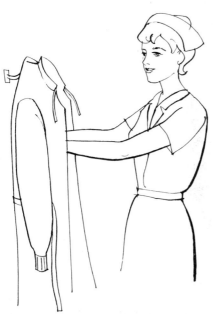

When reusing a contaminated gown, the nurse slips her clean hands inside without contaminating herself with the gown.

sometimes indicated for hospital personnel to wear masks in order to protect themselves from the pathogenic organisms of patients.

Gowning

Gowning is indicated if there is any possibility that the nurse may contaminate her uniform while she is attending a patient with an infection. The gown is long enough to cover the nurse's uniform completely, if a dress, or below the knees of a pantsuit, and generally it is not worn outside the boundaries of the patient's unit.

The simplest and safest practice is to use a clean gown each time it is necessary to protect one's uniform. The gown is put on so that the uniform is completely covered, and when it is taken off it is discarded in a container within the patient's unit. Care is taken that the outside of the gown, which is contaminated, does not touch the nurse's uniform. The nurse washes after she has discarded her gown.

If it is not possible to use a clean gown each time, then the nurse removes the gown *after* she has washed. When she takes it off she hangs it in such a way that the clean side is protected from contamination and the gown can be safely and easily put on later. The neck ties are kept against the clean side so that they do not become contaminated. The next time the nurse uses this gown, she picks it up by the clean side and ties the neck ties before she contaiminates her hands on the outer side of the gown.

For visitors' use, many agencies now provide disposable gowns. These are used once and thrown away.

Barrier Technique

In situations in which the presence of pathogens is suspected or has been proved, medical aseptic practices are observed in order to control their spread and contribute to their destruction. Such medical aseptic practices are called infection precautions. The exact technique employed in a particular situation depends upon the portal of exit, the method of transfer and the portal of entry of the particular pathogen.

In *barrier technique*, mechanical barriers are established to confine the organisms within a given area. The boundaries in a hospital or at home can be the patient's unit or a single room, but all equipment within the designated area is considered contaminated. Barrier technique has the psychological advantage of reminding people of the existence of the pathogenic organisms and the physical advantage of a separate room, which decreases the transfer of organisms by air.

In the past, barrier technique was known as *isolation*. The very word "isolation" describes what can happen to a patient who has an infection. It has been observed that hospital personnel and other patients tend to actually isolate such patients, who then become lonely and feel that they are nuisances. In many instances the words "dirty," "contaminated," and "isolated" have a moral significance for the patient, causing him to feel unworthy and unaccepted. Patients for whom barrier technique is necessary should not be psychologically isolated from others; indeed, physical isolation is often unnecessary when proper precautions are taken. The importance of explanations and support is paramount for these patients; consequently, the nurse needs to understand both her own attitudes and the practices which contribute to her own safety and that of the patient.

Reverse Barrier Technique. In reverse barrier technique, the patient is protected from pathogens in the environment. Instead of keeping pathogens within a defined area, as in barrier technique, the organisms are kept outside the defined area. This is done in a variety of ways, one of which is to place a plastic enclosure around the patient. All air reaching the patient is filtered, and all equipment entering the enclosed area is free of pathogens. Reverse barrier technique is used for patients who are particularly susceptible to infections, for example, people who have severe burns or leukemia. Since these patients do not have normal resistance to pathogenic microorganisms, they are protected within barriers which permit an aseptic environment to be established.

Care of Equipment and Supplies. The increasing use of disposable equipment and supplies has simplified the practice of barrier technique. The wide range of disposables currently available includes dishes, cutlery, medicine cups, syringes, needles, treatment trays, gloves, intravenous sets, drainage sets, bedpans, and bedpan covers. When these articles are used for a patient who requires barrier-technique nursing, concurrent disinfection is considerably easier. There are still some aspects of patient care, however, for which disposables are not applicable. Disposables are also costly and may not be used in all situations. The nurse should, therefore, be familiar with measures that may be used in concurrent and terminal disinfection to control the spread of microorganisms.

Concurrent disinfection refers to the ongoing measures taken to control the spread of infection while the patient is considered infectious. Pathogenic organisms are destroyed continually while the patient requires barrier technique. Measures for concurrent disinfection are detailed later in this section. *Terminal disinfection* comprises those measures which destroy pathogenic organisms after a patient leaves an examining room or a hospital or when he no longer requires barrier technique. In terminal disinfection all equipment within the patient's room is rendered free of pathogenic organisms by appropriate means; for example,

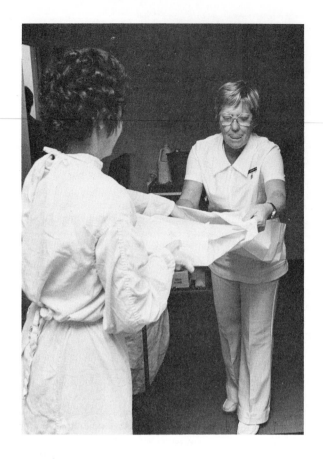

In many agencies contaminated equipment is placed in two heavy paper bags in such a way that the outer bag remains clean.

the walls and floor are washed with a disinfectant, and linen is wrapped and sent to the laundry to be disinfected. If the patient is to remain in the hospital, he usually takes a shower and then goes to another bed unit with clean equipment. The tub or shower is also cleaned with a disinfectant after use.

EQUIPMENT. All equipment used for a patient who has an infection is rendered clean immediately after it is taken from the patient's unit. Equipment such as glass medicine containers, artery forceps, and stainless steel bowls can be autoclaved and thus rendered safe easily and quickly. Many hospitals place such equipment in two heavy paper bags in such a way that the outer bag remains clean. The bag is marked "infectious" and is then autoclaved. If equipment is wet the inner bag should be made of waxed paper in order to contain the moisture and the organisms.

If equipment cannot be rendered safe by autoclaving, it can be exposed to ultra-violet light or soaked in or wiped with a disinfectant solution. Gas sterilization may also be used for some articles. The exact method depends upon the organism of infection and the type of equipment available.

LAUNDRY. Linen bags are generally placed in the patient's unit to hold contaminated linen. When linen has accumulated in the bag, a designated person brings in a clean linen bag, and the contaminated bag is placed in it carefully in order to avoid contaminating the outside of the clean bag. In this way the linen can be transported without danger of contaminating other personnel or equipment. The outer bag is marked "infectious."

The washing methods used in most hospital laundries render most contaminated materials clean. If it is necessary to take special precautions, as with spore-forming bacteria, linen is usually autoclaved prior to laundering.

DISHES. After a patient who has an infection has eaten, his dishes are removed

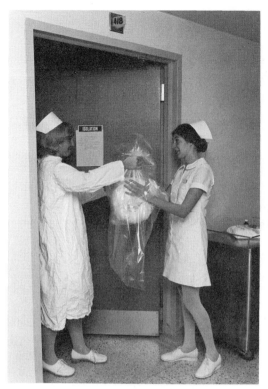

Concurrent disinfection includes the safe disposal of contaminated linen. These nurses are using a "double bagging" technique for the linen which has been taken from the patient's room.

to the bathroom, where the uneaten foods and fluids are disposed of (in the same manner as excreta; see following section); the dishes are then either replaced on the tray and taken to the dishwasher or they are double-bagged and autoclaved prior to washing. Many health agencies have automatic dishwaters which render dishes free of pathogens.

If an autoclave or dishwasher is not available, dishes can be boiled after they have been rinsed or they can be soaked in a disinfectant solution. The latter method is the least desirable, because of the difficulty of immersing the dishes completely and because of the errors that can occur. For example, organic material left on dishes can protect pathogens sufficiently for them to remain active after the normal soaking time.

Disposal of Excreta. Most contaminated excreta can be safely disposed of in the general sewage, where it is subsequently rendered harmless by the sewage treatment facilities of the community. In areas where the treatment of sewage is not considered satisfactory for a particular infectious organism, excreta must be rendered safe before disposal into the sewage system. One method of doing this is to treat the excreta with a prescribed disinfectant, such as chloride of lime, for the time necessary to destroy the pathogens.

Patient Teaching in Barrier Technique. Patients for whom barrier technique is being maintained often have special needs for emotional support. They are frequently physically isolated from other patients, and the hospital staff tends to ignore them, to "leave them until the last." Some patients attach a moral significance to their disease; they feel unworthy and think they are creating extra work for the nurse. If a nurse hesitates in full view of the patient before she enters his room and if she puts on a gown reluctantly or as if it is a bothersome duty, she will only enhance his feeling of unworthiness and lowered self-esteem.

Often a patient will want some recreational activity. Such activities should be designed so that they do not interfere with barrier technique, yet still meet the patient's needs. Materials such as magazines or woodcraft sets can be made safe after they are removed from the contaminated area. Magazines can usually be destroyed, and wood can be sterilized. With a little ingenuity the nurse can usually provide materials which can be either destroyed or sterilized after they have been used.

The explanations provided to a patient who requires barrier technique are crucial to his care. Most people want to participate in their own therapy; moreover, the success of medical asepsis and barrier technique is largely dependent upon the patient's willingness to help. The nurse is guided in her explanations by the needs of the patient to understand the reason for the various precautionary measures, the possible causes of the infection, what it means in terms of his health problem, and how he can help in measures to protect himself from further infection and to help prevent others from acquiring it. The spread of pathogens from the respiratory tract of patients is thought to be best con-

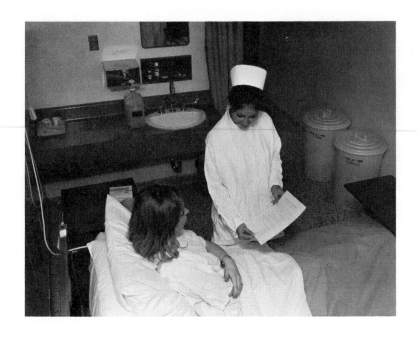

Patients for whom barrier technique is required need an explanation of the various measures involved.

trolled by teaching safe hygiene practices, which include frequent handwashing under running water. A patient with a pulmonary infection is taught to use several thicknesses of paper handkerchief to cover his nose and mouth when he sneezes or coughs. Also, covered, waterproof containers are provided for sputum. Facilities are also made available for the adequate disposal of paper handkerchiefs and sputum containers after they have been used.

Words such as "dirty" and "contaminated" are avoided whenever possible, because of the danger of misinterpretation and the value judgments that the patient may attach to them.

The nurse needs to understand what an infection means to the patient. Frequently a patient acquires an infection as a complication of another disorder after admission to the hospital. Such a complication means a lengthened hospital stay, increased financial cost and perhaps a real threat to life. Some patients react to these stresses with aggression and hostility directed toward the hospital in general or perhaps toward the nursing staff and the doctors. The nurse can offer support by providing an accepting environment in which the patient feels free to work through his feelings. She can also instruct patients in the possible sources of infections. For example, some people acquire

infections because of the manner in which they carry out their daily activities, and some find it difficult to see how faulty hygienic practices could be contributing factors.

The patient with an infection or a communicable disease usually has other problems requiring nursing intervention. Many of these, for example, those associated with fever and wounds, are discussed in later chapters in this text.

PLANNING AND EVALUATING NURSING INTERVENTIONS

The prevention of infection is an integral component of the planning and implementation of all nursing action, whether directly or indirectly concerned with patient care. Adherence to good standards of cleaning and to tested methods of disinfection and sterilization is vital to the prevention and control of infection in a health agency. Adequate handwashing before and after giving patient care to each patient is perhaps *the* most important means of preventing the spread of infection from one patient to another. Combined with strict adherence to good technique and good housekeeping practices, agency-based infections (and all others) can be kept to a minimum, if not completely eliminated.

When patients have a known infection or one is suspected, appropriate precautionary measures are initiated. The specific precautions taken depend on the nature of the infection, the portal of entry of the infectious agent, its exit route from the body, and its mode of transfer. Full barrier technique may be indicated in some cases; in others, precautions with respect to some aspects of care (as, for example, skin and wound care or care with regard to excreta) may be indicated. The specific precautions taken tend to vary according to the policies of the agency, and the nurse needs to be aware of those of the agency in which she is working.

A planned teaching program for the patient, his family, and other visitors is incorporated into the nursing care plan of all patients who are placed on precautionary measures for infections. Evaluations of the effectiveness of the teaching program lies in the acceptance by patient, his family, and other visitors of the need for these precautions, and their understanding of these through their demonstrated careful maintenance of the techniques and procedures recommended.

Some questions the nurse might ask herself to evaluate the effectiveness of her teaching are:

1. Is the barrier technique keeping the organisms within defined areas? How would you know?
2. Are other people in the environment free of the infection?
3. Does the patient have the knowledge and skills he requires to prevent the spread of his infection and to participate actively in his care insofar as he is able?

4. Does he have misconceptions about his infection?
5. Does the patient indicate in any way that he feels isolated? For example, does he complain verbally or show signs of depression?
6. Does he have the contact he wishes with his family, hospital personnel, and other patients without endangering their health?
7. Does he get exercise adequate to meet his needs?
8. Does he demonstrate an active interest in and is he encouraged to participate in his care insofar as he is able?
9. Does he have diversionary materials that interest him?
10. Do the people in the environment know and take the appropriate precautions to prevent their infection?

Evaluation of the effectiveness of nursing intervention is also measured by absence of the infection in other patients, in visitors, and in staff. Many agencies have an infection committee who keep a record of infections in patients in the agency. It is only through the accurate recording and maintenance of statistical records over a period of time that the effectiveness of infection control can be evaluated. Nurses must report signs of infection in a patient promptly. In some agencies nurses must complete an unusual occurrence form on every patient with an infection to facilitate the investigation and follow-up of cases, to evaluate the effectiveness of current practices, and to institute new measures as needed to prevent and control infection.

GUIDES TO ASSESSING THE PATIENT FOR EXISTING AND POTENTIAL PROBLEMS OF INFECTION

1. Is the patient very young? very old? malnourished? tired? weak? generally debilitated?
2. Is there evidence that he has maintained good hygiene practices? Does he need help to maintain them now?
3. Does he have any breaks in the skin or observable mucous membranes? Does he have lesions on the skin? Has he had wounds of any sort? Is he going to have, or has he had, surgery?
4. Has he been exposed to any infectious diseases?
5. Has he been immunized against communicable disease? If so, when were they done and what immunizations has he had?

6. Does he have a health problem(s) or has he had one that reveals a history of infection, causes a present infection, or would make the person more susceptible to infection?
7. Have diagnostic tests for any infectious agents been done? If so, what do the reports indicate?
8. Is the patient showing generalized signs of infection? signs of inflammation?
9. Is the patient coughing, sneezing, or bringing up sputum? Are there secretions from his nose and mouth?
10. Are there exudates from wound or skin lesions? from any of the body orifices?
11. If the patient is on precautionary measures for infection why have these been ordered? What special precautions are being taken?
12. Has the causative agent been identified? If so, what are its usual portal of entry, mode of spread, and exit route?
13. What special precautions are indicated to prevent the spread of the patient's infection?
14. If the patient is on infection precautions, what knowledge and skills does he need to protect himself and others?
15. What measures can you take to minimize his anxiety and prevent sensory deprivation and feelings of isolation?

STUDY VOCABULARY

Antiseptic	Differentiation	Pathogens
Bactericidal	Disinfectant	Secretion
Bacteriostatic	Endogenous spread	Sensitivity
Barrier technique	Excretion	Sterile
Clean	Infection	Sterilization
Concurrent disinfection	Isolation	Surgical asepsis
	Medical asepsis	Terminal disinfection

STUDY SITUATIONS

Mrs. R. Jackson is admitted to a hospital for an operation to remove an ulcer on her left leg. Three days after her surgery, Mrs. Jackson's wound appears reddened and has a purulent discharge. A wound culture has been ordered to identify the infecting organism. Barrier technique nursing is commenced.

Mrs. Jackson, who is 54 years old, is in a room that has four beds and a shared bathroom. Her physician suggests that she move to a private room on the same floor where she will have her own bathroom.

1. What factors would you consider prior to explaining barrier technique to this patient?
2. What should you include in your suggestion to Mrs. Jackson that she move to a single room?
3. Why might she not want to move?
4. Why would it be advantageous for the patient to move?
5. The infecting organism is found to be *Staphylococcus aureus.* What do you need to know about this organism in order to establish a safe environment?
6. Mrs. Jackson's wound is dressed at least twice a day. After this

measure what is done with the (a) old dressing, (b) linen drapes, (c) artery forceps, and (d) unused disinfectant?

7. "The safety of an environment is related to the number of pathogenic organisms in it." What measures in medical asepsis are based on this principle?

SUGGESTED READINGS

Alter, H. J., et al.: Health-Care Workers Positive for Hepatitis B Surface Antigen: Are Their Contacts at Risk? *New England Journal of Medicine, 292*:454–457, 1975.

Brown, M. A.: Adolescents and V. D. *Nursing Outlook, 21*:99–103, February 1973.

Brown, M. S.: What You Should Know About Communicable Diseases and Their Immunization. *Nursing '75*, Part 1, 5:70–72, September 1975; Part 2, 5:56–60, October 1975; Part 3, 5:55–60, November 1975.

Castle, M.: Isolation: Precise Procedure for Better Protection. *Nursing '75*, 5:50–57, May 1975.

Chavigny, K. H.: Nurse Epidemiologist in the Hospital. *American Journal of Nursing*, 75:638–642, April 1975.

Connell, A. D.: Controlling Operating Room-Related Infection in Cancer Patients. *Nursing Clinics of North America, 10*:667–678, December 1975.

Current Immunization Recommendations. Victoria, B. C., Provincial Department of Health, January, 1975.

Dubay, C., and R. D. Grubb: *Infection: Prevention and Control*. St. Louis, C. V. Mosby Company, 1973.

Fox, M. K., et al.: How Good are Handwashing Practices? *American Journal of Nursing, 74*:1676–1678, September 1974.

Hardy, C. S.: Infection Control. *Nursing '73*, 3:18–21, August 1973.

Jenny, J.: What You Should Be Doing About Infection Control. *Nursing '76*, 6:78–79, November 1976.

Maki, D. G., et al.: Infection Control in Intravenous Therapy. *Nursing Digest*, May-June, 1975, p. 5.

McCalla, J. L.: Immunotherapy: Concepts and Nursing Implications. *Nursing Clinics of North America, 11*:59–72, March 1976.

Wylie, H. W., et al.: Immunity Study in New Brunswick 1971–1972. *Canadian Journal of Public Health, 65*:124–126, March-April 1974.

22 WOUND CARE

The nurse should be able to:

Define terms commonly used to classify wounds
Describe the three stages of wound healing
Explain factors affecting wound healing
Apply relevant principles from the biophysical sciences in the
 care of wounds
Place a sterile dressing, using good aseptic technique
Accurately record and report observations about wounds
Demonstrate beginning skill in the application of binders
Demonstrate the five basic turns used in bandaging
Evaluate the effectiveness of nursing interventions in wound care

INTRODUCTION

Possibly no other single aspect of health care has elicited so much controversy over the years as the best method to care for wounds. Although the process of wound healing has been well known and well documented in the literature for many years, there is still no single standardized method of caring for a wound during the process of healing.

Unfortunately, infection of wounds postoperatively is still a major concern in all surgical procedures. The techniques for wound dressing vary from one agency to another, with each agency hoping by its techniques to eliminate all possible sources of wound contamination. The nurse must use all possible care in maintaining strict aseptic technique in the dressing of all wounds. She is guided in this by the procedures that have been developed and tested, and which are recommended by the agency in which she is working. The techniques suggested in this chapter provide general guidelines, utilizing basic principles, to maintain surgical asepsis in dressing wounds, to apply supporting binders, and to bandage various parts of the body requiring protection during the process of tissue healing.

CLASSIFICATION OF WOUNDS

A wound by definition is a break in the continuity of any body structure, internal or external, caused by physical means. Wounds can be classified in three ways: according to the presence or absence of microorganisms, according to the presence or absence of a break in the surface tissue, and according to the cause of the wound.

A wound is said to be clean, contaminated, or infected. A *clean* wound does not contain pathogenic microorganisms, whereas *contaminated* and *infected* wounds do contain such organisms. Normally a wound that is made under aseptic conditions, as for example, a surgical incision, is considered to be a *clean* wound; wounds that occur as a result of accidents are considered *contaminated* until they are proved to be clean. If the pathogenic microorganisms in a contaminated wound are sufficiently virulent and present in sufficient quantity, then an infectious process becomes apparent. The wound is then referred to as an *infected* wound. Frequently the terms "contaminated" and "infected" are used interchangeably although, in the strict sense of the meanings of these words, the two are not the same.

No wound is ever completely sterile. The skin and mucous membranes harbor some microorganisms as normal inhabitants. These are not normally pathogenic; their lack of virulence and their sparsity usually serve to prevent the development of an infectious process.

Wounds are also classified according to the presence or absence of a break in the surface covering. In a *closed wound* there is no break in the skin or mucous membrane. Such wounds are frequently caused by direct blows, traction or deceleration, a twisting or bending force, or direct muscle action. A common example of a closed wound is the fractured femur which so often results when an elderly person pivots or falls. *Open wounds* involve the destruction of skin or mucous membrane, thus exposing the underlying tissue to open air. Cuts, punctures, and surface abrasions are examples of open wounds.

Wounds are classified according to their cause. A *traumatic* or accidental wound is one which occurs by accident. Since it 415 happens under septic conditions, its chances of becoming infected are considerable. An *intentional* wound is one that is produced for a specific purpose, usually under aseptic conditions. For example, the wound made during an operation, generally under ideal sterile conditions, is an intentional wound.

Wounds are further described according to the manner in which they occur.

An *abraded wound* occurs as a result of friction or scraping. It is a superficial wound in which the outer layers of the skin or mucous membrane are damaged or scraped off. An example is the scrape a child gets when he falls on his knees on a cement sidewalk.

A *contused wound* occurs as a result of a blow from a blunt instrument, such as a hammer, without breaking the skin.

An *incised wound* occurs as a result of a cut by a sharp instrument. An example of an incised wound is one made by a scalpel during surgery; the wound edges are smooth.

In a *lacerated wound* the tissues are torn apart and remain jagged and irregular. An example of a lacerated wound is a cut by a saw.

A *penetrating wound* occurs as a result of an instrument which penetrates into the deep tissues of the body. An example is a bullet which enters the chest and lodges in the lung.

A *puncture or stab wound* is a wound made by a pointed instrument, such as a nail or wire. The scalpel is occasionally used by the physician to make a puncture wound so as to promote drainage from tissues. The term "puncture wound" is also used to describe an open wound resulting from a break (or puncture) of the skin surface and underlying tissues by the bite of an animal or the sting of an insect.

THE PROCESS OF WOUND HEALING

A wound, by definition, implies that there has been damage to body tissues. Whenever tissue damage occurs, the localized response of the body is the process of inflammation, described in Chapter 21. The early part of wound healing then shows evidence of this process. The student will note many similarities between the following outline of the process of wound healing and the description of inflammation.

The process of wound healing can be divided into three phases: the lag phase, the fibroplasia phase, and the phase of contraction.

In the *lag phase,* as a result of the injury to the cells, the capillaries become dilated in the injured area. The volume of blood in the area is increased but the speed of the flow of blood is slowed. The blood brings leukocytes and plasma which form an exudate in the injured area. At this time, the injured cells disintegrate and there is some swelling due to the plugging of the lymphatics by fibrin. During this phase, the wound is usually covered lightly by a scab or fibrin network, which is later absorbed.

In the *fibroplasia phase* there is an ingrowth of new capillaries and lymphatic endothelial buds in the wounded area. Fibroplasia results in the formation of granulation tissue (a connective tissue); subsequently there is epithelization (keratinization). The wound appears pink, owing to the new capillaries in the granulation tissue, and the area is soft and tender.

In the third phase, that of *contraction,* there is cicatrization or scar formation by the fibroblasts after the cessation of fibroplasia. The capillaries and lymphatic endothelial buds in the new tissue disappear, and the scar then shrinks.

Open wounds require the formation of more granulation tissue, fibrous tissue and epithelial tissue than closed wounds. During the first five or six days there is little strength in a healing wound; however, during the next 10 days the tissue becomes stronger and better able to withstand tension.

Types of Healing

Healing by First Intention. In healing by first intention the sutured wound heals without infection or separation at the edges. There is minimal granulation tissue present and thus a small scar results.

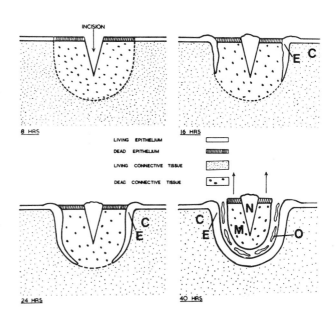

The main histological events in the first 48 hours of wound healing. (a) 8 hours. An area of tissue necrosis extends on either side of the incision. (b) 16 hours. The epithelium is thickened near the line of demarcation between living and dead tissue. A tongue of epithelial cells has begun to invade the underlying tissue at some distance from each side of the incision. (c) 24 hours. Epithelial invasion is well advanced and the two spurs move towards each other. (d) 40–48 hours. The epithelial spurs have met and severed the necrotic tissue (scab) from the underlying tissues. Keratinization of the epithelium is leading to dislodgment of the scab. E, epithelium; C, connective tissue; M, scab; N, blood and necrotic debris in incision track; O, keratin. (From D. Tarin: Wound Healing—a Diagrammatic and Pictorial Account. Nursing Times, 69:1124–1126, August 30, 1973.)

In most surgical incisions, the edges of the wound are sutured closely together and healing occurs by first intention.

Healing by Second Intention. In healing by second intention the edges of the wound are not approximated. As a consequence a large amount of granulation tissue is formed during the healing process, and the scar that results is usually large. The healing of decubitus ulcers illustrates healing by second intention. The crater of the ulcer must be filled in by the growth of new tissue. The process is a slow one and the resultant scar is large.

Healing by Third Intention. This is a combination of the two previously mentioned types of healing. Either the wound is initially left open and later sutured, or it breaks open after an original suturing and has to be resutured. There is considerable granulation tissue formed in this type of healing.

FACTORS AFFECTING WOUND HEALING

Many factors influence the speed and the character of the healing process:

Extent of the Injury. The process of repair and regeneration is naturally longer when tissue damage is extensive.

Nutrition. Nutritional status, specifically the protein and vitamin C levels, affects the healing process. Protein is necessary for the formation of new tissue; vitamin C is involved in the maturation of the collagen fibers (the fibrous tissue) during the later stages of healing.

Age. Healing is more rapid in children than in elderly persons. There are many factors which are felt to retard the healing process in the aged. These include a lessened efficiency of the circulatory system, particularly to surface areas of the body, and an increased likelihood of poor nutritional status among older people.

Blood Supply. The blood supplies the products used in healing. Hence any factor which restricts blood circulation to a wound area interferes with healing. Edema, restrictive bandages and damaged arteries can slow the healing process.

Hormones. It has been demonstrated that large doses of the adrenocortical hormones slow wound healing; for example, cortisone decreases the formation of collagen. This has implications in situations in which prolonged stress stimulates the release of these hormones.

Infection. Infectious processes result

in tissue destruction, which in turn results in a longer healing time. Foreign bodies also interfere with healing.

Edema. Gross edema hinders healing by inhibiting the transport of the building supplies to the area. There is some evidence, however, that a small amount of edema enhances fibroplasia.

Radiation Therapy. It has been shown that five to six days after irradiation (therapy or treatment by exposure to radiation, as, for example, x-ray therapy), the healing process is slowed.

COMMON PROBLEMS IN WOUND HEALING

Two common problems occurring in the process of wound healing are hemorrhage and infection.[1]

Hemorrhage

Hemorrhage has been defined as the escape of blood from the vessel in which it is normally contained. Whenever there is a wound, blood vessels in the area are damaged and bleeding occurs. Bleeding may result from the rupture of small surface blood vessels, or from trauma to larger, deeper-lying ones. The nurse should always be alert to the possibility of hemorrhage occurring during the process of wound healing. It may be caused by spontaneous rupture of a vessel that has been weakened in the process of trauma, by the giving way of sutures that have been used to repair damaged vessels, or by problems in the clotting mechanism resulting from a lack of certain clotting factors in the blood.

Evidence of Hemorrhage. The presence of bright red blood on dressings from a wound that is healing is always a warning to the nurse of the possibility of hemorrhage, and it should be reported, promptly. The beginning nurse should always ask her team leader or instructor to check a wound when she observes fresh

---

[1]In subsequent courses in medical-surgical nursing, the student will be alerted to other problems the nurse may encounter in relation to specific kinds of wounds.

red blood on a dressing. If, in the senior nurse's opinion, the situation is serious, the physician is alerted immediately and the wound checked frequently (every 15 to 20 minutes) to see if the bleeding is increasing. If bleeding becomes excessive, the patient may show signs of shock, which occurs whenever there is any major trauma to the body. Evidence of shock is observed in changes in the vital signs, such as falling blood pressure, a rapid weak pulse, pallor, a cold, clammy skin, weakness, and restlessness. (The subject of shock is discussed in more detail in Chapter 29.) If the nurse detects any of these signs in the patient, the team leader should be alerted at once so that prompt intervention can be initiated.

The Infected Wound

An infected wound is one in which an active infection process is present. All wounds contain organisms; many organisms are present in the air and thus, immediately after a wound is opened, it can be expected to harbor organisms. But the mere presence of microorganisms in a wound does not mean that an infection will necessarily ensue. Other factors are involved in the development of an infection:

The Virulence, Number and Types of Organisms. Certain types and strains of microorganisms are more likely to produce a disease than others. Also, the fewer the number of pathogenic organisms, the less likely they are to produce an infection.

Devitalized Tissue. Unhealthy tissue is less resistant to infection than healthy tissue. Poor circulation, inadequate nutrition, and dehydration all contribute to devitalization of tissue.

Local and General Immunity. Some tissues have a greater immunity than others. Highly vascularized tissue is less prone to infections than tissue nourished by a more limited circulation. Also there is a variability in the general resistance of the tissues of individuals.

Nature of the Wound. The occurrence of infection depends to some extent upon the presence of foreign bodies and organic contamination. Infection is also more likely in extensive wounds and in areas where local resistance is low—for example, in the perineal area. Generally the tissues of the face and neck have high resistance and heal well.

General Condition of the Patient. Anemia, dehydration, and so forth, lower resistance and make any wound more prone to infection.

Organisms Causing Wound Infection

There are several organisms which are commonly found in wound infections. Of the gram-positive group, *Staphylococcus aureus* and *S. albus* are found most commonly. These are spherical asymmetric bacteria that are normally found in the nose, skin, and feces. The α- and β-hemolytic streptococci are also the cause of many infectious processes. It has been stated that 8 per cent of all people carry these bacteria in the nasopharynx.

The toxigenic clostridia are anaerobic spore-forming bacilli. They thrive in airless conditions, being found in the intestinal tracts of animals, in dust, and in soil. *Clostridium tetani,* the cause of tetanus, is a well known member of this family; many physicians automatically give prophylactic doses of tetanus toxoid to patients whose wounds have come in contact with soil.

Of the gram-negative bacteria, the species *Escherichia coli, Aerobacter,* and *Alcaligenes* are frequently found in wounds. These, together with *Proteus* and *Pseudomonas,* are the principal inhabitants of the intestine. They can also often be isolated in the anogenital area, and are frequent causes of urinary tract infections.

Signs of Wound Infection

The patient who has an infected wound is likely to show local and general symptoms of infection. The local symptoms of wound infection are due to an aggravation of the inflammatory process. Typically, the wound area is more reddened, swollen, hot to the touch, and painful than it should be in the normal healing process. In addition, there may be purulent drainage from the wound.

The generalized signs and symptoms of an infection are those we described in Chapter 21 as the body's generalized response to infection (see p. 396). The degree to which a person shows some or all of these symptoms is highly dependent upon the severity of the infection and the resistance of the body.

ASSESSING THE PATIENT WITH A WOUND

In assessing the patient with a wound, the nurse should be aware of the cause of the wound, the type of wound it is, and when the wound took place. If it was the result of trauma, she should be aware of the possibility of foreign objects in the wound or of the presence of infectious agents, as, for example, from the soil. If the wound is a surgical one, she should be aware of the date of operation, the nature of the surgery, the location and extent of the surgical wound, and whether drains or packing were inserted into the operative site.

The nurse should also be aware of the physician's orders regarding wound care. Following some types of surgery, the physician may not want the dressing disturbed for a few days. At other times, the dressing may need frequent changing (for example, several times a day). The physician may also leave specific intructions regarding the ointments to be applied around the wound, or other details for its care.

In addition to these specifics, the nurse should also be aware of the basic nature of the patient's health problem(s) and the physician's overall plan of care for the patient.

The nurse also needs information regarding the patient's age, his general health status, his state of nutrition, the status of his skin and appendages, and his circulatory status. She should also consider whether there is a possibility that the patient has a generalized infection from a cause other than the wound, or a localized infection, as, for example, a boil or other infection involving the skin tissues, in another part of the body. The nurse reviews the nursing history and the initial clinical appraisal of the patient to obtain information on these factors.

She also obtains information about the nature of the patient's health problems and the physician's overall plan of care from his notations on the patient's record. If the patient has had surgery, information on the nature of the surgery, extent of the operative procedure, location of the wound, and insertion of drains (if any were inserted) should be available to the nurse from the operative record on the patient's chart.

If the wound was caused by other than surgical intervention, the cause, nature, and extent of the wound, and interventions such as cleaning or suturing that have been done will be noted in the physician's writeup of the health history of the patient.

The physician's instructions regarding wound care, and any specific precautions to be taken, will be written and included in the doctor's orders.

Finally, the record is supplemented by the nurse's observations of the wound, which include both her objective observations and subjective observations by the patient.

Observation of Wounds

When a wound is examined, as, for example, while a dressing is changed, certain features of the wound itself and the discharge from it are carefully observed. The wound is observed for the approximation of its edges. Some wounds are closed by sutures or skin clips, others by the pressure of a bandage or butterfly tape. A butterfly tape can be made from a strip of adhesive tape narrowed in the middle and placed across the wound so that the adhesive part of the tape sticks to the patient's skin on both sides of the wound and draws the edges of the wound together. The adhesive side of the tape directly over the wound is usually covered so that it will not adhere to the wound itself. Gaping in a sutured or taped wound could delay healing and should be reported. Some wounds are not closed deliberately but are left to close naturally by second intention. A wound is also observed for signs of inflammation and infection, such as redness, swelling, pain, heat, and limitation of function of the part of the body afflicted.

The amount of discharge that is considered normal is dependent upon the site, size, and type of wound. Normally it is not unusual for a wound to exude some *serous drainage* postoperatively. (Serum is the clear portion of the blood.) A wound in the anogenital area can be expected to have more serous discharge than a wound of the face. Serous discharge is amber in color and contains water, blood cells, and some cellular debris.

Sanguineous drainage is red. "Sanguineous" refers to blood. Bright sanguineous drainage is composed of fresh blood; dark sanguineous drainage is composed of old blood.

Infected wounds often have a *purulent discharge.* "Purulent" is defined as containing pus. Pus can be white, yellow, pink, or green, often depending upon the infecting organism. It is usually thick and may have a distinctly unpleasant odor. Other than the three basic kinds of wound discharge there are combinations, which may be described as serosanguineous, seropurulent, and purosanguineous, for example.

An accurate description of a wound's discharge must include the amount. Traditional descriptions, such as gross, moderate, and small, are highly subject to individual interpretation and often relative to the site and type of wound. For example, the amount of drainage that would be considered moderate after perineal surgery would usually be considered abnormally large after an appendectomy. Because the use of these adjectives can be misleading, more exact measures are used. It is the policy in some agencies to describe the amount of drainage by the number of dressings that are soaked and the exact measure of the spread of the drainage upon the dressing. An example of this kind of descriptive charting would be "serosanguineous drainage 7.5 cm. (3 inches) in diameter soaked through two gauze dressings."

In addition to a description of the wound and the drainage other signs and symptoms are recorded—for example, stabbing pain near the wound, evidence of fever, headache, anorexia, or hemorrhage or other subjective symptoms of generalized or localized infection.

PRIORITIES FOR NURSING ACTION

If a patient's wound is causing him discomfort or pain, or if the dressings are soiled, the dressing should be changed promptly. If there are orders not to change the dressings, the original dressing can be covered with a fresh one, and the physician notified so that he can decide on the best course of action.

Two other situations that necessitate prompt action on the nurse's part are hemorrhage and infection of wounds. Hemorrhage is always a medical emergency and the nurse should promptly report her observations if she encounters fresh bleeding or excessive oozing from a healing wound so that action can be taken before the bleeding becomes excessive. If the nurse notes signs of gross bleeding, or signs that the patient is going into shock, immediate action is required. The beginning student should summon help at once, in this case preferably sending someone else for aid and staying with the patient herself. He is usually apprehensive and needs support.

Signs of localized or generalized infection should also be drawn to the attention of the team leader promptly, so that appropriate intervention can be initiated as early as possible in order to arrest the infection in the individual and to prevent its spread to other patients, visitors, and staff.

1. *Skin and mucous membranes normally harbor microorganisms.* In order to decrease the transfer of organisms to a wound, handwashing is indicated before and after attending a patient. In addition, the use of a disinfectant upon and around a wound decreases the number of microorganisms and thus lessens the danger of infection.

2. *Microorganisms are present in the air.* Sometimes a wound is left exposed, particularly if it is a superficial one which has closed itself. The majority of surgical incisions, however, and wounds involving deeper-lying tissues are protected by a sterile dressing. When the dressing is changed, precautions are taken to keep the time the wound is exposed as short as possible and the circulation of the air in the room at a minimum. These precautions have a twofold purpose: to protect the wound from possible contamination by air-borne bacteria in the atmosphere and to minimize the convection of microorganisms from the wound to the circulating air. When a wound is infected, or there is possibility that pathogenic bacteria (such as *Staphylococcus aureus*) are present in the atmosphere, these precautions are particularly important.

3. *Moisture facilitates the growth of microorganisms.* Dressings that are wet with drainage are more likely to foster the growth of organisms than are dry dressings. Often dressings are changed whenever they become soaked through to the top. If there is no order to change the dressing, it can be reinforced with additional dry sterile dressings to inhibit the

---

PRINCIPLES RELEVANT TO THE CARE OF WOUNDS

1. Skin and mucous membranes normally harbor microorganisms.
2. Microorganisms are present in the air.
3. Moisture facilitates the growth of microorganisms.
4. Moisture facilitates the movement of microorganisms.
5. Fluids flow downward as a result of gravitational pull.
6. The respiratory tract often harbors microorganisms, which can be spread to open wounds.
7. The blood transports the materials that nourish and repair body tissues.
8. Skin and mucous membranes can be injured by chemical, mechanical, thermal, and microbial agents.
9. Fluids move through materials by capillary action.

transfer of organisms from the outside to the wound until the physician has been notified.

4. *Moisture facilitates the movement of microorganisms.* When a dressing becomes soaked through to the outside, the movement of microorganisms toward the wound is facilitated because the moisture provides a vehicle for their transport. Because the outside of a dressing is generally highly contaminated, the movement of organisms from the outside inward must be prevented. Maintaining dry dressings inhibits the multiplication and the transfer of organisms.

5. *Fluids flow downward as a result of gravitational pull.* In a draining wound the area of greatest contamination is, in all probability, the lowest part, where the drainage collects. If it is desirable to promote drainage, a drain or packing is usually placed in the lowest part of the wound by the doctor.

6. *The respiratory tract often harbors microorganisms, which can be spread to open wounds.* When an open wound is exposed, measures are taken to prevent the spread of microorganisms from the respiratory tract. It is common practice in many agencies for nurses and physicians to wear masks while dressing wounds, and in some instances patients also wear masks. In any case, as a precautionary measure against contamination, it is advisable not to talk while a wound is exposed.

7. *The blood transports the materials that nourish and repair body tissues.* When dressing and bandaging a wound, care is exercised to ensure that circulation to the area is not restricted in any way. Bandages and dressings are never made restrictively tight, and they are applied starting at the distal portion of the body and proceeding to the proximal portion as a means of promoting venous flow.

8. *Skin and mucous membranes can be injured by chemical, mechanical, thermal, and microbial agents.* The disinfectants and medications used to cleanse and treat a wound and the surrounding tissue should be strong enough to be effective, but they should not irritate healthy tissue. Protective ointments such as sterile petrolatum can be used to protect the skin when it is necessary to use irritating disinfectants upon open wounds.

To avoid mechanical injury at bony prominences which are to be bandaged, padding is provided to prevent irritation due to friction. Adhesive tape must be removed carefully; often, to avoid trauma, specially prepared solvents can be used to loosen the adhesive. Thermal injury can be avoided by the use of solutions at a temperature which is noninjurious to tissue. Room temperature is generally considered to be safe for most tissues.

Microbial injury can be largely avoided by practicing sterile technique in the care of wounds. All solutions, dressings, and equipment that come into contact with an open wound should be sterile.

9. *Fluids move through materials by capillary action.* Loosely woven fabrics such as gauze provide a good surface for capillary action. The fluid is absorbed through the material as each thread in the material conducts the fluid away from the wound by the action of the surface tension of the fluid and the forces of adhesion and cohesion. Adhesion and cohesion refer to forces which draw together.

GOALS FOR NURSING ACTION

The basic goals of nursing action in the care of patients with wounds are:

1. To promote tissue healing
2. To prevent the development of infection in the wound
3. To promote the comfort of the patient.

SPECIFIC NURSING INTERVENTIONS

General Considerations in Wound Care

Just as there is considerable variety in the kinds of wounds, so there is variety in the care that they require. A wound may be closed by sutures, with no drainage resulting. This type of wound is often left with the original dressing in place until it is completely healed. Sometimes wounds are sprayed with a clear plastic material which seals the wound and eliminates the need for any dressings.

Operative wounds are normally sutured with black silk or wire sutures, or they may be held together by metal clips. These wounds do not heal over for the first four or five days postoperatively, and they may or may not require attention. If a wound is expected to drain excessively, a drain or packing is inserted by the physician to facilitate this process. Soft and firm rubber drains as well as plastic drains are used for this purpose. Packing is usually made of a long strip of gauze, often impregnated with a disinfectant or antibiotic. Drains and packing are sometimes withdrawn a little each day to encourage healing from the depth of the wound toward the surface. Considerable drainage can be anticipated from wounds of this nature. Some drains are sutured in place, whereas others are freely movable. Soft rubber drains (Penrose drains) often have a sterile safety pin attached to the distal portion of the drain to prevent it from slipping completely inside the wound.

Wounds that are draining need to be changed whenever the dressings are wet. Not only is the drainage frequently irritating to the skin, but it also serves as a likely site for infection. Wounds that drain urine, feces, or gastric and intestinal secretions necessitate the use of ointments, such as zinc oxide or petrolatum, on the surrounding skin as a protection against irritation. The skin around these wounds should also be cleaned regularly with a mild soap or disinfectant to remove the irritating materials.

Dressings

The frequency with which dressings are changed depends on the needs of the patient and the orders of the physician. An order might state that a wound is to be dressed at regular intervals (for example, twice a day), or it might leave the frequency with which a dressing is to be changed to the nurse's judgment. In the latter situation the dressing is changed when it is wet, but never more often than necessary, because each time a wound is exposed the chance of initiating an infection is increased.

Preparation of the Environment. When a wound is to be exposed to the open air, every effort is made to decrease the number of microorganisms which could possibly come in contact with it. Consequently, windows and doors are closed to eliminate drafts, and curtains are drawn around the patient to provide privacy.

The bed unit is arranged for the convenience of the person changing the patient's dressings. Usually the bedside table or overbed table is cleared beforehand so that the nurse can put the dressing tray in a convenient place. Before wound care, the nurse washes her hands to reduce the number of microorganisms which are normally on her skin (see *Handwashing*, Chapter 21).

Preparation of the Equipment. The specific equipment required depends upon the kind of wound. The safest aseptic technique is carried out by using individual trays containing only the materials and equipment which can be discarded or sterilized after the wound is dressed. By not taking bottles and other articles from one patient to another the transfer of microorganisms by such vectors is eliminated.

For changing most wound dressings it is necessary to have a receptacle for the old dressings and gauze sponges (waxed paper bags permit such contaminated materials to be covered and disposed of easily, while the wax keeps the moisture inside the bag), a container of disinfectant, two or three forceps (tissue and artery forceps are often used), sterile dressings, and gauze sponges. For the care of some wounds it is also necessary to have sterile scissors either to shorten drains or to shape the dressings. The nurse will usually need adhesive tape as well.

After this equipment has been placed on a tray and protected from contamination (by covering it with a sterile towel, for example), it can be safely transported to the patient. Some agencies have standard sets ready for use; it is then necessary only to add the disinfectant and any additional equipment needed by a particular patient. If a mask is to be worn, it is usually put on before the equipment is arranged, and it is kept on until the wound care has been completed.

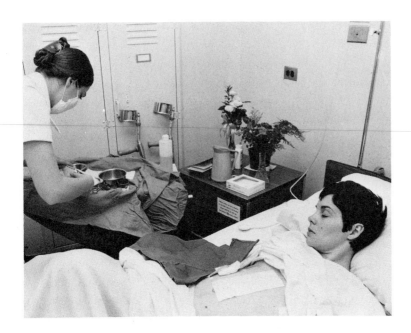

Strict aseptic technique must be maintained throughout the dressing procedure.

Preparation of the Patient. Prior to the dressing of a wound, the needs of the patient for information about the procedure are determined. If the patient will be seeing his wound for the first time, he may want some information about its appearance and what will happen during the dressing change. The details of the explanation depend upon the patient's needs. Often a wound has a meaning for the patient other than the obvious; for example, he might be worried about the appearance of a scar.

The patient can assist by lying still during the procedure in order that the wound and the equipment do not accidentally become contaminated. Some patients need to be advised not to talk and to keep their hands away from the wound area so that sterile technique is maintained. During the explanation, words such as "infection," "contaminated," and "dirty" are used with caution, since they may make the patient feel that something is wrong or may stimulate him to speculate about future complications.

Inexperienced people often ask whether changing a dressing or removing drains and sutures is painful. These people are frequently worried about their ability to cope with pain in a socially acceptable manner. Generally all of these measures are painless, with the exception of removing dressings that adhere to the skin surface. Dressings that do stick to the skin because of dried discharges can usually be removed with little discomfort by soaking them with sterile normal saline or sterile water.

Another possible source of discomfort is the use of a disinfectant with an alcohol base. Such applications may feel cold to the patient and may possibly sting when they come in contact with an open wound. The use of a disinfectant without an alcoholic base is often advisable. Most agencies have a particular type of disinfectant which they recommend using in caring for wounds. If the procedure is going to be uncomfortable, patients are usually better able to cope with it if they have been given some warning so that their responses can be structured in advance.

Prior to the changing of a dressing the patient assumes a position which is convenient and comfortable for him. It may be necessary to provide drapes for adequate warmth and privacy.

Procedure for Donning Sterile Gloves. Some agencies advocate the use of sterile gloves for changing a dressing and cleaning a wound; others prefer a "no touch" technique using sterile forceps. Whichever method is practiced, it is important that all equipment coming in contact with an open wound be sterile. If sterile gloves are to be worn during the dressing procedure, they are usually put on after the soiled dressings are removed. In preparing the dressing tray at the patient's bedside, then, the glove wrapper is laid on a clean, flat surface and unfolded. Many agencies now use disposable sterile gloves; most are now prepowdered. If they are not, the nurse will find a small packet of powder inside the glove wrapper (the powder makes it easier to slip on the gloves).

When the nurse is ready to don the gloves, she carefully lifts the powder packet from the wrapper, opens it, and carefully powders her hands. (If the gloves are prepowdered, this step is not necessary.)

The right-handed nurse usually puts on the left glove first. To do this, she grasps the *inside* of the folded cuff tip of the left glove with her right hand, lifts the glove from the wrapper, and slides her left hand into it. (It is easier if the fingers are kept straight.)

The nurse is then ready to don the second glove. Using the gloved left hand, she slips her fingers *under* the folded cuff edge of the right glove and lifts it from the wrapper. Then, being careful not to touch the skin of her hand or her uniform, she carefully slides her right hand into the glove, pulling the cuff up over the wrist with her left (gloved) hand, which is still under the cuff edge.

The cuff of the left glove may then be pulled up over the wrist (using the same technique of sterile surface to sterile surface), by slipping the fingers of the now gloved right hand under the folded cuff edge of the left glove and carefully pulling it up over the wrist.

When both gloves have been put on, the nurse can adjust the fingers in the same manner she would use in putting on a pair of gloves for street wear.

Procedures for Changing the Dressing. The equipment is arranged in a manner such that it is not necessary to pass soiled dressings and sponges over the sterile field. Generally the old dressing is removed with sterile forceps, the dressing is dropped into the wax paper bag, and the forceps are then placed in a discard container. The wound is then cleansed with a disinfectant. Four rules for cleansing a wound are:

1. Use a sponge only once, cleansing from the top of the wound to the bottom, and then discard the sponge. The cleanest part of the wound is at the top, where there is the least amount of drainage.

2. After cleansing the wound itself, work away from the wound to a distance of about 5 cm. (2 inches). The wound is the cleanest area; the surrounding skin contains more microorganisms.

3. When not wearing sterile gloves, keep the tips of the forceps lower than the handle. Ungloved hands contaminate the handle of the forceps and the solution on the tips will run down to the handle if the tips are held up; then upon lowering the tips the contaminated solution returns to the tips, contaminating the entire instrument.

4. Do not carry contaminated sponges over sterile areas. There is a danger that the contaminated solution will drop on sterile equipment.

After a wound has been cleansed, it is irrigated if this has been ordered. Normally about 500 ml. of a sterile solution at room temperature is used for wound irrigation. If the irrigating solution is irritating to the skin, the surrounding areas should be protected beforehand by an ointment such as sterile petrolatum. During irrigation, the patient lies so that when the nurse administers the irrigating solution with a sterile syringe it flows freely over the wound and then into a receptacle. After an irrigation, the skin is patted dry with sterile sponges.

The new sterile dressing is placed over the wound with sterile forceps. It should be dropped in place rather than moved over the skin so as not to transfer microorganisms from the skin to the center of the wound and to avoid mechanical injury to the wound. When wet dressings are used, they are soaked in the prescribed solution, wrung out with artery forceps, and then placed on the wound. The outer dressing should extend at least 5 cm. (2 inches) beyond an open wound as a precaution against later contamination should the edges be accidentally turned back.

The dressings can be secured by adhesive tape, elasticized tape, waterproof tape, adhesive ties, binders, bandages, or plastic tape. The type of material and the method by which it is secured depend upon the site of the wound and the specific needs of the patient. For the patient who is allergic to adhesive tape, some other type of commercially prepared adhesive bandage can be used. Plastic tape is frequently used on the face because of its nonirritating quality. Waterproof tape keeps a wound dry; thus, it is especially useful next to a draining area. Adhesive ties are used when frequent dressing changes are necessary, since only the tie part needs to be undone when the dressing is changed; the adhesive portion does not have to be removed from the skin unless the tape becomes soiled.

When a dressing is to be secured by adhesive tape, painting the patient's skin with tincture of benzoin beforehand serves to protect the surface epithelium. It is also more comfortable for the patient when areas that have hair are shaved so that the tape does not stick to the hair on removal. Adhesive tape can be readily removed by using a solvent such as acetone to loosen the gum of the tape. Ether and benzene can also be used, but they are highly flammable and for this reason are not often kept near patients.

Binders

Binders can be used to retain dressings, to apply pressure, to support an area of the body, and to provide comfort. Binders are generally made of a heavy cotton material which is strong and durable. Scultetus binders are occasionally lined with flannel, which absorbs moisture and provides additional comfort. When the purpose of the binder is to provide support to abdominal muscles, a two-way stretch type of binder, similar to a girdle, is sometimes used.

Guides for the Application of Binders.
1. Binders are applied in such a manner as to provide even pressure over an area of the body.
2. Binders should support body parts in their normal anatomical position, with slight joint flexion.
3. Binders are secured firmly so that they do not cause friction and thereby irritate the skin or mucous membrane.

Types of Binders. There are five basic types of binders: T binder, straight abdominal binder, scultetus (many-tailed) binder, breast binder, and triangular binder.

THE T BINDER. This binder is made of two srips of cotton attached in the shape of a T. The top of the T serves as a band which is then placed around the patient's waist. The stem of the T is passed between the patient's legs and is then attached to the waistband in front. In some T binders the cotton strip that goes between the patient's legs is split into two tails about 22.5 cm. (9 inches) from the end. These tails provide wider support to the perineal area and add to the comfort of the male patient particularly.

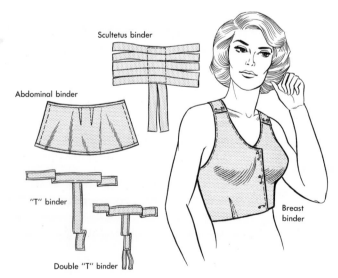

Scultetus binder

Abdominal binder

"T" binder

Double "T" binder

Breast binder

Types of binders.

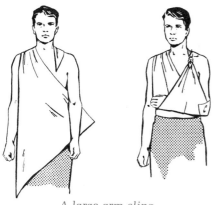

A large arm sling.

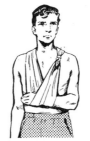

A small arm sling.

T binders are used chiefly to retain perineal dressings. Because of the profuse drainage that often occurs from this area, they are usually changed frequently.

THE STRAIGHT ABDOMINAL BINDER. The straight abdominal binder is a rectangular piece of cotton from 15 to 30 cm. (6 to 12 inches) wide, and long enough to encircle the patient's abdomen and overlap at least 5 cm. (2 inches) in front. This type of binder is used to retain abdominal dressings or to apply pressure and support to the abdomen.

THE SCULTETUS BINDER. Also known as the many-tailed binder, the scultetus binder is a rectangular piece of cotton, usually 22.5 to 30 cm. (9 to 12 inches) wide and 37.5 cm. (15 inches) long, with perhaps 6 to 12 tails attached to each side. It is usually used to provide support to the abdomen, but it can also be used to retain dressings. It can be applied to the chest as well as the abdomen. The advantage of the scultetus binder is that it fits the contours of the body closely.

THE BREAST BINDER. This binder is a rectangular piece of cotton shaped roughly to the contours of the female chest. It usually has straps which fit over the shoulders and pin to the binder in front. Breast binders are used to retain dressings and to apply pressure to the breasts, as when drying up breast milk after the birth of a baby if the mother is not breast-feeding.

THE TRIANGULAR BINDER (SLING). Various forms of the trinangular binder are used to support a limb, to secure a splint (as a first aid measure), and to secure dressings. The triangular binder is made of heavy cotton, is triangular in shape, and has two sides approximately 1 meter (40 inches) in length. It can be applied as a full triangle or, after it has been folded, in a variety of ways.

As a full triangle, the binder is used frequently to make a *large arm sling*. Folded into a broad bandage, it can be used as a *small sling* to support the patient's wrist and hand. A triangular binder can also support a person's arm in such a manner as to elevate the hand. This is called a *triangular sling*.

Triangular binders can also be used to

A triangular sling.

retain dressings on the elbow, hand, shoulder, hip, knee, and foot. For details on the application of binders the nurse should consult a bandaging or first aid book. There are also a number of multimedia aids now available to help students to develop skills in applying binders and bandages.

Problems Related to the Use of Binders. Binders are most often used for large areas of the body, and since they are not secured to skin surfaces, they have a tendency to slip out of position. A binder should be changed or reapplied as often as necessary to maintain its intended function of support, comfort, or the application of pressure. Soiling is also a problem with binders. Because a dirty binder can be a source of both irritation and infection, it is essential to see that soiled binders are changed promptly.

When a binder is applied it should be secured firmly, but the nurse should be careful that there is no interference with normal body functioning. An abdominal or breast binder that is too tight, for example, can restrict movements of the chest wall and interfere with respiration. In postoperative patients this could lead to serious complications. The nurse should be alert for signs of impaired respiration, such as shallow breathing, which could indicate that a binder is too tight and should be loosened.

BANDAGING

A bandage is a piece of material that is used to wrap a part of the body. The purposes of applying a bandage are:

1. To limit movement
2. To apply warmth—for example, to a rheumatoid joint
3. To secure a dressing
4. To keep splints in position
5. To provide support—for example, to the legs to aid venous blood flow
6. To apply pressure in order to control bleeding, promote the absorption of tissue fluids, or prevent the loss of tissue fluids

The type of bandage that is used most frequently in hospitals, physicians' offices, and clinics is the roller bandage. This is a strip of material from 1.8 to 7.4 meters (2 to 8 yards) in length and varying in width from 1.25 to 15 cm. (½ to 6 inches). A roller bandage has three parts: the initial or free end, the body or drum, and the terminal or hidden end.

Materials Used in Bandaging. Gauze is one of the most frequently used materials for bandaging. It is a soft, woven cotton that is porous but not bulky, light in weight, and readily molded to any contour. Although gauze does not wash well and frays with repeated use, it is inexpensive and easily disposed of. The gauze is sometimes impregnated with various ointments such as petrolatum. Gauze is frequently used to bandage fingers and hands and to retain dressings on draining wounds.

Kling is gauze which has been woven in such a manner that it will stretch and thus mold to the body contours. It has a crepe-like texture and tends to cling to itself, an attribute which helps keep it in place after it has been applied.

Flannel makes a soft and pliable bandage. It is heavy and keeps in the heat of the body; therefore it can be used to apply warmth to body joints.

Crinoline is a loosely woven gauze, coarse in texture and strong. Crinoline is impregnated with plaster of paris for use as a base for applying casts. It may also be impregnated with petrolatum for application to an open wound.

Muslin (factory cotton) is a strong, heavy cotton that is not pliable. It is used to provide support, as for splints, or to limit movement.

Elasticized bandages made of cotton with an elastic webbing (Ace bandages) are often used as tensor bandages to apply pressure. They are expensive but can be washed and reused. Patients who require support for their legs immediately following surgery for varicose veins often use tensor bandages.

Elastic adhesive (Elastoplast) is a woven bandage with an adhesive side. It is applied to give support—for example, when dressings are being secured.

Plastic adhesive is a waterproof bandage with an adhesive side. It is somewhat elastic and can be used to apply pressure and at the same time keep an area dry.

Principles Relevant to Bandaging. *Microorganisms flourish in warm, damp and soiled areas.* A bandage is applied only over a clean area; if it is to be placed over an open wound, the wound is dressed aseptically beforehand. Skin surfaces are dry and clean and are not pressed together when bandaging. Adjacent skin surfaces may be kept separated by inserting a 5 cm. by 5 cm. (2 inch by 2 inch) piece of gauze between them. Bandages are removed at regular intervals and the skin surfaces are washed and dried. Soiled bandages are never reused.

Pressure exerted upon the body tissues can affect the circulation of blood. A bandage is applied from the distal to the proximal part of the body to aid the return of the venous blood to the heart. Bandages are always applied evenly so that they do not restrict circulation. They should be checked frequently to make certain that there is no interference with blood supply to the part.

Friction can cause mechanical trauma to the epithelium. A bony prominence of the body is padded before it is bandaged, so that the bandage does not rub the area and cause an abraded wound. Skin surfaces are separated to prevent friction and maceration.

The body is maintained in the natural anatomical position with slight flexion of the joints to avoid muscle strain. Bandages are applied with the body in good alignment to avoid muscle extension, which is fatiguing and produces strain. In particular, adduction of the shoulder and hip joints is avoided.

Excessive or uneven pressure upon body surfaces can interfere with blood circulation and therefore with the nourishment of the cells in the area. Bandage evenly and if possible leave the distal portion of a bandaged limb exposed so that any restriction in circulation can be detected. Signs and symptoms of restricted circulation are pallor, erythema,

cyanosis, tingling sensations, numbness or pain, swelling, and cold.

When a bandage is applied over a wet dressing, allowances are made for shrinkage as the bandage becomes wet and subsequently dries.

Fundamental Turns in Bandaging. There are five fundamental turns in bandaging, and it is these turns that are used to make up the variety of bandages applied to the various parts of the body.

The *circular turn* is used to bandage a cylindrical part of the body or to secure a bandage at its initial and terminal ends. In a circular turn, the bandage is wrapped about the part in such a way that each turn exactly covers the previous one. Two circular turns are usually used to initiate and to terminate a bandage. For comfort the initial and terminal ends are not situated directly over the wound.

The *spiral turn* is used to bandage a part of the body that is of uniform circumference. The bandage is carried upward at a slight angle so that it spirals around the part. Each turn is parallel to the preceding one and overlaps it by two-thirds of the width of the bandage. A spiral turn is

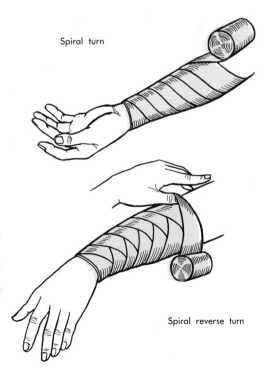

Spiral turn

Spiral reverse turn

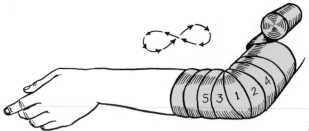

Figure-of-eight turn on the elbow.

used on parts of the body such as the fingers, arms, and legs.

The *spiral reverse turn* is used to bandage cylindrical parts of the body that are of varying circumference, such as the lower leg. To make a spiral reverse turn, the thumb of the free hand is placed on the upper edge of the initial turn, the bandage being held firmly. The roll is unwound about 15 cm. (6 inches) and then the hand is pronated so that the bandage is directed downward and parallel to the lower edge of the previous turn, overlapping it by two-thirds of the width. The roll is then carried around the limb and another reverse is made at the same place so that the turns are in line and uniform.

The *figure-eight turn* is usually used on joints but may also be used for the entire length of an arm or leg bandage. It consists of repeated oblique turns that are made alternately above and below a joint in the form of a figure eight. After the initial circular turns are made over the center of the joint, the next turn is superior to the joint and the next is inferior to the joint. Thus the turns are worked upward and downward, with each turn overlapping the previous turn by two-thirds of the width of the bandage.

The *recurrent turn* is used to cover distal portions of the body, such as the tip of a finger or the toes. After anchoring the

bandage with a circular turn, the roll is turned and brought directly over the center of the tip to be covered. It is then anchored inferiorly, and alternate turns are made, first to the right and then to the left, over the original turn covering the tip so that each turn is held above and below. Each turn overlaps the preceding one by two-thirds of its width. The bandage is secured by circular turns which gather in the ends.

Generally speaking, bandages for the hands, arms, and feet are made with circular, spiral, and spiral reverse turns. Bandages for the joints are made with figure eights, and bandages for the distal portions of the body are done with recurrent turns.

In addition, there are many special bandages, such as the thumb spica, ear and

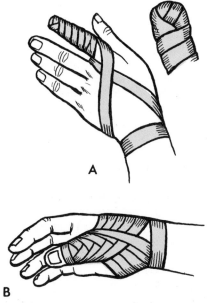

A

B

A, Finger bandage with the tip covered; B, thumb spica.

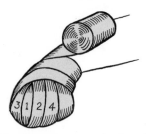

Recurrent turn on the hand.

eye bandages, and skull bandages. It is suggested that the nurse consult a bandaging text for more detailed information.

Guides to Bandaging

1. Face the person who is being bandaged.

2. Start a roller bandage by holding the roll of the bandage upward in one hand, the initial end in the other hand.

3. Bandage from the distal to the proximal and from the medial to the lateral.

4. Do not initiate or terminate a bandage directly over a wound or an area where the patient is likely to exert pressure, as for example, the posterior side of the thigh.

5. Bandage evenly and firmly, overlapping the preceding turn by two-thirds of the width of the bandage.

6. Use the bandage material which best serves the purpose of the bandage.

7. Cover a dressing with a bandage that extends past each side of the dressing.

8. Separate the skin surfaces and pad bony prominences and hollows to prevent friction and to apply even pressure.

9. Check the bandage and look for any signs of restricted circulation.

10. A bandage should be safe, durable, neat, therapeutically effective, and economical.

PLANNING AND EVALUATING NURSING INTERVENTIONS

The specific nursing interventions discussed in this chapter were concerned with changing dressings on a wound, applying binders, and the fundamental techniques of bandaging. The expected outcomes of these interventions are the comfort and safety of the patient. Questions the nurse might ask herself are:

1. Is the dressing, binder, or bandage accomplishing its purpose?

2. Is the patient concerned about his wound? Has his anxiety been allayed?

3. Has the dressing, binder, or bandage been applied so that there is no impairment to circulation?

4. Has the dressing, binder, or bandage been applied so that drainage, if desired, is unimpeded?

5. Has safe sterile technique been maintained?

6. Has each intervention been performed as comfortably as possible for the patient?

Know these

GUIDE TO ASSESSING WOUND HEALING

1. What type of wound does the patient have?
2. What phase of healing would you judge this wound to be in?
3. Is the wound healing normally?
4. Are there factors which might delay healing of the wound? For example, is the patient in poor nutritional status? Does he have an infection?
5. Does the patient show localized or generalized symptoms that would indicate the wound is infected? Signs of bleeding?
6. How would you describe the wound?
7. Does the wound require dressing? If so, how often? Are there special precautions to be taken or additional equipment required for doing the dressing?
8. Does the patient need a binder or bandage? If so, for what reason? What is the best type to use for this patient's needs?

STUDY VOCABULARY

Anorexia	Irradiation	Serous
Clean wound	Infected wound	Virulence
Contaminated wound	Purulent	Wound
Granulation	Sanguineous	

STUDY SITUATION

Mr. John Smith is a law enforcement officer, 30 years old, married, has four children, and is in excellent physical condition. He was admitted to hospital 3 days ago with a bullet wound to his right shoulder. The bullet has been removed, but since there may still be particles of foreign matter present, the physician has not sutured the wound. The physician's orders for Mr. Smith include:

1. Change dressing as necessary
2. Cleanse wound b.i.d. with preferred antiseptic
3. High protein diet
4. Force fluids

When you arrive to change his dressing, Mr. Smith complains of headache and a burning sensation in the region of his wound. You notice a yellow discharge seeping through the previous dressing. Mr. Smith also remarks that he feels hot although there is a fresh breeze coming through the open window beside his bed.

Mr. Smith has been worried that he may not regain full use of his right arm, and since he is right-handed, he fears he may have to resign from active duty.

1. What would you do first when faced with this situation?
2. What might be causing the yellowish discharge from the wound?
3. What other observations might you expect to note in the area of Mr. Smith's wound?
4. What other observations might you note about his general condition?
5. How would you record your observations concerning Mr. Smith?
6. Are there any things you could do to assist in relieving his anxiety?

SUGGESTED
READINGS

Boericke, P. H.: Emergency! First Aid for Open Wounds, Severe Bleeding, Shock and Closed Wounds. *Nursing '75*, 5:40–47, March 1975.

Castle, M.: Wound Care. Clear-cut Ways to Speed Healing. *Nursing '75* 5:40–44, August 1975.

Knight, M. R.: A "Second Skin" for Patients with Large, Draining Wounds. *Nursing '76*, 6:37, January 1976.

LeMaitre, George D., and Janet A. Finnegan: *The Patient in Surgery: A Guide for Nurses.* 3rd edition. Philadelphia, W. B. Saunders Company, 1975.

Manson, H.: Exorcising Excoriation from Fistulae and Other Draining Wounds. *Nursing '76* 6:57–60, March 1976.

Rinear, C. E., et al.: Emergency Bandaging: A Wrap-up of Better Techniques. *Nursing '75*, 5:29–35, January 1975.

Tarin, D.: Wound Healing. A Diagrammatic and Pictorial Account. *Nursing Times*, 69:1124–1126, 1973.

Wagner, M. M.: Injuries to the Chest and Abdomen. *Nursing Clinics of North America*, 8:425–433, September 1973.

UNIT IV

COMMON HEALTH PROBLEMS

23 THE NURSE'S ROLE IN THE DETECTION OF ILLNESS

The nurse should be able to:

Name three component parts of a complete physical examination

List types of information usually included in the health history

Outline the nurse's responsibilities in assisting with the physical examination itself

Name nursing functions related to the collection of specimens

Outline general responsibilities of the nurse when assisting with medical procedures—before, during, and after the procedure.

Describe the purpose and procedure of each of the following diagnostic or therapeutic measures:
1. Lumbar puncture
2. Paracentesis
3. Thoracentesis
4. X-rays
5. Special x-ray examinations
6. Basal metabolic rate
7. Electrocardiography
8. Electroencephalography

Outline specific nursing responsibilities in assisting with each of these interventions

List criteria for the evaluation of the effectiveness of nursing interventions

THE NURSE'S ROLE IN THE 23
DETECTION OF ILLNESS

INTRODUCTION

The curative aspects of the nurse's role are an important part of nursing care. Many of the things that nurses do, in ambulatory and home care settings and in health agencies caring for the sick, are related to the detection of health problems and the restoration to optimal health of the person who is ill, or the provision of palliative measures for those whose illnesses are terminal. (These are in addition, of course, to the provision of comfort and support, which are other aspects of the nursing role.)

The nurse has both independent and dependent functions, as well as interdependent ones, in carrying out the curative aspects of her role. The independent scope of nursing practice in both the detection and the treatment of health problems is rapidly enlarging, as we discussed in Chapter 6. The nursing history and initial clinical appraisal of the patient are important independent functions that assist in determining the nature of the patient's health problem. The nurse also carries out many of the diagnostic tests and procedures needed to determine the exact nature of the problem. These may be undertaken as dependent functions on the orders of the physician or, in many instances today, by the nurse herself on her own initiative.

The therapeutic plan of care for the patient is traditionally the responsibility of the physician, and nurses carry out many of the therapeutic measures prescribed. Nurses working in expanded roles are, however, also accepting more responsibility for developing and implementing therapeutic plans of care for patients. Sometimes the nurse will be practicing alone in a rural or isolated community where there is no physician, but frequently the nurse practices in conjunction with a physician. The nurse in an expanded role may also be responsible for managing the care of patients with long-term, stabilized health problems.

As mentioned also in Chapter 6, the development and implementation of diagnostic and therapeutic plans of care are often nowadays a shared responsibility involving several members of the health team. Each team member has his or her own particular aspects of the total care plan in which he or she is the expert, and these (s)he carries out in coordination with the measures implemented by others involved in the patient's care.

Preparation for expanded role functioning is usually taught in more advanced or postbasic courses to nurses. We will not, therefore, go into these aspects of nursing in this text, but will confine ourselves to helping the beginning student to gain an understanding of some of the measures used in the detection and treatment of illness and her responsibilities in regard to these.

The detection of illness often requires the talents of many different types of health worker. Some of the people who may be involved, in addition to the patient's own physician and the nurse, include: specialist physicians, experts in laboratory procedures, specialists in radiological techniques, and those who have expertise in performing the multitude of specialized diagnostic tests and examinations that seem to be an integral part of today's health care.

These specialists all contribute their talents to the patient's care, but the services of so many workers often confuse

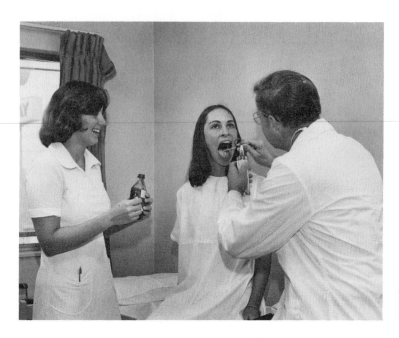

The nurse participates in carrying out many of the tests and examinations used in the detection of illness.

and bewilder the patient and add to his anxiety. The nurse has an important coordinating function in regard to these services; she explains the nature of tests and examinations to the patient, she helps him to participate in carrying them out, she assists in the scheduling of many of these, carries out some herself, and assists other members of the team in carrying out many others.

Examinations and diagnostic tests create a good deal of anxiety in most people. Frequently this anxiety is most directly concerned with the results of the tests, which can mean life or death to the patient. In present ethical practice, the nurse does not give the patient the results of his examinations or tests. This is a responsibility of the physician. The nurse, however, can provide the patient with explanations and reassurance before, during, and after many procedures so as to allay fear and provide emotional support.

Of primary importance to anyone who is undergoing diagnostic tests or examinations is what the results will mean in terms of prognosis and treatment. Some of the questions that may run through a person's mind are: Will the results indicate that he has an incurable disease? that he will be crippled? Will he have to have surgery? These questions preoccupy a patient even with a routine chest x-ray or blood test. People also want to know the reasons for the tests and when they can expect to know the results.

The nurse can provide support by confirming and explaining what the physician has said about "whys" of the test and by giving the patient information which he feels he needs. She explains how the procedure is to be carried out in terms that the patient can understand and answers his questions to the best of her ability. She also assists the patient in his need to help by explaining what he can do before, during, and after the test in order to facilitate the procedure. Moreover, the nurse can communicate her understanding of the patient's anxiety and his need to have confidence in measures being taken in his care.

THE PHYSICAL EXAMINATION

A physical examination is generally carried out by the doctor in an office, clinic, or hospital. Although most people have had a physical examination at some time, it should not be assumed that patients do not require any explanation from the nurse. If a patient does not know the physician, he may be unduly fearful; in such instances the nurse can introduce the doctor and the patient and perhaps explain why the patient requires an examination at this time. Also, since the patient is often fearful about what the physician will find when he examines him, support and understanding from the nurse at this time is particularly important.

There are usually three parts to the examination: the health history, the physical examination itself, and special tests. The *health history* includes both the personal and medical history of the patient. The physician will want to know about the patient's present complaints as well as previous illnesses. The personal history is investigated without using interrogation. It includes the patient's social, religious, educational and economic backgrounds as well as his feelings of achievement and frustration. Habits of nutrition, sleeping patterns, bowel habits, and, for women, the nature of the menstrual cycle are usually included in the history taken by the physician. Habits such as drinking alcohol and smoking also are relevant.

The patient's family history can also be pertinent to his present illness. Some diseases are inherited and some tend to recur in families. Also, with recognition of the multiple causation of illness and an understanding of the reactions of the body to stress, the neuropsychiatric history of the patient has become important (see Chapter 2).

The *physical examination* proceeds from the head to the feet of the patient, with the findings being described in some detail. For the physical examination the physician requires the following equipment: stethoscope, otoscope (for examining the ears and nose), ophthalmoscope (for examining the eyes), percussion hammer, tongue blades, scales, tape measure, sphygmomanometer cuff and dial, and a clinical thermometer. Usually these instruments are kept in a centrally located examining room of an ambulatory care facility or in the nursing unit of the hospital.

The responsibilities of the nurse involve assisting both the patient and the physician with the physical examination. Most patients need some explanation about the examination and its purpose. The patient must undress and may require assistance putting on the gown

provided; the gown is removed during parts of the examination. In a hospital, where the patient generally lies in bed for the examination, a bath blanket is put over him. Patients require privacy and warmth.

Generally, the nurse does not stay during the entire physical examination; however, she should know whether the patient wants her to stay or whether she will be needed to drape the patient. Most agencies and physicians request that a female nurse always be present during a vaginal examination of a female patient when the physician is male. The reason for this is twofold: it contributes to the comfort of the patient and eliminates the possibility of unjust accusations against the physician.

The physical examination includes the taking of vital signs, observation of the general physical and emotional status, and a general inspection of posture, skin, head, eyes, ears, nose, mouth, throat, neck (including thyroid gland and lymph nodes), chest and lungs, heart, breasts, abdomen, genitalia, extremities, back and spine, nervous system, and rectum. When the physician examines the external genitalia and rectum of the male patient, the nurse (if female) usually leaves.

For a rectal examination the patient assumes the Sims position (see Chapter 18) or the knee-chest position.

The *knee-chest position* is frequently used in examinations of the rectum and colon. In this position the patient kneels, with the buttocks upward. The patient's chest and head rest upon the bed surface.

It is important that the patient who assumes this position be adequately draped in order to prevent embarrassment and to provide warmth. Many hospitals have

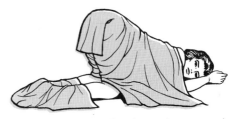

Knee-chest position. The drape is arranged so that the patient is suitably covered and the center fold can be raised to expose the anal area.

special rectal drapes which completely cover the buttocks of the patient except for a circular cutout over the anus. The patient will generally need additional covering for his shoulders and a pillow for his head.

If the health agency does not have special drapes, the nurse can improvise with a cotton drawsheet. The drawsheet is placed across the patient so that the lower edge just covers the buttocks. The corners are tucked around the medial aspect of the patient's thighs. By raising the fold of the sheet, the anal area is exposed.

During this procedure, the physician needs a rectal glove, lubricant, and kidney basin. He (or she) inserts his lubricated gloved finger into the patient's rectum, palpating for abnormalities such as hemorrhoids and fissures.

The *lithotomy position* is used chiefly for examinations and operations involving the reproductive and urinary tracts for both sexes. In this position the patient lies on his back with a small pillow for his head. His hips are flexed and slightly abducted and his knees are also flexed. The patient needs support for his feet if he is to maintain this position for more than a few minutes. The stirrups provide a means for supporting the feet.

Because this position is also embarrassing for most patients, it is important that adequate drapes be provided. One way of draping the patient is to place a drawsheet across the patient so that the lower border is 10 cm. (4 inches) below the symphysis pubis. Then each of the lower corners of the drawsheet are brought to the medial aspect of the patient's thighs and tucked around the patient's legs. When the upper fold of the drawsheet is lifted the patient's perineum is exposed. The nurse should also provide the patient

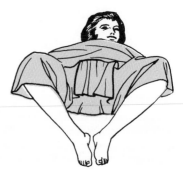

The lithotomy position is modified for treatments such as a urinary catheterization.

with a covering for the upper part of the body. Another method is to place a bath blanket diagonally over the patient. The opposite corners (at each side of the patient) are wrapped around the legs and anchored at the feet. The lower corner can be drawn back and tucked under the top layer of the bath blanket to expose the perineum.

For a vaginal examination the physician requires rubber gloves, lubricant, a vaginal speculum, kidney basin, and a good light. This equipment is sterilized after use in order to prevent the transmission of infection. The physician may also want a tongue blade and a microscopic slide in order to take a sample of the cervical secretions, which are then sent to the laboratory for examination for abnormal cells. This is called a Papanicolaou smear.

The third aspect of the patient's examination comprises the *special tests* and examinations that the patient requires to supplement the findings of the general physical examination.

COLLECTION OF SPECIMENS

Frequently, the nurse is responsible for collecting specimens from patients. These may include specimens of blood, urine, sputum, and drainage from wounds. For these tests, patients usually need explanations as to what they can do to help. Most patients like to be able to assist, and often the success of a test is dependent upon the patient's willingness to provide a specimen or perform some activity at a particular time.

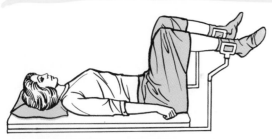

The lithotomy position is often used for urinary and vaginal examinations and operations.

When the nurse collects specimens, her functions include:

1. Explaining the procedure to the patient and gaining his cooperation

2. Collecting the right amount of specimen at the correct time

3. Placing the specimen in the correct container

4. Labeling the container accurately (this usually includes the patient's full name and registration number, the date, the physician's name, and if in a hospital, the number of the nursing unit)

5. Completing the laboratory requisition (this specifies what tests are to be carried out and gives pertinent data about the patient)

6. Recording anything unusual about the appearance of the specimen

Various specimens are sent for microbiological examination in the laboratory. Specimens of a patient's secretions and other excretions are frequently examined in order to isolate and identify an infecting organism. A *secretion* is a product produced by a gland (for example, bile); an *excretion* is a substance excreted or discharged by the body (for example, feces).

For most specimens a sterile container is required, and precautions must be taken to avoid contaminating the specimen with organisms in the environment. A smear or culture may be needed. If a specimen is required for a smear, clean (preferably new) slides and a sterile, cotton-tipped applicator are needed. The specimen is gathered with the applicator, which is rolled over the center of the slide. The smear is covered with another glass slide. The slides are appropriately labeled and sent to the laboratory.

For cultures, the specimen is placed in a sterile container. Urine, blood, ascitic fluid, and the like are usually put in sterile test tubes. For cultures of specimens of wound discharge, many agencies furnish sterile test tubes which are

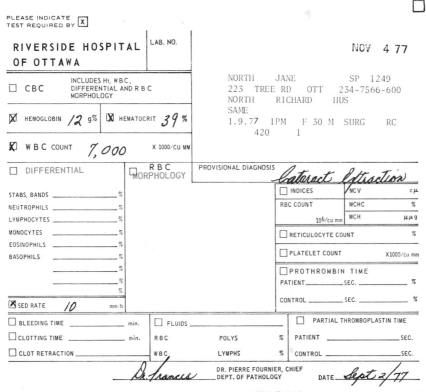

HAEMATOLOGY REPORT

A sample laboratory report for routine blood examination. (Courtesy of the Riverside Hospital of Ottawa.)

equipped with sterile applicators suspended from the cork that seals the tube. When the cork is removed the applicator is removed with it. The applicator tip is touched to the area of discharge and then returned carefully to the sterile container.

Sputum specimens are collected in wide-necked sterile containers or on Petri dishes. Sputum is collected early in the morning, when the patient is most able to cough up sputum from his lungs.

When stools are sent for culture, it is seldom necessary to send the entire specimen. Normally a sterile applicator dipped in the feces is sufficient. If the feces are to be examined for amebae, the specimen is sent to the laboratory while it is warm and it is examined within 30 minutes after it is obtained. Only a small quantity (approximately 3 cc.) of feces is needed for this examination.

It may be necessary to test a culture for differentiation and sensitivity. *Differentiation* is accomplished by means of Gram's stain, which divides bacteria into two classes: gram-negative organisms stain red; gram-positive organisms stain purple. *Sensitivity* refers to the effect of specific antibiotics upon bacteria. The organisms are streaked on nutrient plates, various antibiotics are then added to the plates, and the plates are placed in an incubator. The areas where the growth of the bacteria is inhibited indicate the particular antibiotics to which the bacteria are sensitive.

GUIDES TO ASSISTING WITH MEDICAL PROCEDURES

Before the Procedure

1. Prepare the patient.
   a. Explain the procedure beforehand.
   b. Explain how the patient can help with the examination.
   c. Be guided by the physician in discussing the significance of the test.
   d. Provide privacy.
   e. Drape the patient for his comfort and to facilitate the test.
   f. Help the patient to assume the best position for the test.

2. Prepare the equipment.
   a. Obtain all the equipment for the test.
   b. Maintain the sterility of equipment before and during the test as necessary.
   c. Obtain the containers necessary for specimens and label them.
3. Prepare the environment.
   a. Close the windows and eliminate drafts.
   b. Provide privacy.
   c. Place equipment so that it is convenient for the doctor.
   d. Provide a chair for the doctor when indicated.

During the Procedure

1. Provide emotional support for the patient and help him to cooperate in the test.
2. Provide physical support for the patient while he is maintaining a position.
3. Assist the doctor with the equipment as necessary.
4. Observe the patient for his reactions to the test.

After the Procedure

1. Carry out nursing care measures for the patient's comfort and to prevent complications.
2. Observe the patient closely for untoward reactions.
3. Record the necessary information in the patient's record.
4. Send labeled specimens to the laboratory.
5. Clean and dispose of equipment as necessary.

LUMBAR PUNCTURE

A lumbar puncture is the introduction of a needle into the subarachnoid space for diagnostic or therapeutic purposes. Frequent diagnostic purposes of the lumbar puncture are to obtain a specimen of cerebrospinal fluid for examination, to measure the pressure of the cerebrospinal

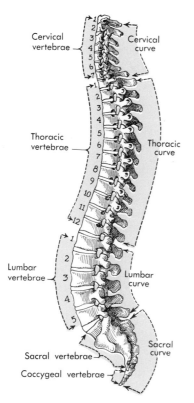

Cervical vertebrae — Cervical curve

Thoracic vertebrae — Thoracic curve

Lumbar vertebrae — Lumbar curve

Sacral vertebrae — Sacral curve

Coccygeal vertebrae —

The sites for a lumbar puncture are the third or fourth intervertebral lumbar spaces.

spinal pressure is between 70 and 200 mm. of water when the subject is in a horizontal position. A person usually has approximately 100 ml. of fluid, which is normally sterile.

In helping a patient prepare for a lumbar puncture, the nurse explains what the patient can expect and what he can do to facilitate the procedure. Since the patient is often anxious about a lumbar puncture, the nurse can reassure him that there is usually very little discomfort. The physician uses a local anesthetic at the site of the entry in order to decrease discomfort. Most frequently the patient is asked to lie on his side with his back near the edge of the bed. His knees are brought up to his chest in order to accentuate the lumbar curve, thus enlarging the intravertebral spaces. It is important that the patient does not move during the procedure because of the chance of dislodging the needle.

The lumbar puncture is a sterile procedure. The equipment that the physician requires usually includes sterile sponges, disinfectant, syringes, needles (Nos. 21 and 24), local anesthetic, mask, sterile gloves, lumbar puncture needles (Nos. 18 and 24), 5 to 12.5 cm. (2 to 5 inches) long, specimen tubes as necessary, manometer to measure spinal fluid pressure, adaptors for needles, and a discard container.

The patient is draped for comfort prior to the procedure. Many doctors' offices and health agencies have sterile fenestrated drapes which the physician puts over the lumbar area, thereby exposing only the site for the puncture. During the procedure itself the nurse can help the patient to maintain the proper position by placing her arms at the back of the patient's neck and behind the knees.

The physician applies a disinfectant and local anesthetic to the area. He or she then inserts the lumbar puncture needle into the intravertebral space. Usually the physician attaches the manometer to the spinal needle in order to obtain a spinal fluid pressure reading. The physician may also perform a Queckensted's test. To assist in this test, the nurse firmly compresses the internal jugular veins on both sides of the patient's neck. Normally the manometer will register a high pressure, because the spinal fluid flow is impeded

fluid, and to inject air or dye into the subarachnoid space preparatory to taking x-rays of the brain and spinal cord. Therapeutically a lumbar puncture is done either to remove cerebrospinal fluid and thereby to reduce the pressure, or to inject medications or anesthetics directly into the subarachnoid space.

The site of the lumbar puncture is usually between the third and fourth or the fourth and fifth lumbar vertebrae. This level is below the spinal cord, and therefore there is no danger of injury to the cord upon the insertion of the needle.

The subarachnoid space normally contains cerebrospinal fluid, which is a clear, colorless liquid. The fluid formed, chiefly by the choroid plexuses in the ventricles or the brain, circulates between the ventricles, the cisterna around the brain and the subarachnoid space. Almost all the cerebrospinal fluid is absorbed into the blood stream through the arachnoidal granulations which project into the subarachnoid spaces. The normal cerebro-

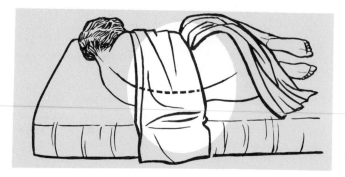

The position for a spinal puncture. Note the curvature of the lumbar region to increase the size of the intervertebral spaces.

temporarily. In conditions in which there is already blockage of the canal, there will be no change in the spinal fluid pressure.

During a spinal puncture the patient is observed for signs of shock, nausea, and vomiting. Shock may be evidenced by sudden facial pallor, accelerated pulse rate, excessive perspiration, and perhaps loss of consciousness. These can occur as a result of the lowering of the spinal fluid pressure or upon the administration of a drug *intrathecally* (into the spinal canal).

After the spinal puncture the doctor advises the patient about what position to maintain. Some physicians have the patient stay in a recumbent position with the bed flat for anywhere from one to 24 hours. Some permit the patient to be up and around. There is a difference in medical opinion as to how long it takes to reestablish normal spinal fluid circulation.

A complication of a lumbar puncture that sometimes occurs is the spinal headache. If the patient does complain of a headache, treatment is instituted.

After the lumbar puncture the nurse records in the chart the time; the procedure; the name of the doctor; the amount, color and consistency of the fluid; the initial and final pressures; the administration of medications; and her observations of the patient.

The *cisternal puncture* is a variation of the lumbar puncture in which the physician inserts a needle into the subarachnoid space at the cisterna magna. The procedure is similar to the lumbar puncture except that the patient's neck is acutely flexed to permit insertion of the needle between the rim of the foramen magnum and the first cervical lamina. A cisternal punture is sometimes done for a

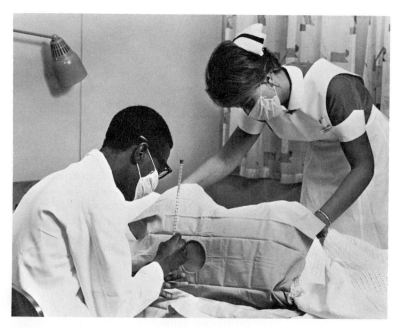

During a spinal puncture a manometer can be used to ascertain the spinal fluid pressure.

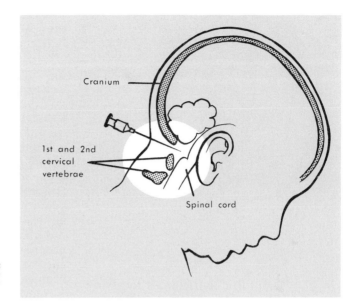

The site for a cisternal puncture is between the foramen magnum and the first cervical vertebra.

ventriculogram, which requires the injection of an opaque medium in order to visualize the ventricles of the brain on an x-ray. The nursing care measures are similar to those involved in a lumbar puncture.

PARACENTESIS

An abdominal paracentesis is the removal of fluid from the peritoneal cavity. When a large amount of fluid accumulates in this cavity, the condition is called ascites and the fluid is called ascitic fluid.

An abdominal paracentesis can be done for either diagnostic or therapeutic purposes. Diagnostically it is performed to obtain a specimen of fluid, which is sent to the laboratory for examination to detect abnormal cells and disease organisms. Evidence of abnormal cells may indicate the existence of a malignancy; the presence of pathogenic microorganisms and the identification of these assists in planning therapy. In therapeutic paracentesis, fluid is usually removed from the peritoneal cavity in order to relieve pressure on the abdominal organs and the diaphragm.

Normally the peritoneal cavity contains just enough fluid to keep the peritoneum lubricated so that the surfaces are not irritated and friction does not result between the peritoneum and other surfaces. The fluid is normally sterile.

Prior to an abdominal paracentesis, the patient requires an explanation of what he can expect and what he can do to help. Most physicians explain the purpose of the test to their patients, and the nurse can be guided by his (or her) explanation in what she says about the purpose of the test. An abdominal paracentesis is usually not a painful procedure, but most physicians use a local anesthetic to minimize discomfort. Before the treatment is started the patient voids in order to empty his bladder. Failure to do this could result in puncturing the bladder with the trochar. If the patient cannot void, the physician should be told in advance of the procedure.

The best position for an abdominal paracentesis is a sitting position so that the force of gravity and pressure from the abdominal organs can assist the outward flow of ascitic fluid. The usual site for the paracentesis is halfway between the umbilicus and symphysis pubis on the midline of the abdomen. An incision to either side is likely to puncture the colon. The patient is screened for privacy and draped for comfort.

Many hospitals have abdominal paracentesis sets which contain all the equipment that is needed for the procedure.

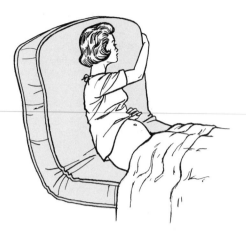

The patient assumes the Fowler's position for an abdominal paracentesis.

The equipment usually includes local anesthetic and a syringe with No. 24 and No. 22 needles, trochar and cannula, rubber tubing (or catheter), which attaches to the cannula and guides the fluid to the container, sterile gloves, mask, disinfectant, sterile gauze sponges, suture material and containers for the specimens. The equipment must be sterile.

After the physician has painted the area with the disinfectant, he anesthetizes the site of entry with a local anesthetic. A small incision is then made and the trochar and cannula are inserted. The rubber tubing is attached to the cannula, the trochar is removed and the fluid is allowed to drain into the container provided (usually a large drainage bottle).

During the paracentesis the nurse observes the patient closely for any signs of shock, such as pallor, sweating, rapid pulse, or syncope (fainting). These can occur particularly when the fluid drains quickly. Many physicians ask that a stimulant such as epinephrine be on hand during the procedure.

After the paracentesis is completed, a small dressing is placed over the incision. The wound may or may not be sutured. If the patient feels faint, an abdominal binder can be applied after the procedure to provide comfort and support. Many complications can occur as the result of a paracentesis; there may be a major circulatory shift of fluids, and it is important to monitor vital signs and observe peripheral circulation frequently both during and for

several hours after the procedure. Deviations from the normal are reported promptly to the physician.

THORACENTESIS

A thoracentesis is the aspiration of fluid from the pleural cavity. Normally there is just enough fluid present to lubricate the pleura so that the lungs can move freely. Pleural fluid is serous. The pleural cavity is a potential space which under normal conditions does not contain any fluid or air except the few milliliters of pleural fluid. The pressure in the pleural cavity is normally negative (−4 mm. of mercury), and because of this the lungs are kept from collapsing.

A thoracentesis may be indicated for either diagnostic or therapeutic purposes. In a diagnostic thoracentesis, a specimen of pleural fluid is obtained in order to identify an infecting microorganism or the presence of abnormal cells. Therapeutically, a thoracentesis is performed to remove fluid that is causing pressure upon the chest organs or to remove air that is inhibiting respirations.

If the patient has not had a thoracentesis previously, he will need an explanation of the procedure beforehand. The patient usually assumes a sitting position so that the fluid collects at the bottom of the pleural cavity. He places his arm over his

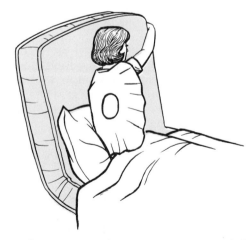

For thoracentesis, the patient assumes a sitting position with her arm across her chest in order to enlarge the intercostal spaces.

head or in front of his chest in order to extend the intercostal spaces. The patient is warned not to cough or to move suddenly during the procedure because of the danger of the needle's becoming dislodged and piercing his lungs.

The equipment that is required for a thoracentesis consists of an aspirating set, an airtight drainage bottle, tubing, suction machine or pump in order to obtain a negative pressure within the drainage bottle, local anesthetic, syringe, sterile gloves, mask, and discard basin.

Before the doctor begins the thoracentesis the nurse establishes negative pressure in the drainage bottle in order to draw the fluid from the pleural cavity. Because there is some negative pressure within the pleural cavity it is necessary to have greater negative pressure in the drainage bottle before fluid can be drained. It is also essential to prevent air from getting into the pleural cavity because it produces pneumothorax (the accumulation of gas or air in the pleural cavity), which causes collapse of the lungs. The thoracentesis needle has an attachable stopcock which can be opened and shut in order to prevent air from getting into the pleural cavity. A syringe can be attached to the stopcock to obtain fluid for laboratory examination.

After the patient assumes a sitting position and is draped comfortably, the physician wipes the area of insertion with disinfectant. The thoracentesis is done below the surface level of the fluid, often in the frontal plane in line with the crest of the ilium. The doctor determines the level of the fluid by percussion. The area is anesthetized locally and then the long thoracentesis needle is inserted through the intercostal space into the pleural cavity. The tubing is connected to the stopcock and to the source of negative pressure, and upon a signal from the doctor the valves are opened to let the fluid flow into the drainage bottle.

During the procedure the nurse watches the patient carefully for any signs of respiratory distress—for example, cyanosis or dyspnea. If the fluid is removed quickly the patient may faint. Puncturing a blood vessel with the needle is a complication which can result in a lung hemorrhage.

After the needle is withdrawn, pressure is applied over the site, collodion is often used to seal the skin over the puncture wound, and a sterile dressing is applied. The patient is observed frequently for several hours after the thoracentesis for any signs of respiratory embarrassment or shock. Damage to the lungs may be indicated by the presence of frothy, blood-tinged sputum (hemoptysis), by excessive coughing, or by difficulty in breathing.

The nurse records on the patient's chart the time; treatment; name of the doctor; amount, color, and consistency of the fluid obtained; and the condition of the patient. If the thoracentesis is successful therapeutically, the patient will probably find breathing easier because the fluid is no longer present to exert pressure upon his lungs.

X-RAYS

X-rays are used as diagnostic and therapeutic measures on almost every system of the body. In this century, with radiation such a highly publicized and emotionally tinged term, some people are afraid that x-rays are injurious. The nurse can safely reassure people that the amount of radiation received in an examination is limited. The nurse herself should be aware that radiation in excess can be dangerous, but it is unusual for patients to receive enough radiation to destroy tissue unless this is done therapeutically. The unit of measurement of x-ray dosage is the roentgen (R).

There are four methods of x-ray examination: visualizing a part of the body on photographic film, visualizing a part of the body on a fluoroscope screen, a combination of these two methods, and cinefluorography.

One of the important factors in taking x-rays is the position that the patient assumes. His position must be such that the part to be visualized is clearly outlined on the film. The nurse can help the patient to prepare for an x-ray examination by explaining that he may find it necessary to assume difficult and perhaps uncomfortable positions for short periods of time.

To x-ray some parts of the body, it is necessary to use a contrast medium so

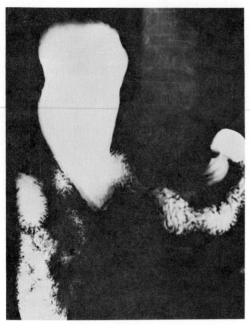

An x-ray showing barium sulfate filling the stomach and the first portion of the small bowel.

time the procedure is completed. Special attention should be given to expulsion of the barium after the x-ray studies are completed. An enema or cathartic may be ordered for the patient following the x-ray series.

Special X-ray Examinations

Intravenous pyelogram. The contrast medium (for example, Diodrast) is injected intravenously and when it is excreted by the kidneys it outlines the kidney pelvices, calices, ureters, and urinary bladder.

Retrograde pyelogram. The contrast medium is introduced through ureteral catheters into the kidney pelvis to outline the urinary tract.

Cholecystogram. This is an x-ray examination of the gallbladder in which a radiopaque contrast medium such as Telepaque is used.

Pneumoencephalogram. This is an x-ray examination of the ventricles and meningeal spaces of the brain in which air or oxygen is used as the contrast medium.

Ventriculogram. This is an x-ray examination of the ventricles of the brain in which air or oxygen is used as the contrast medium.

Myelogram. A myelogram is an x-ray examination of the subarachnoid space of the brain in which a contrast medium such as air is used.

Bronchogram. This is an x-ray examination of the bronchial tree in which an iodized oil is used as the contrast medium.

Hysterosalpingogram. This is an x-ray examination of the uterus and fallopian tubes in which a radiopaque contrast medium such as Lipiodol is used.

Cardioangiogram. In this method, which is an x-ray examination of the heart and great vessels, a catheter introduced into one of the great vessels is used to administer contrast medium such as Hypaque.

Angiogram. This is an x-ray examination of the blood vessels in which a contrast medium is used. It is usually done to outline the vascular system of the brain (cerebral angiogram) or the coronary arteries of the heart (coronary angiogram).

that cavities become radiopaque and thus show on the film or the fluoroscope screen. For the gastrointestinal tract, barium sulfate is the contrast medium used. To visualize the esophagus, stomach, and duodenum, the patient drinks the barium solution; to visualize the colon and rectum, the barium is given as an enema. For x-rays of the ventricles of the brain, oxygen is injected into the spinal canal; organic soluble iodides are used to visualize the gallbladder, urinary tract, and blood vessels.

An x-ray examination of the upper gastrointestinal tract (upper GI series, or barium meal) is done on an empty stomach; therefore, food and fluids are restricted for several hours in advance. Following the examination a laxative or an enema is given to clear the barium from the tract. For a lower GI series, the bowel must be clear of fecal matter. Usually the physician orders castor oil the night before, often followed by a cleansing enema the day of the examination. Patients are often asked not to take food or fluids after midnight of the night before an examination, although breakfast and fluids are sometimes permitted since the food will not have entered the large bowel by the

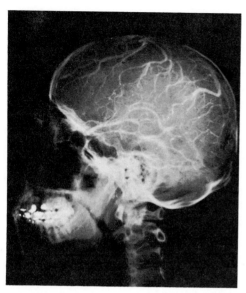

Cerebral angiogram. A radiopaque contrast medium shows the blood vessels of the brain. (J. L. Curry and W. J. Howland: Arteriography: Principles and Techniques. Philadelphia, W. B. Saunders Company, 1966.)

BASAL METABOLIC RATE

The basal metabolic rate (B.M.R.) as a test to reflect thyroid function is gradually being replaced by other tests of thyroid activity, such as the iodine uptake test in which ^{131}I or radioactive iodine is used. Nevertheless, basal metabolic rate tests are carried out in some clinical situations, and therefore patients may need to be prepared for them.

The objective of the basal metabolic rate test is to determine the energy expended by the body at rest. In order to do this, oxygen consumption, which is directly related to the rate of cell metabolism, is measured. In this test, the patient is at rest both physically and psychologically. He does not take food after 9 P.M. or fluid after midnight the night before. Furthermore, he does not smoke prior to the test and he remains in a restful, inactive state.

During the test the patient lies down and breathes in oxygen, which is usually provided through a mask. The amount of oxygen that he uses in a designated time is used in calculating the B.M.R.

ELECTROCARDIOGRAPHY

An electrocardiogram (ECG) is a graphic representation of electrical impulses emitted by the heart. Although electrocardiography is a painless procedure, the idea of heart disease is anxiety producing in many people. Therefore, frequent reassurance and an explanation are necessary.

Electrocardiography is carried out in

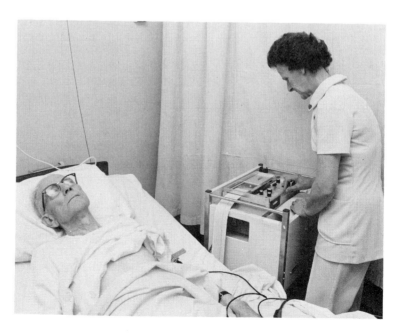

The electrocardiogram (ECG) is a common diagnostic tool used to obtain a graphic representation of electrical impulses from the heart.

hospitals and doctors' offices by a technician, a nurse, or a physician. Small electrodes are strapped on the patient's body in order to pick up the electrical impulses of the heart. A paste is used between the skin and the electrodes to facilitate the transfer of impulses.

ELECTROENCEPHALOGRAPHY

An electroencephalogram is a graphic representation of electrical impulses from the brain. Electroencephalography is similar to electrocardiography in principle, but it is usually done in a laboratory setting. It is generally a painless procedure, but the patient is sometimes sedated beforehand.

The patient assumes a resting position. Tiny electrodes are attached to his scalp and to a machine. These electrodes pick up the electrical potentials produced by the brain cells and record them on a graph. Electroencephalography frequently is used as a diagnostic procedure in patients with neurological conditions. (We mentioned its use also in identifying stages in the sleep cycle in Chapter 18.)

GUIDE TO ASSESSING NURSING NEEDS

1. What tests or examinations have been ordered for this patient?
2. What information should the patient have about these tests or examinations? What other preparation does he need?
3. Is the patient anxious about the test?
4. Does the family of the patient require reassurance or explanations about the tests?
5. What equipment is required for the test?
6. Are there specimens to be collected?
7. Is there a possibility that emergency equipment may be needed?
8. Are there measures to be followed after the test? Does the patient need instructions regarding these measures?

GUIDE TO EVALUATING THE EFFECTIVENESS OF NURSING INTERVENTION

1. Is the patient comfortable?
2. Was the test or examination carried out successfully?
3. Were all specimens sent to the laboratory? Were they correctly labeled and in appropriate containers?
4. Has the test or examination been recorded on the patient's chart? Were pertinent observations noted?
5. Have all after-care measures been instituted? For example, should the patient be in a recumbent position?

STUDY VOCABULARY

Abdominal paracentesis	Lumbar puncture	Pneumothorax
Cisternal puncture	Manometer	Roentgen
Electrocardiogram	Ophthalmoscope	Subarachnoid
Electroencephalogram	Otoscope	Thoracentesis

STUDY SITUATION

You are a nurse in a doctor's office. A patient, Mr. Dawson, has been told by the doctor that he needs to have x-rays taken of his upper and lower gastrointestinal tract before his illness can be determined. Mr. Dawson does not appear to understand the doctor and, apprehensively, he asks you to explain.

Mr. Dawson is 37 years old, has had an eighth grade education and works on a fishing boat. For the past two weeks he has had periods of acute vomiting and diarrhea, which caused him to stop working and come to the doctor. He has a wife and four children at home.

1. What factors about this patient would you consider pertinent to your explanations?
2. What might Mr. Dawson need in the way of an explanation?
3. What should you explain about the x-ray examination?
4. How could you perhaps relieve some of his apprehension?
5. How could you evaluate whether your help has met Mr. Dawson's needs?

SUGGESTED READINGS

Asbury, A. J.: Electronic Equipment in Nursing. *Nursing Times, 69*:861–863, July 5, 1973.

Beaumont, E.: ECG Telemetry. Product Survey. *Nursing '74, 4*:27–34, July 1974.

Bowar-Ferres, S.: Loeb Center and Its Philosophy of Nursing. *American Journal of Nursing, 75*:810–815, May 1975.

Brannon, M.: The Problem-Back Service. *American Journal of Nursing, 75*:1295–1297, August 1975.

Downie, P. A.: Physiotherapy and the Care of the Progressively Ill Patient. *Nursing Times, 69*:892–893, July 12, 1973.

Erikson, R.: Cranial Check: A Basic Neurological Assessment. *Nursing '74, 4*:67–68, August 1974.

Fry, J., et al.: Basic Physical Assessment. *Canadian Nurse, 70*:17–22, May 1974.

Henriques, C. C., et al.: Performance of Adult Health Appraisal Examinations Utilizing Nurse Practitioners, Physician Teams and Paramedical Personnel. *American Journal of Public Health, 64*:47–53, January 1974.

Lynaugh, J. E., and B. Bates: Physical Diagnosis: A Skill for All Nurses? *American Journal of Nursing, 74*:58–59, January 1974.

McGuckin, M.: Improving Your Role in Blood Culture Procedures. Part 2. *Nursing '76, 6*:16–17, January 1976.

Mansell, E., et al.: Patient Assessment: Examination of the Abdomen. Programmed Instruction. *American Journal of Nursing, 74*:1679–1702, September 1974.

Marici, F. N.: The Flexible Fiberoptic Bronchoscope. *American Journal of Nursing, 73*:1776–1778, October 1973.

Maykoski, K.: Nursing Assessment of the Surgical Intensive Care Patient. *Nursing Clinics of North America, 10*:83–106, March 1975.

Neufeld, A. J.: A Ten-Minute Examination to Pinpoint Skeletal Injuries. *ONA J., 2*:273–274, November 1975.

Sana, J. M., and R. D. Judge (eds.): *Physical Appraisal Methods in Nursing Practice.* Boston, Little, Brown & Company, 1975.

Slesser, G.: Auscultation of the Chest—A Clinical Nursing Skill. *Canadian Nurse, 69*:40–43, April 1973.

Stryker, R. P.: *Rehabilitative Aspects of Acute and Chronic Nursing Care.* Philadelphia, W. B. Saunders Company, 1972.

Traver, G. A.: Assessment of Thorax and Lungs. *American Journal of Nursing, 73*:466–471, March 1973.

Watson, E. M., et al.: Clinical Laboratory Procedures. *Canadian Nurse, 70*:25–44, February 1974.

24 MEDICATIONS

The nurse should be able to:

Describe methods commonly used in health agencies for communicating medication orders

Use adequate safety precautions in preparing and administering medications

Compare the advantages and disadvantages of administering medications by the oral, subcutaneous, and intramuscular routes

Prepare and administer medications, using adequate safety measures, by all of the following routes: orally subcutaneously, intramuscularly, intradermally, topically, and by instillations into the ear, eye, nose, throat, and vagina.

Record the administration of medications in the manner used correctly, according to the policy of the agency in which she is working

MEDICATIONS 24

INTRODUCTION

The use of medications as therapeutic agents has been known throughout history. In recent years, however, the number of different medicines that are manufactured commercially for distribution has increased enormously. Although hundreds of new drug products are introduced each year, relatively few of these are new chemical substances. Most new preparations that appear on the market are actually modified forms of drugs previously used, or new dosage forms of the same drug, or new combinations of drugs that have been used for some time. Pharmacists, as well as physicians and nurses, are continually challenged to keep up to date with these constantly changing products.

Sources of information available to nurses about new drugs include the agency pharmacy department, physicians, the professional nursing and medical journals, and information put out by the commercial drug firms. In many health agencies, the pharmacy department maintains an up-to-date *formulary* which lists and describes drugs currently used in the agency. Copies of the formulary are usually distributed to all nursing units, where they are readily available for reference. In addition, many head nurses like to keep a drug file on their nursing units with information about new drugs. The pharmacist is, of course, an excellent reference source, and the nurse should not hesitate to request information from him. Physicians too are usually very willing to explain the nature and purpose of new drugs they have prescribed for patients. With the multitude of new drug products constantly appearing on the market, it is difficult for anyone to keep informed about them all. The nurse should be aware of the sources of information available in her agency about new drugs and should make use of these.

Many drugs are marketed under their trade, or proprietary, names. Each drug usually has at least three names: its trade name, a chemical name, and an official or generic name. The trade (proprietary) name is the name given a drug by the manufacturer. Consequently, one drug may have several trade names, since the same drug may be manufactured by several drug companies, each one giving it a different trade name. The chemical name of the drug is a description of its chemical constituents. The official, or generic, name of a drug is the name under which it is listed in one of the official publications. A generic name is originally assigned by the individual or company which develops the drug. When the drug becomes official, it may be assigned a new generic name, in which case the original one is dropped. Official publications of drugs include the *United States Pharmacopoeia* and the *National Formulary* in the United States. In Canada, the equivalents are the *Vademecum International of Canada* and the *National Formulary* (Canadian); drugs are not termed "official" in Canada, but their generic names appear in these official publications. The World Health Organization publishes a guide, *Specifications for the Quality Control of Pharmaceutical Preparations*, which is an international pharmacopoeia listing important drugs used in many countries.

An increasing number of health agencies are adopting the practice of using the generic or official names of drugs for patient prescriptions. This practice not only eliminates much confusion about the nature of the drug prescribed, but means too that products of different drug companies can be used alternatively, unless the physician specifically requests that one company's product be used.

Drug standards provide for identification, purity, and uniformity of the strength of drugs. The *Pharmacopeia of the United States of America* (U.S.P.) lists drugs and defines the standards according to which a pharmacist in the United States must fill a prescription. The *Vademecum International of Canada* does the same for pharmacists in Canada. In this way the physician can always be assured of the uniform purity and potency of the medications that he or she orders. The World Health Organization publication has been a major step toward establishing international standards for drugs.

The administration of medications is a therapeutic nursing function which is chiefly dependent upon the orders of the physician. Some medication orders state the exact time for administration; others leave the time of administration to the nurse's judgment. For example, it is not unusual for ferrous sulfate to be prescribed three times a day after meals, whereas an order for 15 mg. (¼ gr.) of morphine subcutaneously is often written so that the nurse can give it when, in her judgment, the patient requires an analgesic.

ORDERING AND RECORDING MEDICATIONS

Medications are, in most instances, ordered or prescribed by a physician. In an ambulatory care setting, the physician usually writes the prescription on a form which the patient gives to the pharmacist. The prescription tells the pharmacist what medications the patient is to have, the dosage required, the amount to be supplied, how to prepare it, and the instructions the patient is to be given for taking them. In many places now, the name of the drug and the unit dosage must be included on the label of the medication the patient receives.

In an inpatient facility, the prescription is usually in the form of a written order that is dated and signed by the physician, although some health agencies permit physicians to telephone orders to the nursing staff. In such cases, the physicians are usually required to countersign their orders within a definite number of hours. In an emergency situation medications are given on a verbal order that is later written and countersigned as needed. Generally speaking, written orders are considered to be the safest practice.

There are two types of written orders: the self-terminating order and the standing order. *Self-terminating orders* have a time limit on them. A stat. order is a self-terminating order that is to be carried out only once and immediately, for example, Demerol 100 mg. I.M. stat. (I.M. refers to intramuscularly). It is not repeated unless there are specific instructions to that effect. Another type of self-terminating order is an order in which the time limit is actually specified; for example, the physician writes, aspirin 0.65 g. (gr. $\bar{x}$) for six doses, or digitalis 0.1 g. (gr. $\overline{iss}$) June 12th and 14th. Sometimes a self-terminating order is dependent upon the condition of the patient, as when an order is written, aspirin 0.65 g. (gr. $\bar{x}$) q4h until temperature has remained below 37.8° C. (100° F.) for 24 hours. Some institutions have policies which place a time limit on orders regardless of how they are worded. For example, it is not unusual for a narcotic order to be effective for only three days, after which it is automatically discontinued unless the physician writes another order.

Standing orders are orders which are carried out indefinitely; for example, vitamin C 50 mg. o.d. oral. Some standing orders contain the direction "p.r.n.," which means "as necessary." The administration of a drug under a p.r.n. direction is left to the nurse's judgment. An example of this type of order is Demerol 100 mg. I.M. q4h p.r.n.

An order should always include the name of the drug, the exact dosage, the route of administration, and the frequency of administration. If the physician wishes a medication to be given at a time other than the accustomed distribution time, this should also be specified. The nurse has an obligation to question any order that is ambiguous or which she feels is unsafe for a patient. In health agencies it is a customary practice for all of a patient's orders to be written on a doctor's order sheet, which may be kept in the patient's chart or in a central book. Hospitals employ different ways of flagging charts to indicate that a patient has new orders. The orders are then usually copied in the nursing unit Kardex system or nursing care plan and a medication card may be filled out. A medication card has the patient's full name, the name of the drug, the dosage, the route of administration (in some hospitals if the route is oral it is omitted), the frequency of the administration, and the times of administration. Frequently, the room number or location of the patient's bed is also written on the medication card. If the drug is ordered q.i.d., the exact times are added—for example, 0800 (8 A.M.), 1200 (12 noon), 1600 (4 P.M.), and 2000 (8 P.M.). Medication cards are kept in a central place in the nursing unit and are frequently grouped so that they are easily selected at the time of administration.

Although different methods of posting medication orders are used in various agencies, the nurse should remember that the original written order is the primary source of information. Whenever orders are copied, whether onto a Kardex file, a nursing care plan or a medicine card, the possibility of error is present. The nurse who administers medications should always check the original orders to make certain that communication tools are accurate.

Agencies have different methods of indicating that a medication has been discontinued. In hospitals it is common practice for "discontinued" to be imprinted across the physician's order once it is no longer in force and for the medication card to be discarded. In a public health agency the notation "discontinued" and the date are entered on the nursing care record. Communication tools such as medication cards and nursing care records should be regularly checked against the original orders in order to keep them up to date. In hospitals where orders change frequently this is generally done at least once a day.

Medications are recorded in the patient's chart immediately after they have been administered. They should be recorded by the nurse who administered them. The recording includes the name of the drug, the time it was administered, the exact dosage, the method of administration, and the signature of the nurse administering the drug. Some agencies also require that the status of the person administering the drug also be designated, as, for example, R.N. or S.N. (student nurse).

When a p.r.n. order has been administered a notation is also made as to why the patient took the medicine at that particular time. Recording should also include observations of the effect of the medication when these are, or should be, apparent. In some hospitals the nurse also indicates on the doctor's order sheet that stat. dosages have been administered.

The administration of narcotics and, in some places, barbiturates and other controlled drugs is recorded not only on the patient's chart but also on a special form which is kept separately. Narcotics and other controlled drugs are kept in locked containers in hospitals and their distribution is closely governed. The forms upon which narcotics are recorded vary from place to place, but usually the nurse records the name of the patient to whom the narcotic was administered, the drug and dosage, the date and time, the name of the physician ordering the drug, and the signature of the nurse administering the drug. Any narcotics that are wasted are also recorded with a notation that the drug was wasted. Narcotics, barbiturates, and other controlled drugs are counted at specific times—for example, at the end of each shift—and the number distributed plus the number remaining on hand must tally with the number assigned to the nursing unit or agency. This count is usually done by two nurses, the one coming on duty and the nurse who is "handing over" to her. This practice helps to protect both nurses. Narcotics, barbiturates and other controlled drugs are under strict Federal control. Any losses or inconsistencies in the count must be reported immediately.

GUIDES FOR ADMINISTERING MEDICATIONS

The type of drug preparation often governs the method of administration. Medications are distributed in a variety of preparations, and each type usually requires a specific method of administration. It may be that one preparation can be administered in several ways, but this is specified on the medication label. More often a preparation of a drug has only one method of administration, and if the drug must be administered by some other route, another preparation is required. Drugs are administered only by the route ordered by the doctor and specified on the medication label. For example, penicillin tablets are taken orally, but a special solution of penicillin is given intramuscularly. It is a good practice to read the label carefully and also check the medication card for the route of administration.

The route of administration of the drug affects the optimal dosage of the drug. The optimal dosage of a drug administered by mouth may not be the same as the optimal dosage when the drug is administered subcutaneously. For example, portions of drugs taken orally are excreted through the digestive tract instead of being absorbed into the cells.

The safe administration of medications requires a knowledge of anatomy and physiology as well as a knowledge of the drug and the reason it has been prescribed. A knowledge of anatomy and physiology is particularly important when medications are administered intramuscularly or subcutaneously. For example, when administering a drug intramuscularly, large blood vessels and nerves could be damaged if they are accidentally punctured.

A knowledge of the drug and its effects also helps safeguard against the administration of a medication which could harm a patient. For example, if a patient has very slow respirations (e.g., 10 per minute), morphine can be contraindicated, because it can depress the respirations even more. This knowledge helps the nurse to make intelligent observations which assist in the assessment of the effectiveness of both the medication and the nursing care.

An understanding of the total plan of care for each patient and the desired therapeutic effect of the medications prescribed for him is essential. The nurse should know why the individual patient is receiving each medication so that she knows what to observe in that patient.

The method of administration of a drug is partially determined by the age of the patient, his orientation, his degree of consciousness, and his health problem. It is important for the nurse to report *any* difficulties that are encountered when administering a medication. Perhaps the disoriented patient refuses to swallow his oral medication, or the nauseated patient vomits his medicines after he has taken them. The unconscious patient is unable to take a medication orally, and a child might be too young to swallow a capsule. These observations should be reported to the physician in order that he can assess the specific needs of the individual.

The element of error is a possibility in all human activity. Errors in the administration of medicines can be serious and, because the possibility of error is always present, special precautions are taken to avoid mistakes. If a nurse is ever in doubt about her activity, she should always consult a reliable source before going ahead. Most agencies have literature to which the nurse can refer, and physicians and pharmacies can also be consulted.

If an error is made it is reported immediately to the physician or to the nurse in charge, so that immediate steps can be taken to protect the patient from injury. The error is also analyzed to determine the exact cause in order to safeguard against another such error. Most hospitals also have unusual occurrence forms which the nurse fills out to inform the agency administration of the details of the error (see Chapter 7).

Each patient has his own needs for explanations and support with respect to the administration of medications. Medications are given to *people*, and the nurse will find, as in all of her nursing care, that each individual is different. Some people want to know about their medications; others prefer not to know about them. The amount of knowledge that a person requires is highly dependent upon individual circumstances. The seriously ill patient in a hospital may be too ill to care about any knowledge of the drug. The information that each person should have depends on his intelligence, age, education, illness, and emotional needs. The nurse is guided by both the patient and the physician as to the amount of information she provides.

GENERAL PRECAUTIONS

The administration of medications is a nursing function in most health agencies. In some hospitals the nurse administers all intravenous injections, but in others it is the physician's responsibility to administer specific medications, such as ergotamine, which is used to contract the uterus.

There is a wide variety in the medication policies which guide nursing action. But, regardless of policy, before the nurse administers any medication she must be sure that her action is safe for the patient. A sound basis for safe nursing practice is *knowledge*.

Traditionally the "five rights" have served as guides to the administration of medications: the right drug, the right dose, the right route, the right time, and the right patient. These rights are no less true today than they were years ago; however, sound nursing practice involves more than just a knowledge of these. The nurse's information should extend to an identification of the individual problems of the patient and how she can help the patient resolve these problems. For example, will assisting a patient to change his position and the provision of physical support facilitate the action of an analgesic?

Complementary to the administration of many medications is the provision of nursing care measures that serve to supplement the action of a drug. For example, giving the patient a back rub and straightening his bed might increase the effectiveness of a sedative, and drinking fluids can help prevent the crystallization of some antibiotics in the kidneys.

People vary in their reactions to specific drugs. The patient's reaction to any drug is important and should be recorded. Patients often require information about what reactions to report to the nurse or the physician. This is particularly true for the person who is taking medicine at home and does not have constant contact with health personnel.

A knowledge of the significance of a drug and its prescribed dosage is important for some patients. It is not infrequently heard that "If one tablet is good for me, two tablets are twice as good." Some people also require assistance in order to understand the value of a prescribed dose and its action as well as a realistic explanation of the anticipated results. Not only is this a need of hospitalized patients, but it is also important for people who take medicines in their homes. All people taking medications at home should be aware of the nature of the drugs they are taking, why they are taking them, the dosage they are to take, and possible side-effects of the drug. They should also be alerted to adverse signs and symptoms to watch for when they are taking these medications, and the dangers of altering the dosage or omitting to take medications.

Another area of nursing practice is concerned with idiosyncratic reactions to medications, overdoses of drugs, and the ingestion of poisonous materials. Many medical centers provide immediate information to laymen and physicians about the antidotes and emergency measures for the common poisons. A "Poison Control Center," located in the emergency department of a large metropolitan hospital, is illustrated on page 456. An up-to-date list of the poison control centers can be obtained from the Superintendent of Documents, U.S. Government Printing Office, Washington, D.C. A list of poison control centers in Canada is contained in the *Vademecum International of Canada: Pharmaceutical Specialties and Biologicals* (updated each year) and also the *Compendium of Pharmaceuticals and Specialties of Canada.*

It is also a part of the nursing function to assist in evaluating the effectiveness of a medication and often in making judgments as to when a specific medication should be given. In order to make this evaluation, the patient's problems are considered, as well as the purpose of the therapeutic agent itself.

The need of a patient for some medications varies from time to time and, of

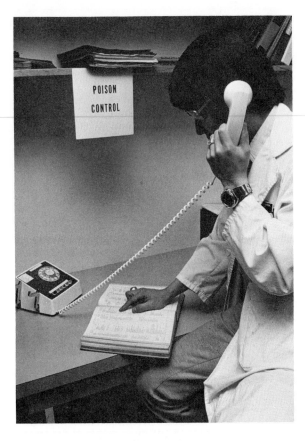

The poison control center is a source of information about the composition, action, and antedotes of poisonous materials. Its services are available to everyone in the community.

course, needs vary from patient to patient. One patient may require frequent sedation, whereas another requires none. Medication orders are based on the patient's specific problems and the action of the drug to facilitate desired therapeutic goals. For example, the physician may want to give a patient a drug that prevents vomiting because of the strain of vomiting upon a freshly sutured wound.

A knowledge of pharmacology includes the actions of drugs, usual dosages and factors which affect dosages, untoward reactions, methods of administration, and drugs that counteract or react with each other. The nurse will find it advantageous, when learning about drugs, to group them according to their systemic action. Many related medicines have similar actions and reactions.

Medications and the Patient

One of the most important factors in the administration of a medication is the iden-

tification of the patient. Any method which accurately identifies a patient is satisfactory. Some hospitals provide each patient with an identification band. Other institutions suggest asking the patient his name before administering a medication. If this is the case, the nurse should not say, "Are you Mr. Smith?" nor should she rely on the patient answering to his name. In both situations, the patient may give an automatic affirmative answer. It is better to say, "What is your name?" The habit of relying upon bed numbers and even room numbers in order to identify people is also dangerous, for patients' rooms are changed and patients move to other units. In situations in which patients are continually reassigned to new rooms, identification is especially difficult.

After the nurse has accurately identified a patient, his need for explanation and support must be met. Often, simple explanations are reassuring to the patient; they can often help provide conditions of acceptance in the patient that can enhance the effectiveness of the drug. At this time the nurse can also provide him with information about the action of the medication as he will perceive it. Patients usually like to feel they are participating in their therapy and have some control over situations. If the physician does not want the patient to receive information about a medicine from the nurse, it can be suggested that he confer with the physician about this subject.

If the administration of a drug is contingent upon some factor, such as the patient's pulse rate, this is assessed first. With few exceptions the nurse stays with a patient until his medication has been completely administered. The exceptions are drugs which have been ordered to be left with a patient, for example, a drug which the patient has for immediate use as needed (such as nitroglycerin for cardiac pain), a cough medicine, or a drug which is contained in an intravenous infusion for gradual administration.

Sometimes people refuse a medication, and often their reasons are valid. If a patient does refuse, the nurse should find out why. Some of the possible reasons are:

1. The medicine is nauseating and makes him vomit.

2. He is allergic to the medicine. A record of the patient's allergies should be noted on admission. Sometimes this is not possible, however; for example, the patient may have been unconscious when he was brought in.

3. The medicine does not help him.

4. He thinks it is the wrong medicine.

5. He believes the physician has changed the order.

6. The needles with which the medicine is administered hurt him.

7. The medicine has an unpleasant taste.

8. He does not want it because of religious or cultural beliefs. For example, a patient of the Hindu religion may refuse a hormonal preparation that contains extracts from cattle; a patient who belongs to the Jehovah's Witness sect may refuse a blood transfusion. Many people who believe in naturopathic remedies will refuse

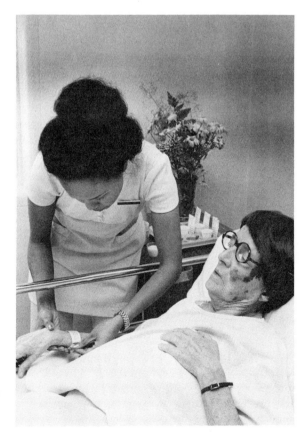

The identification band is one way the nurse can ensure that the right patient receives a medication.

any medicine prepared from inorganic chemicals.

9. He does not understand and is afraid it will harm him.

10. The nurse wants to administer the medication at an inconvenient time, for example, when his visitors are present.

The reason a patient refuses a medicine can often be satisfactorily dealt with by the nurse; for example, if it has an unpleasant taste it can usually be administered in a vehicle such as orange juice. The physician's order should be checked if the patient questions it. Perhaps there is a new order in the chart which has not been transcribed to his medication card. A patient's refusal to take a medication should always be reported to the physician or to the nurse in charge and recorded in the patient's chart. Under some circumstances it is best to notify the physician at once, particularly when a patient's condition is seriously affected by the omission of the medication, as when a patient with heart disease will not take digitalis.

Observing and Reporting

Immediately after a medication has been administered, the fact is recorded on the patient's chart. If the drug was administered at the nurse's discretion, the reason for the administration is also recorded.

After the administration of any therapeutic agent, the nurse observes the patient for his reaction. The criteria by which the nurse judges the effectiveness of a drug depend on the purpose for which it was administered. It can be the alleviation of pain, the reduction of fever, a decrease in swelling, or even the appearance of orange-colored urine. These results are anticipated results and they reflect the effectiveness of the particular medication. The observations are recorded in detail on the patient's chart. Sometimes patients experience untoward reactions as a result of a medication—for example, nausea and vomiting, diarrhea or a skin rash. These observations are always reported promptly. If a reaction is severe, that is, if the patient is acutely uncomfortable or essential body functions

are impaired, the physician is notified immediately so that measures to counteract the adverse symptoms can be instituted. For example, in severe allergic reactions the tissues of the throat may become so edematous that breathing is difficult. Prompt intervention at the earliest sign of an allergic reaction is required. These reactions are also recorded in detail on the patient's chart.

PREPARING MEDICATIONS

The first step in the preparation of any medication is to get the complete order and make sure it is understood. Sometimes agency policies or the orders themselves govern the administration of a specific drug or the special nursing measures which accompany its administration. For example, an order might read "withhold drug if pulse is below 60 beats per minute."

Before administering drugs, the nurse washes her hands to minimize the transfer of microorganisms and then she gathers the equipment she needs. In a hospital all the necessary equipment is usually kept in a medication room near the nursing unit office yet separate from it so that medications can be prepared without disturbance. In the home, such equipment is generally kept in one place, usually in a cupboard which is out of reach of children. Some hospitals use medication carts to deliver the medicines; others use trays, often with special slots so that the medicine card stands upright and can be read easily.

A hospital medication cupboard is usually locked, the key being kept by the head nurse, the nurse responsible for administering medications (if this system is used), or in a designated place in the nursing unit. Adjacent to the medication cupboard are usually a locked narcotic cupboard and a refrigerator. Drugs which lose their potency unless kept cold are kept in the refrigerator.

The nurse selects the medicine that was ordered by the physician. Drugs kept in a hospital are either stock or private (prescription). The former are the more commonly used medicines; the latter are especially prepared for a patient. Stock drugs are frequently grouped according to action; for example, all vitamin preparations are kept together. Another method is to group the drugs alphabetically according to their generic or trade names. Either method facilitates finding a specific preparation quickly.

It has become an accepted safety practice in the preparation of medications to read the label three times on a bottle, tube, package, envelope, or the like. It is read before the container is taken off the shelf, before it is opened, and just before it is placed back on the shelf. Read both the name of the drug and its strength, and pay particular attention to the route of administration by which the particular medicine is designed to be given.

Medications come in a variety of preparations; capsules, Spansules, lozenges, tablets, and liquids can all be given orally. A capsule contains a powder, oil, or liquid within a gelatinous covering; a tablet is a compressed powdered drug. Troches are oral preparations which are sucked. Vials and ampules contain either powdered or liquid medications for injection. A vial is a glass container with a rubber stopper, whereas an ampule is a sealed glass container. A suppository is a medication which is molded into a firm base in order that it can be inserted into a body orifice or cavity. An ointment is a semisolid mixture which is applied topically to mucous membranes or skin.

A medicine must be administered in the exact dose that is ordered by the physician. If small doses are required (for example, for children), the usual practice is to have these doses prepared accurately by a pharmacist. In situations in which the dose must be calculated, the safest practice is for a second nurse to check the calculations made by the first. The nurse should not estimate a dosage on her own initiative; for example, it is not a safe practice to break an unscored tablet to get a dosage. The dose of a drug is ordered by the physician in consideration of the weight, age, sex, and physical condition of the patient. Thus, approximating dosages can be a dangerous practice.

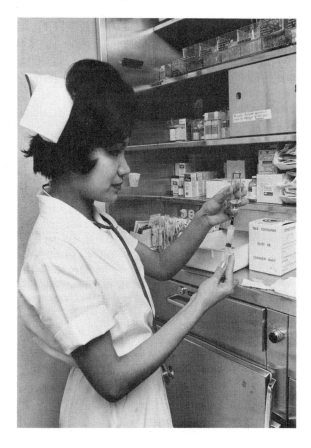

In a hospital, medications are usually prepared in a separate room adjoining the nursing station.

In order to avoid errors the nurse who prepares a medication should administer it herself immediately after she has prepared it. If prepared medicines are left unattended, the chances of the drug being misplaced or taken by another patient are increased. More to the point, the nurse is legally responsible for the medications she administers, and only if she has prepared a medication herself can she testify to the actual constituents of the medication and to its strength. The identification of a medication just by its appearance is a dangerous practice. If it happens that medications are distributed while a patient is in another department, his medication can be returned to the nursing unit and locked in the cupboard with the medication card which serves to identify it.

When a nurse is preparing a variety of medications for a group of patients, the medicines for one patient are separated from the medicines for another. Generally all medicines that are administered by the same route for one patient can be placed in the same container, except for specific drugs whose administration is dependent upon some specified criterion. For example, if digitalis 0.1 g. (gr. $\overline{\text{iss}}$) is to be withheld when the patient's pulse is below 60 beats per minute, this drug is put in a separate container from the other oral medications for that particular patient.

Only a pharmacist should label a container of drugs. Therefore when the nurse finds an unlabeled container or a label which has been partially obscured, the entire container is returned to the pharmacy for clarification. It is also considered a safety practice not to return medications to a container once they have been removed; they should be disposed of by flushing down a toilet or hopper. Some agencies require that a witness be present when narcotics (and sometimes other drugs as well) are disposed of. Drugs should not be transferred from one container to another.

METHODS OF ADMINISTERING MEDICATIONS

The most common method of administering medications is by mouth (orally).

Not only is it simple but it is also the most economical way. Capsules, liquids, tablets, powders, and troches are all administered by mouth. Troches are usually sucked for their local effect. *Sublingual administration* involves placing the drug (for example, nitroglycerin) under the patient's tongue, where it is dissolved and absorbed.

Parenteral refers to the administration of drugs by a needle. Intramuscular, intradermal, subcutaneous, and intravenous injections are common means of parenteral therapy. Intracardiac, intrapericardial, intrathecal (intraspinal), and intraosseous (into bone) injections are less common methods which may be used by physicians. All parenteral therapy involves the use of sterile equipment and sterile, readily soluble solutions. Generally those drugs that are administered parenterally are readily absorbed by the body. Intravenous therapy is discussed in Chapter 29.

Inhalation is the administration of a drug into the respiratory tract. Once the drug is inhaled it is almost immediately absorbed. Volatile and nonvolatile drugs can be inhaled, the latter by means of a vehicle such as oxygen. The administration of medications by inhalation is discussed in Chapter 30.

Instillation is a method of putting a drug in liquid form into a body cavity or orifice, for example the ears, the eyes, and the urinary bladder. Liquid medications can be instilled with a dropper (into the ear), or with a syringe (into the urinary bladder).

Medications are also applied to the skin and mucous membranes; this process is called *topical application*. Antiseptics, astringents, and emollients can be applied as liquids or ointments.

Drugs are generally administered for either their systemic or local effect. *Systemic effect* refers to the actions of the drug upon the entire body, whereas *local effect* is the effect upon one specific area, such as that of an ointment upon a particular area of the skin. Sometimes drugs that are administered for their local effect have systemic actions; for example, an untoward reaction such as a fever may result from the topical application of an ointment to an incision.

A *suppository* is used for insertion into a body cavity or orifice, such as the rectum or vagina. As the suppository gradually dissolves at body temperature, the drug is released and is absorbed through the mucous membrane. Although a suppository is sometimes used to administer drugs when a systemic action is desired, as, for example, a sedative, it is not considered as efficient as a medication administered by other routes. Suppositories are therefore used principally for their local action. They may be used, for instance, to administer an analgesic to the rectal area, or to stimulate peristalsis and bring about a bowel movement.

Oral Administration

Oral medications are absorbed chiefly in the small intestines, although they can also be absorbed in the mouth and the stomach. Medications administered sublingually are absorbed through the capillaries under the tongue. Drugs in liquid form, either upon administration or upon dissolution within the stomach, are absorbed through the gastric mucosa. Absorption of a drug is slowed by the presence of food in the stomach as well as by its administration in concentrated form. Dilution, an alcoholic base, and an empty stomach facilitate absorption.

Advantages and Disadvantages. The oral administration of medications has the advantages of convenience, economy, and safety. It is convenient in that it is a simple method of administration; it is economical in that oral preparations usually cost less to manufacture than many other preparations; it is safe in that its administration does not involve breaking through any of the body defenses—for example, the skin—as is necessary with injections.

The chief disadvantages of the oral administration of medications are their taste, gastric irritation, effect upon teeth, inaccurate measure of absorption, and limited use.

Drugs which are decidedly *unpleasant tasting* can stimulate nausea and vomiting. Drugs in liquid or partially dissolved form activate the taste buds more than drugs in tablet or capsule form; however,

since cold is less stimulating than warmth, the taste buds can be partially desensitized by giving cold fluids or ice chips.

Some medications are particularly *irritating to the gastric mucosa*; others are destroyed by the gastric secretions. The latter are usually manufactured either with an enteric coating so that they do not dissolve in the stomach, or in a form to be given by parenteral administration. Irritation of the gastric mucosa can be minimized by administering a drug after a meal, while food is still in the stomach. Also, the more diluted the medicine is, the less irritating it will be to the mucosa. A medicine which is particularly irritating can sometimes be given in conjunction with another drug or with food, such as bread, in order to modify its undesirable effect.

Some medications are *harmful to the teeth.* Drugs such as hydrochloric acid damage enamel, and liquid iron preparations often discolor the teeth. These undesirable effects can be avoided by giving highly diluted forms and by using a straw in order that the teeth do not come in contact with the liquid. It is also wise to have the patient rinse his mouth with water or a mouthwash after he takes these medicines.

Another disadvantage of the oral administration of medications is the relative inability to *measure their absorption accurately* in the gastrointestinal tract. Certain disorders affect absorption; for example, accelerated peristalsis will decrease absorption because of the drug's speedy propulsion through the gastrointestinal tract. Moreover, some medications are destroyed to a variable extent by gastrointestinal secretions; in addition, the adequacy of the circulation of the blood to the tract affects the rate of absorption. If a person vomits after he has ingested a medicine, the amount of drug retained in his body is questionable. Generally the physician is consulted when this happens in order that he can assess the patient's need for a repeated dose of the medicine.

Oral medications are *limited in use* to patients who are able to swallow and retain them. The unconscious patient, the patient who is unable to swallow, and the vomiting patient are unable to take these medications. Patients who are restricted to taking nothing by mouth cannot be given oral medications. Some patients cannot take oral medications because of gastric suction and some find swallowing difficult because of surgery or paralysis. Frequently it is the nurse who first becomes aware that a patient has difficulty in swallowing a medicine, and her communication of this fact to the physician can result in a change in the order to a more easily consumed drug. Tablets can be crushed and a scored tablet can be broken for easier administration, but the protective coverings of capsules or enteric-coated pills should not be removed to facilitate administration.

Preparation. In the preparation of oral medications for distribution, the nurse follows the general guides outlined earlier in this chapter. Oral drugs are generally distributed in disposable containers. Liquid medications are often given in plastic or waxed paper medication containers. The advantages of using disposable containers are obvious: their cleanliness is assured, and washing and sterilizing are eliminated. Medications should not be handled indiscriminately with the fingers; it is considered a cleaner practice to drop a tablet into the bottle cap or into an empty medicine container before transferring it to the container that the patient uses. If there is any doubt about administering a specific drug, the drug is kept separately from the other tablets for a specific patient.

When pouring liquids, the dose is measured from the bottom of the concave meniscus. Some liquids separate after standing in a bottle and need to be shaken before they are poured. Minims (0.06 cc.) and drops are not interchangeable measures; special droppers or glasses, and, in some agencies, syringes, are used for measuring small amounts of liquid medications.

Administration. After the patient is appropriately identified, the nurse gives him his medications and stays with him until they have been taken. Sometimes the patient needs assistance to sit up or to turn on his side to swallow without choking. Usually people find it easier to take oral medicines with water or juice. If the consistency of a liquid is unpleasant, as, for example, mineral oil, patients often find it easier to take if the medicine has been chilled. With few exceptions drugs are not left at a patient's bedside in hospitals.

Subcutaneous Injection

Advantages and Disadvantages. Some medications are best administered into the subcutaneous tissue by a needle. This route has the advantage of almost complete absorption, provided that the patient's circulation is good; therefore, an accurate measure of the amount of the drug absorbed is possible. Medicines administered in this manner are not affected by gastric disturbances (although it should be remembered that the medicines may themselves cause gastrointestinal disturbances), nor is their administration dependent upon the consciousness or rationality of the patient.

The chief disadvantage of this method is that by introducing a needle through skin one of the body's barriers against infection is broken. It is therefore important that aseptic technique be used for all needle injections.

The Site of Injection. The subcutaneous tissue is just below the cutaneous tissue or skin. It is areolar tissue which has fewer sensory receptors than the skin itself; therefore once a needle is through the skin an injection is relatively painless. Some drugs sting upon injection, but an isotonic solution can usually be administered painlessly. Isotonic refers to a concentration that is the same as a normal saline solution.

The exact site for a subcutaneous injection depends on the need of the specific patient and to some extent upon the policy of the institution. Since drugs administered subcutaneously (hypodermically) are usually given for their systemic effect, the site is irrelevant with respect to any local effect. Areas in the upper arms, anterior and lateral aspects of the thigh, and the lower ventral abdominal wall are suggested.[1] The skin and subcutaneous tissue should be in good condition, that is,

---

[1]Martha Pitel: The Subcutaneous Injection. *American Journal of Nursing,* 71:79, January 1971.

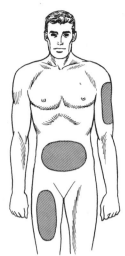

Three sites which are commonly used for subcutaneous injections are the outer aspect of the upper arm, the loose abdominal tissue and the anterior aspect of the thigh.

free of irritation such as itching and free of any signs of inflammation, such as redness, heat, edema, tenderness, or pain. Areas where there is scar tissue should not be used. A common practice is to choose the outer aspect of the patient's upper arm about one-third of the distance down between the shoulder and the elbow. Other sites are the anterior aspect of the thigh, the loose tissue of the abdomen and the subscapular region of the back. Actually the subcutaneous tissue in any area can be injected provided that it is not over bony prominences and is free of large blood vessels and nerves. If a patient is receiving a series of injections the sites are rotated and the site is charted each time so that two consecutive doses are not given in the same area. Sometimes a map is made of the skin areas to be used to indicate the sites for rotating injections, or a chart may be attached to the nursing care plan for the patient.

Equipment. Subcutaneous (hypodermic) injections involve the use of sterile equipment and supplies. These include a syringe, a needle, the medication, and a swab and disinfectant to cleanse the skin. Syringes vary in size from 1 cc. to 50 cc. The 2 cc. syringe, commonly used for subcutaneous injections, is calibrated in cubic centimeters. For the administration of insulin, special 1 cc. syringes are often used. Insulin syringes are usually calibrated in units to correspond to the strength of a particular insulin. Nowadays, the 100 unit scale is most common, although some agencies still use a 40 or 80 unit scale.

A syringe has two parts, the barrel or outer part, and the plunger or inner part. Most syringes are manufactured so that their parts are interchangeable, but if they are not the two pieces of a set bear corresponding numbers on the plunger and barrel.

Syringes are made of glass or plastic. The latter, which are usually disposable, are being used increasingly in hospitals, offices, and clinics. A 2 cc. syringe is usually used for subcutaneous injections. The maximum volume of solution which can be given comfortably by this route is thought to be less than 1.5 cc. (20 minims). Certainly anything greater than 2 cc. (30 minims) will cause pressure on surrounding tissues and therefore be painful.

A needle has a hub and a shaft or cannula. The hub is the larger part that connects to the barrel of the syringe; the cannula is the long narrow part. At the end of the cannula is the bevel (point) or slanted

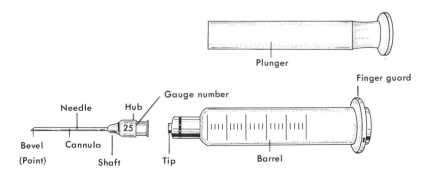

Diagram of needle and parts of a syringe.

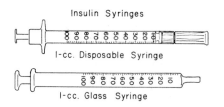

Insulin Syringes

I-cc. Disposable Syringe

I-cc. Glass Syringe

Insulin syringes (disposable or reusable) — U40, U80, U100 (Becton-Dickinson Co.)

(From Lucile A. Wood: Nursing Skills for Allied Health Services. Vol. 3. Philadelphia, W. B. Saunders Co., 1975.)

portion where the fluid is ejected. A short or small bevel is used when there is a danger that a larger bevel would become occluded, as in intravenous injections in which the bevel could rest against the side of the vein. The longer bevel provides a sharper needle and is used for subcutaneous and intramuscular injections.

The needle used for a subcutaneous injection is usually 24, 25 or 26 gauge. The larger the number, the smaller the diameter of the needle. The length that is required varies from 1 cm. (³⁄₈ inch) to 2.5 cm. (1 inch), depending upon the amount of subcutaneous fat and the degree of hydration of the patient. A longer needle is needed for the obese patient, a shorter needle for the dehydrated person. Generally a No. 24 needle 1.5 cm (⁵⁄₈ inch) long is used for the average adult.

The needle used for any injection should be straight and sharp. As disposable needles are increasingly being used, the problem of the bent or dull needle is disappearing. If disposable needles are not used, the needles are checked for sharpness and the presence of barbs before they are sterilized. A needle may be checked for the presence of barbs by passing the tip lightly over a piece of absorbent cotton. If the needle does catch on the cotton, it may have a barb and will be uncomfortable for a patient. Needles that are bent should not be used, because of the danger that they will break off in a patient. The weakest point in a needle is where the cannula joins the hub.

A word of caution on the use of disposable needles and syringes: After use they should be discarded in the designated

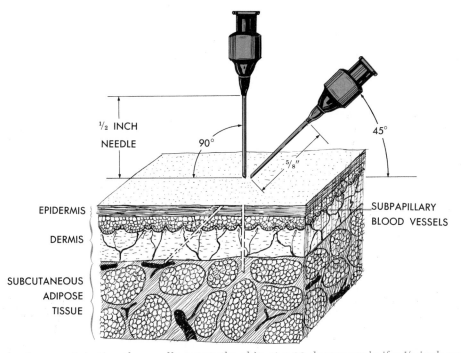

For a subcutaneous injection the needle enters the skin at a 90 degree angle if a ½ inch needle is used, at a 45 degree angle if a ⁵⁄₈ inch needle is used. The bevel of the needle is uppermost. The needle is inserted deeply into the subcutaneous tissue.

containers, never where they can be obtained by addicts. Disposable needles and syringes should be bent after use so that they cannot be used again. These practices also help to protect the housekeeping staff from injury, since the bent needle point will not be as likely to penetrate garbage bags.

Two variations in the traditional means of administering injections subcutaneously are the injector syringe equipped with a spring which releases the needle for rapid insertion, and the jet injector by which the medication is introduced into the subcutaneous tissue by means of high pressure rather than through a needle. Although these methods are preferred in some instances, they have not replaced the usual subcutaneous injection by hypodermic syringe.

Preparation. Medications for injection come in tablet, liquid, and powder forms. All these forms must be kept sterile during preparation and administration. If a drug in tablet form is to be administered subcutaneously, it is first dissolved in a sterile solution. The safest method is to carefully drop the tablet into a sterile container, draw up a measured amount of sterile solution into the syringe (sterile normal saline is less painful to the patient than sterile water), add the solution to the tablet to dissolve it and, finally, draw up the measured amount of medicated solution into the syringe ready for administration. Another method which is being used increasingly is to mix the tablet and the solution directly in the syringe.

Medications in a liquid form generally come in single dose ampules or multiple dose vials. To open an ampule, the nurse first taps it to shake all the medication to the bottom and then obtains a sterile cotton ball which she holds behind the neck of the ampule. Some ampules open directly upon pressure at the neck; others require filing. The cotton ball is used to protect the nurse's fingers when breaking the glass. After the ampule is opened, the needle is carefully inserted, the ampule is inverted, and the solution is drawn into the sterile syringe.

Multiple dose vials of medication have a sealed rubber cap at the top which makes them airtight. The cap is first wiped off with an antiseptic solution, the plunger of the syringe is drawn back to a point which indicates the volume of solution to be withdrawn, and then the needle is inserted through the rubber cap. Air is injected into the vial to equalize the pressure and thus facilitate the removal of the solution. The vial is held upside down with the syringe at eye level in order to obtain an accurate measure of the drug. Incorrect holding of the vial may result in air being drawn into the syringe.

Injectable drugs that come as powders are dissolved in sterile solution before they are administered. Generally there are directions on the label as to the amount and kind of solution that is to be added to a vial. In order to maintain normal pressure inside the vial, air is removed in a volume that corresponds to the amount of solution that is inserted. If a large vial is used, it is often easier to insert a second sterile needle through the rubber cap to allow the free flow of air out of the vial as the fluid flows in.

Some drugs are prepared commercially in two-compartment vials. One compartment contains the powdered medication and the second contains the sterile liquid for dissolving the drug. The insertion of a sterile needle or pressure upon a rubber diaphragm releases the liquid to mix with the powder, which is then ready for injection. Some drugs are packaged this way because they are more stable in a dry state and thus can be kept for a longer period of time than the same drug in liquid form.

Whenever a powder or tablet is prepared for injection it should be completely dissolved before it is drawn into the syringe. Rotating a vial between one's hands is an effective way of mixing a powder and a liquid without creating bubbles on the top of the solution. Bubbles can make it difficult to ascertain an accurate measure of the drug.

Administration. When a subcutaneous injection is to be administered, a site is selected and cleansed with an antiseptic solution. The type of antiseptic used depends on the policy of the agency. Isopropanol in 70 per cent solution is used in many hospitals. The antiseptic solution is allowed to dry on the skin surface prior to insertion of the needle to prevent local irritation at the site of the injection.

When the skin is dry, air is expelled from the needle. The needle is then inserted through the skin. The angle of insertion depends on the size of the needle used. It is recommended that the injection be given deeply into the subcutaneous tissue. Therefore, if a 1.2 cm. (½ inch) needle is used, it is inserted at a 90 degree angle, that is, perpendicular to the skin surface. Injections with a 1.5 cm. (⅝ inch) needle are inserted at a 45 degree angle. Some authorities feel that the skin should not be drawn taut, pinched or pulled into a skin fold for the injection. Rather, it should be left in its natural state.[2] The nurse will find it easier to give the injection, however, if she lightly holds the area around the injection site.

After the needle is inserted, the plunger is drawn back in order to determine whether the needle is in a blood vessel. If no blood appears in the syringe, the solution is injected slowly, after which the needle is quickly withdrawn. If blood does appear in the syringe, the needle is immediately withdrawn and another medication prepared. After the needle is withdrawn the area is massaged gently with an antiseptic sponge to facilitate dispersion of the solution. If there is any sign of bleeding from the site of the injection, firm pressure over the area for a few minutes will usually stop the bleeding and thus prevent bruising.

Recording. A subcutaneous injection is recorded on the patient's record in the same way as any other medication but, in addition, the word "subcutaneous" or the abbreviation "H" follows the dosage of the drug to indicate the route. Sometimes the site of the injection is also recorded.

Intramuscular Injection

Advantages and Disadvantages. Intramuscular injection is the method of choice for the administration of some medications. Drugs which are irritating to subcutaneous tissue are often given by this route. In addition, a larger amount of fluid can be injected into muscle tissue than into subcutaneous tissue. Absorption through a

---

[2]Pitel, op. cit., p. 79.

muscle is faster than through subcutaneous tissue because of the vascularity of the muscle area. The danger of damaging nerves and blood vessels, however, is greater.

The Site of Injection. Regardless of the site chosen, the area must be exposed adequately so that the nurse can see what she is doing. The selection of an area for an intramuscular injection depends on a number of factors: the size of the patient and the amount of muscle tissue available for injection, the proximity of nerves and blood vessels, the condition of the skin around the area, and the nature of the drug to be administered. The site should be anatomically safe; that is, an area should be chosen where the danger of hitting a nerve or large blood vessel is minimal. The tissues in the area should be free of bruising or soreness. There should be no abrasions on the skin, and areas with hardened tissue (such as scar tissue) should be avoided.

Various sites are suitable for intramuscular injections; areas in the buttocks, the thigh, and the upper arm are used most frequently. Generally it is best to rotate the areas when a series of injections is to be given. The gluteal muscles are thick and permit the injection of larger quantities of fluid. Also, the use of these muscles in many normal daily activities aids in the absorption of drugs administered by this route. Two sites in the gluteal muscles are commonly used: the dorsogluteal site and the ventrogluteal site.

The *dorsogluteal site* uses the gluteus maximus muscle. The site may be located by dividing the buttock into quadrants. The crest of the ilium and the inferior gluteal fold act as landmarks for describing the buttock. The injection is given in the upper outer quadrant of the buttock, 5 to 7.5 cm. (2 to 3 inches) below the crest of the ilium. By using this area, large blood vessels and the sciatic nerve are avoided. Another method for locating a safe gluteal site is to draw an imaginary line from the posterior superior iliac spine to the greater trochanter of the femur. This line runs lateral and parallel to the sciatic nerve, and consequently an injection lateral and superior to it is in a safe area.

When the *ventrogluteal site* is used the

injection is made into the gluteus min-imus and the gluteus medius muscles. To locate the ventrogluteal area, the nurse has the patient lie on his back or his side. She then places her hand on the patient's hip with her index finger on the anterior superior iliac spine, and stretching her middle finger dorsally, palpates the crest of the ilium and presses below the iliac crest. The injection site is the triangle that is formed by her index finger, middle finger, and the crest of the ilium. The ven-trogluteal site is being used increasingly because there are no large nerves or blood vessels in the area; also there is usually less fatty tissue than in the but-tocks. If the patient's gluteal muscles are tense, he can flex his knees to relax them for the injection.

The *vastus lateralis* muscle on the lateral aspect of the thigh is also being used more frequently for intramuscular injec-tions. The area is free of major blood ves-sels and nerve trunks, and the vastus lat-eralis muscle provides a good long area when numerous injections have to be given. The muscle extends the full length of the thigh from mid-anterior to mid-lat-eral and is approximately 7.5 cm. (3 inches) wide. The injection may be given anywhere from approximately 10 cm. (4 inches) above the knee to approximately 10 cm. (4 inches) below the hip joint.

The *deltoid muscle* of the arm is also used for intramuscular injections. This site is two to three fingerbreadths down from the acromion process on the outer aspect of the arm. In most people this is a smaller muscle than the gluteal muscle and therefore is not capable of absorbing as large a volume of medicine comfort-ably. The essential danger in this area is that of harming the radial nerve.

Equipment. The equipment required for an intramuscular injection is similar to that used for a subcutaneous injection. The quantity of solution to be adminis-tered varies from 2 to 10 cc. In many agencies, however, nurses are permitted to inject no more than 5 cc. in any one in-jection; therefore, if more than 5 cc. is or-dered, the amount is given in two injec-tions. A 2 cc., 5 cc., or 10 cc. syringe is used with a No. 19 to 22 gauge needle 2.5 to 5 cm. (1 to 2 inches) long. The gauge of

the needle to be used depends on the vis-cosity of the drug and the sensitivity of the patient. The length of the needle depends on the size of the patient's mus-cle and the amount of adipose tissue that is present. It is desirable to inject the drug into the center of the muscle. A No. 22 needle 3.75 cm. (1½ inches) long is commonly used for an adult.

Preparation. The drug is prepared for administration in the same way as for a subcutaneous injection. Some authorities recommend that a small air bubble be left in the syringe to force the last of the drug out of the needle into the muscle and thus prevent any solution from being left in the subcutaneous tissue when the needle is removed. There is probably consider-able merit to this practice, particularly with drugs that are known to be irritating to subcutaneous tissue.

Administration. For an intramuscular injection to the gluteal muscle, the patient lies in a prone position with his toes inter-nally rotated in plantar flexion. In this position the gluteal muscles are relaxed and there is good visualization of the in-jection site.

The selection of the area for an injec-tion is determined by four factors: Is it an-atomically safe? free of bruises or sore areas? free of hardened areas? free of abrasions on the skin?

The muscle is palpated and the skin is wiped as for a subcutaneous injection. The skin is held taut and the needle is in-serted at a 90 degree angle to the distance required to reach the center of the mus-cle. When the needle is inserted smoothly and firmly, this is a relatively painless procedure. The skin is then released and the plunger is withdrawn in order to make sure the needle has not entered a blood vessel. Keeping the needle in place, the solution is injected slowly into the muscle tissue. The needle is then removed quickly and the area massaged gently with the disinfectant sponge to aid in dispersion of the solution.

In the air bubble method mentioned, it is common practice to draw a small bub-ble of air into the syringe before the solu-tion is injected. The bubble rises to the top of the solution when the syringe is in-verted for the injection. The air then

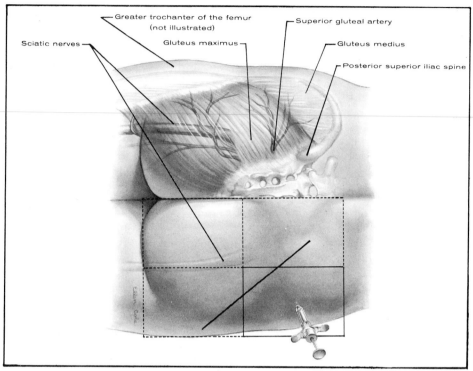

Intramuscular injection. With the patient lying in a prone position, the nurse can establish the dorsogluteal site as indicated. (Courtesy of Wyeth Laboratories, Philadelphia, Pa.)

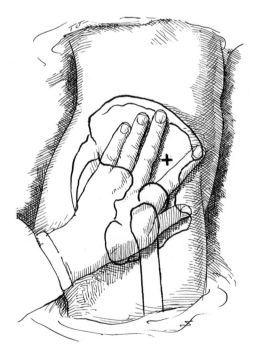

Locate the triangle for injection by placing the left index finger on the anterior iliac spine and the middle finger just below the iliac crest. (From What's New. Abbott Laboratories, No. 211, Spring, 1959.)

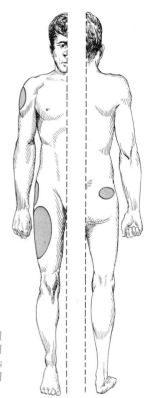

Four sites used for intramuscular injections are the deltoid muscle, the ventrogluteal site of the gluteus minimus and gluteus medius muscles, the dorsogluteal site of the gluteus maximus muscle, and the vastus lateralis muscle on the lateral aspect of the thigh.

helps to clear the needle of fluid before the needle is withdrawn. This prevents dripping of the fluid as the needle is being withdrawn through the subcutaneous tissue.

When administering particularly irritating drugs into muscle tissue, the Z track method is used. In this method the site is selected and then the skin is pulled firmly toward the lateral aspect of the buttock. The injection site is reassessed, cleansed with disinfectant solution, and then the needle is inserted at a 90 degree angle to the desired depth. The plunger is then pulled back slightly to determine whether the needle has entered a blood vessel. If

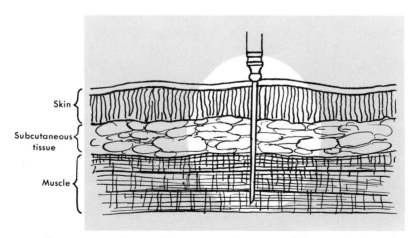

Skin

Subcutaneous
tissue

Muscle

For an intramuscular injection the needle is inserted at a 90 degree angle into the center of the muscle.

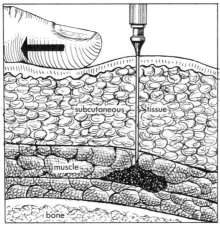
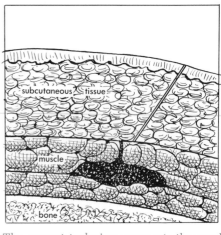

Diagram of Z track method of intramuscular injection. The correct technique converts the needle track into a zig-zag which prevents leakage into tissues.

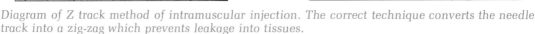

blood appears, the needle is withdrawn and another site is selected. If no blood appears, the solution is injected slowly. After injecting the solution, the nurse waits for 10 seconds to allow the medication to disperse. She then withdraws the needle and allows the stretched skin to return to its normal position. Then the area is massaged with a cotton ball. This method helps keep the drug in the muscle and away from the subcutaneous tissue.

With careful technique, complications from intramuscular injections can be avoided. Abscesses, nerve injuries, cysts and necrosis of tissue do occur as a result of intramuscular injections; however, the use of aseptic technique, individual establishment of landmarks for injection sites, and the alternating of sites help to avoid these unpleasant results.

As more research is done in the field of intramuscular injections, the nurse may well find traditional techniques being modified in many agencies in the light of new research findings.

Recording. After the administration of an intramuscular injection, the drug, dosage and method of administration are recorded. The abbreviation "I.M." is frequently used to indicate the route. The site of administration is often recorded also.

Intradermal Injection

An intradermal injection is the injection of a small amount of fluid into the dermal layer of the skin. It is frequently done as a diagnostic measure, as in tuberculin testing and allergy testing. The areas of the body commonly used are the medial aspect of the forearm and the subscapular region of the back.

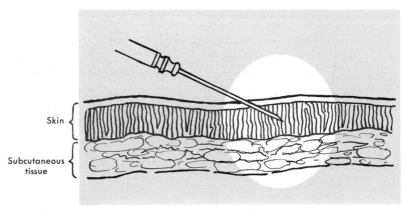

For an intradermal injection the needle is held at a 15 degree angle, bevel upward, and inserted into the dermal layer of the skin.

A 1 cc. syringe (or a tuberculin syringe) and a 26 gauge needle 1 cm. (³/₈ inch) in length are commonly used. A tuberculin syringe is calibrated in tenths and hundredths of a cubic centimeter in order that minute doses can be measured. The needle is inserted at a 15 degree angle with the bevel up, and the fluid is injected to produce a small bleb just under the skin.

Topical Application

Medications may be applied to the skin or mucous membranes in the form of lotions, ointments, or liniments. Lotions are liquid preparations which are usually applied to protect, soothe, or soften surface areas, to relieve itching, or to check the growth of microorganisms. Ointments are preparations with a fatty base, such as lard, petroleum, jelly, or oils. They may be applied to the skin or mucous membranes where they are melted by the heat of the body and absorbed. Ointments are frequently used for antiseptic or antimicrobial purposes. Liniments are liquids which are applied to the skin by rubbing. They are frequently used to warm an affected area; this dilates the superficial blood vessels and also helps to relax tight muscles.

Lotions or Liniments
EQUIPMENT. The application of lotions or liniments is often a clean, rather than a sterile, procedure in a home situation. In a hospital, or other inpatient facility, however, it is advisable to use sterile cotton balls or gauze to apply the liquid and to use a sterile glove on the hand being used for the application. The nurse will then need a medicine tray, the bottle of lotion or liniment, packages of sterile 5 × 5 cm. (2 × 2 inch) gauze, or sterile cotton balls, and a sterile glove for this procedure.

ADMINISTRATION. The area where the lotion or liniment is to be applied is exposed, making sure that the patient is kept warm and not unduly exposed. The bottle is opened and the cap placed upside down on the tray. The package of gauze or container of cotton balls is opened and the nurse then puts on the sterile glove. Using the gloved hand, she picks up the gauze or cotton ball. Then, holding the bottle of lotion in her un-gloved hand, she pours the required amount onto the gauze, being careful not to spill the liquid over the label. (It is wise to hold the label facing outwards to avoid this.) The lotion or liniment is then applied to the affected area. Lotions are not rubbed in; liniments are. The procedure is repeated until all of the affected area is covered. The nurse observes the area carefully for changes in color, swelling, the appearance of a rash, or other observable signs.

Ointments
EQUIPMENT. As with lotions and liniments, it is advisable in an institutional setting to use sterile equipment for the application of an ointment. A sterile glove is not needed since the ointment is applied with a sterile tongue depressor. The equipment required is a medicine tray, the jar or tube of ointment, sterile tongue depressor(s), sterile gauze, and tape, if the area is to be covered after application of the ointment.

ADMINISTRATION. The area is exposed; the jar or tube is opened and the cap placed upside down on the tray. The nurse then removes the tongue depressor from its wrapper, being careful to keep the distal end sterile. The ointment is then squeezed or scooped onto the tongue depressor and applied to the area with gentle but firm strokes. The tongue depressor is never returned to the jar for additional ointment. A new one is used instead. The nurse again observes the skin for changes such as color, rash, or swelling. A sterile dressing is applied as indicated to keep the ointment from soiling the bed or patient's linen.

RECORDING. After the administration of a lotion, a liniment, or an ointment, the drug and the method of administration are recorded. The nurse also records her observations of the condition of the area to which the medication was applied and any changes she noted (as described above.

Instillations

Ear Instillations. Liquid medications are instilled into the ear cavity usually for one of two purposes: to insert a softening agent so that earwax can be removed easily or to introduce an antibiotic suspension in cases in which the ear canal or the eardrum is infected.

EQUIPMENT. The medication to be inserted should always be warmed before being inserted into the ear. A temperature of 40.6° C. (105° F.) is recommended. Cool solutions are uncomfortable and may cause dizziness or nausea because the equilibrium sense receptors in the semicircular canals are stimulated. The bottle of ear drops may be placed in a small open container of warm water for a few minutes before it is to be used. The temperature of the solution may be tested by dropping a small amount on the inner aspect of the wrist. If it feels comfortable (that is, neither hot nor cool), the solution should be comfortable for the patient.

The nurse will need a medicine tray, a sterile medicine dropper, the bottle of medication, and some sterile cotton balls. Many preparations for individual use come with an attached dropper.

ADMINISTRATION. This procedure is best done with the patient in a sitting position with the ear in which the drops are to be instilled nearer the nurse. The medication is drawn up into the medicine dropper. The nurse then straightens the auditory canal. One method of doing this is as follows: With her left hand on the lobe of the ear, the nurse grasps the upper portion of the auricle between her middle and index fingers and pulls gently with an upward and backward motion to straighten the auditory canal of an adult. For a child, the lobe is pulled downward and backward. The tip of the dropper is inserted into the external ear canal, taking care not to injure the delicate ear tissue. The medicine is injected by compressing the bulb on the dropper. The external meatus is plugged with a sterile cotton ball to keep the medicine from escaping, unless drainage from the ear is being promoted, in which case the meatus is not plugged.

RECORDING. After the administration of the medication, the time, the medication, the amount instilled, and the affected ear are recorded, with a notation also made if a cotton ball was inserted.

Eye Instillations. Liquid medications in the form of eye drops, or eye ointments, are instilled into the eye for any one of

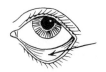

The desired site for instillations of a medication into the eye is midpoint of the lower fornix. (From Lucile A. Wood: Nursing Skills for Allied Health Services Vol. 3. Philadelphia, W. B. Saunders Co., 1975.)

several reasons: to soothe the eye if it is irritated, to dilate the pupil for an eye examination, to apply an anesthetic, or to combat infection.

EQUIPMENT. The administration of eye drops or an eye ointment requires a medicine tray, the bottle of medication with an eye dropper (most eye medications come in bottles with their own dropper) or the tube of ointment, and cotton balls or tissues. Medications for the eye are ordered individually for each patient; they should never be used for another patient.

ADMINISTRATION. The patient may be in a sitting position or supine position for this procedure. If the patient is sitting up, the nurse will find it easier to stand behind the patient to instill eye drops. The nurse asks the patient to look upward; this helps to keep the dropper from touching the cornea if the patient blinks and also helps him to keep his eye from moving while the drops are being instilled. The nurse pulls the lower eyelid down towards the cheek, using her left index finger and thumb (if she is right-handed), to expose the lower fornix. The medication is dropped onto the lower fornix (spot indicated on the diagram above). Excess drops may be wiped off the cheek with a cotton ball or tissues. In removing the eye dropper from and returning it to the bottle, the nurse takes care not to touch the outside of the bottle with the dropper, to avoid contaminating it.

If an ointment is to be applied, a thin ribbon of the ointment is laid along the entire length of the fornix. Ointment that is at room temperature is easier to apply. To end the ribbon cleanly, the tube is twisted with a lateral movement of the wrist. The patient's eyelids should be closed gently after the application. Having the patient roll the eyeball around with the lid closed helps to ensure that the medication covers the entire exterior eyeball. The eyelid is gently dried with a cotton ball or tissue to remove excess medication.

In the case of some medications, such as atropine, care must be taken that it does not get into the lacrimal (tear) duct. To avoid this possibility, the nurse can place her thumb over the inner canthus.

RECORDING. When the eyedrops or ointment has been instilled, the nurse records this on the patient's record, noting the time, the amount, and strength of the medication, and which eye (right, left, or both) received the medication.

Nose Instillations. The usual purpose of instilling medication into the nose are either to heal infections or to shrink swollen membranes.

EQUIPMENT. For this procedure, the nurse needs a medicine tray, the medication, a dropper (most nose drops come in a bottle with attached dropper) or an inhaler or atomizer, and disposable tissues or a towel.

ADMINISTRATION. The dorsal recumbent position is considered the best position for the instillation of nose drops. A pillow under the shoulders permits the head to drop back, allowing the medication to flow deep into the nasal cavity. The patient may also be positioned with his head over the edge of the bed; if this position is used, the nurse supports the patient's head with one hand to avoid undue strain on his neck muscles. The patient's head may be positioned either in a straight line from the neck (Proetz position), or with the head deflected to one side (Parkinson position). The former is usually advised if the medication is being used to treat the ethmoid and sphenoid sinuses; the latter is used in treating for the frontal and maxillary sinuses.

To avoid touching the outer or inner surfaces of the nose, the nurse holds the dropper slightly above the nostril to inject the drops, directing the tip toward the midline of the superior concha of the ethmoid. This deflects the medication towards the back of the nasal cavity. The patient is instructed to lie in a recumbent position for 5 to 10 minutes to allow the medication to be absorbed.

When an inhaler or an atomizer is used

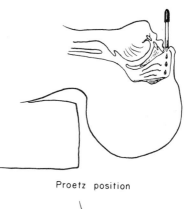

Proetz position

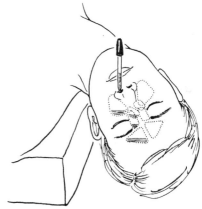

Parkinson position

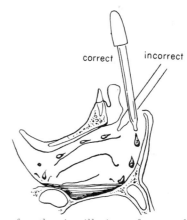

correct   incorrect

Positions for the instillation of nose drops. (From Lucile A. Wood: Nursing Skills for Allied Health Services. Vol. 3. Philadelphia, W. B. Saunders Co., 1975.)

instead of a dropper, the same procedure is used. The patient is instructed to breathe through his nose while keeping his mouth open during the treatment.

Throat Instillations. The throat may be either sprayed or painted in applying an antiseptic or an anesthetic.

EQUIPMENT. For spraying or painting a throat, the nurse will need a medicine tray, a tongue depressor, the bottle of medication and, if the medication is to be painted on the tissues, cotton-tipped applicators.

ADMINISTRATION. The best position for this procedure is for the patient to be sitting up and the nurse standing directly in front of the patient, so that she can look down into the throat. A good light is essential for this procedure.

The nurse asks the patient to tilt his head backwards (or she helps him to do this) and to open his mouth. She uses her left hand to hold down the tongue with a tongue depressor, and applies the spray or medication, using either an atomizer for spraying or cotton-tipped applicators for painting the tissues.

RECORDING. After the throat has been sprayed or painted, the nurse records the time, the name and strength of the medication used, and the method of administration.

Vagina Instillations. Medications are usually instilled into the vagina to combat infection. They may be applied in the form of a suppository or an ointment. Ointments for use in the vagina usually come in a narrow tube with an attached plunger.

EQUIPMENT. For this procedure, the nurse needs a medicine tray, sterile or one-use gloves, the medication, and a perineal pad and binder.

ADMINISTRATION. The patient is positioned in the dorsal recumbent or side-lying position with the legs spread far enough apart to enable the nurse to see the vaginal opening. The patient is draped so that only the perineal area is exposed. Using her left hand to hold open the vagina, the nurse inserts the suppository or tip of the tube applicator into the vagina. If a tube applicator is used, the plunger is pressed down to expel the ointment. A perineal pad is applied to keep the medication from soiling the patient's clothes.

TOLERANCE AND ADDICTION

When some medications are taken over a long period of time, the effect of the drug diminishes and the patient requires continually larger doses. This reaction to a medicine is called tolerance. Narcotics are among the drugs for which patients frequently develop such a tolerance.

Addiction refers to the habitual use of a drug. Usually the person is physically and psychologically dependent upon the drug. As we mentioned earlier, drug addiction is a major health problem, particularly among young people. For more information on this topic, the nurse is directed to some of the articles in the *Suggested Readings* at the end of Chapter 4.

Addiction may also become a problem when people are ill and receive narcotics or barbiturates over a prolonged period of time.

An awareness of which drugs are most likely to result in tolerance and addiction is important. At the first indication that a drug is not acting as it did previously, or at the first indication of dependency upon a particular medication, the physician should be notified. Often alternative medicines can be administered as a preventive measure.

| GUIDE TO SAFE MEDICATION ADMINISTRATION | 1. Does the patient have any allergies?
2. What medications have been prescribed for the patient?
3. Why is the patient receiving these medications?
4. What observations should the nurse make relative to the effect of these medications on the patient?
5. Are there specific nursing measures indicated because of the action of drugs contained in these medications? |

6. How are the patient's medications to be administered?
7. What precautions should be taken in administering these medications? Are there special precautions that should be taken because of the patient's age, physical condition, or mental state?
8. Do any of the medications require special precautionary measures in their administration?
9. Does the patient have learning needs relative to his medicinal therapy?
10. Does the patient or his family require specific skills or knowledge in order to continue medicinal therapy at home?

GUIDE TO EVALUATING THE EFFECTIVENESS OF MEDICATIONS

1. Is the patient taking the medicines that have been prescribed?
2. Have the medications been administered safely?
3. Does the patient show signs or symptoms which indicate that the medications are effective (or ineffective)?
4. Has the administration of the medications been accurately reported on the patient's record? Have pertinent observations been recorded and reported to appropriate personnel?

STUDY VOCABULARY

Addiction	Isotonic	Sublingual
Ampule	Local	Suppository
Enteric coating	Minim	Systemic
Inhalation	Oral	Topical
Intradermal	Parenteral	Vial
Intramuscular	Subcutaneous	

STUDY SITUATION

In the health agency in which you are having clinical experience, find out the following information:

1. The method by which medications are ordered for patients.
2. Communication tools used to facilitate the execution of these orders by nurses, e.g., Kardex file, medication cards, etc.
3. The location of medications on a nursing unit, storage facilities, and system for arranging medications.
4. The equipment used for preparing and administering medications.
5. Safety precautions taken in the preparation and administration of medications.
6. The approved method of recording medications by various administration routes, including narcotic and controlled drugs.
7. Reference material on drugs.
8. Pertinent agency policies regarding the administration of medications.

SUGGESTED
READINGS

Asperheim, M. K., and L. A. Eisenhauer: *The Pharmacological Basis of Patient Care.* 3rd edition. Philadelphia, W. B. Saunders Company, 1977.

Drugs and Alcohol. *American Journal of Nursing,* 76:65, January 1976.

Errors in Insulin Doses Due to the Design of Insulin Syringes. *Pediatrics,* 56:302–303, August 1975.

Falconer, M. W., A. S. Ezell, H. R. Patterson, and E. A. Gustafson: *The Drug, The Nurse, The Patient.* 5th edition. Philadelphia, W. B. Saunders Company, 1974.

Geolot, D. H., et al.: Administering Parenteral Drugs. *American Journal of Nursing,* 75:788–793, May 1975.

Hays, D.: Do It Yourself the Z-Track Way. *American Journal of Nursing,* 74:1070–1071, June 1974.

Herbst, S. F.: A New Approach to Parenteral Drug Administration. *American Journal of Nursing,* 75:1345, August 1975.

Irving, M.: Going International in Metric. *Hospital Administration in Canada,* August 1974, p. 20.

Lambert, M. L., Jr.: Drug and Diet Interactions. *American Journal of Nursing,* 75:402–406, March 1975.

Lang, S. N., et al.: Reducing Discomfort from IM Injections. *American Journal of Nursing,* 76:800–801, May 1976.

Laugharne, E.: Insulin Goes Metric: A Time for Review. *Canadian Nurse,* 71:22–24, February 1975.

Lenhart, D. G.: The Use of Medications in the Elderly Population. *Nursing Clinics of North America,* 11:135–144, March 1976.

Levine, D., et al.: A Special Program for Nurse-Addicts. *American Journal of Nursing,* 74:1672–1673, September 1974.

Lowenthal, W.: Factors Affecting Drug Absorption. Programmed Instruction. *American Journal of Nursing,* 73:1391–1408, August 1973.

Moggach, B. B.: Drug Administration Times Should Be Reexamined. *Canadian Nurse,* 71:17–19, January 1975.

Morgan, A. J.: Minor Tranquilizers, Hypnotics and Sedatives. *American Journal of Nursing,* 73:1220–1222, July 1973.

Smith, S. E.: How Drugs Act. Parts 1–7. *Nursing Times,* 71:26–32, June 26, 1975 to August 7, 1975.

CHAPTER 25

Fever, Hypothermid, and the Therapeutic Application of Heat and Cold

25 FEVER, HYPOTHERMIA, AND THE THERAPEUTIC APPLICATION OF HEAT AND COLD

The nurse should be able to:

Define terms commonly used to describe disturbances of body temperature

Explain in simple terms the heat-regulatory mechanisms of the body

Explain factors affecting body temperature

Identify common problems of disturbed temperature regulation with regard to variations in body temperature

Apply relevant principles in planning and implementing appropriate nursing interventions in the care of patients with disturbances of body temperature

Identify and intervene appropriately in emergency situations with regard to temperature variations

Evaluate the effectiveness of nursing interventions in the care of patients with disturbances of body temperature

Apply relevant principles in planning and implementing therapeutic interventions involving heat and cold applications

478 Evaluate the effectiveness of nursing interventions

INTRODUCTION

Usually the heat-regulating mechanism of the body maintains a precise balance between heat production and heat loss. In this way the internal body temperature is kept within a very narrow range, usually varying not more than a degree or so in a day. The heat-regulating mechanism, as we mentioned in Chapter 9, is one of the body's most important homeostatic mechanisms.

Every once in awhile, however, the balance is upset and deviations outside the normal range of body temperature occur. Many people who are ill have an elevated temperature. It is, indeed, one of the cardinal signs of illness, often being one of the first observable indications that there is a disturbance of body function. The maintenance of a higher than normal temperature puts considerable stress on the body's adaptive mechanisms, and is very debilitating.

The balance may also be upset in the opposite direction from fever. Mild degrees of lowered body temperature apparently do not do as much harm to the body as fever does. Everything simply slows down and when the body warms up, it will commence to function at the normal levels again. However, the problem of accidental *hypothermia* (excessively low body temperatures due, in most cases, to prolonged exposure to cold environmental temperatures) has been receiving increasing attention. It appears to be more common than was once thought. *Frostbite*, which involves freezing of the skin tissues in one area of the body, such as exposed earlobes, the tip of the nose, fingers, or toes, has always been a problem in cold climates. This and *chilblains*, which are a mild form of frostbite, are a common source of discomfort, particularly to older people who live in cold, damp climates where homes are not always equipped with central heating.

Applications of both heat and cold have been used for centuries to treat various disorders of the human body. Both have systemic and localized effects on body tissues and are still frequently utilized in therapy.

THE BODY'S MECHANISMS FOR TEMPERATURE REGULATION

Body heat results from the energy released by foods in the process of cellular metabolism. Heat is lost from the body through a variety of means: direct contact with cooler objects in the immediate environment (principally air) by the process of *conduction,* which is enhanced by the *convection* (movement) of air currents circulating around the body; the *evaporation* of moisture from the surface of the body; and the transfer of heat, in the form of electromagnetic waves, from the body to cooler objects in the environment by *radiation.*

The regulatory mechanisms controlling body temperature are located in the preoptic area of the hypothalamus. Neurons in this area respond to changes in the temperature of the blood circulating through the area by sending impulses either to the anterior heat-losing center 479 (in the hypothalamus) or to the posterior heat-promoting center. These centers have a reciprocal effect on each other; when one is activated, the other is depressed.

The body has various adaptive mechanisms either to promote heat if body temperature falls too low, or to lose excess heat if the temperature goes too high.

Stimulation of the heat-producing center increases wakefulness and stimulates muscular activity. If the individual does not engage in some form of exercise in response to this, the body will initiate its own muscular activity involuntarily in the form of shivering, which can produce a considerable amount of heat within the body. Concomitantly, stimulation of the sympathetic nervous system (which results in the release of norepinephrine directly into body tissues) facilitates the release of both epinephrine and norepinephrine into the blood stream. Consequently, cellular metabolism is speeded up, which increases heat production.

Stimulation of the sympathetic nervous system also results in the phenomenon of piloerection, which means that the hairs literally stand on end. In human beings, this can actually occur but most often a milder reaction takes place, evident in the "gooseflesh" appearance of the skin. In animals with long hair, this mechanism serves to entrap a layer of warm air next to the skin. In human beings, the mechanism is not so effective in providing insulation, but it occurs nonetheless. Cessation of sweating usually occurs as well, to reduce the amount of heat lost through evaporation of water from the body surface.

Concomitantly, vasoconstriction occurs and blood is drawn from surface vessels to minimize the amount of heat lost through conduction, convection, and radiation. The individual becomes pale and his skin is cold to the touch; he also feels cold.

With prolonged exposure to colder temperatures than normal, as in cold climates in the wintertime, the thyroid gland is stimulated to increase production. This increases the metabolic rate, thereby increasing heat production. However, this is a slower process, which occurs over a period of weeks.

Stimulation of the heat-losing center, on the other hand, has an inhibitory effect on the mechanisms for heat production, and the reverse effect is seen. Muscular activity is decreased; metabolism is slowed down; circulation to the skin is increased; and the rate of production of thyroxin by the thyroid gland gradually decreases.

The body also has two other mechanisms to facilitate heat loss; these are sweating and panting. In lower animals, rapid shallow breathing (panting) increases the amount of heat lost by evaporation of moisture from the respiratory tract or tongue. In human beings the principal mechanism for cooling the body is by increasing perspiration. This greatly facilitates the loss of heat from the body through the process of evaporation of moisture from the skin.[1]

FACTORS AFFECTING BODY TEMPERATURE

Under conditions of good health, a number of normal activities and physiological processes affect body temperature. Any factor which increases the metabolic rate will raise the temperature of the body; conversely, a decreased metabolic rate will lower body temperature. In exercise, the muscular activity increases body temperature as a result of heat production by body muscles. Heavy muscular exercise may increase the body temperature by as much as 2.2° C. (4° to 5° F.). Usually an elevated temperature due to exercise quickly returns to normal with the cessation of exercise.

Strong emotions, such as anger, will also raise body temperature because of stimulation of the sympathetic nervous system. The "heat of anger" and "feverish with excitement" expressions we use can, indeed, be physically true. One notices this particularly with children, whose body temperatures are more labile (that is, they fluctuate more easily) than those of adults.

Disturbances in the production of thyroxin by the thyroid gland also affect body temperature. An excess production of thyroxin (an overactive thyroid gland)

[1]Arthur C. Guyton: *Function of the Human Body.* 4th edition. Philadelphia, W. B. Saunders Company, 1974, pp. 397–407.

increases the basal metabolic rate, thereby stimulating heat production. People with a thyroid deficiency, on the other hand, have a lower metabolic rate, and consequently a body temperature that is usually at the low end of the normal range.

An increase in body temperature itself will stimulate the cells to increase the rate of cellular metabolism and heat production. For each 1° C. rise in temperature, the rate of heat production increases 13 per cent, and the metabolic rate may be forty times as much as normal. As a result, an increased temperature by itself tends to heighten a fever. A lowered body temperature has the reverse effect of decreasing metabolism which will, in turn, lessen body temperature still further.

The specific dynamic action of foods also affects body temperature. The body's metabolic rate is stimulated by the intake of food and remains elevated for several hours after a meal. Foods differ in their specific dynamic qualities. Proteins increase the metabolic rate much more than fats and carbohydrates do, and the increase remains high over a longer period of time. This is the basis for the sustaining powers of a breakfast with high protein content.

Besides the factors which increase the metabolic rate, a number of other factors, some of which were discussed in Chapter 9, will also influence body temperature.

For example, the environment has a pronounced effect upon body temperature. Not only permanent changes, such as those encountered when moving to a hot or cold climate, but also temporary changes, such as a brief hot spell, affect the body by raising or lowering its temperature. The body's ability to withstand high environmental temperatures is dependent on the humidity of the atmosphere. When the air is dry and there are sufficient air currents to carry away heat from the body by convection, an individual can stand very high temperatures with little or no increase in body temperature. If on the other hand, the humidity is high, body temperature begins to rise very quickly. This explains why one feels so uncomfortable on hot, "muggy" days.

Similarly, a cold environment decreases body temperature. Cold, damp weather is much more chilling than cold dry weather, and when there is considerable amount of air movement, increasing amounts of heat are carried away from the body. The "wind chill" factor can then produce the effect of a temperature much lower than that which is registered on the outdoor thermometer.

Environmental changes have a greater effect on the body temperatures of infants and elderly people than of others. In infants, the heat regulating mechanism is immature. For the first year of life, the body temperature is highly dependent on the temperature of the environment. In older people, the peripheral circulation is decreased owing to changes in the aging skin, which lessens their ability to adapt to changing environmental temperatures.

Clothing, of course, decreases the effects of environmental temperatures on body heat. The insulation of the body by adequate, warm clothing lessens the impact of cold temperatures. In warm climates, cottons and linens are more comfortable to wear because they absorb moisture. Synthetic fibers and wool do not absorb as well; hence, they inhibit the removal of perspiration from the body.

It has been observed that during the menstrual cycle there is a fall in the early morning temperature of most women just after the onset of menstruation. The temperature remains at this lower value until ovulation takes place. Then there is an abrupt rise of 0.3° to 0.4° C. (0.5° to 0.75° F.), which continues until the start of the next menstrual period.

Early in pregnancy there is a slight rise in the temperature of most women, which continues until about the fourth month. There is then a gradual fall in the temperature, which usually remains slightly below normal levels throughout the remainder of the pregnancy.

Although normal processes can cause mild fluctuations in body temperature, fever is a typical manifestation of many illnesses. The most common of these are infections, diseases of the central nervous system, neoplasms, and metabolic disorders. The prolonged use of some drugs, among them morphine and LSD, may also give rise to fever.

The physiological mechanisms responsible for fever are not known for all disease processes. It is generally felt that fever may be caused by abnormalities in the brain itself or by toxic substances that affect the heat-regulating mechanisms.

A number of stimuli may activate the hypothalamic centers. Important among these are the substances called *pyrogens*, which are secreted by toxic bacteria or released by degenerating tissue. It is believed that these substances stimulate the release of a second substance, *endogenous pyrogen*, from the leukocytes which have been drawn to the diseased area. The endogenous pyrogens then act on the thermoregulatory centers.[2]

There is evidence to support the belief that fever caused by pyrogens has some beneficial effects in helping the body to combat infection. It is felt that the fever acts in two ways: (1) It creates an undesirable temperature for the survival of bacteria; and (2) the increased rate of metabolism in the cells increases their production of immune bodies and also their ability to phagocytize foreign bodies, thus impeding bacterial invasion.

Dehydration can also affect the hypothalamic centers directly so that the temperature rises to febrile levels. Part of the elevation is due to lack of fluids for sweating, which deprives the body of one of its principal mechanisms for losing excess heat.

Fever may occur postoperatively owing to any one of a number of causes. It may be due to excessive heat production, as in the case of pathogenic infection, but is usually thought to be due to inadequate heat elimination.[3]

Fever frequently accompanies a head injury and is often seen in patients with spinal cord injuries. In these cases, it is felt to be caused by pressure on, or injury to, the hypothalamus or the tracts leading to and from the heat-regulating centers.[4]

The most common cause of hypothermia is prolonged exposure to cold environmental temperatures, although a lowered body temperature may be induced artificially sometimes for the purpose of cardiac or vascular surgery, or in the treatment of some poisons.

People vary considerably in ability to withstand cold temperatures. Persons with darkly pigmented skin, aged people, and those in poor physical condition are more affected by the cold than others. The amount and type of clothing worn for insulating the body are also important. Multiple layers of lightweight clothing serve to entrap warm air close to the skin and have been found to be more effective than fewer layers of bulky, heavy clothing for keeping the body warm. Water acts as a heat conductor, and damp clothing therefore conducts heat away from the body. The "wind chill" factor, as we mentioned, considerably increases the effect of cold environmental temperatures on the body. Rarefied atmospheres, as experienced by mountain climbers, also magnify the effect of cold on the body.

COMMON PROBLEMS

The body temperature can swing in either direction outside the normal range; *fever* is the term commonly applied to temperatures above normal and *hypothermia* to temperatures below normal.

A term that is frequently used synonymously with fever is *pyrexia*. *Hyperpyrexia* and *hyperthermia* are used interchangeably to designate an abnormally high fever—that is, 40.6° C. (105° F.) or over. *Habitual hyperthermia* refers to a condition in which the average daily temperature is slightly above normal limits.

Although prolonged fevers are not seen as commonly today as in the years before antibiotics, it is well for the nurse to know the technical terms used for different types of fevers. The terms are descriptive and explain the nature of the fever.

An *intermittent* or *quotidian* fever is one in which the temperature rises each day but falls to normal sometime during the 24 hour period, most usually during the early morning hours. A *remittent* fever is one which shows marked variations in the temperature readings during a

[2]Arthur C. Guyton: *Textbook of Medical Physiology.* 5th edition. Philadelphia, W. B. Saunders Company, 1976, p. 966.
[3]American College of Surgeons: *Manual of Preoperative and Postoperative Care.* Philadelphia, W. B. Saunders Company, 1967, p. 266.
[4]Cyril M. MacBryde and Robert S. Blacklow (eds.): *Signs and Symptoms: Applied Pathologic Physiology and Clinical Interpretation.* 5th edition. Philadelphia, J. B. Lippincott Company, 1970, p. 462.

24 hour period, the lowest reading, however, always being above the patient's normal level. In a *relapsing* fever, the patient's temperature may be normal for one or two days, then elevated for varying periods. These periods of normalcy are interspersed irregularly throughout the course of a relapsing fever. The term *hectic* or *septic* may be used to describe an intermittent fever in which there are wide fluctuations in daily temperature readings. It is not unusual for the temperature to vary as much as 2.2° C. (4° F.) within a 24 hour period in this type of fever. Another type of fever is called a *constant* fever. In this type, the patient's temperature remains at essentially the same level over a period of days or weeks.

The Stages of a Fever

The typical stages of fever occur in response to the physiological processes that are taking place within the body. There are three distinct stages to a fever: (1) the chill phase, or period of rising temperature; (2) the course of the fever, when the temperature is maintained at an elevated level; and (3) the termination, or period when the temperature falls to normal. During the three stages, different sets of mechanisms are operating, giving rise to the signs and symptoms characteristic of each stage.

The Chill Phase. During the onset of a fever, it is thought that there is a resetting of the body's internal "thermostat" at a higher level.[5] This may be a response to the presence of pyrogenic substances, or to any one of the other causes listed in the section on the etiology of fever. The resetting of the internal thermostat brings the body's heat-producing mechanisms into play as an attempt is made to bring the temperature up to the "desired" level. The person experiences what is known as a *chill*. Muscular activity is increased, in the form of shivering, which may vary in severity from merely a feeling of being cold, with slight shivering, to violent muscular contractions (shaking chills).

At the same time as the shivering mechanism is induced, the rate of cellular metabolism increases, and the waste products of metabolism, carbon dioxide and water, are formed in greater quantities. The increased carbon dioxide level in the blood stimulates the respiratory center and the person breathes faster and more deeply. This leads to extra fluid loss, and the patient feels thirsty. Also, as metabolism is accelerated, there is an increased demand by the cells for more oxygen and glucose. The heart beats more rapidly (in response to this demand), and the nurse will note that the patient's pulse rate is higher than normal.

Concomitantly, heat-conserving mechanisms are instituted. Vasoconstriction occurs and the patient becomes pale, and his skin is cold to the touch. He also feels cold and may ask for extra blankets. Often, there is a "gooseflesh" appearance to the skin as "piloerection" takes place. Sweating usually also ceases.

During the chill phase, the rectal temperature rises steadily, although the elevation is usually not evident by oral thermometer until the end of a chill. Body temperature may be increased by as much as 1.1° to 4° C. (2° to 7° F.).[6] A chill may last for a few minutes or as long as an hour. In mild cases of fever, such as one sees with the common cold or in light cases of influenza, the chill phase is usually brief.

The Course of a Fever. During the second stage of a fever, or when the fever is "running its course," the temperature has reached the preset level and there is a balance between heat production and heat loss. Because of the increased body temperature, the skin feels warm to the touch and there is usually a generalized flushing of the skin. The increased metabolic rate required to maintain the elevated temperature puts heightened demands on the body for more oxygen and glucose. The heart and respiratory rates remain high, and water loss through respiration increases the patient's feeling of thirst. The elevated temperature also increases nervous irritability. Headache, photophobia (sensitivity to light), and restlessness

---

[5]Guyton, *Textbook of Medical Physiology*, p. 965–966.

[6]MacBryde and Blacklow, op. cit., p. 460.

or drowsiness (or both) are not uncommon symptoms. An abnormally high fever is often accompanied by a state of mental confusion, which may progress to *delirium*. The patient becomes disoriented as to time and place. He may not know where he is or, often, what day it is. Sometimes the patient may have *hallucinations*. He may become quite irrational and combative. Finally, prostration (collapse) may ensue. In young children, a convulsion not infrequently accompanies fever, usually at the outset.

The maintenance of an elevated temperature is very debilitating to the patient. During the first week or so of a fever, there is always some destruction of body protein and albuminuria is usually noted in the laboratory findings of the febrile patient.[7] The patient often complains of a generalized weakness and he is not inclined to much activity. Aching of the muscles and joints is also frequently present. In addition to the destruction of tissue protein, it is believed that the parenchyma of many cells begins to be damaged when the body temperature rises above 40° C. (105° F.).[8] In sustained high fevers there may be permanent damage to nervous tissue, since this tissue does not regenerate. The upper limit for survival has been estimated by various experts to be a body temperature of 46° C. (114.8° F.).[9]

Febrile patients usually lose weight. Although the increased metabolic rate maintained during the course of a fever increases the body's need for nourishment, most patients have little interest in food. This loss of appetite (anorexia) may give way to nausea and vomiting as the fever progresses. The combination of increased need for food and lack of interest in it leads to a loss of weight.

Usually, during the course of a fever, the temperature does not remain at a constant level but tends to fluctuate. Thus, periods when body temperature is rising are usually interspersed with periods when it is falling, even though the lowest temperature reached may always be above normal. When the temperature is falling, mechanisms for additional heat loss are dominant. Vasodilatation occurs and the skin becomes flushed and warm. Sweating (diaphoresis) is usually present to maximize heat loss through evaporation. The body thus loses more fluids, and the possibility of dehydration presents a problem.

When fever is prolonged, the problem of dehydration is more likely to occur. This is due to a number of factors including the greater loss of water through increased respirations and the further loss of fluids from sweating during periods when the body temperature is falling. There is often a lessening in the output of urine as more than the usual amount of fluid is lost through the skin and lungs. Other evidences of dehydration may be noted. The skin and mucous membranes may appear parched and dry. The patient's lips may become cracked and sore, and lesions may occur at the corners of the mouth. These lesions are termed *herpes simplex*, but are often referred to as "fever blisters" because they are so frequently seen in patients with fever. The nurse may note other signs and symptoms of dehydration, as discussed in Chapter 29. It is well to remember that young children, in particular, become dehydrated very quickly if there is a sustained fever.

The Termination of a Fever. When the cause of the elevated temperature has been removed, as for example, when antibiotics have "taken hold" and removed the cause of infection, the body's thermostat is reset at its original level. The mechanisms for increased heat production cease to operate, and mechanisms for increased heat loss are instituted. These are the same mechanisms which have already been described as operating during the course of a fever when the temperature is fluctuating and there is a temporary drop. The patient's temperature may drop to normal quickly, over a period of hours (by crisis), or gradually over a period of days or weeks (by lysis).

Hypothermia is the term applied to body temperatures below the normal range. A body temperature below 36.1° C. (97° F.) is generally considered subnormal. The most common problems of subnormal core or surface body temperature

---

[7]Guyton, *Textbook of Medical Physiology*, p. 967.
[8]Ibid.
[9]MacBryde and Blacklow, op. cit., p. 456.

are those we mentioned in the introduction, that is, accidental hypothermia, frostbite, and chilblains.

ASSESSING FOR DISTURBANCES IN BODY TEMPERATURE

It is important to observe all patients for the signs and symptoms of fever. Many agencies have specific policies for the taking of temperatures. Some institutions require that all patients have their temperature taken once, or sometimes twice, a day to screen for fever. If once a day, it is usually considered that early evening is the best time, since in many patients with a fever, this is time when the temperature is most elevated. If temperatures are taken in the morning, it should be an hour or so after the patient wakens and the body temperature is stabilized. When a patient has a fever, the temperature should be taken at more frequent intervals. If it is abnormally elevated, as often as every 15 minutes is sometimes indicated. All newly admitted patients should have a temperature taken, as well as all preoperative and postoperative patients. Postoperatively, the temperature is usually taken every four hours for the first 48 hours. In addition to these general guidelines, the nurse should be alert to signs and symptoms indicating the presence of fever and should take the patient's temperature if, in her judgment, it should be taken. The temperature should be evaluated in relation to such factors as the patient's usual normal temperature, the time of day, the environmental temperature, and the normal physiological processes that may affect body temperature. Details on the methods of taking body temperature are given in Chapter 9.

The pulse and respirations should be checked, for both rate and quality. The color of the patient's skin should be noted, since it is relevant to heat elimination. Heat loss is proportional to the amount of blood circulating to the body surface. A reddened, flushed appearance indicates a high proportion of blood near the surface. It is usually seen when a fever is established and the body is attempting to rid itself of excess heat. On the other hand, pallor may indicate the onset of a chill and a rising body temperature. The nurse should note if the patient complains of any physical symptoms such as headache, malaise, or other discomfort.

An accurate assessment of the patient's nutritional status is important. In this regard, the nurse should determine the patient's ability to tolerate food and fluids. The patient should also be observed for signs of weakness and fatigue.

The nurse should be alert to signs of dehydration in the patient. She should note the presence or absence of sweating. Both the amount and the color of the urine should be observed. When there is an inadequate intake of fluids, or an excessive amount is being lost through sweating or other means, the body attempts to balance this through the excretion of a more highly concentrated urine. The urine may then be scanty in amount and darker (more brown) in color than normal, straw-colored urine.

The nurse should also be alert to the patient's mental condition. The patient who has a fever is often irritable. He may complain about the details of his care and manifest anxiety and irritation in ways which are often annoying to nursing personnel. His need to be understood and to be helped in handling his anxieties must be recognized by the nurse. In patients with a high fever, as we mentioned, there may be mental confusion, which may progress to delirium. The nurse should be alert to the increased need to protect the safety of these patients.

Lowered temperatures of parts or all of the body surfaces, or of its internal core, are usually seen in people who have been exposed to very cold outside temperatures. In these people, the nurse should be alert to objective and subjective observations as these are described below.

PRIORITIES FOR NURSING ACTION

In determining priorities for nursing action, the nurse must assess the severity of the patient's condition. If the patient's temperature is abnormally high, there is an immediate need to lower it. The patient should be put to bed, if he has been up and around, and the physician notified promptly. There are a number of measures which may be used to bring about a rapid reduction in body temperature. These include the use of antipyretic drugs which have a systemic action and various techniques for "surface cooling" of the body.

Other disturbances in the body's homeostatic heat balance that require prompt intervention include heat cramps, heat exhaustion, heat stroke, chilblains, frostbite, and accidental hypothermia.

Heat cramps may occur in hot climates or hot weather as a result of prolonged, excessive sweating. This depletes the sodium chloride in body fluids and results in pallor, extreme thirst, nausea, and dizziness. The body temperature may be normal or slightly elevated, and, if the salt depletion is excessive, severe muscular cramps result. Putting the person in a cool room and giving fluids with salt added (as, for example, lemonade with salt in it), salt in the form of tablets, or a hypotonic solution of table salt and baking soda (1 level teaspoon of salt and $1/2$ teaspoon of baking soda in 1 liter of water) will relieve mild cases. (A good first aid measure is lemonade with salt added.)

Heat exhaustion may result from lengthy exposure to heat, especially if combined with high humidity. The person usually becomes very pale, with a cold, clammy skin and lowered blood pressure. The person shows signs of shock (pale, cold and clammy skin, lowered blood pressure, rapid, weak pulse, generalized weakness, and often nausea and vomiting). Generally moving the person to cooler and less humid surroundings and giving fluids will relieve this condition. Stimulants, such as strong black coffee, may also help.

Heat stroke, a condition of severe prostration, may be caused by prolonged exposure to high environmental heat temperatures. It is most frequently seen in the elderly and is believed to be due to failure of the heat regulatory centers in the brain. The condition is characterized by very high fever, coma, and the absence

of sweating. It requires immediate action to lower the body temperature as quickly as possible. Prompt medical intervention is needed and the individual should be hospitalized.[10]

On the other side of the temperature spectrum, the common priority problems are chilblains, frostbite, and accidental hypothermia.

Chilblains, which are a mild form of frostbite, are evidenced by itching, swelling, and redness of the skin, most commonly in the fingers, toes, and earlobes. The condition tends to recur in susceptible people. Because of decreased efficiency of the peripheral vascular system, elderly people are more afflicted by this uncomfortable problem than younger adults. Many people are successfully treated by diet and exercise; people with this problem should be under medical care. One word of warning—neither excessive heat nor excessive cold should be applied to chilblains.

Frostbite is an actual freezing of skin tissues. The area becomes very white and cold to the touch, and the sensory receptors in that part are anesthetized so that the person is unable to feel any sensation in the frostbitten part of the body. Rapid rewarming of the part with moist heat is advocated after the person has been taken to a safe place. The area should *not* be rubbed with snow or ice; friction of any kind increases the possibility of damaging tissues. Dressings or ointments should be applied, and the person should be kept from using the affected part if at all possible. Analgesics may be given if the pain is severe. If the person has been badly frost-bitten, prompt medical intervention is indicated.[10]

In cases of *accidental hypothermia*, the body temperature has been known to go down as low as 69.8° C. and the person survived.[11] The individual in this case was a 24 year old woman in Tennessee, so

[10]Thomas Flint, Jr., and Harvey D. Cain. *Emergency Treatment and Management.* 5th edition. Philadelphia, W. B. Saunders Company, 1975, pp. 629–636.

[11]Heather Carswell: Accidental Hypothermia: A Matter of Turning the Scoreboard Around. *The Medical Post*, p. 15, November 12, 1974.

PRINCIPLES RELEVANT TO DISTURBANCES OF BODY TEMPERATURE

1. The maintenance of a temperature above normal level requires the expenditure of an increased amount of energy by the body.
2. Body cells are damaged by excessively high temperatures.
3. A high body temperature may in itself stimulate further heat production.
4. Body tissues freeze when exposed to excessively low environmental temperatures.
5. Irreparable tissue damage can result if prompt intervention is not taken.
6. Heat is lost from the body through the mechanisms of radiation, conduction, convection, and evaporation.

it is not always the elderly who are the victims (although they are more vulnerable), nor does accidental hypothermia only occur in cold, northern climates or in people who have been caught in a snowstorm in the mountains. The condition requires prompt medical intervention and hospitalization. For this condition, there have been many new developments in treatment; warming of the body by internal means—that is, by warming the blood rather than applying external heat—is now being advocated by many authorities.

GOALS FOR NURSING ACTION

The principal goals of nursing action in the care of the patient with a fever are:
1. To reduce the amount of heat produced within the body
2. To facilitate heat elimination from the body
3. To minimize the effects of fever on the body

The goals of nursing action for the patient with excessive lowering of surface or core body temperature, depending on the severity of the problem, are:
1. To thaw tissues
2. To prevent tissue damage
3. If necessary, to obtain medical intervention as soon as possible

SPECIFIC NURSING INTERVENTIONS

General Measures

The patient who has an elevated temperature needs rest. Rest and inactivity

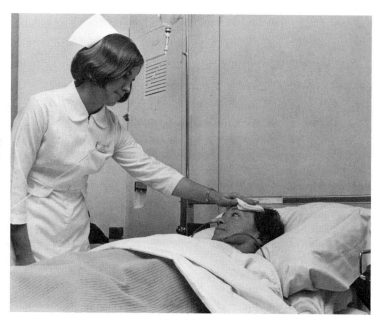

Sometimes a cool, moist cloth on the forehead helps the patient to feel more comfortable when he has a fever.

decrease the rate of the metabolic process and also muscular activity and thereby decrease the amount of heat produced in the body. Usually, the patient is restricted to bed in order to curtail his activities. Rest, however, involves more than restrictions of physical activity; it also means mental rest. Sometimes the simple act of taking a patient's temperature may itself give rise to anxiety on the part of the patient. An elevated temperature may mean that surgery is postponed, or that a much anticipated return to home and family is delayed. The patient needs to be assured that all is being done for his welfare and that he is in competent hands. Anticipating the needs of the patient helps him to relax. Very often, a simple explanation of procedures and treatments can alleviate many anxieties.

The febrile patient needs a cool, quiet environment. The patient with a fever is often irritable and may be hypersensitive to stimuli. An effort should be made to minimize noise and provide the patient with the opportunity for rest. A cool, comfortable room increases heat elimination and helps the patient to rest more easily. Sometimes a fan is used to increase the circulation of air in the room and facilitate the removal of heat from the body through conduction and convection. Care should be taken, however, that the patient does not become chilled. The bedclothes of the febrile patient should be light and comfortable, since heavy coverings inhibit heat elimination.

Measures to Minimize the Effects of Fever on the Body

The presence of a temperature above the normal level places stresses on the body's adaptive mechanisms. The patient is usually uncomfortable; he is losing more than the normal amount of fluids and using more energy than usual to maintain the elevated body temperature. Nursing action should then be directed toward relieving discomfort, maintaining hydration, and maintaining the patient's nutritional status.

Comfort Measures. Good hygiene is important to the patient's health and com-fort. Profuse diaphoresis (sweating), a common accompaniment of fever, is uncomfortable. Bathing the patient and assisting him to change his gown and bedding so that he is clean and dry are important contributions to his physical well-being. Because sweat glands are more numerous in the axilla and around the genitalia, these areas need particular care when the patient is bathed. Flannelette sheets, because of their greater absorbency, are often used in place of ordinary cotton (muslin) ones on the beds of patients who are perspiring profusely.

Maintaining Hydration. The hydration of the patient is of primary importance. Diaphoresis and the loss of additional fluids through increased respirations increase the amount of fluid eliminated from the body, and this fluid needs to be replaced. In addition, during a fever, there is increased production of metabolic waste products, which must be eliminated. The necessity for removing these products from the body, together with any toxic substances that may be present, emphasizes the importance of fluids. Generally 3000 cc. per day is considered a desirable fluid intake. If the patient is unable to take fluids orally or in sufficient amounts, parenteral fluids may be ordered.

An accurate record of the patient's fluid intake and output must be maintained. Intake records should include all fluids taken orally and those given parenterally. In computing output, urine should be measured accurately and a note made of the extent of sweating and the loss of any fluids through vomiting or diarrhea. Suction returns should also be included in the output calculations.

The patient should be observed carefully for signs of dehydration. When a patient becomes dehydrated during the course of a fever, his skin often becomes dry and scaly. The application of creams helps to keep the skin in good condition. Dehydration frequently results also in cracks in the patient's lips, tongue, or mucous membrane lining of the mouth. Good oral hygiene is imperative to prevent infection from developing and also to contribute to the patient's comfort. There is a need to cleanse, hydrate, and lubricate the mouth and lips. If the patient is unable to clean his own teeth with a toothbrush, he may be helped by the nurse, who uses a toothbrush or a tongue depressor with gauze and mouthwash. If ordinary mouthwash is ineffectual, the nurse may need to use a stronger solution, such as half-strength hydrogen peroxide or milk of magnesia.

Frequent intake of fluids helps to maintain hydration of the oral cavity. Rinsing the mouth with water (or mouthwash) and chewing gum also help to preserve hydration. If the patient is unable to take fluids orally, to rinse his mouth, or to chew gum, the nurse may meet this need for the patient by cleaning the mouth with swabs. Glycerin and lemon swabs, or swabs dipped in milk of magnesia, are used in many places for this purpose.

Lubrication may be accomplished by the application of creams or petrolatum to the lips. If the patient is unable to apply lubricating cream himself, the nurse can meet this need by applying sterile petrolatum to the lips. The petrolatum should be sterile because there are frequently splits or cracks in the lips due to the fever, which provide a portal of entry for infection.

Maintaining Nutritional Status. The old adage of "feed a cold and starve a fever" has been proved wrong. Indeed, because of the body's increased metabolic rate and the increased destruction of tissues that are so often a concomitant of fever, there is a need for both proteins and carbohydrates. Proteins aid in the formation of body tissue; carbohydrates supply the body with much-needed energy. Frequently these products are supplied in the liquids taken orally or given parenterally. The patient's weight should be checked at frequent intervals, and the physician should be kept informed of the patient's nutritional status so that appropriate therapy may be instituted.

Rest is essential to minimize the patient's energy requirements. Physical activity should be kept to a minimum. During the convalescent stage, activity should be increased gradually to prevent tiring the patient unduly.

An important function of the nurse is the communication of her observations to other members of the health team. Any elevation in the patient's temperature is considered significant and should be evaluated and reported accurately and promptly. If the temperature is markedly elevated, the physician should be informed immediately so that appropriate therapy can be instituted.

Measures to Reduce Heat Production and Facilitate Heat Loss

Antipyretic Drugs. Antipyretic drugs, such as aspirin, are often ordered to reduce a patient's fever. These drugs have a specific action on the heat-regulating centers but do not eliminate the cause of the fever. Their administration may be designated at specific times or the order may leave the time of their administration to the nurse's judgment. It is not unusual for antipyretic drugs to be given when a patient's temperature reaches 38.9° C. (102° F.). When a patient who has a fever is receiving antibiotics, these are usually administered at regular intervals in order to maintain a therapeutic drug level in the patient's body. The use of antibiotics for patients with infections reduces the fever by eliminating the cause of it—that is, the infection within the body.

Tepid Sponge Bath. When it is considered desirable to lower the patient's temperature rapidly, a tepid sponge bath may be given. This is a simple and reliable nursing measure that can be employed either in a home situation or in the hospital. It is carried out on the order of a physician. The technique is based on the principle that the body loses heat through the mechanisms of conduction to a cooler substance, in this case the tepid water, evaporation of water from the surface of the body, and convection of the heat away from exposed body surfaces during the bathing process.

Prior to the bath, the temperature, pulse, and respirations are taken. These observations are important for the subsequent evaluation of the effectiveness of the bath. There are many ways of giving a tepid sponge bath. One way is described here.

The equipment required for the tepid

sponge bath consists of a basin of water 30° C. to 38° C. (85° to 100° F.), towels, wash cloth, bath blanket, and isopropanol rubbing compound. To initiate this nursing care intervention the top bedclothes are fan-folded to the foot of the bed, and the patient is draped with his bath blanket. Then his gown is removed and his body is sponged. Heat is lost from the body as water is sponged onto the body surface and some of it is permitted to evaporate. Large areas are sponged at a time, for example, one side of the leg, one side of the arm, the chest and the abdomen. Long strokes are used on the legs and on the back. Because the blood vessels are close to the body surface in the axilla, the wrists and the groins, the cooling effect of the bath is enhanced by applying the wet cloths there for an extended period of time, that is, by slowing down the bathing process in these areas. A gentle patting motion is used to dry each area; brisk rubbing increases the activity of the cells and therefore the rate of heat production. The back of the patient is then gently rubbed with the isopropanol rubbing compound before the gown and covers are replaced.

The temperature, pulse, and respirations are taken 20 minutes after the sponge bath. The bath is usually repeated until the patient's temperature has reached the level designated by the physician. If the physician's order does not include the temperature at which treatment is to be discontinued, the bath should be stopped before the normal temperature is reached. A further drop in temperature may be expected to occur after it is discontinued.

Sometimes an alcohol bath is ordered, because alcohol evaporates at a lower temperature than water and thus hastens the cooling process. In this case, isopropanol is substituted for the water or, in some instances, may be added to the water. If alcohol is used, the procedure is always terminated before the temperature reaches normal.

A nursing intervention which is somewhat similar to the tepid sponge bath is the use of a wet sheet and a fan to increase heat elimination from the body. The patient is covered only by a sheet which has been dampened with water. A fan is so directed that there is constant movement of air over the sheet. This measure promotes evaporation and convection and thereby increases heat loss from the body. This is a rather drastic measure and is used only in exceptional circumstances.

Hypothermia Machines. Many hospitals now have a hypothermia machine which is used for rapid surface cooling of the body. This machine[12] may be used for patients who have temperatures of 39.4° C. (103° F.) and over when it is felt that it is essential to bring the body temperature down quickly or when there has been brain damage to the heat-regulating centers and it is necessary to maintain artificial cooling of the body over a prolonged period of time.

This technique uses the mechanisms of radiation and conduction. The patient is placed on or between cooling blankets, which are attached to a refrigerating machine. The blankets contain coils in which a refrigerant circulates. A considerable amount of heat is lost from the body through direct conduction to the cooling substance and through the radiation of heat waves from the body to the cooler blankets.

Because some people shiver in response to the application of the hypothermia blanket, drugs are sometimes given to minimize shivering. Patients receiving hypothermia treatment frequently need a great deal of reassurance and explanation about the treatment.

Applications of Heat and Cold

Applications of heat and cold as therapeutic measures are probably well known to the student before she commences her nursing education. Applying a hot water bottle or a heating pad to cold feet is a comfort familiar to many, particularly to those who live in cold climates. The application of ice as a means of stopping

---

[12]A more detailed account of hyperthemia and hypothermia equipment may be found in Estelle Beaumont: Hypo/Hyperthermia Equipment. *Nursing '74,* 4:34–41, April 1974.

nosebleed (epistaxis) is a common therapeutic measure carried out in the home. In addition, rubbing the chest with a decongestant ointment or a liniment is a traditional remedy for the treatment of colds in many families. The student herself has probably already had firsthand experience with many of these therapeutic measures.

Generally speaking, applications of heat and cold are used in the hospital and the home as therapeutic measures. In the hospital, these measures are carried out at the direction of the physician. Occasionally heat and cold also serve as comfort measures. If this is the sole reason for their use, it is often left to the judgment of the nurse and patient whether and how to apply them. The nurse therefore needs a knowledge of the physiological reactions resulting from these measures and of the untoward reactions which may occur. If the nurse is ever in doubt about the use of heat or cold, she should consult the physician before she applies these measures.

Applications of heat and cold are also used in the course of physical medicine as part of rehabilitation programs. In these instances physical therapists use such measures as paraffin baths and whirlpool baths on the advice of the physician.

Types of Applications. Heat and cold are relative degrees of temperature dependent to some extent upon the perception of the individual. The temperature at the surface of the skin of the torso is generally 33.9° C. (93° F.).

Applications at this temperature are usually undifferentiated as either cold or hot, but applications that are 11.1° C. (20° F.) below or 8.3° C. (15° F.) above this level excite cutaneous nerve fibers. Local tolerance is thought to range between 4.4° C. (40° F.) and 43.3°C. (110° F.) Generally any application that is above or below these levels can be the cause of tissue damage.

Temperature is perceived in gradations: cold to cool tepid, indifferent, and warm to very very hot. Different areas of the body have varying sensitivity to changes in heat and cold. For example, the back of the hand is not particularly sensitive to changes in temperature. Also, people perceive the temperature more acutely when the temperature of the skin is changing. That is why a hot bath feels hotter at first than it does after the skin becomes adjusted to it. Extremes in temperature, both hot and cold, are perceived as painful (see Chapter 31).

Many different types of hot and cold applications can be used as therapeutic measures. Both heat and cold can be applied as dry treatments or as moist treatments, and the source can be varied according to the purpose. Moreover, irritants and counterirritants are quite similar in action to applications of heat. An *irritant* is a substance which, when applied to a patient's skin, produces a local inflammatory reaction through its chemical action. An irritant becomes a *counterirritant* when the purpose of its application is a reflex action in underlying tissues, that is, when the purpose of the treatment is to initiate a physiological reaction in tissues underlying the skin. Mustard is a common example of a counterirritant that has had a long history of use as a local application (mustard plaster) to relieve congestion in the chest.

The choice of the kind of application that is to be used is dependent upon a number of factors:

1. The purpose of the application
2. The age of the patient and the condition of his skin
3. The general physical health of the patient
4. The area of the body that is affected
5. The duration of the treatment
6. The availability of equipment

Principles Related to the Application of Heat and Cold. The principles given serve as guides to the use of hot and cold applications.

Reasons for the Application of Heat. Heat is applied to the body for any of several reasons. It can be applied to produce a local or systemic effect or both. A local effect is one that is specific to a defined area of the body, for example, to relieve local muscle spasm. A systemic effect is one that is reflected in the body as a whole — for example, general warmth felt throughout the body.

Heat is known to relieve pain. Thus

PRINCIPLES RELATED TO THE APPLICATION OF HEAT AND COLD

1. Heat is distributed throughout the body by the circulating blood and by direct conduction throughout the tissues.

2. Heat is lost from the body chiefly through conduction, convection, and evaporation at the surface of the skin.

3. The amount of heat that is lost from the body is directly proportional to the amount of blood that is circulating close to the surface of the skin.

4. The amount of blood that circulates close to the surface of the skin is influenced by the dilatation and constriction of peripheral arterioles.

5. Applications of heat and cold influence the dilatation and constriction of peripheral blood vessels.

6. Moisture conducts heat better than air.

7. People vary in their ability to tolerate heat and cold. People at both extremes of the age spectrum—that is, the very old and the very young—are particularly sensitive to heat and cold.

8. People become less sensitive to repeated applications of heat and cold.

9. The length of time of exposure to extremes in temperature affects the body's tolerance of the temperature.

---

pain that is caused by the contraction of muscle fibers is relieved when the muscle spasm is reduced by heat. Heat also increases circulation to an area and can thereby relieve the pain of ischemia (lack of blood). Sometimes the collection of fluid in an area can cause pain because of the increased pressure. The swelling can be reduced by the application of heat. As blood circulation improves, fluid is more easily absorbed from the tissues and consequently swelling or edema is reduced. Frequently hot applications to a swollen area, such as the ankle, are alternated with cold applications, because heat and cold are most effective while the temperature of the area is changing. The cold in this instance reduces the flow of fluid to the swollen area.

Toxins and waste products are also thought to be causes of discomfort which can be relieved by an increase in blood circulation to the irritated tissues.

The fact that heat helps to alleviate many types of pain does not mean that it is indicated for all instances of pain. Heat can hasten the suppurative (pus-forming) process, and in the case of an inflamed appendix it could cause the appendix to rupture. Although the physician supplies the directions regarding the application of heat, the nurse must always be aware of the purpose of the treatment and alert to possible untoward actions. There is, for instance, always a danger that a burn may result from the local application of heat, or that deeper-lying tissues may be affected and, for example, an inflammatory process may be aggravated. Inflammation is the reaction of tissues to injury; it is characterized by pain, swelling, redness, and local heat.

Heat increases circulation to the area of the body to which it is applied. It therefore can be applied to improve the oxygenation and nourishment of tissues, thus aiding tissue metabolism and subsequent healing. For example, heat applied to an infected surgical incision not only hastens suppuration, but it also increases the nourishment of the tissue cells and the healing process. Improved circulation in this case also enhances the elimination of toxic and waste substances via the blood stream.

A hot drink is known to have the effect of intensifying peristalsis. Peristalsis is the wavelike contraction of the muscles of the digestive tract which propels its contents along. This increased peristalsis can be utilized to help a patient establish regular bowel habits. For example, one-half hour after drinking coffee for breakfast the patient is encouraged to try to defecate so as to utilize the mass peristalsis stimulated by the hot fluid.

Another purpose of applying heat locally is to soften exudates. An exudate is a discharge produced by the body tissues. Sometimes the discharge from an open wound forms hardened crusts over the area. Hot moist compresses are often used to soften these crusts so they can be easily removed. It has already been mentioned that heat is also used as a comfort measure. It can be used to promote the relaxation of skeletal muscles and thereby to promote general comfort and rest.

Reasons for the Application of Cold. Cold is applied to the body for both systemic and local effects. For systemic purposes, cold is applied to slow the basal metabolic rate. This is indicated in certain kinds of heart surgery, because a low basal metabolic rate results in a lessened demand of the body tissues for oxygen and nourishment and thus decreases the work of the heart. For a similar reason a patient's limb may be packed in ice prior to amputation. The cold slows the speed of the circulation of the blood and thus enables the surgeon to control bleeding more easily during the operation.

Cold can also be applied to stop hemorrhage, since it constricts the peripheral arterioles and increases the viscosity of the blood, in addition to contracting the muscles and depressing cardiac action. The nurse often sees ice bags applied routinely to patients after a tonsillectomy as a prophylactic measure against hemorrhage.

Cold applications slow the suppurative process and the absorption of tissue fluids. They also reduce swelling, such as that in epididymitis (an inflammation of the testis), and slow other inflammatory processes, for example, inflammation of the eye.

Because cold contracts the peripheral blood vessels, it raises the blood pressure. This is more usually a side effect than the sole reason for cold applications.

Pain can also be relieved through the use of cold applications. Cold restricts the movement of the blood and tissue fluids; therefore it relieves pain caused by an increased amount of fluid moving into the tissues, as in the case of a sprain. In addition, intense cold numbs pain receptors. As a result cold is used as a local anesthetic. There is, however, a danger in the prolonged use of intense cold: it interferes with the supply of oxygen and nourishment to the tissues and may result in tissue death.

Local Applications of Heat. Heat can be applied to a patient as radiant heat, conductive heat, or conversive heat. Radiant heat is heat whose wavelength is in the infrared portion of the electromagnetic spectrum.[13] Conductive heat is heat transferred by direct application—for example, by a hot water bottle or hot compresses. Conversive heat is heat converted from primary sources of energy—for example, from short wave or ultrasound wave energy. The application of this latter type of heat is classified as medical diathermy; it is utilized to provide heat to deep tissues. Radiant and conductive heat provide heat to the superficial tissues only.

Both moist and dry forms of heat can be applied to the skin or mucous membranes. Usually it is necessary to apply superficial heat for 20 to 30 minutes in order to obtain the desired effect.

Since patients become accustomed to heat after prolonged applications, they should be cautioned against turning up a heating pad or refilling a hot water bottle without checking the temperature. All patients are observed closely for any untoward reactions to heat applications, such as a prolonged erythema (redness), blister formation, or discomfort.

THE HOT WATER BOTTLE. The hot water bottle has long been a vehicle for applying dry heat to the body. It is used as both a therapeutic and a comfort measure, although therapeutically its use is being surpassed by the electrical heating pad. Some hospitals and other inpatient health agencies have prohibited the use of hot water bottles because of the ever-present danger of burns to patients.

The water for a hot water bottle is tested for its exact temperature. It has already been explained that 58° C. (135° F.) is generally considered to be a desirable temperature for an adult whose sensations and circulation are intact. A temperature of 50° C. (120° F.) is considered safe for children and for adults who are uncon-

---

[13] Howard A. Rusk: *Rehabilitation Medicine.* 2nd edition. St. Louis, C. V. Mosby Company, p. 79.

scious or debilitated or who have impaired circulation. The water for a hot water bottle can usually be obtained from the hot water tap; its temperature is checked by the thermometers that most hospitals provide for measuring the temperature of unsterile solutions.

The hot water bottle is filled one-half to two-thirds full, and the air is expelled from the remainder of the bottle by pressing the sides together before the top is applied. In this way the hot water bottle remains fairly light and is easily molded to the patient's body.

After the outside of the hot water bottle has been dried, it is tested for leakage and then placed in a cloth cover before it is taken to the patient. The cover slows the transmission of heat, absorbs perspiration, and thereby lessens the danger of burning. The stopper of the hot water bottle is well covered, because it can become sufficiently hot that on direct contact it will burn a person's skin.

The hot water bottle is placed on the desired area and molded to the patient's body. If the hot water bottle is given to a person who burns easily, it is wise to place a sheet or blanket between the person and the bottle. When continuous heat is to be applied, it is usually necessary to change the hot water bottle every one and a half to two hours in order to maintain the desired temperature.

When hot water bottles are not in use they are hung upside down with the top unscrewed. This allows the bottle to dry inside and prevents the sides of the bottles from sticking together.

THE ELECTRIC PAD. Electric pads and electric blankets are frequently used as a means of providing dry heat. They have the advantages of being light, of being easily molded to the patient's body and of providing constant heat. Their disadvantages are related to cleaning and to the danger of short circuits, particularly when they are used with oxygen equipment. The heating pads that are used in hospitals are frequently covered with a plastic material that can be easily and effectively cleaned. It is often possible to lock the mechanism for setting the temperature of the heating pad so that it cannot be changed without the nurse being aware of it.

THE INFRARED LAMP. The infrared lamp, which supplies radiant heat, is used to provide heat to a localized area of the body. Infrared radiation penetrates 3 mm. of tissue at the most; thus it provides surface heat only.

The action of infrared heat is to increase blood circulation (hyperemia), thereby increasing the supply of oxygen and nourishment to the tissues. An infrared lamp is frequently used in the treatment of decubitus ulcers. It is also often used in obstetrical and gynecological cases to promote the healing of a suture area on the perineum.

Before applying heat from an infrared lamp, the nurse observes that the patient's skin is dry and clean. This lessens the danger of burning the skin. A small infrared lamp is placed 45 to 60 cm. (18 to 24 inches) from the area of skin that is to be treated; a larger lamp is placed 60 to 75 cm. (24 to 30 inches) away. The heat is provided for from 15 to 20 minutes, but the patient is checked after the first five minutes to make sure that he is not being burned. At the end of the treatment the patient's skin is generally moist, warm, and pink.

The danger in the use of the infrared lamp is that the patient will be burned. The nurse should frequently observe the patient's reaction to the application of infrared heat and terminate the treatment at the first sign of reddening or pain. In addition the patient should be warned that the lamp will become hot after it has been on for a few minutes. Placing an infrared lamp under the bedclothes is inadvisable because of the danger of fire.

THE "BAKER" (HEAT CRADLE). The "baker" is another means of providing radiant heat. In this case the heat is less localized; it is often applied to large areas, such as the abdomen, chest, or legs. The baker is a metal cradle into which are installed several electrical sockets for luminous bulbs. The metal acts to reflect the heat from the bulbs toward the patient. Often the baker is covered by the top bedding in order to hold in the heat and to prevent cooling by the circulating air. The temperature of the baker should not exceed 52° C. (125° F.).

STEAM INHALATIONS. In the care of patients with respiratory conditions,

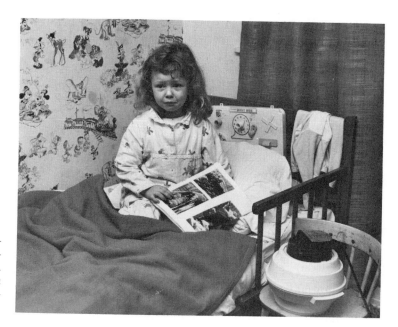

Heat in the form of steam inhalations is often used to relieve the congestion of a cold. This little girl does not seem too happy about the treatment.

steam inhalations are frequently used to loosen congestion and to help liquefy secretions. Both hot and cold steam are used. The topic of inhalations is discussed in Chapter 30.

THE HOT COMPRESS.   Hot compresses, which utilize the principle of heat conduction, can be either sterile or unsterile moist applications. Generally gauze is soaked in the solution ordered, the excess fluid is wrung out of the gauze, and the gauze then applied to the specified body surface. The compress should be moist but not so wet that the solution drips from it. Sterile precautions are indicated when the compress is to be applied to an open wound or to an organ such as the eye. In such cases, sterile gauze is soaked in a sterile or antiseptic solution, and sterile forceps or sterile gloved hands are used to wring out the compress. The compress is applied at the hottest temperature that the patient can tolerate. Frequently an insulating waterproof cloth is placed over the compress in order to hold in the heat. In some situations heating pads or hot water bottles are placed over the compress to provide additional heat.

Hot compresses are often indicated to hasten the suppurative process and to improve the circulation of blood to the tissues. Normal saline and antiseptic solutions are frequently ordered by the physician.

Compresses generally retain heat poorly, the length of time that they remain hot being somewhat dependent upon the thickness of the material, the temperature of the solution, and the use of insulating materials. Ordinarily compresses are ordered every hour or every two hours; however, if constant applications of hot moist compresses are ordered, the nurse or the patient should change them every 10 to 15 minutes.

THE HOT PACK.   A hot pack, which is sometimes referred to as a hot fomentation or foment, is a piece of heated moist flannel or similar material that is applied to a patient's skin in order to provide superficial moist heat. It is used for a larger area than the hot compress. Because intense heat can be applied in this manner there is a danger that the patient may be burned. This danger is minimized if the hot pack is sufficiently dry that water does not drip from it.

A hot pack can be prepared by boiling or steaming pieces of flannel or by heating commercially prepared packs. If the flannel is boiled it is necessary to wring it out before applying it. There are hot pack machines available which steam the flannel to prepare it for application. Once the foment has been heated it is applied directly to the patient as hot as he can tolerate it. If the hot pack is shaken slightly before it is applied there is little danger of burning the patient and it is more comfortable for him. Sometimes petrolatum is applied to the skin beforehand to serve as a protective coating and to slow the transfer of heat. The hot foment is covered with an insulating waterproof material and then secured to the patient with a towel or binder. Often a hot water bottle or heating pad is applied over this to provide additional heat.

A hot pack usually keeps hot for 10 to 15 minutes. Once it has cooled it is removed and, if continuous heat is required, it is replaced with another pack. If the patient does not need another application for some time, his skin is dried.

Hot packs are frequently indicated to relieve muscle spasm, as when a patient has poliomyelitis. They are also applied to hasten the suppurative process and to decrease muscle soreness.

Upon the application of a hot pack, an erythema of the skin is to be expected as a result of the vasodilatation of the local blood capillaries. Blistering of the skin should be avoided.

BODY SOAKS. Body soaks and arm and foot soaks are therapeutic measures ordered by the physician to provide warmth or to apply a solution to cleanse an area of the body. Generally they are indicated to hasten suppuration, to cleanse an open wound, or to apply a medicated solution to a designated area.

Special portable containers, including both arm and foot baths, are available commercially for this purpose. These containers can be sterilized in order to provide a sterile environment when one is indicated, as when burned areas need to be soaked.

The solution for a body soak is ordered by the physician. Often sterile normal saline or sterile water is used. The temperature of the solution should be 47.2° C. (115° F.) unless otherwise ordered by the physician for a specific reason.

The patient's dressings are removed and his limb is immersed gradually into the solution. The dressings may need to be soaked before removal to avoid trauma to the tissues. The limb is immersed slowly in order to acclimatize the patient to the temperature of the solution. The patient assumes a comfortable position during the treatment to avoid fatigue and muscle strain. The length of the treatment is usually 20 minutes. The temperature of the solution is checked every five minutes, and additional solution is supplied when necessary. After the soaking is completed, the patient's limb is dried and dressings are replaced as necessary.

If the patient has an open wound, aseptic technique is carried out. The container, the solution, and the towels are sterile. In some agencies, the nurse wears a mask when carrying out this procedure. Sterile dressings are applied after the soak (see Chapter 22).

During and after soaking an area of the body the nurse observes the condition of the patient's wound and the amount and character of any discharge. It is expected that the heat of the solution will cause some vasodilatation and erythema and that the solution itself will cleanse and soften exudates. These observations are then recorded.

THE THERAPEUTIC BATH. Therapeutic baths are provided to supply warmth, to cleanse, and to apply a medication. They are indicated chiefly for people who have skin diseases or who have had certain kinds of perineal or rectal surgery.

The solutions that are used are ordered by the physician; the most common are saline, tap water, sodium bicarbonate, starch, and oatmeal. The last three, often called colloid baths, can now be purchased commercially in special preparations.

The temperature for the therapeutic bath can vary from 4.4° C. to 47.2° C. (40° F. to 115° F.). The temperature ranges of the baths are generally classified as follows:

Hot bath   40.6–47.2° C. (105–115° F.)
Warm bath   38.9–40.6° C. (100–105° F.)
Tepid bath 36.7° C.   (98° F.)
Cold bath   4.4–21.1° C. (40–70° F.)

Unless otherwise ordered, the bath is

generally given at a temperature of 36.7° C. (98° F.) — a tepid bath.

A bathtub contains approximately 30 gallons of fluid when it is two-thirds full. The nurse may need this information in order to calculate the correct amount of medication to be added to a bath. For example, a normal saline solution requires 40 g. of sodium chloride to 4 liters of water (1½ ounces to 1 gallon). The following quantities of medication are for a bathtub two-thirds full.

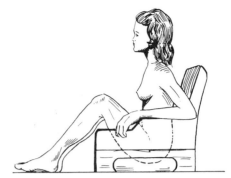

Adequate support aids the patient in being as comfortable as possible in a sitz bath. (From Lucile A. Wood and Beverly Rambo, eds.: Nursing Skills in Allied Health Services. Vol. 1. Philadelphia, W. B. Saunders Co., 1977.)

Medication	Amount or Strength
Sodium bicarbonate	250 g. (8 ounces)
Potassium permanganate	1:20,000
Sodium chloride	1200 g. (45 ounces)
Tar	60 cc.

Once the patient's bath is drawn, the ordered medication is added and the temperature is checked. Then the patient is assisted into the tub. Generally a male patient prefers an orderly or male nurse to help him. Usually the patient remains in the bath for 15 minutes, and he is checked regularly for any untoward reactions. If the patient complains of vertigo (dizziness) or syncope (fainting) the bath should be terminated at once. The water should be drained off and the patient assisted from the tub as soon as he is over the attack. The nurse should not attempt to move the patient when he is feeling dizzy or faint. She should always obtain assistance as needed to ensure the patient's safety.

The patient's skin is patted dry with a soft towel after a medicated cutaneous bath. If dressings are necessary, new ones are applied.

The *sitz bath* is a special bath the purposes of which are chiefly to provide warmth, to cleanse, and to provide comfort to the patient's perineal area. It is often indicated after rectal or perineal surgery.

There are several commercially manufactured sitz baths available. Some models fit over toilets, on chairs, or on beds. There are also comfort seats that can be placed in bathtubs, as well as separate sitz bath units.

The sitz bath is generally ordered with saline solution or tap water. The temperature is 38.9° to 40.6° C. (100° to 105° F.), and the patient stays in it for 10 to 20 minutes. The nurse observes that the perineal region of the patient is immersed if he is seated in a bathtub or that his perineal area is being irrigated if he is seated in a commercial sitz bath.

Usually patients who require sitz baths have recently had rectal or perineal surgery and therefore comfort is an important concern. Adequate support during the bath is also essential. The patient may require help during the bath, particularly if there is any doubt about his ability to tolerate the bath. The patient's pulse is taken five minutes after the start of the bath; if it is unduly accelerated or irregular, he should return to bed, and the nurse then reports this to the physician.

In recording a sitz bath on the patient's chart, the nurse records the appearance of the patient's wound, the amount and character of the discharge, and any untoward reactions experienced by the patient, as well as the time of the treatment and the nature of treatment itself.

DIATHERMY. Medical diathermy is the provision of heat to the deep tissues of the body by transforming certain kinds of physical energy into heat in the deep tissues. It is usually done in a physical therapy department under the direction of a physician.

Various types of high frequency currents are used: short wave, microwave, and ultrasound. The treatment is painless, the patient's chief perception being one of warmth. It is used for much the same reasons as superficial heat.

THE ULTRAVIOLET LAMP. Ultraviolet radiation is also used clinically to treat wounds and skin diseases. The sun is a natural source of ultraviolet light, but artificial sources are used therapeutically. The hot quartz mercury lamp, the carbon arc lamp and, of course, the sun lamp are all used.

Generally, ultraviolet radiation is carried out in a special department, such as the physical therapy department. The normal skin reaction produces an erythema, tanning, and a proliferation of the cells of the epidermis.

If the patient needs ultraviolet treatments the physician generally orders them every other day for maximum effect. Fair-skinned people are more sensitive to ultraviolet radiation than dark-skinned people. Sulfanilamide medications increase this sensitivity.

Local Applications of Cold

THE ICE BAG. The ice bag or ice cap and the ice collar are commonly used means of applying dry cold to the body. An ice collar is a long narrow rubber or plastic bag which fits around the neck.

Ice bags are usually made with an opening through which small pieces of ice are inserted. Once the ice bag is filled the air is expelled before the top of the ice bag is secured. The air is removed in order that the ice bag can be molded to the patient's body.

Before the flannel cover is put on, the bag is dried. The cover retains cold for more gradual application and it absorbs the water formed by atmospheric condensation. The bag is placed on the area of the body to be cooled.

Generally, ice bags need to be refilled when all the ice has melted or as ordered. If continuous ice applications are ordered, the ice bag is checked once an hour to see that the cold is maintained.

When an ice bag is in place, the pressure of the bag should not cut off circulation. At the first sign of tissue numbness and a mottled bluish appearance, the bag should be removed and the physician notified. These signs could be the result of either the cold or pressure upon the tissues.

Cold applications are often alternated with hot applications, or the cold applications are spaced in such a way that the tissue warms between applications. The alternate contraction and dilatation of the blood vessels is a highly effective method of inducing hyperemia and increasing tissue fluid absorption.

When ice bags are not in use they are

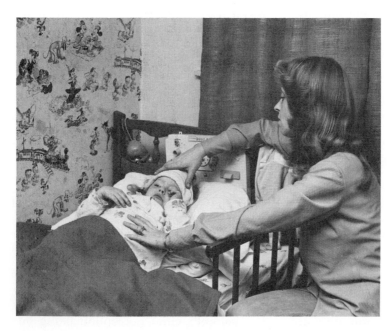

A moist cold compress is used by this mother to soothe her feverish child.

stored with the tops removed so that the air will dry the inside and prevent the sides from sticking together.

THE ICE COMPRESS. Moist cold can be applied by means of ice compresses. These are frequently used to terminate a nosebleed (epistaxis) or to supply moist cold to the eye.

An ice compress is usually made of gauze or other cloth material. The gauze is cooled over ice chips, wrung out, and then applied. It is replaced as it becomes warm. Another method of applying a moist cold compress is to place some chipped ice in a cloth bag, which is then placed directly over the area to be cooled. The disadvantage of this is that as the ice melts the water drips on the patient.

Just as in the application of the ice bag, the patient's skin is observed for any signs of untoward effects of the cold. Prolonged vasoconstriction can result in venous congestion and subsequent tissue anoxia. If the patient's skin maintains a bluish, mottled appearance for several hours, there is danger of permanent damage to the cells.

Most hospitals have ice-making machines and ice crushers to break the ice into small pieces. The chips of ice are used in ice applications because they mold easily to the body and are more comfortable.

THE ICE PACK. Ice packs are used occasionally to lower the body temperature or to lower the temperature of a patient's limb prior to surgery. Hypothermia refers to lowering the body temperature artificially. It is done in some types of open heart surgery, and it is usually carried out in the operating room.

On a hospital nursing unit the nurse occasionally sees a patient's limb packed in ice in preparation for amputation. A special container is available commercially for this purpose. The patient's leg (or arm) is wrapped in cloth and placed in the container. Chips of ice are then packed around the limb. It is important that the patient be given the explanation of the procedure that he requires and that the ice be kept around the limb for the prescribed length of time.

Applications of Irritants and Counterirritants. Many kinds of preparations are available for administration as irritants. The purpose of some irritants is merely to

cause hyperemia through surface vasodilatation (rubefacients), whereas others have been used to produce blisters (vesicants) or abscesses (pustulants). The latter two kinds of irritants are rarely used tody.

An irritant is applied gently to the designated surface area. Following its application the area is observed every five minutes, the irritant being left on for 20 minutes unless otherwise specified. Irritants are washed off gently with warm water and soap and the skin is patted dry.

An irritant becomes a counterirritant when its primary purpose is to relieve underlying congestion or pain. Goodman and Gilman state that the afferent nerve impulses from the skin area upon which the counterirritant is applied are relayed via the cerebrospinal axis to efferent vasomotor fibers that supply the internal organ. As a result, there is a relief of congestion of the internal tissues by redirection of the blood toward the surface.[14]

Of the many counterirritants that were used in the past—for example, the linseed poultice, flaxseed poultice, and mustard plaster—the mustard plaster is the one still used occasionally today. The mustard plaster (mustard sinapism) is a mixture of mustard, flour, and warm water. Hot water is not used because it inactivates enzymes in the mustard. The proportions vary according to the age of the individual:

Infant: 1 part mustard, 12 parts flour
Child: 1 part mustard, 8 parts flour
Adult: 1 part mustard, 3 parts flour

The skin is observed after the application has been on for five minutes; if it is reddened it is removed. At the end of the treatment (20 minutes) the skin should appear reddened but not blistered. People with fair skins tend to burn easily. After the mustard plaster has been removed and the patient's skin has been washed and dried, petrolatum or olive oil is applied to the skin to soothe it.

Mustard plasters can be purchased commercially. The precautions just mentioned should also be followed when using these preparations.

[14]Louis S. Goodman and Alfred Gilman: The Pharmacological Basis of Therapeutics. 3rd Ed. New York, Macmillan Company, 1965, pp. 981–983.

GUIDE TO ASSESSING DISTURBANCES OF BODY TEMPERATURE

1. What is the patient's temperature? His pulse and respiratory rate?
2. Are these abnormal in view of the time of day, the patient's activities, and other physiological factors that might cause a slight or temporary deviation from the normal TPR?
3. Has the patient had prolonged exposure to excessively hot or cold environmental temperatures?
4. Is immediate nursing or medical intervention indicated?
5. Does the patient show signs that he is having a chill?
6. What is the color of the patient's skin? Does it feel warm? cool to the touch? or cold?
7. Is the patient perspiring?
8. Does he complain of any physical symptoms such as headache or fatigue? pain? absence of sensation in any part of the body?
9. Is the patient able to tolerate food and fluids?
10. Is the patient losing excessive amounts of fluid through perspiration or increased respirations? Is his urine normal in color and amount?
11. Does he appear dehydrated?
12. Is the patient restless, irritable? Are there signs of mental confusion?
13. What medications have been prescribed for this patient?

GUIDE TO EVALUATING THE EFFECTIVENESS OF NURSING INTERVENTION

1. Has the patient's temperature come down? Is it within safe limits?
2. Is his fluid intake adequate for his needs?
3. Is his nourishment adequate?
4. Is the patient comfortable?
5. Is he getting sufficient rest?
6. Is his skin in good condition? His mouth?

GUIDE TO ASSESSING THERAPEUTIC APPLICATION OF HEAT OR COLD

1. Does the patient understand the purpose of the treatment?
2. What precautions need to be taken to protect the patient from harm?
3. Is he aware of the dangers?
4. Does the patient require added safety precautions because of his age, his general physical condition, the condition of his skin or his mental state?
5. Is the patient able to participate in his treatment? Is this desirable?
6. Are there specific skills that the patient (or his family) needs to learn or knowledge that he needs to gain in order to carry out the treatment at home?

GUIDE TO
EVALUATING THE
EFFECTIVENESS OF
NURSING
INTERVENTION

1. Is the patient safe during the application?
2. Is he comfortable?
3. Is the hot or cold application producing the desired physiological effect, for example, increased circulation to the part, or relief of pain?

STUDY
VOCABULARY

Chill	Exudate	Irritant
Conductive heat	Hectic fever	Ischemia
Constant fever	Hyperemia	Prostration
Conversive heat	Hyperthermia	Pyrexia
Counterirritant	Hypothermia	Pyrogen
Delirious	Inflammation	Relapsing fever
Epistaxis	Intermittent fever	Remittent fever
Erythema		

STUDY SITUATION
(1)

Mrs. S. James is a 34 year old woman who works as an aide in one of the city hospitals. She is married and has a five year old son. Mrs. James is admitted to the hospital with an elevated temperature of unknown etiology. Her temperature at admission was 39.1° C. (102.4° F.), her pulse 100, and her respirations 24. The patient had a chill during her first evening in the hospital, when her fever rose to 40° C. (104° F.). The following morning she felt improved, but she still perspires profusely and in the evening appeared restless and flushed.

The doctor left orders that Mrs. James was to have a tepid sponge bath and aspirin gr. $\bar{x}$ if her temperature rose above 39.4° C. (103° F.). He also asked the patient to drink at least one glass of fluid every hour of the day.

1. What factors are relevant to your explanation of a tepid sponge bath to this patient?
2. How can the patient's production of body heat be minimized?
3. How can the loss of body heat be facilitated?
4. What is the action of aspirin gr. $\bar{x}$?
5. How should you evaluate the effectiveness of the nursing care?
6. Why did the doctor want Mrs. James to drink at least one glass of fluid every hour?
7. What observations would indicate to the nurse that the patient is taking insufficient fluid?
8. Describe an environment which would be therapeutic for this patient.

STUDY SITUATION
(2)

Mrs. J. Watson has an infected cut on her right hand. She is at home and the physician has ordered hot soaks for her hand. As the public health nurse you have been asked to assist Mrs. Watson. This patient is 75 years old and she has poor blood circulation.

1. What are the specific problems of this patient in relation to her infected cut?
2. What factors should you take into consideration in helping to plan this patient's care?
3. What physiological reactions are to be expected as a result of the hot soaks?
4. How could the effectiveness of the soaks be evaluated?
5. What specific precautions should be taken? Why?
6. Outline the objectives and a plan of care for this patient.

SUGGESTED READINGS

Alderson, M. J.: The Effect of Increased Body Temperature on the Perception of Time. *Nursing Research,* 23:42–49, January-February 1974.

Blake, J.: Accidental Hypothermia in Fit Young Adults. *Nursing Mirror,* 141:46–49, August 21, 1975.

Everall, M.: Cold Therapy. *Nursing Times,* 72:144–145, January 29, 1976.

Glor, B. A. K., and Z. E. Estes: Moist Soaks: A Survey of Clinical Practices. *Nursing Research,* 19:463–465, September-October 1970.

High Body Heat Possible Complication of Surgery. *AORN Journal,* 22:862, December 1975.

Moore, J., et al.: The Case of the Warm, Moist Compress. *Canadian Nurse,* 71:19–21, March 1975.

O'Dell, A. J.: Hot Packs for Morning Joint Stiffness. *American Journal of Nursing,* 75:986–987, June 1975.

Petrello, J. M.: Temperature Maintenance of Hot Moist Compresses. *American Journal of Nursing,* 73:1050–1051, June 1973.

Pinel, C.: Accidental Hypothermia in the Elderly. *Nursing Times,* 71:1848–1849, November 1975.

Stallings, J. O., et al.: Malignant Hyperpyrexia Anesthesia Complication. *AORN Journal,* 21:642–645, March 1975.

CHAPTER 26

Anorexia, Nausea, and Vomiting

26 ANOREXIA, NAUSEA, AND VOMITING

The nurse should be able to:

Discuss the significance of *anorexia, nausea,* and *vomiting* as
problems affecting a person's nutritional status
Describe the anatomical structures and physiological mechanisms
involved in these problems
Discuss factors causing these problems
Describe signs and symptoms that commonly accompany anorexia,
nausea, and vomiting
Assess patients with these symptoms
Determine priorities for nursing action
Apply relevant principles in planning and implementing
appropriate nursing interventions, including measures to:
prevent these symptoms
assist in maintaining hydration and nutritional status
provide the patient with comfort and support
Evaluate the effectiveness of nursing interventions

INTRODUCTION

Loss of appetite is part of the "just feeling sick" phenomenon that may be the body's general reaction to stress of any kind. A slightly elevated temperature, which is another aspect of the same syndrome, is frequently the first objective indication that something is wrong with body functioning. A loss of interest in food is often the first thing noticed by the individual.

An adequate intake of food and fluids is essential for survival. In addition, the partaking of nourishment is inextricably bound to so many aspects of our daily lives and, for the normal healthy person, it is a source of pleasure as well as an essential ingredient of living. Any disturbance in the desire for food, or interference with the ability to eat and to drink, is therefore of vital importance to the optimal health of an individual.

A loss of the desire for food often leads to nausea and vomiting, if the source of stress is not removed and the body's normal equilibrium is not restored. The inability to take in food and fluids, or the body's rejection of them, poses a serious threat to homeostasis and involves all areas of functioning of the human body.

Gastroenteritis, which is a common cause of anorexia, nausea, and vomiting, is, as we have mentioned earlier, a major cause of death in many parts of the world. It still remains one of the most common causes of short-term illness in North America. It is a distressing problem for many international travelers, whose gastrointestinal tracts are exposed to foods and fluids that are not a part of their normal diet. In addition, anorexia, nausea, and vomiting frequently accompany so many health problems that the nurse should be acquainted with the physiological mechanisms involved in these disturbances, and be able to take appropriate interventions to assist patients with these problems.

THE PHYSIOLOGY OF ANOREXIA, NAUSEA, AND VOMITING

Anorexia, nausea, and vomiting refer to varying degrees of distress of the upper gastrointestinal tract. *Anorexia* means loss of appetite, or lack of the desire for food, and it involves the subjective perception of a distaste for food. The individual often expresses this by saying "I don't feel like eating." This may be the first indication of a disorder of the gastrointestinal tract. Anorexia may precede nausea. In *nausea*, not only is there a distaste for food but the mere thought of food becomes repelling and, in addition, the individual usually complains of an uncomfortable sensation in the region of the stomach. This uncomfortable sensation is frequently described as "feeling sick," a lay term often used for nausea. In most cases, nausea precedes vomiting. *Vomiting* is the forceful ejection of the stomach's contents.

Anorexia, nausea, and vomiting are commonly seen in conjunction with a great many health problems. They can indicate disturbances of the gastrointestinal tract itself or of almost any system of the body. They can reflect the body's reaction to emotional stress. Situations which the individual perceives as stressful, whether these are pleasant or unpleasant, can, and often do, produce these symptoms. Cultural values can also affect a person's reaction to food. Eating habits, personal likes and dislikes, and the social significance of food in different cultures, can all be related to these symptoms (see Chapter 16).

Anorexia, nausea, and vomiting are considered by many to be sequential stages of the same physical phenomenon, although any one of the three may occur by itself in the absence of the other two.

Anorexia has been defined as a loss of appetite. Appetite is the pleasant sensation of a desire for food. Although appetite and hunger frequently occur together, they are not the same, hunger being an uncomfortable sensation which indicates a physiological need for nourishment, whereas appetite is a learned response. As such, appetite is closely related to cultural and social values. To a large extent, one's appetite is conditioned by previous pleasant experiences with food. A number of different stimuli will arouse the appetite. These include olfactory stimuli, such as the pleasant odor of something cooking; visual stimuli, such as an attractively served meal; auditory stimuli, including the clatter of pots and pans in the kitchen as dinner is being prepared; or gustatory stimuli. One may taste a sample of food, for example, find it agreeable, and the appetite is whetted for more.

Appetite, or the feeling of a desire for food, is accompanied by certain visceral changes. These include increased gastric tone and accelerated hydrochloric acid secretion in the stomach. The individual frequently experiences an increase in salivation also as the mouth "waters" for food.

When a person loses his appetite, or suffers from anorexia, it has been noted that specific visceral changes occur. There is usually a hypofunctioning of the stomach; gastric tone is lessened, and the secretion of hydrochloric acid is decreased. It has also been observed that the stomach of the anorectic patient is pale in comparison with those of people with normal appetites.

These same physiological findings have been observed in individuals suffering from nausea, except that, in the case of the nauseated person, they are more pronounced. In nausea, there is a relaxation of the walls of the stomach, and gastric secretions and muscular contractions cease. Because of this relaxation, the stomach is usually situated lower in the abdominal cavity than it normally is. At the same time as the muscles of the stomach are in a relaxed state, the muscular wall of the intestine shows increased contractility, and contents from the duodenum may be regurgitated back into the stomach.

Most people locate the sensation of nausea as being in the epigastric region. The uncomfortable feeling in this area is usually accompanied by other symptoms of a distressing nature. Frequently there are increased perspiration and greatly increased salivation. Beads of perspiration may be evident on the person's forehead or upper lip, and he may state that his mouth is full of saliva. The individual's blood pressure usually drops and his pulse and respirations are rapid. An increased pulse rate may be followed by a decreased one. Some people feel faint, some complain of vertigo (dizziness) and headache. *Retching*—that is, an unproductive attempt at vomiting—may occur several times before vomiting actually takes place.

The act of vomiting involves a sequence of events which culminates in the forceful ejection of the stomach's contents. Initially there is a relaxation of the upper portion of the stomach, including the cardiac sphincter. This is followed by strong contractile waves in the lower portion of the stomach, which effectively close off the pyloric sphincter and prevent the stomach contents from passing into the duodenum. Subsequently, the diaphragm and the abdominal muscles contract. The strong contractions of these muscles during the act of vomiting account for the feeling of "soreness" which many people experience as an after effect of vomiting. With the simultaneous contraction of the diaphragm and the abdominal muscles, intraabdominal pressure is greatly increased and the stomach is literally squeezed between the two sets of muscles. The contents in the relaxed upper portion of the stomach are then forced upward through the esophagus and out through the mouth. Normally, the glottis is closed and respirations cease during the act of vomiting in order to prevent the vomitus from being aspirated (entering the lungs).

FACTORS CAUSING ANOREXIA, NAUSEA, AND VOMITING

The primary center controlling vomiting is located in the medulla oblongata. It is thought that stimulation of this center may give rise to anorexia, nausea, or vomiting, depending on the degree or intensity of the stimulus. Thus, a person who does not feel like eating may become nauseated at the sight of food and may vomit if he tries to eat it. However, vomiting is not always preceded by nausea, and it is believed, therefore, that only certain areas in the vomiting center are directly involved with nausea. The vomiting center may be stimulated by a number of factors. These include chemical stimuli (drugs), impulses from the cerebral cortex (strong emotions), and impulses arising from receptors in the viscera (internal factors).

Drugs

A number of different chemical agents may give rise to anorexia, nausea, and vomiting. Among these are many common drugs such as digitalis (frequently used in the treatment of people with heart conditions); a number of the narcotics, such as morphine; and many drugs used as anesthetics. When giving a patient any medication, in fact, it is important to note whether nausea and vomiting are listed as possible side effects of the drug, and, if so, to watch for these symptoms in the patient. The drug apomorphine, because of its specific action on the vomiting center, is often administered when it is considered desirable to rid the stomach of its contents—if, for example, the individual has ingested a poisonous substance. Other toxic substances, such as bacterial toxins, that are circulating in the blood stream may also stimulate the vomiting center. It is believed that circulating toxic chemical agents activate a chemoreceptor trigger zone, which is located in the fourth ventricle. When this zone is excited, it transmits impulses to the primary vomiting center, where the symptoms of anorexia, nausea, and vomiting are initiated.

Motion Sickness

A disturbance in motion, such as those one experiences with the rolling motion of a ship at sea or with any rapid change in direction of the body, stimulates receptors in the labyrinth of the ear. These receptors send out impulses that are carried by the vestibular nerve to the cerebellum, and thence to the chemoreceptor zone in the fourth ventricle. Impulses from this zone are then transmitted to the vomiting center in the medulla.[1]

Strong Emotions

It was mentioned in the introduction to this chapter that stressful situations may give rise to anorexia, nausea, or vomiting. The event or situation need not necessarily be unpleasant. An individual may be "too excited to eat" and, in countless poems and romantic novels, the person in love is described as someone with no appetite (among other symptoms). However, it is in connection with unpleasantly stressful situations that the symptoms of anorexia, nausea, and vomiting are most often noted. Worry over a pending examination, pain, anxiety, and fear may all give rise to these symptoms. Similarly, other psychic factors such as the sight of something particularly abhorrent, unpleasant odors, or even extremely loud noise can also take away one's appetite, make one feel nauseated, or cause vomiting. It is thought that these stimuli originating in the cerebral cortex activate the vomiting center directly, rather than being transmitted through the chemoreceptor trigger zone.

Internal Factors

The parts of the body containing receptors which initiate vomiting are the stom-

---

[1] Arthur C. Guyton: *Textbook of Medical Physiology*. 5th edition. Philadelphia, W. B. Saunders Company, 1976.

ach, duodenum, uterus, kidneys, heart, pharynx, and semicircular canals of the ear. The gag reflex is a familiar example of a reaction to stimulation of the receptors in the pharynx. The stimuli which give rise to anorexia, nausea, and vomiting include irritation of the receptors, as, for example, the tickling of the back of the throat to induce vomiting; the eating of irritating foods; stretching of the organ, as occurs as when a child stretches his stomach by overeating and promptly vomits; or pressure on the receptors. Irritation of the gastrointestinal tract by infectious, chemical or mechanical agents, and distention of or trauma to other viscera are also believed to affect the vomiting center directly, rather than being relayed through the chemoreceptor zone.

ASSESSING FOR ANOREXIA, NAUSEA, AND VOMITING

In assessing the individual suffering from anorexia, nausea, or vomiting, the nurse may gather information from both the patient and his family. Pertinent information includes the nature of the patient's discomfort, the length of time the person has had these symptoms, the severity of the symptoms, and their relationship to eating habits, personal lifestyle, and emotional stress. Specific causal factors should be identified, if possible. For example, has the patient eaten something that disagreed with him? Is he taking any medication which may have gastrointestinal side-effects? Is he under emotional stress? The patient or his family can often explain many of his cultural or religious beliefs that may affect his appetite and eating habits. Thus, the orthodox Jewish patient may not want to eat dairy products and meat at the same meal. The Chinese person may prefer rice and tea with his meals, and may leave the standard hospital food untouched.

From the nursing history and the initial clinical appraisal, the nurse can gather much pertinent information about the person's usual food habits and his current nutritional status at the time of his admission to the health agency. The nurse should note particularly the patient's normal appetite, his attitudes towards eating, and cultural or religious affiliations that might affect his eating patterns. The nurse should also be alert to information about the patient's ability to take foods and fluids orally. What is the state of his mouth (for example, his teeth)? His state of consciousness is also important, as is his ability to swallow. If he is not able to take nourishment orally, the nurse should be aware of the non-oral methods of feeding that are being used with this patient. Is he receiving intravenous therapy? gastric feedings?

The nurse should also be aware of the patient's health history, any current health problems he has, and the physician's diagnostic and therapeutic plans of care. These will be on the patient's record, and the nurse may also find there reports from diagnostic tests and examinations that have already been done.

Subjective Observations

Anorexia and nausea are subjective feelings; hence, their identification is highly dependent on the individual's ability to express his discomfort. "I'm not hungry" or "I don't feel like eating" are ways of expressing a reluctance to eat. The person who says "I feel sick" or "I feel sick to my stomach" is usually putting into words his feeling of nausea. The nurse can supplement the patient's observations by noting his reactions to food. Does he seem to anticipate and enjoy his meals? Does he simply toy with food, and actually eat very little? Or, does he push the food away at mealtimes without touching it? Such behavior can indicate that a person is anorectic and perhaps nauseated. Sometimes concomitant with a lack of interest in food are listlessness and apathy.

Objective Observations

As noted in the section on physiology, the person with nausea may show outward signs of his distress. The nurse should observe the individual for such signs as pallor, excessive perspiration, and increased salivation. Usually a person who is nauseated becomes pale and obviously uncomfortable. Beads of perspiration may show on the upper lip, or excessive perspiration be noted on other parts of the body. The nurse may note, if she takes the person's pulse, a marked acceleration in pulse rate.

Vomiting is usually preceded by nausea. Prior to vomiting a person frequently becomes very pale and perspires profusely. He may complain of neurological symptoms, such as vertigo and tingling sensations in his fingers and toes. He may also describe pain in the epigastric region.

In projectile vomiting the impulse to vomit is very sudden, occurring with little or no warning (that is, with no symptoms of nausea beforehand). Moreover, the ejection of the stomach's contents is more forceful than in ordinary vomiting. This type of vomiting is often seen in patients with head injuries.

Vomiting should be assessed in terms of both the nature of the vomiting and the characteristics of the vomitus (material vomited). In relation to vomiting, the nurse should determine its type—that is, whether it is projectile or regurgitated (ordinary vomiting); whether it is preceded by feelings of nausea; its frequency; and its occurrence in relation to intake of food, the administration of drugs, and the individual's emotional state. Characteristics of the vomitus which should be noted are: amount; color; consistency (that is, watery, liquid, or solid); the presence of undigested food, blood or other foreign substances; and odor.[2]

Gastrointestinal disturbances quickly result in deterioration of the patient's nutritional status. Food and fluids, especially the chloride ions, are lost as a result of vomiting of gastric juices. Prolonged deficiency in nourishment and in fluid intake results in malnutrition and dehydration; dehydration, in turn, can cause constipation. The patient can be expected to be constipated because of the fluid withdrawn from the feces in an effort by the body to compensate for the lowered fluid intake or fluid loss. There will probably

also be a decrease in the amount of urine excreted, and the urine is more concentrated.

A person who suffers from anorexia or nausea over a period time loses weight and, in addition to showing signs of dehydration and malnutrition, will become weak and listless owing to inadequate intake of nutrients. The individual who has experienced prolonged vomiting will show more pronounced effects due not only to the lack of intake but also to the loss of food and fluids through vomiting. This individual may show a marked weight loss and rapidly progressive signs of weakness and prostration, as well as signs of fluid and electrolyte imbalance (see Chapter 29). Prolonged vomiting in children is more serious than in adults because of the relatively greater loss of fluids and electrolytes in proportion to body weight.

Diagnostic Tests

Specific diagnostic tests may be ordered by the physician. It is quite usual for a specimen of the vomitus to be sent to the laboratory for examination. Frequently it is examined for blood. Microscopic examination may reveal occult blood, that is, blood which is present in the specimen but hidden to the naked eye. The nurse's responsibility includes seeing that a correctly labeled specimen is sent to the laboratory in the designated container.

Blood chemistry tests can also be significant. The patient who is vomiting is losing hydrochloric acid (HCl) and therefore H^+ ions. He is in danger then of developing alkalosis. An examination of the blood gases may be ordered to determine the acid-base balance (see Chapter 29). A decrease in blood chlorides (hypochloremia) is also likely to occur as Cl^- ions are lost along with the H^+ ions. Prolonged vomiting may cause severe sodium depletion as well.

PRIORITIES FOR NURSING ACTION

In determining priorities for nursing intervention, the immediate situation must

---

[2] Madelyn T. Nordmark and Anne W. Rohweder: *Scientific Foundations of Nursing.* 3rd edition. Philadelphia, J. B. Lippincott Company, 1975, p. 106.

PRINCIPLES RELEVANT TO ANOREXIA, NAUSEA OR VOMITING

1. A healthy body requires a balanced diet, which includes the intake of sufficient nutrients as well as approximately 2100 to 2900 cc. of fluid in every 24 hour period.

2. Factors in the individual's external environment and within the body itself can cause anorexia, nausea, and vomiting.

3. Anorexia, nausea, and vomiting can often be prevented by the elimination of unpleasant environmental stimuli.

4. Normally, 100 to 200 cc. of fluid is lost directly from the gastrointestinal tract in a 24 hour period.

5. The loss of food and fluids through vomiting can seriously disturb the body's fluid and electrolyte balance.

be assessed and appropriate action instituted. The patient who is vomiting, for example, needs prompt attention, directed primarily at relieving the symptom, providing him with comfort and support, and preventing complications.

With most patients who are anorectic or nauseated, the immediate problem is usually to prevent the aggravation of the symptoms. The nauseated individual usually feels better lying down in a cool and quiet room with adequate ventilation. If this is not possible, the person should be encouraged to sit quietly and take a few deep breaths. This helps to relax the diaphragm. Measures to take the person's mind off his gastrointestinal problems may also help.

GOALS FOR NURSING ACTION

Nursing action in the care of patients with anorexia, nausea or vomiting is directed towards three basic goals:

1. The prevention of these symptoms, whenever possible

2. The maintenance of hydration and nutritional status

3. The maintenance of the patient's comfort and hygiene

SPECIFIC NURSING INTERVENTIONS

Preventive Measures

The prevention of anorexia, nausea, and vomiting involves a consideration of both the patient and his environment. The nursing care measures that are effective in preventing these problems are often specific to the causes which have been discussed. The nurse can often assist the patient to identify situations and stimuli which induce these symptoms, and she can then modify or eliminate these from the patient's environment. Frequently the patient is aware of events or subjective experiences, such as pain, which cause nausea and vomiting.

An environment that is clean and pleasant is helpful in stimulating the appetite and preventing nausea and vomiting. If the patient eats while he is in bed, the nurse can provide him with a clean table that is free of equipment. The emesis basin should be kept out of sight. If the patient feels more secure with it nearby, it can be kept within easy reach.

Unpleasant odors, sights, and sounds are noxious stimuli which may contribute to anorexia, nausea, or vomiting. To dissipate unpleasant odors, a well-ventilated room is important, and the use of deodorants may be necessary at times. Vomitus is always removed immediately and treatment trays are covered and placed as inconspicuously as possible. Bedpans and urinals are kept covered and out of sight; for esthetic and hygienic reasons they are not placed on the patient's bedside table. Unpleasant sounds are avoided whenever possible.

It is important to allow for personal hygiene prior to meals. Most people like to wash their hands and freshen up before they eat. In this regard, sick people are no different from those who are well, and personal cleanliness is perhaps more important in the case of the person who has anorexia or a tendency to become nauseated. Personal hygiene should include the use of the washroom or the bedpan, and an opportunity for the patient to wash his hands (and face) and clean his teeth or rinse his mouth if he so desires.

Other measures which stimulate a person's appetite and prevent nausea are those which provide physical comfort. These include the prevention or elimination of pain; appropriate positioning; exercise or inactivity, whichever an individual needs, just prior to a meal; good oral hygiene; reduction of fever; a comfortable temperature and adequate ventilation within the room; and refraining from unpleasant nursing measures just prior to eating. Emotional discomfort can also affect a person's appetite. Worry, fear, and excitement can inhibit the desire for food and also delay the passage of food through the gastrointestinal tract. This latter point is important to remember with preoperative patients, since it may be a contributing factor in postoperative nausea and vomiting. Explanations and psychological support help the patient to deal with anxieties and cope with life situations.

In discussing measures which prevent anorexia, nausea, and vomiting, the use of tonics to improve the appetite and of antiemetic drugs to control nausea and vomiting must be included. Most physicians have their own preferences about tonics to improve the appetite. These are usually ordered 20 to 30 minutes before meals or may be given once or twice daily. Antiemetic drugs have a specific action on the vomiting center, and they may be given 20 minutes to half an hour before mealtimes or otherwise as ordered. Many people who are susceptible to motion sickness travel much more comfortably if they take an antiemetic medicine shortly before embarking on a plane trip or other journey. It is well to remember that these drugs usually produce some drowsiness as a side-effect.

Many people find the isolation of the sickroom lonely. They are much more likely to anticipate their meals with pleasure when they have pleasant company. Some hospitals have dining rooms where patients can eat together in a situation analogous to dining at home. For the patient at home or confined to bed in hospital, someone to chat with at mealtime often makes for a pleasant interlude that encourages the patient to eat.

Comfort and Hygiene Measures

The nurse can assist the vomiting patient by holding a curved basin (emesis basin) under his chin to catch the vomitus, and supporting his head and shoulders. Most people find it easier to vomit when they are in a sitting position with the head bent over the basin. If the patient is lying down, his head should be turned to one side and his body placed in a side-lying position if possible. Again, the head should be supported. The patient who is in a dorsal recumbent position can choke and aspirate vomitus unless his head is raised and supported so that the vomitus can drain out of the mouth. In postoperative vomiting, the patient will find it less painful if the nurse supports his incision with her hands while he vomits.

The nurse should stay with the patient while he is vomiting. Vomiting is an unpleasant experience. Not only is it physically distressing but there is a loss of control and dignity which most people find embarrassing. The nurse can do much to reassure the patient by a calm acceptance of the situation and sympathetic yet efficient ministrations. For the patient's own feelings of dignity, and because most people find it distressing to watch someone vomiting, the patient should be screened from the view of others. Curtains can be quickly drawn around the patient's bed, or the door of his room closed to ensure privacy.

While the patient is vomiting, the nurse should provide him with tissues and help him to wipe his mouth. After he has stopped vomiting, mouth care and a hand and face wash will help him to feel more comfortable and relaxed. Any linen that has been soiled should be changed. The room should be aired and the patient allowed to rest.

If the patient is unable to tolerate food

or fluids, frequent mouth care is essential to prevent complications (see Chapter 19).

Maintenance of Hydration and Nutritional Status

Helping the patient to maintain a satisfactory hydration and nutritional status is an important nursing function. Encouraging the individual to take fluids regularly helps him to attain adequate fluid intake. If he has difficulty in retaining fluids, giving him small amounts of fluid at frequent intervals is preferable to giving a large volume all at once. Patients who have been vomiting are usually permitted clear fluids only until vomiting subsides. Ginger ale and clear tea are frequently tolerated much better than other fluids when the stomach is upset. When other fluids are introduced into the patient's diet, those that are high in carbohydrate and protein are preferable because of the body's need for energy and tissue-building nutrients.

People who are anorectic or nauseated may become more so when confronted with large servings of food. Small portions, attractively served, are usually more appealing. It is often necessary to cater to the individual's particular food preferences to encourage him to eat. Patients should also be assisted with their meals if they are unable to manage alone. Today when hospital meals are frequently served by someone other than a nurse, it is perhaps more important than ever for the nurse to visit each patient at mealtime and offer whatever assistance is needed. All too often meals are left untouched or little is consumed because the patient could not cut his meat, butter his bread, or open one of the numerous cartons and containers that are used nowadays in meal service.

For patients who are unable to tolerate food and fluids by mouth or are taking an insufficient quantity, parenteral fluids may be prescribed. In some cases the patient is fed through a tube which is inserted into the stomach. This latter method of feeding is called a *gastric gavage*.

Many patients with gastrointestinal problems require gastric suction. This is a method of removing the gastric contents by means of suction apparatus. Patients on gastric suction are usually maintained with intravenous feedings to provide them with fluids and nourishment.

In some instances, it may be necessary to cleanse the stomach before further food and fluids can be taken, particularly if the individual has ingested some noxious substance. The procedure for washing out the stomach is called *gastric lavage*. This procedure is also frequently carried out prior to gastric surgery.

The description of a technique for carrying out each of these nursing measures is detailed below.

In maintaining fluid and electrolyte balance, the accurate recording and reporting of fluid intake and output is essential. Both parenteral and oral intake must be accurately assessed. The patient can often help in recording the amount of fluid he drinks. If the patient is receiving gastric tube feedings, the amount given must be recorded accurately. On the output side, the amount of emesis should be measured or estimated when measurement is not feasible. In addition, drainage and suction returns should be included in the total output.

When the patient is receiving supplementary fluids, such as intravenous or interstitial therapy, the nurse is also responsible for the care specific to this therapy (see Chapter 29).

Gastrointestinal Intubation. The primary reasons for the insertion of a tube into the stomach or the intestine are:

1. To establish a means of draining the stomach or intestine by suction; this is often done when a patient has an obstruction of the gastrointestinal tract or has undergone surgery of the tract

2. For diagnostic purposes—for example, to identify malignant cells or microorganisms such as the tubercle bacillus in the gastric washings

3. To aspirate the stomach contents, as when a person has taken poisonous materials

4. To establish a route for feeding the patient who is unable to take nourishment by mouth

KINDS OF TUBES. There are many kinds of tubes used for gastrointestinal intubation. The Miller-Abbott tube and the

Cantor tube are commonly used for decompression of the intestine. The *Miller-Abbott tube* has a double lumen and a weighted tip with a balloon attached. The tube is inserted by a physician into the stomach and passed through the pylorus into the intestine. Once it is positioned in the intestine, the balloon is blown up with air, and the tube is subsequently propelled onward by the peristaltic waves of the intestine. An adaptation of this tube is the addition of a bag containing 4 cc. of mercury, which weights the tube and facilitates its passage into the small intestine. The modified tube is called the *Harris tube.*

The *Cantor tube* also has a bag of mercury at its tip. It is a single lumen tube with a number of holes on the sides which allow suction to be applied along the intestinal tract.

The *Levin tube* is commonly used for gastric intubation. The tip of the tube is solid, but there are several holes on the side. It is normally passed through the nose of the patient into his stomach. The insertion of a Levin tube is usually the physician's responsibility; however, when there is no gastric disease and the patient is conscious, the nurse often inserts the Levin tube.

THE INSERTION OF A LEVIN TUBE. Before the insertion of a Levin tube, the procedure is explained to the patient. Not only do most patients want to know how they can help, but explanations frequently allay fear. The passage of a tube is painless, but it sometimes stimulates the gag reflex as it passes over the nasopharyngeal area. If the patient breathes deeply at the first sign of gagging, he is less likely to become nauseated and vomit.

In the preparation of the equipment, the rubber Levin tube is placed in a bowl of chipped ice. This makes the tube more rigid (because cold causes contraction) and thus more easily directed on insertion. It also lubricates the tube. Usually a plastic Levin tube is sufficiently rigid for insertion, but it must also be lubricated with water.

In addition to the ice and the Levin tube, a protective covering, a kidney basin, tissues, a syringe, a cup, a straw, and a stethoscope (optional) are required.

The syringe is used to withdraw the stomach's contents after the Levin tube has been inserted. This also determines that the tube is positioned in the stomach. The cup and straw are to give the patient a drink of water to facilitate swallowing the tube.

If it is possible, the patient assumes Fowler's position. In this position the passage of the tube is facilitated by the pull of gravity; it also makes it easier for the patient to spit out vomitus if this becomes necessary during the insertion of the tube.

The kidney basin and tissues are required because the patient may vomit. As noted previously, stimulation of the glossopharyngeal nerve endings in the posterior pharynx transmits impulses to the vomiting center in the medulla of the brain.

As a guide to the distance to which the tube is to be inserted, the nurse measures the distance from the patient's nose to an earlobe and then to the umbilicus. This distance is roughly equal to the distance from the lips to the stomach. The nurse then marks this distance on the tube with a piece of adhesive tape.

As a lubricant for the Levin tube, water has two advantages: (1) it moistens the tube and thus permits smoother passage of the tube over the mucous membranes, and (2) if the tube enters the lungs, the water is not likely to become a focus of irritation. Some agencies suggest that a water-soluble lubricant be used; such lubricants are less dangerous to the lungs than oil base lubricants.

The Levin tube is never forced upon encountering an obstruction. Not only is force unpleasant to the patient, but the mucous membrane that lines the gastrointestinal tract is easily damaged and provides a likely site for infection.

To facilitate the passage of the tube, the patient is given a mouthful of water to swallow as the tube is inserted into the esophagus. Swallowing helps to pass the tube down the esophagus into the patient's stomach by setting up peristaltic waves.

The stomach is never empty; it always contains at least a little gastric juice, which is secreted by the glands in the walls of the stomach. Therefore the position of the tube can be ascertained by aspirating with the syringe. The obtaining of gastric contents verifies that the tube is positioned in the patient's stomach. If gastric juice cannot be obtained, the following tests should be performed:

Place the free end of the tube in a container of water. Rhythmic bubbling usually indicates that the tube is in the patient's lungs.

Hold the end of the tube to the ear. A crackling sound usually indicates that the tube is in the patient's lungs.

Ask the patient to hum. If the tube is in the patient's lungs he will not be able to do this.

Another technique is to inject a small amount of air with the syringe and then listen to the epigastrium with a stethoscope.

If the patient coughs during the insertion of a tube, it should be removed immediately. Cyanosis and dyspnea often indicate that the tube has entered the trachea. Once it has been ascertained that the Levin tube is in the patient's stomach, the tube is secured to the patient's face with a small piece of adhesive tape.

THE IRRIGATION OF A LEVIN TUBE. The purpose of the irrigation of a Levin tube is to wash the lumen of the tube in order to maintain a clear passage. Usually this is not a sterile procedure unless the patient has just had stomach surgery. (If the patient has had surgery, it is important to maintain aseptic technique in all procedures involving the operative area.) The order to irrigate the Levin tube is issued by the physician. Irrigations are ordered for regular intervals, or they are done only when the tube becomes blocked. In either case it is important to watch the patient closely and note whether the tube becomes occluded. If the patient is on gastric suction, the most obvious sign of blockage is a lack of gastric returns from the tube. In addition, the patient is likely to feel uncomfortable and his abdomen will be distended.

After the nurse has provided the explanation that the patient requires and has reassured him that this is a painless measure, she assembles the necessary equipment. She requires a syringe, usually a 20 cc. or 30 cc. syringe, or an Asepto syringe; the irrigating solution specifically designated by the physician (often water or

normal saline), and a receptacle for the returned irrigation fluid.

Between 15 and 30 cc. of fluid is injected into the tube before the plunger is gently drawn back to withdraw the fluid. Because the mucous membrane lining of the stomach is easily damaged, the fluid is injected and withdrawn very gently. This measure is repeated until the tube is cleared. If fresh blood appears as a result of the irrigating, the measure is terminated and the information is reported to the physician. During the irrigation the nurse observes the color and consistency of the returning fluid. This is recorded on the patient's chart.

Gastric Suction. The purpose of gastric suction is to remove the contents of the patient's stomach. It is indicated as a measure to prevent or relieve distention and vomiting, to remove blood postoperatively, and to remove the stomach contents of patients who have gastrointestinal obstructions. It may also be used as a measure to cleanse the stomach prior to gastric surgery.

Generally speaking, there are two types of gastric suction: continuous and intermittent. Continuous suction is applied continuously; intermittent suction is turned on and off as the patient requires or, usually, on the physician's order.

There are four basic ways of supplying suction. First, there is the electric suction machine, which is a portable machine that can be brought to the patient. It is run by electricity and the amount of suction can usually be regulated. The second method of supplying suction is by means of suction apparatus built into the wall. Many modern hospitals have suction outlets at the head of the patient's bed. The pressure of these systems can also be regulated by the nursing personnel.

The third method of supplying suction is by the use of the principle of displacement of water. Systems based on this method do not require electricity and are simple to construct. There are both two- and three-bottle systems. Simply explained, the water falls by gravity from bottle *B* to bottle *A* (see the accompanying illustration). This creates a vacuum in bottle *B*. If bottle *B* is connected directly to the patient's gastric tube, the vacuum is transmitted to his stomach, with the result

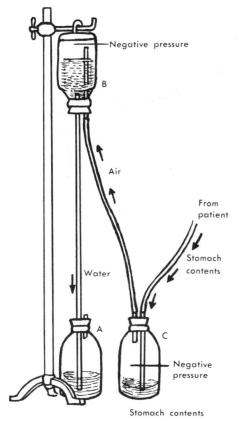

The water displacement method of producing suction.

portant part of the patient's fluid output, the nurse measures the amount of drainage accurately, and she notes the clarity, color, and consistency of the drainage. These observations are reported on the patient's record. Any untoward changes in the patient's suction returns, such as bright red returns, or in the patient's condition, such as an accelerated pulse, are reported promptly so that the physician can be notified.

Gastric Lavage. Gastric lavage is the washing out of the stomach. It is done prior to some types of gastric surgery and as a means of removing noxious substances which have been ingested. The latter is often an emergency procedure, carried out in the emergency department of the hospitals or in the doctor's office.

For a gastric lavage a special tube frequently is used. It has a larger lumen than the Levin tube, and it may have a funnel at one end to facilitate the administration of the fluid for washing the patient's stomach. Because the lavage tube has a larger lumen than the Levin tube, it is usually inserted through the patient's mouth into his stomach by the physician. When a Levin tube is used, it can be inserted through the patient's nose or through his mouth.

The equipment required for a gastric lavage consists of the lavage tube and funnel, the solution ordered by the physician, a pail to receive stomach contents, ice in which to place the tube (see *Gastrointestinal Intubation*), a kidney basin for vomitus, and a protective covering for the patient.

The physician usually administers 500 cc. of solution into the patient's stomach, and he then inverts the funnel to allow the stomach's contents to empty into the pail. To create a siphon, the tube is pinched while some of the fluid is still in it, and then it is lowered and inverted below the level of the patient's body and held inside the pail. Gravity drains the fluid from the tubing, and the vacuum thus established in the tubing draws the liquid from the patient's stomach. The washing is repeated until the physician considers that the stomach is satisfactorily cleansed.

During the lavage the nurse notes the reaction of the patient, the amount and

that the stomach's contents flow to bottle *B*, that is, from a high pressure area to a low pressure area. If, on the other hand, bottle *B* is connected to bottle *C*, and bottle *C* is connected to the patient's gastric tube, the stomach contents will be received in bottle *C*.

A fourth means of supplying suction is by the Gomco Thermotic pump, which is electrically operated but is motorless. This pump provides intermittent suction through the alternate contraction and expansion of air.

When a patient requires gastric suction, he will probably find the gastric tube irritating to his throat, and it is likely that he will not be able to take fluids by mouth. Therefore, he requires special care for his mouth and nose so that they do not become dry, cracked, and subsequently infected. To ease the irritation by the tube on the patient's throat, the physician may order anesthetic lozenges.

Since gastric suction returns are an im-

kind of solution used, and the amount, color, and consistency of the returns. These observations are reported in the patient's record. Following gastric lavage, the patient usually needs a mouthwash.

Gastric Gavage. A gastric gavage is a feeding given to a patient through a tube which is inserted either through his nose or through his mouth into his stomach. It is done when the patient is unable to take food orally. The feeding can be given in two ways: at intervals ordered by the physician (for example, every four hours), or as a continuous drip over the 24 hour period. The latter method is usually indicated when the patient has diarrhea, gastric irritability, or a reflex bowel disturbance.

The food used for a gavage feeding is usually given as a thick liquid. A typical tube feeding might include powdered milk, cream, cereal, strained meats and vegetables, orange juice, corn oil, sugar, iodized salt, vitamin compounds, and water. The feeding may be made up using different amounts of various nutrients in order to meet the patient's dietary needs.

It is the physician's responsibility to order the type of nourishment that the patient requires. In some health agencies a regular house diet is mixed in a blending machine so that it can be fed by gavage tube.

Often the patient who is to receive a gavage feeding has a Levin tube already inserted. If this is not the case, the physician usually inserts the tube (see *Gastrointestinal Intubation*). The nurse explains to the patient that feeding through the tube is painless and will provide him with adequate water and nourishment.

The nurse heats the feeding to room temperature. Sometimes the physician requests that the stomach be aspirated prior to a new feeding to determine if the food is being passed into the intestinal tract. Before commencing the feeding the nurse should raise the head of the bed, unless this is contraindicated. She then injects a small amount of water into the tube to make sure that the lumen is clear. A disposable feeding bag may be used or the feeding may be injected by syringe. If a disposable bag is used it may be hung on an intravenous standard, and the rate of flow adjusted as desired. If the syringe method is used, care is taken to allow as little air as possible to be injected into the patient's stomach. The feeding should always be given slowly. Usually the gavage feeding flows through the tubing by gravitational force; however, if it does not do this readily, slight pressure can be applied on the plunger of the syringe. After the completion of the feeding, a small amount of water is again inserted into the tubing in order to clear the lumen of the tube of the gavage feeding. This prevents souring of any formula in the tube. Some patients learn to administer their own gavage feedings.

The nurse records the amount of the gavage feeding that the patient has taken, as well as the amount of water that was administered. Should the patient start to gag or vomit during the gavage feeding, the feeding is terminated, and the situation is reported to the physician and recorded in the patient's record.

If the patient is to have a continuous gavage, a Baron food pump or a burette (glass or plastic container) and tubing may be used. The burette is hung to the side of the patient at a level just above him. The nurse adjusts the rate of flow of the gavage feeding as the physician has ordered. She also maintains a level of gavage fluid in the burette. The patient is observed at frequent intervals for any untoward signs resulting from the feeding.

Hyperalimentation. When the body is seriously depleted of nutrients, it is often necessary to replace these by giving more than optimal amounts. If the person is unable to take these orally, they are frequently given by intravenous infusion. The term "parenteral hyperalimentation," often referred to simply as "hyperalimentation," is used for the intravenous administration of such nutrients as amino acids, dextrose, fructose, and so forth. The subject of hyperalimentation is usually covered in detail in courses in medical-surgical nursing, and the student will learn more about it in these courses.

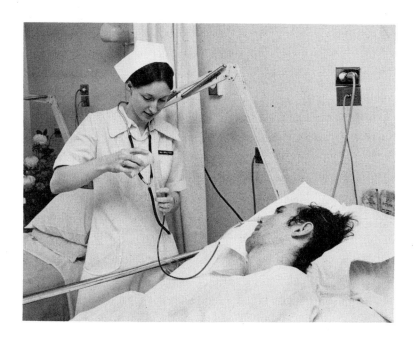

A gastric gavage or tube feeding is frequently given when the patient is unable to take food orally.

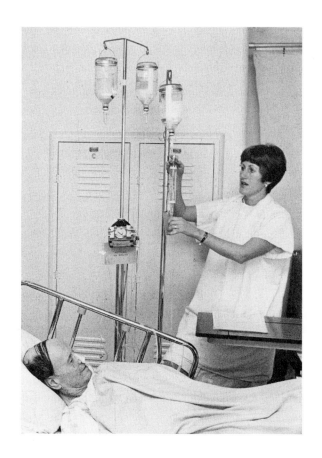

Hyperalimentation is a method of giving large amounts of nutrients via the intravenous route to patients whose nutritional reserves have been seriously depleted.

GUIDE TO
ASSESSING FOR
ANOREXIA,
NAUSEA, AND
VOMITING

1. What is the nature of the patient's problem? Is he anorectic, nauseated, or has he been vomiting?
2. How long has he had this problem? Is it related to a specific cause, such as particular foods, medications, or stressful situations?
3. Does the patient have other distressing symptoms, such as headache or pain?
4. If the patient is vomiting, what is the nature of the vomitus? its amount? How often does he vomit?
5. How much food and fluid is the patient taking?
6. Does he show signs of poor nutritional status? of dehydration?
7. Have specific laboratory tests been ordered? If so, what are the nurse's responsibilities relative to these? What learning needs does the patient have with regard to them?
8. Have specific diagnostic or therapeutic measures been prescribed? If so, what is the nurse's responsibility relative to these? What are the patient's learning needs with regard to these?
9. Are there factors in the environment which contribute to the patient's discomfort? Can these be modified?
10. What nursing measures can contribute to the patient's comfort and hygiene?

GUIDE TO
EVALUATING THE
EFFECTIVENESS OF
NURSING
INTERVENTION

1. Is the patient comfortable?
2. Is he obtaining adequate food and fluids for his nutritional needs?
3. Do laboratory tests reflect adequate hydration? For example, does the level of blood chlorides and blood pH indicate electrolyte balance, and does the specific gravity of the urine indicate hydration?
4. Have the distressing symptoms been alleviated? That is, has vomiting stopped? Is nausea less troublesome? Is the patient beginning to regain his appetite?

STUDY
VOCABULARY

Anorexia	Hunger	Projectile vomiting
Appetite	Hypochloremia	Retching
Cachectic	Hypoglycemia	Vertigo
Emesis	Nausea	Vomitus

STUDY SITUATION

Mrs. W. Stanley had her appendix removed three days ago. Since she returned from the operating room, she has been nauseated continually and vomits after every meal. Mrs. Stanley says she has severe pain in her operative area, and she is reluctant to eat and to get out of bed. The doctor has ordered that she get up and walk to the bathroom at least three times a day and that she eat a normal diet, with adequate fluids in between meals.

1. What are the possible reasons for this patient's nausea and vomiting?
2. What nursing interventions might alleviate her?
3. What specific observations should the nurse make about the patient?

4. When the patient says she does not want to get out of bed, what should the nurse do?
5. How could the nurse possibly increase Mrs. Stanley's appetite?
6. What dangers and complications can be concomitant with vomiting?
7. By what criteria can the nurse evaluate the effectiveness of her nursing care?
8. What is an adequate intake of fluid for this patient, and how could you best gain her cooperation in taking this amount?

SUGGESTED READINGS

Armer, D.: Two Students Study Opposite Ends of the Weight Problem... Anorexia Nervosa. Part 1. *Journal of Practical Nursing, 25*:18–19, February 1975.

Baldwin, W.: Anorexia Nervosa. *Nursing Times, 71*:134–135, January 23, 1974.

Melton, J. H.: A Boy With Anorexia Nervosa. *American Journal of Nursing, 74*:1649–1651, September 1974.

Naish, J.: Discomfort After Food. *Nursing Times, 71*:2060–2062, December 25, 1975.

Schmidt, M. P. W., et al.: Modifying Eating Behavior in Anorexia Nervosa. *American Journal of Nursing, 74*:1646–1648, September 1974.

Snell, B., et al.: Whetting Hospitalized Preschoolers' Appetites. *American Journal of Nursing, 76*:413–415, March 1976.

When Vomiting Signals a Geriatric Emergency. *Nursing Update, 6*:12–13, June 1975.

27 CONSTIPATION AND DIARRHEA

The nurse should be able to:

Discuss the importance of adequate normal fecal elimination to
    the health and well-being of the individual
Discuss normal and abnormal functioning in regard to fecal
    elimination
Discuss factors which may cause disturbances in bowel function-
    ing
Assess a patient's status in regard to fecal elimination
Identify situations requiring immediate nursing intervention in
    the care of patients with problems of bowel functioning
Apply relevant principles in planning and implementing nursing
    interventions for problems of bowel functioning, including
    measures to:
    reestablish normal bowel functioning
    relieve distressing symptoms
    maintain fluid and electrolyte balance
    maintain adequate nutritional status
    maintain comfort and hygiene
Evaluate the effectiveness of nursing intervention

CONSTIPATION AND DIARRHEA 27

INTRODUCTION

The other side of the problem of disturbed functioning of the gastrointestinal tract is interference with the elimination of wastes from the tract. Elimination is, of course, as vital to the healthy functioning of the human body as the intake of food and fluids.

The human body has four mechanisms for the removal of waste products: from the gastrointestinal tract as feces, from the urinary tract as urine, through the lungs in expired air, and through the skin as perspiration. Each mechanism has its specific function in clearing the body of wastes resulting from the processing of nutrients and their subsequent utilization in the cells. Wastes eliminated from the gastrointestinal tract contain primarily the food residues and gases that result from the digestion of food.

Interference with the normal functioning of gastrointestinal elimination has serious repercussions on the body's total functioning. The individual is usually uncomfortable and often distressed. If normal functioning is not restored all body systems will eventually be affected. Complete stoppage of bowel functioning is a medical emergency and surgical intervention is usually necessary to overcome the problem.

Constipation is a very common problem among normal, otherwise healthy people. Diarrhea is a frequent manifestation of stress, as we discussed in Chapter 12 on anxiety. Bacterial diarrheas are a part of the problem of gastroenteritis, which we mentioned in the last chapter. The loss of essential nutrients and electrolytes by this route makes the problem one of major significance. It is particularly serious in infants and young children, whose nutritional reserves can soon be depleted by excessive losses from the gastrointestinal tract.

NORMAL AND ABNORMAL BOWEL FUNCTIONING

Diarrhea and constipation are abnormal variations in the evacuation of feces. Diarrhea is the discharge of loose, watery stools due to excess rapidity in the passage of waste products of digestion through the gastrointestinal tract. Constipation is the passage of hard, dry stools due to undue delay in the evacuation of feces.

The variation in the consistency of feces is explained by the fact that as the waste products of digestion pass through the large intestine, water is absorbed from them. Consequently, the consistency of the stool depends to a certain extent on the length of time the food is in the gastrointestinal tract. Normal feces consist of approximately three-fourths water and one-fourth solid materials. In diarrhea, the feces are soft and watery, whereas in constipation, the feces usually have increased solid content.

There is a wide variation in the normal frequency of evacuation of waste products; consequently diarrhea and constipation must be considered in relation to a person's normal habit. The person who has four or five bowel movements in one day is not necessarily suffering from diarrhea, nor is the person who has one bowel

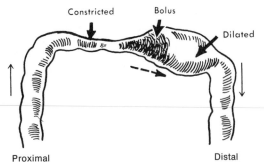

Constricted   Bolus   Dilated

Proximal   Distal

Waste products pass through the large bowel as shown here.

movement every three days necessarily suffering from constipation.

During the process of digestion, waste products pass through the large intestine in wavelike propulsions called *peristalsis.* In this movement, the part of the colon that is distal to the bolus (waste products) relaxes while the portion of the colon that is proximal to the bolus contracts. Thus, the waste products are propelled forward. Peristalsis occurs in the large intestine at infrequent intervals. It is stimulated by the intake of food and fluids into the gastrointestinal tract. Usually the food or fluid remains in the entire tract from eight to 72 hours after ingestion. When the food enters the duodenum, approximately a half hour after ingestion, there is a mass peristaltic action in the large intestine called the gastrocolic reflex. This is an opportune time for defecation.

Although the rectal reflex is stimulated by the presence of waste products in the rectum, the act of defecation itself is controlled voluntarily. Therefore, a person may or may not respond to the stimulus. If he ignores the urge to defecate and the waste products remain within the rectum, he may become constipated. In some patients, spinal cord injuries destroy the rectal reflex, which is normally transmitted from the rectum to the sacral area by the parasympathetic nerves. These patients may also lose control of the voluntary muscles concerned with defecation. With special training, however, they can often achieve a certain regularity of bowel habits.

The large intestine, in addition to having its own intrinsic innervation, also responds to stimulation of the sympathetic and parasympathetic nervous systems. The parasympathetic nerves promote peristalsis and increase muscle tone; the sympathetic nerves inhibit peristalsis and decrease muscle tone. Consequently, emotions may affect the functioning of the bowels. For example, anxiety may be mediated either through the parasympathetic nerves, with resultant diarrhea, or through the sympathetic nerves, with resultant constipation. This helps to explain the role of emotions as contributing or causative agents in diarrhea and constipation.

FACTORS AFFECTING BOWEL FUNCTIONING

Constipation

Any factor that causes undue delay in the passage of feces is a cause of constipation. *A breakdown in the conditioned reflex for defecation* is by far the most common. In man, the act of defecation is under voluntary control and is conditioned to time and activity. When the urge to defecate is overcome by voluntary muscle contraction, the rectum adjusts itself to the increased tension or may even return stools to the sigmoid. If this is habitually done, the normal conditioned reflex is lost. This may be due to habits developed in early childhood or to failure on the part of adults to respond to the normal defecation urge because of the pressures of time and daily activities. Pain on defecation, such as that associated with hemorrhoids or rectal surgery, will also interfere with the normal conditioned reflex. *Hemorrhoids* are enlarged veins in the rectal area.

Another common cause of constipation is *excessive tone of the circular muscle of the intestines*, which is thought to be due to an imbalance of the autonomic nervous system. Strong emotions, as discussed earlier, are believed to cause constipation through the increased production of epinephrine, with resulting inhibition of peristalsis. Some drugs, among them morphine and to a lesser extent codeine, decrease motility in the small intestine and the colon because of their action on the central nervous system. Constipation may also result from injury to or diseases of the central nervous system.

Disturbances in reflex peristalsis may be due simply to the lack of sufficient fluids or bulky foods in the diet. An inadequate intake of foods such as cereals and vegetables may result in insufficient bulk in the residue of waste products to stimulate the reflex for defecation. The excessive use of laxatives may cause constipation, due to overstimulation of the bowel and a "wearing-out" (accommodation) effect on the nerves initiating the reflex action. People who habitually use laxatives frequently have to change the type taken to overcome this effect. Disease processes, such as inflammation of the pelvic or abdominal viscera, or tumors, may also cause a disturbance in reflex peristalsis.

Mechanical disturbances that can also cause constipation include weakness of the intestinal muscles as a result of disease processes, old age, or lack of essential vitamins (notably the B group) or electrolytes (particularly potassium). Weakness of the voluntary muscles controlling defecation may also cause constipation. The abdominal, the pelvic, and the diaphragmatic muscles are all important in initiating and completing defecation. Weakness in any of these will make defecation difficult. Obstruction in any part of the gastrointestinal tract will also delay or prevent the passage of feces. Obstruction may be caused by disease processes or may be the result of congenital abnormalities.

Diarrhea

The causes of diarrhea are numerous. Some diarrheas are due to *direct stimulation or irritation of the central or autonomic nervous system*. Diarrhea resulting from tension is an example. Diarrhea may be the most obvious manifestation of anxiety in a stable individual. Pre-examination diarrhea is a fairly common occurrence among students, as is pre-battle diarrhea among soldiers. Certain drugs, as, for example, reserpine (used for the treatment of hypertension), may also cause hypermotility of the intestine by acting on the autonomic nervous system, with resultant diarrhea.

Probably the most common set of causes of diarrhea, however, is the group due to *irritation of the gastrointestinal tract*. These result in a reflex type of diarrhea, the reverse of the mechanism that occurs in constipation. The irritation may be mechanical, as that caused by dietary indiscretions such as eating coarse foods or an excessive amount of seasonings; it may be chemical, as in some food and drug poisonings; or it may be, in some individuals, an allergic reaction to certain foods. Shellfish is a well-known allergen to many people. Inflammation of the intestinal mucosa due to pathogenic infection is a very common cause of diarrhea. It is believed that the diarrhea experienced by many international travelers is caused by changes in the normal bacterial flora of the colon. Certain drugs, termed cathartics, cause formation of loose stools through irritation of the intestinal mucosa.

There are a few conditions producing diarrhea which may be considered to be *defects in the anatomical processes necessary for defecation*. Some disease conditions may cause an increase in the neuromuscular excitability of the intestine. Certain "malabsorption syndromes" also exist, in which the problem is one of failure on the part of the intestines to reabsorb water as the digestive products pass through it.

ASSESSING FECAL ELIMINATION STATUS

In assessing the patient with problems of constipation or diarrhea, it is essential to know if the condition is acute or chronic. Initially the nurse needs to know about the bowel habits and the normal patterns of defecation of the individual. People vary in their frequency of defecation, and what is normal for one person may not be normal for another.

A knowledge of the patient's pattern of fecal elimination includes the frequency of defecation and a description of the consistency of stools (hard, soft, liquid), as well as their color and odor. Feces may contain foreign matter which the patient may be able to describe, such as blood, worms, pus, or mucus. Most people become anxious if they think there is blood in the stools. Black stools may indicate the presence of old blood, and red stools, fresh blood; however, certain foods and medications can also discolor feces. For example, beets can color feces red and iron (in a medication) can color feces black.

The nurse should also determine whether the patient takes laxatives regularly and, if so, what medications are used. It is not uncommon for some people to give themselves a daily enema if they are habitually constipated. On the other hand, some people feel that a "good purge" or "cleaning out" every once in a while is beneficial to the system, and they will use a strong cathartic for this purpose, even if they are not constipated.

Food habits are also pertinent in assessing the needs of the patient with constipation or diarrhea. Failure to ensure that the diet has sufficient bulk may lead to constipation. The ingestion of irritating foods may cause diarrhea. It is important to know then what the individual's dietary intake has been in the immediate past and also what his normal food habits are.

Since emotions play such an important role in the causation of many cases of diarrhea and constipation, it is helpful to determine if the patient has been under any particular stress.

Much of this information will have been gathered during the taking of the nursing history and the initial clinical appraisal. The nurse also needs to be aware of the nature of any health problems the patient has which may affect bowel functioning, and of the physician's plans of care for the patient. She supplements these data with her observations.

Subjective Observations

Control over defecation and urination is taught in early childhood and may be associated with values of good and bad. In some cultures, control over bladder and bowel functioning is expected early, and there may be much tension and anxiety associated with the early teaching. Moreover, lack of control over urination or defecation represents a loss of independence.

Many people are embarrassed to talk about their elimination problems. In discussing these problems, then, the nurse should ensure privacy, since it is often difficult for patients to talk about their bowel habits in the presence of other people. The nurse, too, may find it hard to ask the personal questions that are necessary. Questions should be phrased in simple, nontechnical language that assists the patient to give pertinent information in his answers and yet maintain his own feelings of personal dignity in doing so.

The constipated patient may complain of headache, or state that he has a bloated feeling, anorexia (loss of appetite), or nausea. The person with diarrhea often complains of pain, and it is important to find out whether it is generalized abdominal pain or pain of a spasmodic, gripping nature.

Flatus results from swallowed air, the consumption of gas-forming foods, or bacterial action within the large intestine. The air accumulates in the intestine and often causes generalized discomfort and crampy pain. The patient who is constipated may also complain of headache, nausea, and anorexia. These usually disappear upon evacuation of the rectal contents.

Another frequent complaint of the constipated patient is that of *tenesmus,* that is, frequent painful straining in attempts at defecation which are unproductive of stool. If the stool remains in the rectum for a long period of time, it may develop into a large, hardened mass which is difficult to expel. Sometimes there is seepage around the mass, with a resultant discharge of small amounts of liquid stool. This is important to remember, particularly in bedridden patients, because there is the possibility that constipation may be overlooked when it has been noted that the patient has had a bowel movement.

The person who has diarrhea often complains of generalized abdominal pain. This is usually caused by flatus, which distends the large and small intestines. He may also have pains of a piercing, gripping nature. These are usually spasmodic and are caused by the strong peristaltic contractions of the intestinal musculature as the waste products are propelled precipitously through the gastrointestinal tract. These pains are frequently accompanied by a feeling of urgency in the need to defecate. Although frequency in the number of stools is not always an indication of diarrhea, it often occurs with diarrhea. Again, as in constipation, there may be frequent, painful straining, which in the case of the patient with diarrhea may produce a small watery discharge rather than formed stool.

Objective Observations

The patient with constipation may not be able to communicate his discomfort verbally to the nurse. She should, therefore, be alert to the signs and symptoms that indicate this discomfort. The patient may have had no bowel movement for several days; he may have abdominal distention, and he may be passing large amounts of flatus by rectum or by mouth. The hospitalized patient is particularly prone to constipation because of lack of exercise and the alterations in daily activity and, often, in diet that are imposed by being confined to hospital. These interfere with the normal conditioned reflex for defecation.

In observing the feces of the constipated patient, it is important to note consistency, color, size, shape, and odor of the fecal matter. The presence of foreign matter, as described earlier, should also be noted.

The person who is constipated may exhibit signs and symptoms other than the passage of hardened feces. Abdominal distention when the bolus remains in the large intestine is frequently apparent in patients who are constipated. The distention is caused by the air which remains in the large intestine and the fluid which moves back into the large intestine when the waste products have been there for a long time. These two, air and fluid, result in abdominal distention. The patient appears to have a swollen abdomen which on palpation feels hard and unyielding.

Pertinent observations in the case of the patient with diarrhea include the frequency and consistency of the stools, as well as their odor and the presence of foreign matter. Undigested food is sometimes present in the feces because of the speed with which it is propelled through the gastrointestinal tract. If the diarrhea is prolonged, the patient will show signs and symptoms of fluid and electrolyte loss. They include poor tissue turgor, weight loss, and thirst. The patient with prolonged diarrhea may appear thin and emaciated. He complains of fatigue, weakness, and general malaise. Nausea and vomiting frequently accompany diarrhea and further aggravate the loss of fluids and electrolytes.

It is essential that an accurate record of the patient's intake and output be maintained. This will include the number of bowel movements and the approximate amount of fluid lost through the feces. The nurse should also note the patient's ability to tolerate foods and fluids. It is very important to determine the patient's nutritional status and to observe signs of weakness and fatigue. Signs of localized irritation around the anus may be present. These include redness and pruritus (itching), which add to the patient's discomfort.

Diagnostic Tests

Among the diagnostic tests for diarrhea and constipation is the laboratory examination of a specimen of feces. It is often the responsibility of nursing personnel to collect the specimen and send it to the laboratory, where it is examined for such substances as blood, microorganisms, fat, undigested food, or *urobilin*. Blood from the lower gastrointestinal tract is usually bright red, whereas old blood from the upper tract may appear black. On the other hand, blood may be present but *occult*, that is, hidden to the naked eye.

In order to identify infectious agents such as parasites which may be present in the gastrointestinal tract, it is not necessary to keep the specimen warm unless mobile forms (for example, amebae) are suspected. Ova and cysts can be identified in cold specimens.

Excess fat in the stools can be indicative of gastrointestinal disease, as can the presence of undigested food and urobilin. Normally there is a considerable amount

PRINCIPLES RELEVANT TO CONSTIPATION AND DIARRHEA

1. Normal fecal elimination is essential to efficient body functioning.
2. The body's fluid and electrolyte balance can be seriously affected by disturbances in fecal elimination.
3. The act of defecation is normally under voluntary control.
4. The oral intake of food and fluids can stimulate the gastrocolic reflex.
5. Control of defecation is an important area of independence to most individuals.
6. Strong emotions can affect the functioning of the gastrointestinal tract.

of the latter in feces, but in cases of an obstruction in bile flow the feces may be clay-colored and negative for urobilin.

X-ray and fluoroscopic examinations of the gastrointestinal tract may also be necessary (see Chapter 23).

Sigmoidoscopy is the inspection of the sigmoid portion of the colon with a lighted instrument. After enemas are given, the patient assumes the knee-chest position and the physician inserts the sigmoidoscope in order to visualize the lining of the sigmoid. Usually this examination is embarrassing and uncomfortable. The nurse can assist the patient by draping him comfortably and assuring him that the discomfort is of short duration.

PRIORITIES FOR NURSING ACTION

In determining priorities for nursing action in the care of patients with either diarrhea or constipation, the nurse must take into account the acuteness of the condition. In the severely constipated patient, there may be an immediate need to end the patient's discomfort through bringing about a bowel movement. With the patient who is acutely distressed with diarrhea, nursing intervention will be directed first toward controlling the discharge of stools. There may also be an urgent need to replace lost fluids and electrolytes.

GOALS FOR NURSING ACTION

The basic goals of nursing action in the care of patients with constipation or diarrhea are:

1. Reestablishment of normal bowel functioning
2. Relief of distressing symptoms
3. Maintenance of fluid and electrolyte balance
4. Maintenance of adequate nutritional status
5. Maintenance of comfort and hygiene

SPECIFIC NURSING INTERVENTIONS

Measures to Reestablish Normal Fecal Elimination

Constipation. Constipation is a problem for many people, both sick and well. It is almost always a problem for patients confined to bed, and care should be taken to direct nursing action toward its prevention in patients who are ill. Because bowel and bladder habits are learned early in childhood and each individual's pattern of elimination is different, the nurse should develop a plan of care in conjunction with the patient, taking into consideration the individual's previously established pattern.

Important factors to consider in preventing constipation or in overcoming a long-standing problem of constipation include: regularity of time for defecation, prompt attention to the urge to defecate, a diet that contains sufficient laxative foods as well as a sufficient intake of fluids, and exercise.

The gastrocolic reflex is stimulated by mass peristaltic action which occurs most frequently after meals and is usually strongest after breakfast. Immediately after the morning meal is therefore a good time to encourage the patient to move his bowels. Affording the patient privacy is important. Sufficient time should be allowed for the process, and the patient should not be hurried. If his condition permits, the individual should be allowed to go to the lavatory to have a bowel movement or to use a bedside commode. Most patients find it awkward to use a bedpan to have a bowel movement. If a bedpan has to be used, the patient should be in a sitting position unless this position is contraindicated.

The patient may need to be helped to increase his sensitivity to the stimulus for defecation. Providing hot fluids helps to activate mass peristalsis, and some people find that a cup of hot tea or coffee, or a glass of hot water (some like hot water with lemon) taken before breakfast helps to stimulate the rectal reflex. The patient should be given an explanation of the process of elimination with stress placed on the importance of responding to the urge to defecate. The individual can sometimes be helped to defecate by massaging the abdomen in a circular motion, moving downward over the descending colon on the left side of the abdomen. Slight pressure on the side of, or posterior to, the anus sometimes helps expel feces. Nursing personnel use cotton gauze or digital pads for this measure.

Through repetition of these measures at the same time each day or as frequently as the patient is in the habit of having a bowel movement, regular habits can often be established. Glycerin suppositories or enemas are also used in some situations to facilitate defecation, particularly when regularity is being established. Their use is then gradually withdrawn as a regular pattern is set. Laxative drugs and stool softeners, such as mineral oil, may also be used sometimes to help in developing regularity, their use again being gradually terminated as the patient gains improved colonic functioning.

The individual may require help also in establishing dietary patterns that give him a sufficient amount of laxative foods and adequate fluids for normal bowel functioning. Fluid intake, it is usually suggested, should be 2000 cc. to 3000 cc. per 24 hour period. The diet should contain sufficient bulk to stimulate reflex activity, as well as other foods which the individual finds have a laxative effect on him. Usually, fruits and fruit juices in sufficient quantity have the desired effect. Prunes and prune juice have particularly good laxative effects.

Constipation is aggravated by inactivity and poor muscle tone. A regular program of activity designed for the individual can be planned and the patient assisted to carry it out. Strengthening of the abdominal muscles is particularly important.

Bowel training for patients with spinal cord injuries or for patients who are incontinent of feces for other reasons may be accomplished through systematic and repeated efforts, using the methods just described. Many agencies have developed their own specific regimen for bladder and bowel retraining, and descriptions of some of these may be found in the recent nursing literature. Articles on the subject are included in the *Suggested Readings* at the end of the chapter.

Diarrhea. In attempting to reestablish normal bowel functioning in the patient with diarrhea, it is important to know the cause of the diarrhea. The most common cause is irritation of the gastrointestinal tract; removal of the irritant will in most cases therefore stop the symptoms. If the diarrhea is psychological in origin (for example, if it is caused by anxiety or tension), it will often disappear when the stressful situation is over. If, however, it is a chronic problem, medical intervention is usually necessary to help the patient to resolve his problems. Some diarrheas are the result of defects in the anatomical processes necessary for defecation. These conditions require medical therapy.

Measures to Relieve Distressing Symptoms

Patients who suffer from constipation or diarrhea are uncomfortable. They often have distressing symptoms accompanying their condition such as abdominal distention, excess flatus, and pain (see the section on signs and symptoms earlier in the chapter).

The constipated patient is usually relieved of his discomfort and concomitant distressing symptoms when a satisfactory bowel movement is effected. This may be brought about by the administration of a laxative or by the use of a rectal suppository, an enema, or a colonic irrigation. At times, manual extraction of feces is necessary. If laxatives are ordered, these are usually given at bedtime so that they will act after breakfast the following morning.

Medications to coat and soothe the lining of the intestines (emulsive drugs) or to reduce muscular spasm (antispasmodic) are often prescribed for patients with diarrhea. Some of these drugs are taken at regular intervals during the day; others are taken after each bowel movement. If the diarrhea is caused by an infectious agent, appropriate therapy to combat the infection is prescribed by the physician.

Relief of abdominal distention and excess flatus can often be accomplished through the insertion of a rectal tube. Sometimes an enema may be ordered for this purpose also.

The Enema. An enema is the injection of fluid into the rectum. Generally its purpose is to aid in the elimination of feces or flatus from the colon. This may be done to relieve constipation or remove fecal impaction, to cleanse the rectum and colon prior to examination, or as a safety measure to prevent possible infection in patients who are undergoing surgery or who are about to deliver. It may, however, be used for other purposes, as, for example, to reduce cerebral edema (magnesium sulfate enema).

Enemas may be divided into three groups according to their mode of action: those that stimulate evacuation by distention, those that stimulate peristalsis by irritation, and those that lubricate.

CLEANSING ENEMAS. Cleansing enemas are given chiefly to remove feces from the colon. There are many kinds of cleansing enema: The *soapsuds enema* usually contains 1000 to 1500 cc. of soap solution. The *saline enema* contains 1000 cc. of normal saline. A third kind of cleansing enema that is often used is the *tap water enema,* which contains 1000 to 1500 cc. of tap water.

These enemas, because of the volume of fluid used, serve to distend the rectum and lower colon, thereby stimulating the evacuation reflex. The soapsuds enema also has an irritating effect, due to the chemicals contained in the soap, and this enhances the action of the enema.

Today, disposable enemas are commonly used in many home and hospital situations. These contain hypertonic solutions, usually of sodium phosphate and biphosphate compounds. Their action is predominantly irritating, although the distention produced by the injection of the fluid also helps to stimulate peristalsis.

OIL ENEMAS. An oil enema may be given in cases in which there is severe constipation or the patient has a painful anal condition. The oil acts principally as a lubricant to make evacuation easier. Various oils, such as mineral, olive, or cottonseed oil, may be used. The amount given is small, usually 150 to 200 cc., and it is usually intended that the patient retain the enema for approximately an hour. Often a cleansing enema is ordered following an oil retention enema.

CARMINATIVE ENEMAS. The carminative enema is given to help expel flatus from the colon. There are several kinds of carminative enema. The *2, 2, 2 enema* contains 60 cc. of glycerin, 60 cc. of magnesium sulfate (50 per cent solution), and 60 cc. of water. The *milk and molasses enema* contains 240 cc. of milk and 240 cc. of molasses. It also is used to remove flatus from the colon. The *Mayo enema* contains 240 cc. of water, 60 cc. of white sugar, and 30 cc. of sodium bicarbonate. The sodium bicarbonate is mixed with the water and sugar and administered while the solution is still bubbling.

OTHER TYPES OF ENEMAS. Other enemas are given for a multiplicity of purposes. The *anthelmintic enema,* consisting of 15 cc. of Quassia chips and 250 cc. of water, is used to remove parasitic worms from the colon. The *astringent enema,* one form of which consists of 60 cc. of alum and 1000 cc. of water, is used to contract tissue and to stop hemorrhage. The *emollient enema* is used to coat the mucous membrane of the colon and to soothe irritated tissue; 180 cc. of starch solution is commonly used for this purpose. *Sedative* and *stimulant enemas* are also given. Paraldehyde is commonly

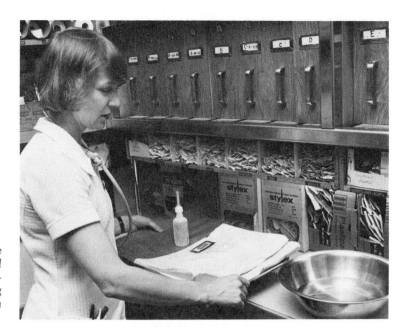

Today many hospitals use disposable equipment and commercially prepared solutions for enemas, making this nursing intervention easier.

used for sedative enemas, whereas 90 to 180 cc. of black coffee is a common ingredient of the stimulant enema. *Magnesium sulfate solution* and *ice water* are also used for enemas. Magnesium sulfate, 120 cc. of a 50 per cent solution, reduces cerebral edema. Ice water is used as an enema to reduce fever.

EQUIPMENT AND SUPPLIES. Enema equipment and solutions are obtainable in disposable sets. If these sets are not available, the patient requires certain clean equipment. Rectal tubes are usually made of rubber; however, plastic rectal tubes are also available today. Rectal tubes vary in diameter; they are measured on the French scale. A No. 22 or No. 24 French is the size commonly needed by an adult. Also needed are a container for the enema solution, tubing to connect the rectal tube to the container, a clamp, a small receptacle for extra fluid, and a lubricant for the rectal tube. The patient will also need a bedpan if he cannot use a toilet.

ADMINISTRATION. Before the enema equipment is taken to the patient, he will probably require some explanation about this measure. The patient's active help is important to the effectiveness of the enema. For maximum results he should try to hold the solution for 10 minutes. If the patient is in bed the head of the bed is lowered to make the bed level so that the fluid will flow in by force of gravity. It may not always be possible to have the bed completely flat; for example, if the patient is short of breath, the head of the bed should be no lower than is safe for him.

The top bedding is fan-folded to the foot of the bed and the patient is provided with a drape for warmth and comfort. For the administration of the enema, the patient is usually placed on his left side with both knees flexed, the top leg slightly higher than the lower one. It is felt that in this position, the descending colon being on the left side, the injection of fluid is facilitated by the force of gravity. However, this position may be varied according to the patient's condition and his wishes.

The usual temperature of a solution for an enema is 40.6° C. (105° F.). This temperature is not harmful to the mucous membrane lining the colon and rectum. The rectal tube is well lubricated (usually with a water soluble lubricant) in order to facilitate its insertion into the rectum and to lessen the irritation of the mucous membrane. Prior to the insertion of the tube the equipment is connected and a small amount of fluid is run through the tubing to expel the air. Then the tubing is

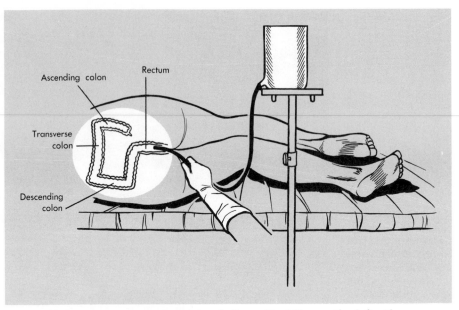

To have an enema administered, the patient lies on the left side.

clamped, and the rectal tube is inserted approximately 10 cm. (4 inches) into the rectum. The rectum of the average adult patient is 17.5 to 20 cm. (7 to 8 inches) in length. If the patient takes a deep breath while the tube is being inserted, the anal sphincter relaxes and the rectal tube can be inserted more easily. The tube must be inserted beyond the internal sphincter. If any obstruction to the insertion is encountered, the tube is withdrawn and the physician is notified. A rectal tube should never be forced because it might damage the mucous membrane or aggravate a disease process.

The solution for an enema is released slowly for the patient's comfort and to avoid damage to the mucous membrane. The higher the solution container is held, the greater is the pressure exerted. Hence, the solution container should not be more than 60 cm. (2 feet) above the level of the bed. For gynecological patients, the container is suspended at the patient's hip level in order to lessen the pressure on the adjacent reproductive organs. If the patient complains of discomfort while the solution is flowing, the flow is stopped for a few minutes and then recommenced cautiously. Any further discomfort demands the termination of the measure.

Following the administration of the solution, the rectal tube is pinched and removed. The patient retains the enema for 10 minutes if possible. In the case of an oil retention enema, the length of time for retention of the fluid is usually one hour.

When the enema is expelled, the nurse makes certain observations. She observes the color and consistency of the feces, the approximate amount of fluid returned, the general amount of flatus that is expelled (large, small), and the general reaction of the patient. All these observations are recorded in the patient's chart. The nurse also takes particular note of any unusual findings in the enema returns, for example, blood, mucus, pus, or worms. Following the expulsion of the enema, the patient is made clean and comfortable. The equipment is then rinsed in cold water and washed in hot soapy water. In hospitals, equipment is sterilized after each use to avoid the transfer of organisms. Disposable equipment is placed in a paper bag or other suitable container for removal.

SIPHONING AN ENEMA. If the patient cannot expel the enema within a half hour after its administration, it is usually necessary to siphon off the enema. This is generally a nursing decision. To siphon off an enema is to withdraw the enema solution from the patient by using positive-negative pressures and the force of gravity. The equipment and supplies required include a rectal tube and water soluble lubricant, a small amount of tap water (40.6° C. or 105° F.), a receptacle for the enema solution, and a funnel.

The patient lies on his right side with his hips drawn to the edge of the bed. In this position the descending colon is uppermost, a situation that facilitates the removal of the enema solution by force of gravity. The receptacle for the enema solution is placed at a level lower than the patient's hips, often on a chair at the side of the bed.

The rectal tube is first connected to the funnel and then well lubricated with the water soluble lubricant. The funnel is then half filled with water while the tubing is pinched to prevent leakage. The rectal tube is inserted into the patient in the same manner as for an enema. The pressure on the tubing is released and a small amount of fluid allowed to run into the rectum. Then the funnel is quickly inverted and lowered over the bedpan. The negative pressure of the fluid in the tube and funnel produces a siphon, which draws the enema fluid from the patient's colon.

After the removal of the enema fluid, the patient may require assistance regarding his comfort and hygiene. The enema fluid is observed for its color and consistency, and these observations are charted on the patient's record.

The Rectal Tube. The purpose of the insertion of a rectal tube is to facilitate the expulsion of flatus. The equipment required for this measure includes the rectal tube, a receptacle for the end of the tube, a lubricant, and adhesive tape. The adhesive tape is used to hold the rectal tube in position.

After the patient's need for information about this measure has been met, he is asked to lie in the same position as for an enema. The rectal tube is lubricated and inserted 10 cm. (4 inches) into the rectum. It is then taped in place, and the free end of the tube is put in a container placed near the patient's buttocks. A rectal tube is usually left in place for half an hour.

After the tube has been removed and the patient has received any needed assistance, the approximate amount (large, small) of flatus that was expelled is noted. Usually the patient can describe this. In addition, since the patient who has flatus usually has a hard distended abdomen, the nurse can palpate his abdomen to note any change. These observations are then recorded on the patient's chart.

The Manual Extraction of Feces. The manual extraction of feces is the removal by hand of impacted feces from the rectum. A fecal impaction is a large hardened mass of feces which has accumulated in the rectum, usually owing to prolonged constipation. The equipment required for manual extraction includes a rectal glove, a container for the glove, a lubricant, and a bedpan. After the measure has been explained to the patient, he lies on his left side.

The nurse puts on the rectal glove and thoroughly lubricates her second or third finger. She inserts this finger carefully into the rectum and manually breaks the impacted feces. The lubricant is used to facilitate the insertion of the nurse's gloved finger and to protect the rectal mucosa from abrasion. When the feces have been broken, they are removed by hand to the bedpan. The manual extraction of feces is often followed by a cleansing enema. This is ordered by the physician or the nurse in charge. After this nursing measure, the nurse charts the amount, color, and consistency of the feces. She also notes the presence of any flatus and the patient's general reaction (pallor, fatigue, and the like).

The Rectal Suppository. A medicated rectal suppository is administered for many reasons: it is used as a local irritant to facilitate elimination, as a vehicle for the administration of a sedative, or as an antispasmodic. The equipment needed for the insertion of a rectal suppository consists of a rectal glove, lubricant, the suppository, and a container for the suppository. The patient may need information about the function of the suppository and its insertion as well as the nursing techniques that are involved. The patient lies in the same position as for an enema.

With a gloved hand, the suppository is inserted one fingerlength, approximately

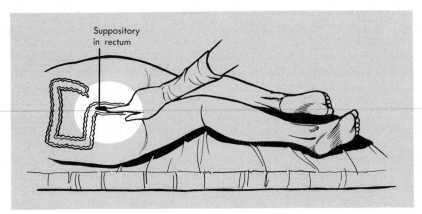

The insertion of a rectal suppository.

7.5 to 10 cm. (3 to 4 inches) into the rectum. It is usually possible to tell when the suppository is in place because the rectal sphincter "grabs" or "sucks" it in and closes. If the purpose of the suppository is to aid in the expulsion of the rectal contents, the patient should try to retain the suppository for about 20 minutes. If the suppository is administered for other purposes, it is retained indefinitely. When inserting the suppository, care must be exercised to be certain that the mucosa of the rectum is not torn and that the suppository is not forced when any resistance in the rectum is met. The suppository must contact the bowel wall; it should not be inserted into a bolus of stool.

After the suppository has been administered, this fact is recorded, as are the effects of the suppository. These can often be observed 15 to 30 minutes after administration, depending upon the medication.

Care of the Colostomy

IRRIGATION OF A COLOSTOMY. A colostomy is the surgical formation of an artificial anus through the abdomen into the colon. The purpose of a colostomy is usually to divert the feces from the intestinal tract through this artificial opening. A colostomy may be permanent or temporary.

In a permanent colostomy there is usually only one opening (stoma); in a temporary colostomy there may be two. The one closer to the stomach is called the proximal stoma; it is from this opening that the feces are discharged. If there is a second stoma it is farther from the stomach (closer to the anus) and hence is referred to as the distal stoma. There should be some direction in the nursing care plan as to how the nurse may distinguish between the proximal and distal stomas. An irrigation is generally prescribed for the functioning proximal stoma; only occasionally is a solution (an antiseptic solution, for example) instilled into a distal stoma.

The purpose of a colostomy irrigation is to cleanse the colon of fecal matter by injecting fluid into the colon through the colostomy opening. The equipment required for this nursing measure is similar to that needed for an enema, with the addition of a small rectal tube, a large glass Y connector, and unsterile waste gauze. The person who has a colostomy often needs careful instruction with regard to both the colostomy dressing and the colostomy irrigation. Most people can, with guidance, assume the responsibility for carrying out these measures themselves. There are several methods of irrigating a colostomy. One method is detailed here.

The nurse's approach to these nursing measures is extremely important. The patient is often anxious about his adjustment to the change in his life pattern as a result of this surgery, and any revulsion on the part of the nurse could be particularly disturbing to the patient and his family. Patients often feel embarrassed and find the colostomy hard to accept. They may not want to watch the nurse irrigate it at first, or they may be angry that this has happened to them. The nurse may also have strong feelings of dislike at doing this procedure which may show in her facial expression. Her calm acceptance of the situation and her care to protect the patient's feelings of dignity can do much to reassure the patient.

At the commencement of a colostomy irrigation, the patient lies on the side toward which the colostomy opening has been made, or sits upright so that the expulsion of feces is more easily accomplished. If he is in bed, the lower bedding is protected by a waterproof towel and the top bedding is fan-folded down to expose the colostomy opening. A bedpan is placed conveniently at a level lower than the colostomy opening. The container for the irrigating solution is placed not more than 30 cm. (1 foot) above the patient's pelvis in order to keep the pressure of the fluid low enough not to damage the mucous membrane of the intestine. A narrow rectal tube is connected to the irrigating container and a small amount of the irrigating solution is permitted to run through the rectal tube in order to expel the air in it.

The rectal tube is lubricated, and then inserted gently into the colostomy stoma.

The irrigating fluid is allowed to run slowly into the colon. After a small amount is administered, the intake tubing is clamped and the output tubing is released so that the return flow drains into the bedpan. This process is repeated until the returns from the colostomy are clear.

The returns of the irrigation are observed for color and consistency of the fecal matter. The condition of the operative area is also noted. Throughout this nursing measure the patient should be encouraged to participate actively. Most patients learn to carry out a colostomy irrigation while they are in the hospital so that they can eventually do this independently.

Especially designed for colostomy irrigations are the Binkley and Stockley apparatuses. Each consists essentially of a plastic cup which fits over the colostomy stoma. The cup has a hole for the catheter and a detachable plastic sheath which guides the fluid and feces into a receptacle. One of the advantages of these is the complete enclosure of the fluid and feces during the irrigation.

DRESSING THE COLOSTOMY. The colostomy dressing is a clean procedure rather than a sterile one. The dressing on the colostomy stoma is changed as often

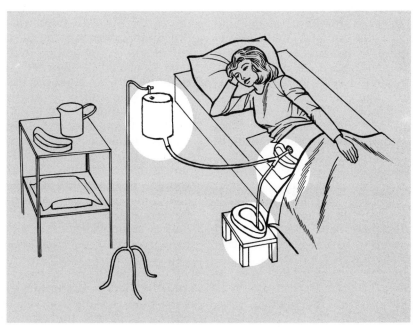

The administration of an irrigating solution to a colostomy by means of a Y tube.

as necessary in order to keep the the patient clean and his skin free from fecal matter. It is important that the skin surrounding the stoma be protected from irritation. Usually a protective lubricant, such as zinc oxide, is used for this purpose.

The equipment that is needed for a colostomy dressing includes unsterile gauze, unsterile dressings, lubricant, a tongue depressor, and a container for the disposal of the soiled dressings. Nursing personnel may use rubber gloves if they desire. As with the colostomy irrigation the nurse's approach to this task is important. Most people require considerable reassurance and a calm acceptance of the task. The patient can be helpful; in fact most people learn to change their own dressings. Therefore, each time the nurse dresses a colostomy she should be conscious of the learning needs of the patient.

The patient sits in a comfortable position for changing his dressing. If he is in bed, the bottom bedding is protected with waterproof material and the bedclothes are fan-folded to expose the colostomy stoma. The patient is draped for warmth and comfort. The soiled dressings are removed and the skin around the colostomy stoma cleansed with soap and water. A protective substance is then applied generously to the skin around the stoma, and a clean dressing is applied. The first layer of dressing usually consists of gauze, then unsterile surgical dressings are applied. Adhesive ties are used to hold the dressing in place. The color, the consistency, and the amount of fecal matter on the old dressing are recorded. The nurse also records the appearance of the colostomy stoma and the presence of any excoriated areas. (Excoriation is the loss of superficial tissue, such as epidermis.)

Plastic colostomy bags are also available commercially. They have attachable, specially designed belts that are worn around the waist or bags that stick directly to the skin. These bags are disposable and are changed whenever they become soiled.

Colonic Irrigation. A colonic irrigation (enteroclysis) is a measure designed to wash out the lower colon. Its purpose may be merely to cleanse the large intestine, or it may be to stimulate peristalsis and relieve distention. Other uses of the colonic irrigation are to relieve inflammation and to reduce body temperature. In the latter two instances the temperature of the solution is usually cooler. The equipment required for a colonic irrigation consists of the solution, a solution container, a colonic irrigation tube (No. 30 French is suggested), a lubricant, a catheter (No. 20 French is suggested), and a bedpan.

Initially the colonic tube is marked 5 to 7.5 cm. (2 to 3 inches) from the tip; adhesive tape can be used for this purpose. The catheter is marked 12.5 cm. (5 inches) from the tip in the same manner. These marks serve as a guide to the distance to which the tubes should be inserted. The type and temperature of the solution are prescribed by the physician.

This is not a painful measure, but patients usually require information about it. The patient turns on his right side with his hips toward the edge of the bed. This position facilitates the drainage of fluid from the colon. He is provided with drapes. The tubing and the catheter are connected to the solution container and the solution is allowed to run through the tubing before it is clamped. Both the colonic tube and the catheter are lubricated; the tip of the catheter is then placed in the opening or eye on the side of the colonic tube. The other end of the colonic tube is placed in a receptacle at the patient's bedside. Holding the two tubes together the nurse gently inserts them into the rectum up to the 7.5 cm. (3 inch) mark on the colonic tube. Next the catheter is drawn back sufficiently to free its tip from the colonic tube and it is then inserted to the 12.5 cm. (5 inch) mark. The solution is allowed to flow gradually and continuously so that the inflow and outflow are equal. If the patient has pain, the flow is stopped for a few minutes. If the pain persists, the irrigation is discontinued and the discomfort is reported.

When the irrigation returns are clear, the irrigation is discontinued, but the colonic tube is kept in place until drainage ceases. If at any time the colonic tube becomes blocked, it must be removed and cleansed, then reinserted.

The character of the return flow is observed. Particular note is made of the presence of mucus, blood, pus, or feces. The observations are recorded on the patient's chart.

Maintenance of Fluid and Electrolyte Balance

Adequate fluid and electrolyte balance is necessary to normal body functioning. Patients who have diarrhea need extra fluid intake to compensate for the fluid lost through the gastrointestinal tract. In diarrhea, fluids and electrolytes are lost because of hypersecretion of mucus from the membrane (due to irritation) and because of lack of reabsorption by the bowel of fluids ingested and of fluids secreted into the bowel. Normally, 8 liters of fluid are secreted into the bowel in a 24 hour period. Most of this fluid is reabsorbed. Severe diarrhea depletes the body's potassium level and lowers the amount of sodium chloride. The initial effect of this electrolyte loss is acidosis as a result of the loss of base; however, with prolonged potassium loss, alkalosis is eventually accompanied by a chloride loss.

In constipation there is a need for additional fluid intake both as an aid in activating peristalsis and to keep the feces soft. Often merely ensuring that the patient is taking enough fluids is sufficient to relieve constipation.

Maintenance of Adequate Nutritional Status

Maintaining adequate nutrition can be a particular problem for the patient who has diarrhea. Because the food moves quickly through the gastrointestinal tract, many food constituents are not absorbed. The ingestion of small amounts of nonirritating food at frequent intervals is often helpful in preventing diarrhea and facilitating absorption. Usually a bland diet is ordered to prevent further irritation of the gastrointestinal mucosa.

The constipated patient, on the other hand, may be anorectic and need help to stimulate his appetite. The diet for the constipated patient should be planned to meet his needs for fluids, extra bulk, and for foods that have a laxative effect. (See section on reestablishment of normal bowel functioning, p. 526.)

Maintenance of Comfort and Hygiene

Meeting the comfort and hygiene needs of the patient with elimination problems is a valuable contribution to his sense of well-being. Cleanliness is essential. The sight and odor of fecal material is repugnant, and the high bacteria count in feces makes it a possible source of contamination. The patient should be given the opportunity to wash his hands after he has had a bowel movement (as he would normally do at home). The rectal area should be cleansed and the patient assisted with this if he is unable to do it himself. Soiled linen should be removed immediately.

Some patients with diarrhea feel more secure if the bedpan is close at hand. In these cases, the pan can be kept covered and placed inconspicuously within reach. Care should be taken that the pan is emptied and cleaned after each use.

After the patient has defecated, his room may require ventilating and freshening to eliminate unpleasant odors. Since such matters can be embarrassing to the patient, the nurse should take the initiative in these measures.

Many patients with defecation problems develop irritation of the skin and mucous membranes in the anal area. Cleanliness is important to prevent infection, and emollient creams help to keep the skin intact and to soothe the irritated area.

An important factor to consider in the care of patients with constipation or diarrhea is the nurse's reaction to these patients and their problems. It is helpful if the nurse can accept her own feelings and not communicate these to the patient.

GUIDE TO ASSESSING FECAL ELIMINATION

1. Does the patient have constipation or diarrhea? How long has he had this condition? Has he been eating any irritating food?
2. Does he require immediate medical or nursing intervention to relieve these symptoms?
3. What is the patient's normal pattern of defecation? Is he in the habit of taking laxatives or enemas?
4. Is he under stress?
5. What is the consistency of the patient's feces? their color, odor, and frequency? Do the feces contain foreign matter such as blood or pus?
6. Is the patient able to communicate his discomfort to the nurse? If so, does he complain of accompanying signs and symptoms such as anorexia, headache, abdominal pain, or distention? Does he have pain on defecation?
7. Are there signs of fecal impaction as, for example, the passage of small amounts of seepage instead of formed stool?
8. Is the patient's nutritional status satisfactory? Is his fluid and electrolyte balance normal? Is he taking sufficient exercise?
9. Does the patient's diet contain a sufficient amount of bulky foods to ensure stimulation of the defecation reflex? Is he taking enough fluids?
10. What are the patient's learning needs in relation to the reestablishment of a normal pattern of defecation? in relation to hygiene measures with regard to defecation?

GUIDE TO EVALUATING THE EFFECTIVENESS OF NURSING INTERVENTION

1. Is the patient comfortable? Is he free from distressing symptoms?
2. If the patient has been constipated, has a successful bowel movement been accomplished? If he has had diarrhea, have the stools returned to normal in consistency and frequency?
3. Has a normal pattern of elimination been established?
4. Is the patient aware of his dietary and fluid needs to ensure adequate fecal elimination? Does his selection of foods and his fluid intake indicate this?
5. Does the patient practice good hygiene? For example, does he wash his hands after defecation?

STUDY VOCABULARY

Cathartic	Feces	Peristalsis
Colostomy	Flatus	Sphincter
Constipation	Impaction	Stool
Defecation		

STUDY SITUATION

Mr. S. Norris is a 70 year old man living at home who has abdominal pain. He has been retired for five years after an active life as a house painter, and he now spends most of his time watching television. Mr. Norris lives alone in a small house just outside the city. He has three grandchildren who live a few miles away and he visits them on Sundays.

Mr. Norris has been increasingly uncomfortable because of constipation during the past few years. He says he never took medicines when he worked but now has to take a laxative every day. Because he does not like to cook, he generally eats toast and jam. His doctor has asked you to assist Mr. Norris to regulate his bowel habits.

1. What factors should you take into consideration before assisting Mr. Norris?
2. What observations should you make regarding Mr. Norris's bowel habits?
3. For what reasons might Mr. Norris be constipated?
4. Outline the expected outcomes of nursing interventions for Mr. Norris.
5. What should you include in your teaching program for this patient?
6. Mr. Norris's physician has ordered a Fleet enema for the patient. How would you explain this measure to him?
7. Describe the position most desirable for the administration of an enema and why it is desirable.
8. What observations should you record regarding the enema?
9. How would you evaluate the effectiveness of your teaching?

SUGGESTED READINGS

Baker, R. B.: Constipation and the Geriatric Patient. *Nursing Care,* 8:21, October 1975.

Connors, M.: Ostomy Care: A Personal Approach. *American Journal of Nursing,* 74:1422–1424, August 1974.

Corman, L., et al.: Cathartics. *American Journal of Nursing,* 75:273–279, February 1975.

Curtis, C.: Colonoscopy: The Nurse's Role. *American Journal of Nursing,* 75:430–432, March 1975.

Dudas, S. (Guest Ed.): Symposium on the Care of the Ostomy Patient. *Nursing Clinics of North America, 11*:389–478, September 1976.

Given, B. A., and Simmons, S. J.: *Gasteroenterology in Clinical Nursing.* 2nd edition. St. Louis, C. V. Mosby, 1975.

Keusch, G.: Bacterial Diarrheas. *American Journal of Nursing,* 73:1028–1032, June 1973.

Lewin, D.: Care of the Constipated Patient. *Nursing Times,* 72:444–446, March 25, 1976.

McIntosh, H. D., et al.: Turista—It's Not a Single Disease. *Heart and Lung,* 5:636–640, July/August 1976.

Schauder, M. R.: Ostomy Care: Cone Irrigations. *American Journal of Nursing,* 74:1424–1427, August 1974.

Schultz, C. M.: Nursing Care of the Stroke Patient. Rehabilitative Aspects. *Nursing Clinics of North America,* 8:633–641, December 1973.

Sheridan, J. L.: Obstructions of the Intestinal Tract. *Nursing Clinics of North America, 10*:147–155, March 1975.

Willington, F. L.: Incontinence. 5. Training and Retraining for Continence. *Nursing Times, 71*:500–503, March 27, 1975.

URINARY PROBLEMS 28

The nurse should be able to:

Discuss the importance of adequate urinary elimination to the
 health and well-being of the individual
Describe the body processes involved in voiding
Describe normal functioning with regard to urinary elimination
Discuss factors which may cause disturbances of urinary
 functioning
Outline the process of assessment of a person's urinary
 elimination status, indicating likely subjective and objective
 findings
Identify common problems of urinary elimination
Apply relevant principles in planning and implementing nursing
 interventions for urinary problems
Identify priorities and take appropriate action in regard to patient
 problems in urinary elimination
Evaluate the effectiveness of her nursing interventions

INTRODUCTION

In order to maintain effective functioning, the human body must rid itself of wastes. Most of the nitrogenous wastes of cellular metabolism are excreted in the urine. In addition, the urinary system plays an important role in maintaining the fluid and electrolyte balance of the body. Both of these functions are essential in the maintenance of physiological homeostasis.

The act of voiding is also an important area of independent functioning for an individual. Control over voiding is learned early in childhood, and actual or potential loss of independence in regard to this vital function constitutes a serious threat to the individual's social and emotional well-being. If such a loss occurs, he fears it will mean a return to the dependent state of infancy, and his feelings of self-esteem are markedly jeopardized.

Most people have difficulty in discussing urinary functioning and problems they may have in connection with it. In our culture, there are social taboos about the subject of elimination and, once a child has been toilet-trained, he is taught that this topic is not talked about in polite company. The act of voiding is also done privately in our society. Then, too, the intimate anatomical relationship between the urinary and the reproductive tracts contributes to making urinary functioning a sensitive topic. Necessary intervention is a potential source of embarrassment for both the nurse and the patient, particularly if one is male and the other female. If the nurse can discuss urinary elimination and carry out necessary nursing measures matter-of-factly, without showing signs of embarrassment herself, this can go a long way towards putting the patient at ease.

ANATOMY AND PHYSIOLOGY OF THE URINARY TRACT

The urinary tract consists of the kidneys, the ureters, the bladder, and the urethra. Normally, a person has two kidneys. These are situated in the back part of the abdominal cavity, behind the peritoneum and just below the diaphragm, one on either side of the spinal column.

The kidneys are complex organs whose chief functions are the elimination of waste products of body metabolism and the control of the concentration of the various constituents of body fluid, including the blood. These functions are accomplished through an efficient filtering system that removes the excess water, acid, and other wastes from the blood as it passes through the kidney. The blood retains the essential elements needed by the body through selective reabsorption. Blood comes to the kidney through the renal artery and is filtered in the glomeruli of the nephrons. The filtrate contains water, the waste products of metabolism, electrolytes, and glucose. These products pass along the nephron's tubules, where some solutes and water are reabsorbed. The tubules also secrete substances such as drugs into the urine.

The body can continue to function effectively even though a considerable amount of kidney tissue has been damaged—indeed, even if one kidney is absent or does not function at all.

The ureters are long, narrow muscular tubes which serve to transport urine from the kidneys to its storehouse, the bladder.

The chief function of the bladder is to retain urine until it can be excreted. The average adult bladder holds from 300 to 500 ml. of urine; however, the bladder has been known to hold from 3000 to 4000 ml.

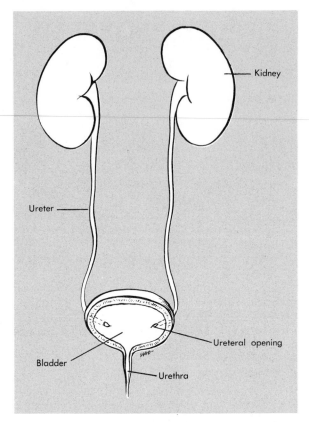

The urinary system.

of urine. The bladder is a hollow muscular organ whose efficient functioning is dependent upon the maintenance of muscle tone in the bladder wall and upon the integrity of the nervous system innervating the bladder.

The bladder, when empty, lies in folds in the pelvic cavity. As urine enters it in rhythmic spurts from the ureters, the walls of the bladder expand and it expands into the pelvic cavity, thrusting upwards into the abdominal cavity. When a sufficient amount of urine has accumulated in the bladder, normally 300 to 500 ml. in the adult, sensory impulses are sent to the spinal cord and thence to higher centers in the brain. The individual becomes aware of the urge to void. If there are no inhibiting factors, the muscle of the bladder wall contracts and the internal sphincter at the base of the bladder relaxes, allowing urine to flow into the urethra. The stimulus allowing this act is a stretch reflex that is evoked by increase in pressure as the bladder fills with urine. The action is essentially a cord reflex, although it may be facilitated or inhibited by higher centers.

Micturition—the act of voiding—is normally under voluntary control after about the age of three years. This control is exerted via a second external sphincter muscle. The external sphincter is located about the middle of the urethra—in men, just as the urethra enters the glans penis.

The urethra itself is a short, muscular tube whose function is to carry urine from the bladder to its exit point from the body. In women, the urethra is approximately 3 to 5 cm. (1¼ to 2 inches) long; it opens just above the vagina. In men, the urethra is about 20 cm. (8 inches) long from its origin in the bladder to its external opening in the glans penis. It crosses the length of the penis and carries the products of both the urinary tract and the reproductive tract in the male. Meatus is the term used for the external opening of the urethra in both men and women.

The entire urinary tract is lined with a continuous layer of mucous membrane that stretches from the meatus to the pelvis of the kidney.

NORMAL URINARY FUNCTIONING

The average adult usually excretes between 1000 and 1500 cc. of urine in a 24 hour period. The total volume varies with the amount of fluid intake and also with the amount of fluids lost through other routes, such as sweating, vomiting, or diarrhea.

The pattern of voiding—that is, the number of times a person voids during the day and the amount eliminated each time—is highly individualized. It depends on a number of factors, such as early childhood training, habitual response to the urge to urinate (nurses are noted for delaying their response to this impulse in themselves), amount of fluids consumed, and the capacity of the individual's bladder, among other things. Most people void first thing in the morning, possibly four to six times during the day, and again before retiring. A person does not usually have to get up at night to void unless he has consumed a large amount of fluids prior to bedtime.

In appearance, normal urine is clear and straw-colored or light amber. The darker the color, the more concentrated it is. The specific gravity of urine has a normal range of 1.0003 to 1.030. Usually, the first urine voided in the morning is more concentrated than that excreted at other times of the day.

Normal urine has a pH of 4.8 to 8.0; it is usually slightly acidic (with a pH around 6) in people on normal diets. When left to stand, urine gradually becomes alkaline, owing to the disintegration of its constituents, and a cloudy sediment develops.

Freshly voided urine has a faintly aromatic odor, which becomes stronger on standing. Normally urine contains creatinine, uric acid, urea, and a few white blood cells. It does not normally contain bacteria, red blood cells, sugar, albumin, acetone, casts, pus, or calculi (stones that form in the urinary tract).

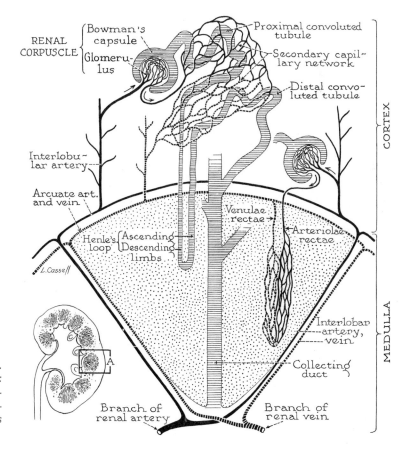

A nephron. (From B. G. King and M. J. Showers: Human Anatomy and Physiology. Sixth edition. Philadelphia, W. B. Saunders Company.)

FACTORS AFFECTING
URINARY ELIMINATION

Under conditions of good health, a number of factors may affect the volume of urinary output and the pattern of voiding, as well as the characteristics of the urine excreted. These factors should be taken into consideration in the nurse's assessment of an individual's urinary elimination status.

Urine carries away most of the body's excess water. Hence, as mentioned earlier, both fluid intake and the amount of fluids lost through other routes will affect the volume and usually also the frequency of urinary output. Age also affects the volume and frequency of urinary elimination. In children, a proportionately larger amount of body weight is in a fluid state than in adults. Children, therefore, excrete a greater volume of urine in proportion to body weight and, because of their smaller bladders, need to void more frequently than do adults. A generalized loss of muscle tone and lessening efficiency on the part of the kidneys contribute to the need on the part of many older people to void more frequently and in smaller amounts than younger adults, usually also with increased feelings of urgency.

Then, too, because of inborn differences in anatomical structure and physiological functioning, some people have a larger bladder capacity than others or a seemingly more efficient urinary system. They may not, then, need to void as often as others. Early childhood training also plays its part in an individual's response to the urge to urinate. Because voiding is under voluntary control, however, people may alter their voiding patterns because of situational factors, such as the availability of toilet facilities, the pressures of work, mealtimes, and the like. During pregnancy, women often complain of having to void more often than usual. This is caused by pressure of the expanding uterus on the bladder wall, thereby causing the individual to more easily feel the urge to void.

A person's diet may affect the constituents of urine. A vegetarian diet, for example, will cause the urine to be alkaline. Drugs will sometimes change the appearance of urine. For example, Mandelamine, a urinary antiseptic, when given in conjunction with a sulfonamide (an anti-infective) will cause the urine to be turbid.[1]

Emotional factors may also cause urinary disturbances. Anxiety, for example, often stimulates the urge to void more frequently (as in a nervous person waiting in an airport for his plane to depart, or a student waiting for an examination to begin). Strong fear may cause a person to void involuntarily. Pain, on the other hand may inhibit voiding.

In addition to the normal factors which may affect urinary elimination, a number of abnormal conditions may cause dysfunctioning of the urinary system.

Infection is one of the most common causes of urinary disturbances. Because the entire urinary system is lined with a continuous mucous membrane, an infection that initiates in one part of the system can travel rapidly to all parts of the tract. Bacteria commonly found in the large intestine (colibacillus, for example) are common causes of urinary tract infection. The proximity of the outlets of the gastrointestinal and the urinary tracts contributes to this transfer. Women in particular are prone to bladder infections because of the shortness of the female urethra. Stasis of urine in the bladder as a result of retention is another factor predisposing to infections and also the formation of bladder stones.

Disturbances in the circulatory system also can have an effect upon kidney function. Heart disease and diseases of the venous and arterial systems often interfere with the circulation of blood to the kidneys. Normally, 170 liters of blood are filtered through the adult kidneys in one day. From this filtration process approximately 1 to 1.5 liters of urine are formed and excreted. Any disease that interferes with the circulation of blood through the kidney can result in the impairment of kidney functioning.

Obstructions may occur in almost any part of the urinary tract. Most commonly they are seen in the pelvis of the kidney,

---

[1] Mary W. Falconer et al.: *The Drug, the Nurse, the Patient.* 5th edition. Philadelphia, W. B. Saunders Company, 1974, p. 369.

in the ureter, and, in the male, in the prostatic section of the urethra. Blockage of the urinary tract, whether by a malignancy or stones, hinders the excretion of urine.

Hormone disturbances, such as those resulting from dysfunctioning of the adrenal or pituitary glands, can also have an adverse effect upon the kidneys. Antidiuretic hormone, aldosterone, and possibly norepinephrine affect the reabsorption of fluid within the kidney tubules.

A *generalized trauma* to the body, such as hemorrhage, burns, or shock, or a systemic infection can also affect the kidneys. For example, in severe dehydration there is a depletion in the amount of fluid within the body, which can severely disturb kidney function, even to the point of failure.

Any *generalized muscular disturbance* can also affect urinary tract function. Specific dysfunctions of the muscles of the bladder, the ureters, or the urethra can cause urinary symptoms, such as retention of urine or poor urinary control.

Neurologic factors can interfere with normal kidney and bladder function. Drugs which depress the central nervous system, for example, can cause a loss of voluntary control over micturition. Hence, patients under heavy sedation and those undergoing general anesthesia may void by reflex action when the bladder is full. Damage to the spinal cord or to the pathways that transmit impulses from the spinal cord to the brain may also result in the loss of voluntary control over voiding, as may damage to the brain itself.

COMMON PROBLEMS

Dysfunction of the urinary system may manifest itself in localized disturbances in the passage of urine or in generalized problems resulting from impairment of elimination of waste products from the body.

Localized Problems

Of the localized problems, the following are among those most commonly seen: urinary incontinence, dysuria, burning, frequency, urgency, nocturia, poly-uria, urinary retention, oliguria, renal anuria, and foreign substances in the urine.

Urinary incontinence, or involuntary voiding, is a common urinary problem, particularly among the ill. Sometimes there is a complete inability to control the flow of urine and, as a result, a constant dribbling occurs. Not only is this demoralizing and embarrassing to the individual, but the urine can also be a source of irritation to the skin in the anogenital area. Urinary incontinence sometimes occurs temporarily after an operation. It can also result from diseases of the nerves and muscles of the bladder. Women in whom the muscles of the pelvic floor have been weakened by childbirth and other people with poor muscular control sometimes have problems with *stress incontinence* – that is, they may excrete small amounts of urine involuntarily with exertions such as coughing or laughing.

Dysuria is another common problem; it refers to difficulty in voiding or pain on voiding and may be caused by a number of factors. It can result from a blockage in any part of the urinary tract, from trauma, from muscular abnormalities of the bladder, ureters, or urethra, from infection of the urinary tract, or from psychogenic factors. In older men, hypertrophy (increase in size) of the prostate gland, which surrounds the urethra, is a common cause of difficulty in voiding.

A *burning* (or *scalding*) sensation on voiding may be caused by the excretion of a more highly concentrated urine than normal; it is also a frequent problem in people with infections of the urinary tract.

Frequency – that is, voiding more often than usual – may be caused by very benign factors such as drinking an excessive amount of fluids. As mentioned earlier, it is a common problem during pregnancy and, while inconvenient, is usually not indicative of serious urinary dysfunction. Anxiety, as also noted above, can stimulate voiding and cause distressing frequency, at times with loss of control. On the other hand, frequency, particularly combined with urgency, is also commonly seen in people with infections of the urinary tract.

Urgency, the urge to void in a hurry, is an embarrassing problem. Its most common cause is infection of the urinary tract, although it may also be due to the same causes that produce frequency.

Nocturia refers to the need to get up from sleep in order to void. It may be due simply to drinking a large amount of fluids prior to bedtime, but it may also be caused by disturbed kidney functioning, particularly with regard to the kidney's inability to concentrate urine. Nocturia is not to be confused with *enuresis*, or bed-wetting, which is a fairly common childhood and sleep disorder (see Chapter 18).

Polyuria (diuresis) is the passage of an increased amount of urine. It can be caused by failure of the tubules to reabsorb water or by disturbances in the hormonal balance of the body. Certain drugs, called *diuretics*, are often given to increase urinary elimination in people who suffer from fluid retention; these drugs cause a temporary polyuria.

Urinary retention is another common problem. In retention, the urine is formed in the kidneys, but the person is unable to excrete it from the bladder. As a consequence, his bladder becomes distended and he feels increasingly uncomfortable. Some patients have retention with overflow; they void small amounts of urine frequently but continue to have distended bladders. Urinary retention predisposes a person to bladder infection (cystitis).

Oliguria is the passage of a lessened amount of urine. This condition can be caused by dehydration or by an impairment of the circulation of blood to the kidney. A lowered efficiency of the kidney or a blockage within the urinary tract can also result in oliguria.

Renal anuria (suppression of urine) is a condition in which there is an absence of urinary excretion from the kidneys. It is usually indicative of serious kidney impairment. If this condition is prolonged, toxic substances build up within the body and the patient eventually dies. In both renal anuria and urinary retention, the patient is unable to void; however, in urinary retention the urine is retained in the bladder, whereas in renal anuria, the urine never reaches the bladder.

Foreign substances in the urine may be found upon examination in the laboratory. Blood in the urine *(hematuria)* may be due to kidney damage or to infections of the urinary tract. The presence of pus *(pyuria)* and of albumin in the urine *(albuminuria)* is also frequently caused by infections. The presence of protein in the urine *(proteinuria)* is usually due either to tissue disintegration or to an increase in glomerular permeability. *Casts,* on the other hand, are coagulated protein from the lumen of the kidney tubules. Sugar in the urine *(glycosuria)* is seen when the body is unable to utilize all the sugar which is ingested.

Generalized Problems

In addition to the localized problems related to urinary dysfunctioning, generalized problems occur. When there is severe reduction in the ability of the kidneys to function, the patient usually develops *uremia.* This condition may result from trauma or infection, for example, or because of a chronic kidney disorder. The impairment in renal functioning has several effects on the body, in addition to a lessened amount of urine excretion (oliguria), which progresses (if not checked) to complete urine suppression (anuria). Water is retained, and there is a resultant edema of body tissues. The acid-base balance is disturbed, and the patient may develop acidosis owing to failure of the kidneys to remove the acidic products of metabolism. Potassium excretion is impaired, with a resulting high concentration of potassium in body fluids. This may give rise to neuromuscular irritability, as evidenced by an irregular pulse, for example. There is usually retention of the nonprotein nitrogenous waste products of metabolism as well, particularly of urea, whence the condition derived its name.

Thus, there are significant changes in blood chemistry. The concentration of urea in the blood (blood urea nitrogen, or BUN) may be increased from a normal value of 15 to 25 mg. per 100 ml. to as much as 200 mg. per 100 ml. in severe cases of uremia. Similarly, the blood creatinine level may rise from a normal value of 1.2 mg. per 100 ml. to 13 mg. per 100 ml. The extent of the increase in blood levels of these substances provides an indication of the severity of the kidney impairment.

Other problems may also accompany impaired kidney functioning as a result of the body's attempts to rid itself of wastes normally excreted in the urine by utilizing other channels. Perspiration is increased and deposits of salts may accumulate on the skin (urea frost); the skin becomes pale and powdery, and the patient may have problems such as itching (pruritus) and an offensive odor on the skin due to the urea deposits.

When the kidneys are inhibited in the elimination of excess acid from the body, the lungs attempt to compensate for this; there are respiratory changes involving the character and depth of respirations. The respirations become deeper, the rate of respirations increases, and sometimes the patient's breath has the odor of urine.

ASSESSING URINARY ELIMINATION STATUS

In assessing the patient's urinary elimination status, the nurse needs information about the patient's usual voiding pattern (bladder habits) and any deviations from the normal that he is having at the time he was admitted to the health agency. She considers these in terms of the patient's age, his usual food and fluid intake, and disturbances that he has now with regard to taking sufficient food and fluids to maintain optimal urinary functioning.

She takes into consideration the patient's mental status: Is he confused? What is his level of consciousness? She also considers the possibility of potential or actual sources of anxiety he may have, which might cause or contribute to disturbances in urinary functioning.

Most of this information will be available from the nursing history and the clinical appraisal. In addition, the nurse needs to be aware of the nature of the patient's health problem(s) (if identified), and the physician's diagnostic and therapeutic plans of care for the patient. If diagnostic tests or examinations have been carried out, the nurse will find these reports very helpful in her assessment of the patient. Information from these sources is supplemented by the subjective and objective data she gathers in her observations.

Subjective Observations

People who have urinary problems are usually considerably distressed; their symptoms are often uncomfortable, sometimes inconvenient, and occasionally embarrassing. Often people are reluctant to talk about their urinary problems, and they may need encouragement in order to verbalize them. It is important to minimize the individual's feelings of embarrassment by ensuring privacy and a quiet place for discussion.

The patient may describe sensations of pain related to voiding, for example, or he may have noted disturbances in the normal pattern of voiding. The patient may be distressed by frequency or urgency in the need to void, or conversely, he may find micturition difficult. Patients are usually aware, too, of changes in the amount of urine. When there is either suppression of urine formation in the kidneys, or retention of urine in the bladder, the amount of urine voided may be small. On the other hand, in some types of disease conditions, there may be copious amounts of urine formed and excreted. Some patients find that their sleep is disturbed because of the need to urinate. This may happen when kidney function is impaired and there is a loss of the normal ability of the kidneys to vary the concentration of urine. The patient may also be the first to notice abnormalities such as the presence of blood or pus in the urine.

Objective Observations

The nurse also makes specific observations from which she gathers objective data. The characteristics of the patient's urine (color, odor, consistency, amount, and the presence of abnormal constituents) are observed; these should be checked against the normal ones. If the urine is lighter than normal in color, this may be due to either an abnormally high intake of fluids or a diminution of the concentrating power of the kidneys. A dark, brownish color usually indicates a more concentrated urine. Urine may also be almost orange in color in some conditions owing to the presence of bile salts. Drugs

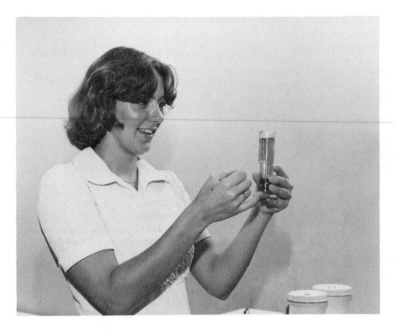

Often nurses are called upon to perform various diagnostic tests on urine.

may also change the color of the urine. Urine sometimes has a sweetish odor, often described as "fruity," which is characteristic of the presence of acetone. Blood in the urine may be observed as bright red, or the urine may be smoky in color. Another abnormal constituent which may be noted by visual observation is pus, which often gives a cloudy appearance to the urine.

The nurse should also note carefully the patient's intake and output and relate these to her other observations about the patient's voiding pattern and the characteristics of the urine. Urinary retention, for example, can be identified by checking the amount and frequency of voiding. If the patient voids 30 to 50 ml. of urine every 1 to 2 hours, he is probably retaining urine. In addition, a distended bladder can often be palpated. With the patient in the dorsal recumbent position, palpation just above the symphysis pubis reveals a firm distention, and percussion with the fingers causes the dull sound indicative of a full bladder.

In addition, the nurse should be alert to manifestations of generalized problems in relation to urinary dysfunctioning as these have been described earlier in this chapter.

One of the primary responsibilities of the nurse in caring for patients with urinary problems is the observation and recording of pertinent facts. The early detection of edema, of changes in the pigmentation of the skin, or of signs of central nervous system or neuromuscular dysfunction can contribute significantly to the total plan of care for the patient.

An important part of the nurse's responsibility is often to take exact measurements of the patient's fluid intake and output. These fluids are usually measured in cubic centimeters and recorded on a fluid balance sheet on the patient's chart. Occasionally it is also necessary to record the amount of fluid ingested as a part of the patient's food and the amount lost in perspiration and feces, but these are rare situations. Normally fluid output includes all liquid drainage (for example, gastric suction, vomitus, bleeding, or diarrhea) and urine excretion.

Numerous diagnostic laboratory tests are performed on urine to evaluate kidney function. Some tests indicate the rate of glomerular filtration, tubular reabsorption, and excretion by the kidneys.

A routine *urinalysis* is probably the most common urine examination. It includes microscopic examination and tests of pH, specific gravity, albumin, and sugar.

A sample laboratory urinalysis report form. (Courtesy of Vancouver General Hospital.)

Urine Test	Normal Results
pH	4.8 to 8.0
Specific gravity	1.003 to 1.030
Albumin	Negative
Sugar	Negative
Microscopic examination	(Female) few red blood cells; few casts
	Straw to light amber in color

Blood in urine may be obvious or hidden. Laboratory tests can detect red blood cells and dissolved hemoglobin (hemoglobinuria).

Nurses are frequently called upon in the clinical areas to perform some of the more routine laboratory tests on urine. Thus, a nurse may be requested to carry out a test for specific gravity or to test the patient's urine for the presence of sugar or acetone.

Tests of renal function include the phenolsulfonphthalein test, the Fishberg concentration test, concentration and dilution tests, and the urea clearance test. Generally speaking, most of these tests have special requirements for the food and fluid intake of the patient, the hours when urine specimens are to be collected, and, perhaps, definite times when blood specimens are to be collected. It is important that the patient understand what he should do to prepare for these tests and how he can help with them.

Urine cultures are done to determine the presence of pathogenic microorganisms. A catheter specimen may be required for culture, but usually a midstream specimen will suffice. Urine is normally sterile.

When a midstream specimen from the male patient is needed, the patient cleanses the urinary meatus with an antiseptic solution. He voids some urine, which is discarded, and then collects the midstream urine in a sterile container. The remainder of the stream is also discarded.

Obtaining a midstream specimen from a female patient is more difficult. The labia and vestibule should be thoroughly cleansed with soap and water or antiseptic solution. If soap is used, it must be rinsed off. The patient then voids. The first part of the stream is discarded, the midstream specimen is caught in a sterile container, and the remainder of the urine

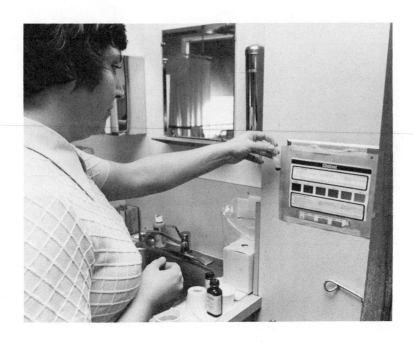

This nurse is checking the sugar content in her patient's urine by comparing its color to the color chart provided in a Clinitest set.

is also discarded. Most female patients find it easier to obtain this specimen when the toilet is used for discarded urine.

Some blood tests are also indicative of kidney function. The nonprotein nitrogen test (NPN) measures the ability of the kidney to remove urea, creatine, and so forth, from the blood. The blood urea nitrogen (BUN) test is a more sensitive test of kidney function. For each of these tests, 5 cc. of venous blood is collected.

There are many examinations of the urinary tract. A cystoscopy is the examination of a patient's bladder with a lighted instrument which is inserted up the urethra. The intravenous pyelogram and retrograde pyelogram outline the pelves, calices, ureters, and urinary bladder by means of a contrast medium which is visible on x-ray.

PRIORITIES FOR NURSING ACTION

When a patient has an impairment in kidney functioning, the body's ability to eliminate the nitrogenous waste products of protein metabolism is decreased. The accumulation of these waste products within the body constitutes a serious threat to the patient's life. One of the most important aspects of nursing care for patients with renal disorders is the constant monitoring of fluid intake and output. If there is a decrease in fluid loss below the levels considered safe, this fact should be reported promptly so that appropriate therapy can be instituted. In assessing the safety levels for the patient, the nurse is guided by the physician's estimate for this particular patient, but it is helpful for her to remember that the normal urine output in an adult is approximately 1000 to 1500 cc. per day. An output of less than 25 cc. per hour (600 cc. in a 24 hour period) is considered inadequate for a normal adult.

If the patient's problem is one that causes interference with the excretion of urine from the bladder, it is important that he be watched for signs of urine retention. Although some adult bladders have been known to hold up to 3000 to 4000 cc. of fluid, not all bladders will contain this quantity and there is a danger of rupture when the bladder content is considerably below this point. The early detection of urinary retention is therefore vitally important. (The identification of urinary retention is discussed in the section on signs and symptoms of urinary problems earlier in the chapter.) It should be reported promptly so that appropriate medi-

PRINCIPLES RELEVANT TO URINARY PROBLEMS

1. Most of the nitrogenous wastes of cellular metabolism are eliminated by the kidneys.

2. The kidneys play an important role in maintaining the fluid and electrolyte balance of body tissues and fluids.

3. The average adult loses approximately 1000 to 1500 ml. of fluid from the kidneys in a 24 hour period.

4. Awareness of the need to void normally occurs when the bladder contains from 300 to 500 ml. of urine.

5. Mucous membrane lines the urinary tract.

6. Previous learning influences an individual's attitudes and behavior with regard to elimination.

7. The excretion of urine is normally an independent function in the adult.

cal or nursing intervention can be started. Frequently, it is left up to the nurse to initiate action; that is, the physician may leave an order for catheterization of the patient every eight hours as needed (p.r.n.). When catheterization is needed, it should be done promptly. A patient should never be left with a distended bladder.

GOALS FOR NURSING ACTION

The goals of nursing care of the patient with urinary problems depend to a large extent on the nature of the problem. If there is impairment of kidney functioning, nursing measures are directed toward assisting to reduce the workload of the kidneys until such time as they are able to resume normal activity, and assisting to minimize the effects of impaired kidney functioning on the body. In this, the nurse is guided by the physician's plan of therapy for the patient.

If the problem is one of interference with the elimination of urine, rather than impaired kidney functioning, nursing measures are directed toward facilitating the elimination of urine from the bladder and assisting in the reestablishment of a normal voiding pattern.

In all types of urinary problems, an important aim of nursing care is to provide emotional and physical comfort measures which the patient finds supportive.

SPECIFIC NURSING INTERVENTIONS

Assisting With Measures to Reduce the Workload on the Kidneys

The principal functions of the kidneys are to control the concentration of the various constituents of body fluid and to eliminate the waste products of metabolism, chiefly the nitrogenous wastes of cellular metabolism. When kidney function is impaired, various measures may be instituted to relieve them of some of their workload. Often the patient is put to bed to minimize activity and, hence, lessen cellular metabolism. Unless the patient is losing large amounts of protein in the urine (which occurs in some conditions), he is usually given a low-protein diet, again to minimize the amount of nitrogenous wastes from protein metabolism which need to be eliminated. There may also be restrictions placed on the sodium and potassium in his diet, since sodium contributes to fluid retention, and the accumulation of potassium, which a damaged kidney cannot excrete (or has a lessened ability to excrete), may cause serious neuromuscular disturbances. The patient's fluid intake may be limited to prevent or lessen edema. It is important for the nurse to see that instructions regarding both food and fluid intake for the patient are followed exactly. Patients with renal disorders often suffer from anorexia and may need encouragement to eat their meals. The patient should be made aware of the importance of adhering to the diet and fluid intake that has been ordered for him, since this is part of his therapy. Many patients can help to keep track of their fluid intake; by encouraging them to participate in their care in this way, the nurse can often gain their cooperation.

Sometimes, in order to put the kidneys at rest and give them a chance to recover when there has been extensive tissue damage, or to maintain patients whose kidneys are no longer functioning, an artificial kidney is used. In the artificial kidney, blood is continually removed from an artery and allowed to circulate through a channel with a thin membrane through which a *dialyzing fluid* removes the impurities from it before it is returned to the patient through a vein. This process is called *renal dialysis*. There are several different types of machine for renal dialysis now available on the market, including a unit for home use. Some patients require renal dialysis for a short period of time, to tide them over an acute episode, but many people without functioning kidneys have been maintained over a period of years with an artificial kidney. Frequently, these patients come into an outpatient department or a clinic for dialysis every few days. In addition to renal dialysis, other methods of removing impurities from body fluids are occasionally used, such as peritoneal or gastrointestinal dialysis. In these techniques, large amounts of dialyzing fluid are injected into the peritoneal cavity or inserted into the gastrointestinal tract and later removed. Dialysis occurs in these cases through the mucous membrane. For additional detail on the use of the renal dialysis machine, the nurse is referred to Symposium on Renal Disease, *Nursing Clinics of North America, 10*:411–516, September, 1975.

The experience of undergoing renal dialysis can be very frightening for the patient. Often the individual is very ill, and the large and complicated machinery that is used can provoke much anxiety. Usually there are a number of people involved in operating the machine, in taking samples for laboratory analysis, and in supervising technical details, and this too can be alarming to the patient. A simple explanation of the procedure frequently helps the patient to understand what is happening to him. The nurse should always be mindful of the patient's needs for encouragement and supportive care. The presence of someone who is interested in him as an individual as well as in the technical aspects of his care can be very reassuring.

Measures to Minimize the Effects of Renal Impairment on the Body

When there is impairment of kidney function, the individual's fluid and electrolyte balance is disturbed. There is usually a retention of fluid in the tissues, and the patient's fluid intake is frequently restricted to minimize this tendency. When edema is present, the nurse should remember that edematous tissue is more prone to break down than normal tissue is, and therefore nursing measures to maintain the integrity of the skin are especially important. Patients who are confined to bed require particular attention to prevent the development of pressure areas. Fluids tend to collect in dependent parts of the body, such as the sacral area in bed patients, and also the lower limbs. These areas should be carefully watched for signs of impending tissue breakdown, and measures should be taken to prevent this. (See Chapter 19 for a discussion of measures to prevent the formation of decubitus ulcers.)

Meticulous skin care is important in the care of patients with renal impairment, not only as a factor in maintaining skin integrity, but also to cleanse the skin of perspiration. When the body is hampered in the elimination of waste products through the kidneys, increased amounts of nitrogenous wastes are excreted through sensible and insensible perspiration. This may cause a crystal-like product to gather on the skin, which can create an unpleasant odor. As a result, bathing is particularly important for the patient's cleanliness and comfort.

To compensate for the lessened ability

of the kidneys to excrete excess acid, an increased amount of carbonic acid is eliminated through the respiratory tract. Measures to facilitate breathing are therefore important. When the patient is in bed, his position should be such that maximum expansion of the chest is possible. The room should be well-ventilated, and an adequate supply of oxygen ensured. (See Chapter 30 for a discussion of measures to facilitate respiration.)

The accumulation of nitrogenous wastes due to the kidneys' lessened ability to excrete these may cause disturbances in neuromuscular functioning. Headache and lethargy are not uncommon, and in severe cases of renal impairment, the patient may become disoriented and subsequently comatose. In these cases, the safety needs of the paient must be especially kept in mind. Although the sensorium usually remains clear even in patients with considerable kidney damage, it is always wise to watch for signs of mental confusion, particularly in older patients. Measures such as siderails to protect the confused patient from injuring himself and the application of mitts to prevent him from pulling at catheters or other tubing are frequently needed. (See Chapter 20 for a discussion of the safety needs of confused patients.)

Weakness of the muscles may result from the retention of potassium ions, and the patient usually fatigues easily.

Because the heart is a muscular organ, it is usually affected by potassium retention. Readings of the apical heart beat are frequently ordered to assist in monitoring cardiac function in patients with renal disorders.

Measures to Facilitate the Elimination of Urine From the Bladder

Maintenance of adequate urinary elimination is important to physiological functioning. For the patient who has difficulty in voiding, there are certain nursing measures which can be provided to assist him. In addition to urinary catheterization, which is carried out as ordered by the physician, there are also measures to stimulate the act of micturition. Some ways in which this is done are:

1. Helping the patient to assume a natural position for voiding
2. Providing a commode or, preferably, assisting the patient to the bathroom if this is possible (male patients frequently find it easier to void when they are standing rather than sitting or lying down)
3. Running water within the patient's hearing
4. Providing water in which he can dangle his fingers
5. Providing privacy and setting aside a time for voiding
6. Providing a warm bedpan or urinal
7. Applying a warm hot water bottle to the patient's lower abdomen (this may require a doctor's order)
8. Pouring warm water over the perineum (the water must be measured)
9. Relieving pain

It has long been accepted that warmth applied to the bladder and perineal areas will help to relax the muscles used in voiding and therefore facilitate this process.

Unless the physician has expressly ordered the insertion of a urinary catheter, the foregoing measures are tried before catheterization is considered.

Patients who cannot void or those who void without control are usually embarrassed as well as anxious. The nurse can offer support by providing explanations of the reason for the problem. The patient should be encouraged to respond to the urge for voiding promptly, rather than waiting. It is important, in this regard, for the nurse to answer the patient's call signal promptly also that the patient is not kept waiting for a urinal or a bedpan. At no time should the nurse show impatience or a lack of understanding of the patient's distress.

Urinary Catheterization of the Female Patient. A urinary catheterization is the introduction of a narrow tube, called a urinary catheter, through the urethra into the bladder in order to remove urine. It is ordered by the physician, although it is usually carried out by a female nurse for the female patient and by a male nurse, an orderly, or the physician for the male patient. This does not mean, however that a female nurse might not find it necessary to catheterize a male patient on occasion.

The purpose of urinary catheterization may be to obtain a sterile urine specimen for laboratory examination or to empty a patient's bladder preoperatively so that the danger of incising the bladder is lessened. A urinary catheterization is also ordered postoperatively for a patient who is unable to void. Normally the act of voiding is a spinal cord reflex subject to voluntary control by the cerebrum. After surgery, however, some patients have difficulty in voiding. This is particularly true when anxiety is mediated through the hypothalamus and the sympathetic nervous system to the nerves which supply the bladder muscles.

Another reason for a urinary catheterization is to insert a retention or indwelling catheter in order to prevent uncontrollable voiding or voiding upon an operative area. A patient who has surgery on her perineum will probably have an indwelling catheter inserted postoperatively in order to prevent the urine from irritating the operative area.

EQUIPMENT. A catheter is a hollow tube made of rubber, plastic, glass, metal, or silk. Plastic catheters are becoming increasingly popular. Catheters are graded in size according to the French scale; No. 14 and No. 16 catheters are commonly used for the catheterization of the adult female patient. The larger the number, the larger is the lumen of the catheter. It is, of course, safest to use the correct size of catheter for each patient, but should the nurse be unsure about which size to use, she should use a smaller size in order not to harm the mucous membrane of the urethra or to cause the patient discomfort. The larger the lumen of the catheter, the more quickly will urine flow from the bladder, but usually this is not of great importance unless the patient's bladder is greatly distended. In any case, a clamp can be used to regulate the flow of urine according to the physician's order.

There are many kinds of catheters available. Retention or indwelling catheters are inserted into the patient's bladder and are kept in place by an inflated balloon or a rubber ring which is larger than the bladder orifice. These catheters may have a single lumen, as in the mushroom catheter, a double lumen, or even a triple lumen, as in the Foley-Alcock catheter. The latter type of catheter is used for continuous irrigations, in which the fluid flows continuously up one lumen to the bladder and down a second lumen into a receptacle. The third lumen is connected to the inflated balloon which keeps the catheter in place. A straight catheter is usually used when the purpose of the catheterization is to remove urine rather than to have the patient retain the catheter.

The equipment for a urinary catheterization should be sterile. Because the mucous membrane lining the urinary tract is continuous and because the warm mucous membrane is a likely place for the propagation of bacteria, an aseptic technique is carried out throughout the entire catheterization procedure. Disposable, prepackaged catheterization sets are available, but if these are not used, the set that is to be used is checked to make sure that it is sterile.

A catheterization set contains, at a minimum, the catheter, a receptacle for the urine, and materials for cleansing the labia and urinary meatus of the patient. Some agencies suggest that the nurse use sterile rubber gloves during the catheterization procedure, whereas others suggest that sterile forceps may be used for the insertion of the catheter. In either case it is important that the catheter remain sterile during its insertion up the urethra into the patient's bladder.

The nurse needs to have a good light in order to visualize the urinary meatus and prevent contamination. Either an extension lamp or an extendable lamp can be used to illuminate the perineal area.

Since urinary catheterization can be an embarrassing measure, it is important that the nurse protect the patient from unnecessary exposure. The positions that are most often used for the catheterization are the dorsal recumbent or lithotomy positions, although some authorities are now advocating that a side-lying position be used, with the patient's knees flexed and the upper leg higher than the lower. Once the patient assumes the position that is to be used, she is covered with drapes in such a way that her legs and body are adequately covered. Then only the perineal area is exposed. In her explanation to the patient, the nurse assures her that the catheterization is usually painless but that the patient may experience a feeling of pressure and of wanting to urinate because the catheter irritates the urethra. Discomfort is minimized if the patient is relaxed.

PREPARATION OF THE PATIENT. In explaining a urinary catheterization, the nurse must be guided by the needs of the patient. Some patients want a detailed explanation; others simply want assurance that it is a painless measure. From inexperience many patients want to know whether it will hurt, how long it will take, and where the tube goes. The nurse should rarely assume a knowledge of anatomy on the patient's part; indeed, she may be surprised at some of the beliefs people have. That sterile technique is maintained is important to the patient's safety, but the patient probably has little awareness of this.

If the patient needs a retention catheter, she probably requires reassurance that she will be able to move about freely in bed and, very often, will still be able to get out of bed. The length of time a retention catheter remains in place depends upon the reason for its insertion; this matter is left to the physician's judgment. Points which can prove helpful to the patient with a retention catheter are:

1. Usually the patient should drink a large amount of fluid, approximately 3000 cc. per day

2. The patient may move freely in bed

3. The patient should not lie on the catheter tubing

4. It is normal to have a feeling of wanting to void for a while while the catheter is in place

After the patient has been properly draped, a sterile towel is placed between the patient's legs to make it easier to maintain sterile technique. The receptacle for the urine is then placed on the towel near the urinary meatus. It is advantageous if this receptacle is lower than the patient's bladder so that the urine will flow easily from the bladder to the receptacle by the force of gravity. All the equipment is placed conveniently.

CLEANSING THE PERINEAL AREA. Trauma to the mucous membrane of the urinary tract and the admission of bacteria to the urinary tract can result in a local or a generalized infection. Therefore, the patient's perineal area is cleansed thoroughly. There are many different ways suggested to do this; soap and water and a variety of antiseptics are used. Regardless of the method used, the patient's labia must be as clean as possible, and the urinary meatus as free from bacteria as possible.

The following are guides to cleansing the perineal area:

1. If the area is obviously soiled wash with soap and water and then dry; all soap is carefully removed, because it can inactivate some disinfectants

2. Use a mild, nonirritating disinfectant

3. Use each swab just once, cleansing from the cleanest area (near the symphysis pubis) toward the most contaminated area (near the rectum)

4. Cleanse the outer labia, the inner labia, and then the vestibule of the peri-

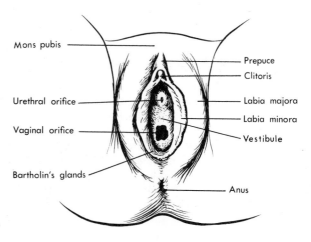

Mons pubis —
Urethral orifice —
Vaginal orifice —
Bartholin's glands —

— Prepuce
— Clitoris
— Labia majora
— Labia minora
— Vestibule
— Anus

The female perineum.

neum; a minimum of five sponges is needed

5. Once the vestibule has been cleansed, the labia must not touch it until the catheter has been inserted. It is necessary to keep the labia separated with the fingers for adequate visualization and to prevent unwanted contamination of the catheter.

INSERTION OF THE CATHETER. The catheter used in a urinary catheterization should be smooth so that it will not damage the mucous membrane of the urethra. In order to facilitate the passage of the catheter up the urethra, a water soluble lubricant is used. The lubricant is applied to the catheter prior to its insertion into the urethra.

With sterile forceps, sterile gloves, or sterile gauze, the urinary catheter is picked up approximately 10 cm. (4 inches) from the tip and inserted gently into the urethra. The catheter should be inserted 3 to 5 cm. (1¼ to 2 inches) into the urethra—that is, the distance from the urinary meatus to the bladder. If any resistance is met during the passage of the catheter, it is withdrawn and the situation is reported to the physician.

The other end of the catheter lies in the sterile receptacle between the patient's legs and is held in place until the patient's bladder is empty or until the urine specimen has been obtained. If the patient has a large amount of retained urine, the distended bladder should be emptied gradually. Not all fluid should be drained off at once or there is danger of decompressing the bladder too quickly. The sudden release from pressure may result in injury to the organ itself or may cause a generalized reaction within the body, characterized by chills, an elevated temperature, and, occasionally, shock. These complications can be avoided by clamping off the catheter at intervals to allow time for the bladder to adjust to the changes in pressure caused by withdrawing the urine from it. Once the urine has been obtained, the catheter is pinched and withdrawn slowly. The patient is assisted with drying the perineal area and assuming a comfortable position before the equipment is removed.

A description of the urine is recorded. This includes the amount, the color, the clarity, and any unusual characteristics. If the urine has an unusual odor, if the nurse encountered any difficulty during the urinary catheterization, or if the patient experienced any unusual discomfort, these observations are also recorded.

Urinary Catheterization of the Male Patient. Usually this measure is carried out by the physician, orderly, or male nurse; however, on occasion a female nurse may have to catheterize a male patient. This can be particularly embarrassing to the patient, but he will be helped by an understanding, competent manner on the part of the nurse. The equipment that is necessary is similar to that used for a female urinary catheterization. The use of sterile rubber gloves is advised to facilitate the maintenance of sterile technique.

The downward curvature of the prepubic urethra of the male can be straightened by lifting the penis and, with slight traction, holding it perpendicular to the patient's body. The patient lies in the dorsal recumbent position, his knees flexed and his legs slightly rotated externally to expose the penis. The draping and placing of the equipment are similar to that used for a female catheterization.

After the catheter and the urethral orifice are lubricated, the penis is extended vertically as described and the catheter is then inserted to a distance of approximately 20 cm.—that is, into the patient's bladder. When, in the course of the insertion, the catheter meets the resistance of Guérin's fold or the pouch of the fossa navicularis, the resistance can be bypassed by twisting the catheter. If the catheter encounters resistance at the vesical sphincters, it should not be forced, but held firmly until the sphincters relax. Once the catheter is in place the procedure is similar to that for a female catheterization.

Insertion of a Retention Catheter. If a patient requires an indwelling catheter, a syringe, sterile water for the inflation of the balloon of the catheter, connecting tubing, and a receptacle for the draining urine are needed, in addition to the equipment used in a simple catheterization. After the indwelling catheter is inserted into the patient's bladder, the balloon is filled with the amount of sterile water that it is designed to hold. After the water has been injected, slight tension is placed upon the catheter to make sure that it is in place and that it will not come out of the patient's bladder easily. If the balloon is in the patient's urethra, the nurse will encounter considerable difficulty in filling the balloon and the patient will complain of discomfort. In such cases, the catheter is inserted a little farther into the bladder and the fluid is again injected into the balloon.

Once the indwelling catheter is safely in the patient's bladder, it is attached to the connecting tubing, the other end of which is in a receptacle, which is often attached to the patient's bed. Sterile technique is maintained while connecting the tubing.

The receptacle for the urine is situated at a level lower than the patient so that the urine flows readily by force of gravity. The tubing should not loop below the receptacle, because a kink may be formed which occludes the lumen. In addition, the urine then would have to flow against gravity. The tubing is pinned to the bed in such a manner that the lumen of the tubing is patent. This can be accomplished by pinching a piece of sheet on either side of the tubing and pinning the sides over the tubing. The tubing that lies on the top of the bed should be kept flat to facilitate drainage. Sometimes the catheter tubing is taped to the patient's thigh to avoid pulling on the catheter as the patient moves about in bed. The nurse should make sure that the patient's leg is never resting on the tubing, since this

will occlude the lumen. Also, the lowest point of the tubing should always be above the level of urine in the drainage bottle, or, as already stated, the urine is forced to run uphill, against the force of gravity.

For the patient with an indwelling catheter, the physician may order continuous or intermittent drainage. If he orders continuous drainage, the catheter is attached to the tubing, and the urine is allowed to drain freely into the receptacle that is provided. If intermittent drainage is ordered, the tubing is clamped at designated intervals.

Urine receptacles are available commercially which attach to the upper leg and can be used to receive urine from a catheter while the patient is walking around. These leg bags are usually disposed of when they accumulate urine and are replaced by clean, sterile bags.

When the patient requires continuous or intermittent drainage, many agencies now use disposable closed drainage sets. When these are used, the urine bag is simply emptied when full, or at regular intervals, and the tubing is left untouched until the entire set is either removed or changed. If closed drainage sets are not used, it is necessary to change the tubing and urine receptacle regularly to prevent the accumulation of salt deposits and the development of unpleasant odors. Often the urine receptacle is changed daily and the tubing every few days.

When tubing is changed or the catheter is disconnected from the tubing for a

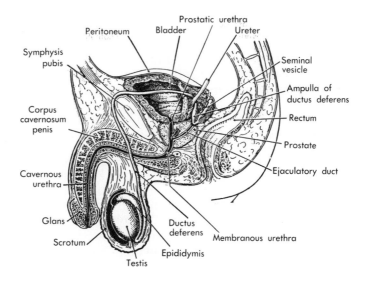

The male urogenital system.

period of time, for example, when the patient is to be up and walking around, or when a bladder irrigation is to be done, it is vitally important that the sterility of both the catheter and tubing be maintained. Small disposable urinary adaptor protectors are now available. These provide a sterile cover for both tubing and catheter when these are disconnected.

Urinary catheters are usually changed at the physician's order. They are never changed without good reason because of the danger of infection to the patient. If there is any obstruction to urine flow which is not cleared by an irrigation, the catheter should be replaced. Other signs that a catheter may need to be changed are:

1. Insufficient urine in the drainage bottle in comparison with the fluid intake of the patient

2. Abdominal distention just above the symphysis pubis, which on palpation indicates a full bladder (see discussion of urinary retention, p. 544)

Male External Drainage. An external urinary appliance is often used for men instead of a retention catheter for patients who are unable to control voiding. (Protective pants may be used for women; these have a nonabsorbent plastic or rubberized lining. They can be worn over an absorbent pad.) The external appliance for men is a rubber condom with a short tube that can be connected to a drainage bottle or bag. Known by various names, such as urosheath or "Texas condom," it provides a convenient and relatively safe method of collecting urine from patients who are incontinent. It is considered much safer than risking the chance of infection through the use of a retention catheter. It also makes bladder retraining easier, since the condom can be left off for gradually increasing periods of time so that the patient feels more "normal." This psychological effect in itself is important for the patient.

The condom is disposable, relatively inexpensive, and easily applied so that it can be changed frequently. It is rolled over the penis so that the narrow tube opening at the end is over the urinary meatus at the tip of the penis. The tube is then connected to a drainage tube and attached to a bottle or other container for the urine.

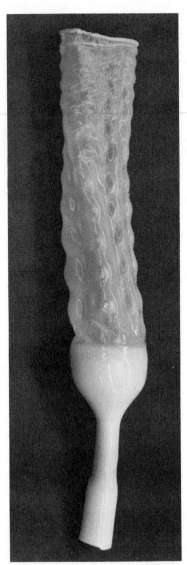

Male external drainage appliance. (From Ruth Stryker Gordon: *Rehabilitative Aspects of Acute and Chronic Nursing Care.* 2nd Ed. Philadelphia, W. B. Saunders Co., 1977.)

Urinary Bladder Irrigation ("Internal"). The procedure of bladder irrigation is not used as commonly today as in times past. It is now felt by many physicians that the danger of introducing infection into the bladder during the course of the irrigation is sufficiently great to offset many of the benefits. When a bladder irrigation is ordered, the importance of maintaining sterile technique during the procedure cannot be overstressed.

A physician might order urinary bladder irrigations for a patient who has an indwelling catheter. The purpose of the irrigations is to cleanse the bladder or to apply an antiseptic solution to the lining of the bladder.

This nursing measure is a sterile procedure similar to urinary catheterization. The equipment required includes a container for the irrigation solution, a receptacle for the returned irrigation solution, and a syringe with a tip that fits into the urinary catheter. The solutions that are used for irrigations vary considerably; sterile water, sterile normal saline, and many antiseptic solutions are used. The irrigating fluid is usually administered at room temperature unless the physician orders otherwise.

Sterile equipment is used for the bladder irrigation, and sterile technique is maintained throughout this nursing measure. The end of the catheter and the end of the tubing are kept sterile while the bladder is irrigated. Frequently they are put in a sterile container placed close to the patient's leg.

After the tubing has been disconnected from the catheter, a small amount of sterile solution is introduced into the bladder. This is done by using either a funnel or an Asepto syringe. The amount of solution that is recommended for insertion varies in different agencies, with many suggesting that no more than 50 cc. be introduced at any one time for an "internal" bladder irrigation, 30 cc. for an irrigation done through a retention cath-

eter. The solution is always administered gently in order not to damage the mucous membrane lining. The fluid should be allowed to run in slowly and the syringe or funnel should be kept low to prevent exerting undue pressure on the walls of the bladder. The catheter is pinched off before the syringe (or funnel) is completely empty to prevent the introduction of air into the bladder. The fluid is then withdrawn by permitting it to drain from the catheter into a basin. This procedure—the administration of fluid and its return—is repeated until all the solution ordered has been used or until the return flow is clear.

In recording this nursing measure the nurse notes and records the strength and kind of solution used in the bladder irrigation and the character of the return flow. Was the return flow cloudy or colored? These observations are reported in the patient's record.

Measures to Assist in the Reestablishment of a Normal Voiding Pattern

Some patients with urinary problems have difficulty in voiding; others may suffer from urinary incontinence. For those patients whose ability to control voiding has been lessened, the nurse can often assist them to train their bladders to func-

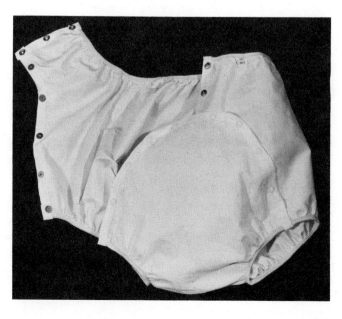

Protective pants with a nonabsorbent plastic or rubberized lining may be used for women patients who are incontinent. (From Ruth Stryker Gordon: Rehabilitative Aspects of Acute and Chronic Nursing Care. 2nd Ed. Philadelphia, W. B. Saunders Co., 1977.)

tion at regular and predictable times. For the nurse to be able to assist the patient in this, she should know his normal pattern of voiding. What are the times when he voids and when is he usually dry?

The patient is encouraged to assume as natural a position as possible for voiding and to void at regular times, preferably at his normal voiding periods. There is considerable debate whether the effort involved in getting on and off the bedpan exceeds that involved in getting out of bed and using a commode. Many women patients find it easier to void when they use a bedside commode, and male patients find it easier if they stand at the side of the bed to use a urinal. If permissible, these measures often help the patient in regaining a normal pattern of voiding.

The patient can be assisted to void by the various means just described. In addition to those already mentioned, digital pressure at the side of the urinary meatus or a circular movement over the bladder can often stimulate urination. If the patient has had a catheter in place over a period of time, he will need to have it clamped for intervals of two to three hours in order to increase the muscle tone before bladder training is initiated. The patient can expect accidents during a bladder training regimen; nevertheless, many people do develop a regular voiding pattern.

It has already been mentioned that the patient should be encouraged to void as soon as he feels the urge to do so. The importance of having nursing personnel answer the patient's call signal promptly cannot be overemphasized. The patient should not be kept waiting or allowed to become incontinent because his request for a bedpan or a urinal went unheeded.

If an accident does occur, the patient's bedding should be changed at once. If it is not allowed to stay wet this has the psychological advantage of encouraging the patient to keep his bed dry. Changing wet linen also helps to prevent skin irritation and the development of unpleasant odors.

In a bladder retraining program, it is essential that the patient have an adequate intake of fluids to stimulate the secretion of sufficient urine to distend the bladder enough so that the micturition reflex is initiated at regular times. The provision of fluids at regular intervals helps to ensure an adequate intake; under normal circumstances, a minimum of 3000 cc. should be maintained, preferably more if the patient can tolerate a larger amount.

Patients on a bladder retraining regimen have much need for both physical and emotional support. They usually require physical assistance from nursing personnel when they need to use a bedpan, commode, or toilet. The dependence on others and the lack of control over such a basic function as voiding can be very distressing to the patient. Since both the patient and his family will probably need help, the nurse must understand the meaning that urinary problems have for them. Sympathy, tolerance, and patience are all required of the nurse in helping patients with urinary problems.

GUIDE TO ASSESSING URINARY ELIMINATION STATUS

1. What is the patient's usual voiding pattern? present pattern?
2. Is he having problems with voiding? If so, what are they?
3. Is he voiding an amount of urine that is normal in relation to his intake and sufficient to promote health?
4. Are there any factors that might be affecting his voiding pattern?
5. Does he have difficulty in discussing his urinary problems?
6. Does the patient need help in reestablishing a normal voiding pattern?
7. Does he need help with his diet and fluid intake?
8. Does he need an explanation of laboratory tests and nursing care measures?
9. Does the patient or his family need skills or knowledge in order to prevent a recurrence of his problem to improve his health?

GUIDE TO EVALUATING THE EFFECTIVENESS OF NURSING INTERVENTION

1. Is the patient taking the required amount of fluids to maintain adequate fluid balance?
2. Are the laboratory test results showing improvement?
3. Is the patient's skin in good condition?
4. Is he getting sufficient rest?
5. Is he taking an adequate diet?
6. Is he comfortable—free from pain, restlessness, and anxiety?

STUDY VOCABULARY

Albuminuria	Edema	Pyuria
Anuria	Glycosuria	Renal dialysis
Calculi	Hematuria	Retention
Casts	Hemoglobinuria	Suppression
Catherization	Micturition	Urea frost
Cystitis	Nocturia	Uremia
Cystoscopy	Oliguria	Urinalysis
Diuresis	Polyuria	Voiding
Dysuria	Proteinuria	

STUDY SITUATION

Mrs. Smith needs an indwelling catheter prior to her surgery tomorrow. Mrs. Smith is an intelligent person; she understands the purpose of her surgery but she has never had a urinary catheterization. The catheter is to be inserted the next morning.

That afternoon Mrs. Smith's husband comes to the nursing unit desk greatly disturbed. His wife has told him that she has to have a tube inserted and he does not understand why. In talking with Mr. Smith, the nurse learns that his mother had had a tube inserted and she died two days later.

1. What factors should the nurse consider in her explanation?
2. What should the nurse include in her explanation to Mr. Smith? Why?
3. What principles guide the nurse regarding a urinary catheterization?
4. Why is a urinary catheterization a distressing measure?
5. What nursing care interventions would be essential for Mrs. Smith as a result of the indwelling catheter?
6. How can the nurse evaluate the effectiveness of her nursing care after the catheterization?

SUGGESTED READINGS

Beaumont, E.: Urinary Drainage Systems. *Nursing '74, 4*:52–60, January 1974.

Garner, J.: Urinary Catheter Care. Doing It Better. *Nursing '74, 4*:54–56, February 1974.

Garrett, J. J.: Oliguria in Postoperative Patients. *Nursing Clinics of North America, 10*:59–67, March 1975.

Maney, J. Y.: A Behavioral Therapy Approach to Bladder Retraining. *Nursing Clinics of North America, 11*:179–188, March 1976.

McGuckin, M.: Microbiologic Studies: Urine Cultures—Key to Diagnosing Urinary Infections. Part 1. *Nursing '75, 5*:10–11, December 1975.

O'Neill, M. (Guest Editor): Symposium on the Care of Patients With Renal Disease. *Nursing Clinics of North America, 10*:411–516, September 1975.

Santopietro, M. C. S.: Meeting the Emotional Needs of Hemodialysis Patients and Their Spouses. *American Journal of Nursing, 75*:629–632, April 1975.

Walser, D.: Behavioral Effects of Dialysis. *Canadian Nurse, 70*:23–25, May 1974.

Watt, R. C.: Urinary Diversion. *American Journal of Nursing, 74*:1806–1811, October 1974.

Willington, F. L.: Incontinence. 5. Training and Retraining for Continence. *Nursing Times, 71*:500–503, March 27, 1975.

29 FLUID AND ELECTROLYTE PROBLEMS

The nurse should be able to:

Describe the distribution of fluid and the major electrolytes in the
body
Discuss the normal methods of fluid and electrolyte intake and
output to and from the body
Explain the principal mechanisms that maintain the body's acid-
base balance
Identify factors in a patient that may affect or be affecting his fluid
and electrolyte imbalance
Assess patients for problems of fluid and electrolyte balance
Apply relevant principles in planning and implementing
appropriate nursing interventions in the care of patients with
actual or potential problems of fluid and electrolyte
imbalance, including measures:
to maintain fluid and electrolyte balance
to assist in restoring balance if a disturbance has occurred
Evaluate the effectiveness of nursing interventions

INTRODUCTION

Water has been called the indispensable nutrient. Approximately 50 to 70 per cent of the total body weight of an adult is made up of water and its dissolved constituents; 70 to 80 per cent of the total body weight of the infant is similarly in a fluid state. The fluid system plays an essential role in the body. Its principal functions are (1) the transportation of oxygen and nutrients to the cells and the removal of waste products from them, and (2) the maintenance of a stable physical and chemical environment within the body. Important in the latter function are the *electrolytes.* You will recall from your chemistry courses that electrolytes are compounds which in water solution separate into particles, each capable of carrying an electrical charge. Sodium (Na^+), for example, carries a positive charge; it is therefore a cation. Chlorine (Cl^-), with which it combines to form salt ($NaCl$), carries a negative charge; it is an anion. The electrolytes in body fluids are important in the chemical reactions that occur within the cells. They also help to regulate the permeability of cell membranes, thus controlling the transfer of various materials across the membrane. They are vital to the maintenance of the body's acid-base balance and are also essential in the transmission of electrical energy within the body. Without the calcium ion, for example, muscle contraction could not occur.

Under normal circumstances, the body maintains a very precise fluid and electrolyte balance. Both the volume and the constituents of body fluids vary but little from day to day, and usually return to a state of equilibrium within a very few days following any minor disturbance.

Serious fluid and electrolyte balance may occur as a result of a number of *health problems.* The nature of the imbalance may be either an excess or an insufficiency. An individual may retain an excess amount of fluid in the tissues and become edematous. On the other hand, he may lose an inordinate amount of fluids (through persistent vomiting, for example) and become dehydrated. Whenever fluids are lost or retained in excessive amounts, there is an accompanying loss or retention of electrolytes so that both fluid and electrolyte balances are disturbed. Disturbances in fluid and electrolyte balance can cause serious repercussions within the body. Both the transportation and regulatory functions of the fluid system are likely to be affected. The cells may not get sufficient nourishment, for instance, or there may be an accumulation of waste products due to inefficiency of the mechanism for their removal. The body's acid-base balance may be upset and temperature regulation impaired (see Chapter 25) . There may also be interference with the transfer of materials across the cell membrane so that a shift occurs in the distribution of fluids and electrolytes. Activities within the body that depend on the transmission of electrical energy, such as muscle contraction and the relay of nerve impulses, may also be impaired.

Whenever there is a disturbance in fluid and electrolyte balance, the body attempts to compensate for the lack or the excess, whichever the case may be, by bringing into play various adaptive mechanisms. A very common example of this occurs in the person who perspires heav-

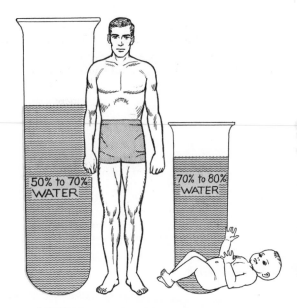

The Distribution of Fluid and Electrolytes

Fluid within the body is generally considered to be distributed in what may be termed two basic compartments. First, body fluids are found within the cells of the body. This type, termed *intracellular fluid*, accounts for approximately 40 to 50 per cent of the total body weight. Second, fluid occurs outside the cells of the body; this is *extracellular fluid*. There are two kinds of extracellular fluid. One is the fluid in the spaces between the cells; called *interstitial fluid*, this component accounts for approximately 15 per cent of the total body weight of an adult. The other component, *intravascular fluid*, is the fluid in the blood and lymph vessels; it makes up approximately 5 per cent of total body weight in an adult.

There is a constant shift of fluid from one compartment to another as it performs its function of transporting nutrients and oxygen to the cells and removing wastes and manufactured products from the cells. In health, the amount of fluid in the circulating blood and the total amount of fluid within the cells must be maintained at a fairly constant volume. In cases of dehydration the body fluid is drawn from within the cells and routed into the blood

ily on a hot day and then finds that he is thirsty for extra fluids to replace those he has lost through sweating. The body has a number of adaptive mechanisms in addition to thirst; these are discussed later in this chapter.

If the imbalance is too great, however, or persists over a prolonged period of time, the body's adaptive mechanisms may not be able to cope. In this event, the body's defenses collapse and prostration ensues. This may happen, for example, when there is a continuous loss of fluids with no replacement, or a very sudden large loss, as in massive hemorrhage.

THE PHYSIOLOGY OF FLUID AND ELECTROLYTE BALANCE

In order to understand the physiological processes involved, it is perhaps easier to consider different aspects of fluid and electrolyte balance under separate headings:

1. The distribution of fluid and electrolytes within the body
2. The modes of transport of fluids and electrolytes
3. The balancing of fluid intake and output
4. Mechanisms regulating fluid and electrolyte balance
5. Maintenance of the body's acid-base balance

	EXTRACELLULAR FLUID	INTRACELLULAR FLUID
Na^+	142 mEq/l.	10 mEq/l.
K^+	5 mEq/l.	141 mEq/l.
Ca^{++}	5 mEq/l.	<1 mEq/l.
Mg^{++}	3 mEq/l	58 mEq/l.
Cl^-	103 mEq/l	4 mEq/l.
HCO_3^-	28 mEq/l.	10 mEq/l.
Phosphates	4 mEq/l.	75 mEq/l.
SO_4^{--}	1 mEq/l.	2 mEq/l.
Glucose	90 mgm.%	0 to 20 mgm.%
Amino acids	30 mgm.%	200 mgm.%?
Cholesterol Phospholipids Neutral fat	0.5 gm.%	2 to 95 gm.%
Po_2	35 mm.Hg	20 mm.Hg ?
Pco_2	46 mm.Hg	50 mm.Hg ?
pH	7.4	7.0

The electrolyte content of body fluids. (From Arthur C. Guyton: Function of the Human Body. 4th Ed. Philadelphia, W. B. Saunders Co., 1974.)

vessels. This explains why a patient who is unable to retain fluids owing to prolonged vomiting soon loses the elasticity of his subcutaneous tissue, his skin becoming loose and flabby.

The principal electrolytes and their concentrations in extracellular and intracellular fluid are given in the accompanying illustration. It can readily be seen that the electrolyte composition of the two types of fluid is quite different. The fluid contained within the cells is essentially a potassium solution, whereas extracellular fluid is high in sodium ions. Both types of fluid also contain specified quantities of other electrolytes, as shown in the illustration.

The electrolyte composition of the two types of extracellular fluid (that is, interstitial and intravascular) is essentially the same insofar as principal electrolytes are concerned. The fluid within the blood vessels does, however, contain a much greater concentration of protein than is found in the interstitial fluid.

Modes of Transport

In the process of body functioning, fluid and electrolytes are constantly moving from within the cells to the extracellular compartments and vice versa. This transfer is accomplished by several different means, the three most common being osmosis, active transport, and diffusion.

Osmosis is the movement of a solvent, such as water, through a partition separating solutions of different concentrations. The solvent tends to pass from a solution with a lesser concentration to one with a higher concentration to equalize the concentrations of both solutions. This movement is possible when a semipermeable membrane separates the two solutions. Cell membranes and the walls of capillaries are examples of semipermeable membranes. However, some of the dissolved substances in body fluid do not move between the membranes as readily as water. Electrolytes are examples of this.

Therefore, when it is necessary for the body to transfer electrolytes from the cells to the extracellular fluid—to achieve a balance, for example—an *active transport mechanism* is brought into play. Although this mechanism is not yet completely understood, it is believed that a substance known as *adenosine triphosphate (ATP)* is released from the cell. This substance appears to give the electrolytes the energy required to pass through the semipermeable membrane. The transfer of sodium, potassium, and a number of other ions, including amino acids, is believed to take place via this mechanism.

Diffusion is a process whereby molecules and ions tend to distribute themselves equally within a given space. When used in connection with gases, it refers to the process by which the molecules of the gases interpenetrate and become mixed; this occurs because of the incessant motion of the molecules. The exchange of oxygen and carbon dioxide that occurs in the alveoli and capillaries of the lungs takes place through a process of diffusion.

Balancing of Fluid Intake and Output

A person derives fluid and electrolytes from three main sources: the fluid that is ingested in liquid form, the fluid content of the various foods that are eaten, and the water that is formed as a byproduct of the body's oxidation of foods and body substances. The total daily intake of water under normal circumstances is approximately 2100 to 2900 ml. The average amount of fluid gained by an adult in a 24 hour period from each of the sources listed above is:

Ingested fluids	1000 to 1500 ml.
Ingested food	900 to 1000 ml.
Metabolic oxidation	200 to 400 ml.
Total	2100 to 2900 ml.

Water is lost from the body through the skin by perspiration, through the lungs in expirations, and from the kidneys in the urine. In addition, a small amount of fluid is excreted in the feces. The total daily loss of water from the body in normal circumstances is approximately 2100 to 2900 ml., depending largely upon the amount of fluid intake. It is lost as follows:

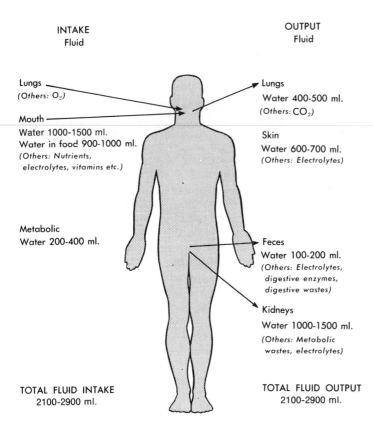

INTAKE
Fluid

Lungs
(Others: O_2)

Mouth
Water 1000-1500 ml.
Water in food 900-1000 ml.
(Others: Nutrients,
electrolytes, vitamins etc.)

Metabolic
Water 200-400 ml.

TOTAL FLUID INTAKE
2100-2900 ml.

OUTPUT
Fluid

Lungs
Water 400-500 ml.
(Others: CO_2)

Skin
Water 600-700 ml.
(Others: Electrolytes)

Feces
Water 100-200 ml.
(Others: Electrolytes,
digestive enzymes,
digestive wastes)

Kidneys
Water 1000-1500 ml.
(Others: Metabolic
wastes, electrolytes)

TOTAL FLUID OUTPUT
2100-2900 ml.

Normally the body maintains a precise balance between fluid intake and fluid output. The average daily intake of fluids from various sources and output via various routes are shown here. (From Mary W. Falconer, Annette Schram Ezell, H. Robert Patterson, and Edward A. Gustafson: The Drug, The Nurse, The Patient. 5th Ed. Philadelphia, W. B. Saunders Co., 1974.)

In urine	1000 to 1500 ml. daily
In feces	100 to 200 ml. daily
From the skin	600 to 700 ml. daily
From the lungs	400 to 500 ml. daily[1]

The balance between the fluid taken in and the fluid excreted is maintained within a very narrow range. The intake usually equals the output over a three day period even though it may not always be equal over a single 24 hour period.

Mechanisms Regulating Fluid and Electrolyte Balance

The main forces at work in holding water within the various compartments of the fluid system of the body are generated by proteins and electrolytes. In the intra-

vascular compartment (blood vessels) the force is generated largely by the serum albumin, in the intracellular fluid by the sodium ion, and within the cells by protoplasm. Water passes freely through the capillary walls and membranes, but the protein molecules and the sodium ions do not move as freely. These substances exert an osmotic pressure which tends to hold water in the respective compartments. Osmotic pressure is that pressure exerted by particles which tends to draw a solvent toward it. A patient who has lost a great deal of serum albumin through malnutrition tends to become edematous, since fluid is drawn from the blood plasma into the intercellular spaces. This happens because the main force holding the water in the blood vessels has been lost.

By far the most important regulatory mechanism operating to maintain the body's fluid balance is the *kidneys*. When the intake of fluid is insufficient or when there is an excessive loss of fluid from the body, the amount of urine that is excreted

[1]Mary W. Falconer, Annette Schram Ezell, H. Robert Patterson, and Edward A. Gustafson: *The Drug, the Nurse, the Patient.* 5th edition. Philadelphia, W. B. Saunders Company, 1974, p. 146.

is decreased. Conversely, when an excess amount of fluid is ingested, urine output increases. This is accomplished through the selective reabsorption of water in the tubules of the kidney.

The kidney also exerts the main control over the sodium and potassium balance of the body through the selective reabsorption of these ions in the tubules. When sodium and potassium need to be retained, increasing amounts are reabsorbed. Excess sodium and potassium are excreted in the urine. If there is an acute shortage of sodium in the body, the excretion of this ion through the urine may be cut to almost zero. In the case of potassium, however, there appears to be an obligatory excretion of a certain amount in the urine.[2] Thus, there is always some potassium in the daily urine output, even though the body reserves may be dangerously low. This factor is taken into account by the physician when he is planning replacement therapy.

The control of fluid and electrolyte balance by the kidneys is influenced by two sets of hormones. The *antidiuretic hormone* (ADH), which is produced primarily in the anterior hypothalamus and stored in the pituitary gland, is a major factor in controlling water reabsorption. When the body takes in an insufficient quantity, or there is water deprivation from other sources, the secretion of ADH is stimulated. This in turn causes increased reabsorption of water in the kidney tubules and a lessened volume of urinary output. *Aldosterone*, one of several steroid hormones produced in the adrenal cortex, exerts a major influence in promoting the retention of sodium and the excretion of potassium. Aldosterone secretion appears to be stimulated by such factors as a lessened sodium intake, an excess of potassium, muscular activity, trauma, and emotional tension.[3]

The gastrointestinal tract also helps to regulate fluid and electrolyte balance. The manner in which this is done is similar to the action of the kidneys — that is, through the selective reabsorption of water and solutes, the reabsorption taking place principally in the small intestine. Although the volume of digestive juices secreted into the gastrointestinal tract each day is considerable (approximately 8200 ml.), all but about 100 to 200 ml. of fluid is reabsorbed. Under normal circumstances, only a small amount of the body's daily fluid loss is from the gastrointestinal tract in the feces, and the loss of electrolytes by this route is normally negligible. Both fluid and electrolytes may be lost in considerable quantity, however, in such conditions as vomiting and diarrhea.

Thirst is another of the regulatory mechanisms operating to maintain fluid balance. Thirst is the desire for more fluids. It usually indicates a basic physiological need for water, although it may sometimes occur as a result of dryness of the mucous membranes of the mouth and throat from other causes, such as mouth-breathing. In cases in which thirst is due to a simple dryness of the oropharynx rather than a basic lack of water in the body, it may be relieved by measures to keep the mucous membranes moist. Good oral hygiene can usually relieve this dryness.

"True thirst," due to a basic lack of water, usually occurs when body cells are dehydrated, extracellular volume is lessened (as in a hemorrhage), or certain centers in the hypothalamus are stimulated.[4] It is thought that the thirst mechanism is closely related to the control of water balance by the antidiuretic hormone (ADH). When the body is suffering from a lack of water, the thirst mechanism operates to increase the intake of water, while ADH restricts the loss of water through urinary output.

The lungs are also important in the regulation of fluid and electrolyte balance. Ordinarily, the amount of water lost from respiration is quite small. Whenever respirations are increased in rate and depth, however, the amount of water lost via this route is also increased and may become a significant factor to consider. This may occur, for example, with strenuous muscular exercise, in fevers or any condition

[2]Cyril M. MacBryde and Robert S. Blacklow (eds.): *Signs and Symptoms: Applied Pathologic Physiology and Clinical Interpretation.* 5th edition. Philadelphia, J. B. Lippincott Company, 1970, p. 787.

[3]Ibid., p. 774.

[4]Ibid., p. 757

in which respirations are considerably increased, or when the air that is breathed is very dry. This last point is important to remember in the administration of inhalation therapy. Oxygen or other substances given by inhalation should always be humidified in order to counterbalance the loss of water through expiration. The loss of electrolytes through respiration is normally minimal, although the lungs can play an important role in maintaining the acid-base balance of the body, as discussed later.

Maintenance of Acid-Base Balance

Intimately connected with the fluid and electrolyte balance of the body is the maintenance of acid-base (or H⁺) balance. You will recall from your chemistry courses that acids carry hydrogen ions which can be released to combine with other substances. Alkalis (base substances) do not carry hydrogen ions, but can combine with the hydrogen ions released by an acid. The relative acidity or alkalinity of body fluids is expressed in terms of pH, which refers to the concentration of hydrogen ions in the fluid. The pH is measured on a scale of 1 to 14. Water, which is considered a neutral substance (being neither acid nor alkaline) has a pH of 7.0. The pH scale is based on a negative logarithm, and acidic solutions have a pH lower than 7 and alkaline solutions a pH higher than 7.

Normally, the acid-base balance (or H⁺ concentration) of body fluids is maintained by means of four mechanisms. A local small buildup of extra acid or base may be corrected by a simple process of *dilution*—that is, the circulating fluid picks up the extra ions and takes them away from the trouble spot; they become diluted in the total volume of fluid circulating. The excess acid accumulated in a muscle after exercise, for example, may be removed in this way. The body also has a system of *buffers*, which operate within the fluid system to correct a tendency toward either acidity or alkalinity. Buffers are pairs of substances consisting of a weak acid and its salt, which act as sponges to absorb extra hydrogen or base ions, as required. The principal buffering agents in body fluids are the carbonic acid-bicarbonate system, which operates mainly in the extracellular fluid; the phosphate buffer system, which operates predominantly in the intracellular fluid; and the protein buffer system, which operates in both (proteins can act as either acids or bases as needed). If the first two mechanisms fail to effect a balance, the body has two other regulatory mechanisms which may be brought into play—namely, the *kidneys* and the *lungs*. The kidneys can vary the acidity of the urine in response to the body's need to throw off excess acid or base. They act principally by controlling base bicarbonates. The lungs aid in maintaining acid-base balance through their control of carbonic acid. They can eliminate either more or less carbonic acid (in the form of carbon dioxide and water), thus either ridding the body of excess acid or conserving it. When you have engaged in strenuous exercise, for example, you may find that you are breathing more quickly and more deeply than usual, as the body attempts to rid itself of the extra acid from the waste products of muscle cell metabolism.

When large amounts of fluids are lost or retained in the body, there can be disturbances of acid-base balance. The balance can swing in the direction of a higher concentration of either acid or base. The term *acidosis* refers to a swing towards the acid side, either through a retention of excess acid (H⁺ concentration) in the body, or a depletion of the body's alkaline reserves. The normally basic state of body fluids becomes more acidic; a pH below 7.35, the lowest point on the normal range for blood, is generally considered to indicate acidosis. *Alkalosis* is the opposite of acidosis; there is either a lessening of the acid (H⁺ concentration) of body fluids or an excess of alkaline reserves. When the pH of the blood exceeds 7.45, the highest point in the normal range, the condition is called alkalosis.[5] When acidosis or alkalosis results from disturbances in metabolism the term metabolic acidosis or metabolic alkalosis is used; when it results from disturbed respiratory functioning, it is called respiratory acidosis or respiratory alkalosis.

---

[5]For a more detailed description of acid-base (hydrogen ion) balance, the reader is directed to Joan Luckmann and Karen C. Sorensen, *Medical-Surgical Nursing*. Philadelphia, W. B. Saunders Company, 1974, pp. 218–232.

FACTORS AFFECTING FLUID AND ELECTROLYTE BALANCE

There are many factors which will disturb the body's fluid and electrolyte balance. It is perhaps helpful here to group them under five general headings.

Insufficient Intake

The sources of water and electrolytes for the body are the food and fluids ingested. Any disturbance in the source of nourishment is reflected in the body. Sometimes people who are anorectic and nauseated also show a disturbed fluid and electrolyte balance, particularly when these symptoms are prolonged.

Disturbances of the Gastrointestinal Tract

A very large volume of fluid in the form of digestive juices is secreted into the gastrointestinal tract each day. Almost all of this fluid is reabsorbed during the process of digestion. Interference with the normal processes of secretion and reabsorption can result in serious fluid and electrolyte imbalance. The nature of the imbalance depends to a large extent on the portion of the gastrointestinal tract affected. In order to appreciate the significance of this point, it is helpful to keep in mind the volume, the pH, and the electrolyte composition of the various digestive juices. The approximate volumes and pH of the principal digestive juices per day are as follows:

	Daily Volume	*Usual pH*
Saliva	1500 ml.	6.7
Gastric secretion	2500 ml.	1.0–2.0
Intestinal secretion	3000 ml.	7.8–8.0
Pancreatic secretion	700 ml.	8.0–8.3
Bile	500 ml.	7.8
	Total 8200 ml.[6]	

---

[6]Norma M. Metheny and W. D. Snively, Jr.: *Nurses' Handbook of Fluid Balance.* 2nd edition. Philadelphia, J. B. Lippincott Company, 1974, p. 195.

The major components that are involved in electrolyte and acid-base balance are found in the gastric and intestinal secretions. Gastric juice contains large quantities of hydrochloric acid and a significant amount of sodium. Gastric mucus contains a high proportion of sodium and chloride, small but significant amounts of potassium, and a relatively small amount of carbonate. Thus, when fluids are lost from the stomach through vomiting, there may be a significant loss of acid as well. Prolonged vomiting may cause severe sodium depletion and loss of the chloride ion also. The body's reserves of potassium may be lessened also. Gastric suction removes hydrochloric acid and fluids; gastric washings can severely deplete the store of chloride ions, particularly if these washings are done with water rather than normal saline. All gastric tube irrigations as well as gastric washings should therefore be done with isotonic saline to prevent the depletion of these electrolytes.

Pancreatic juice, bile, and the intestinal secretions are predominantly basic and contain relatively large amounts of carbonate, as well as sodium and chloride. In addition, a large proportion of the total volume of potassium excreted from the body daily is via the gastrointestinal tract in the feces. Thus, diarrhea generally results in the loss of fluids, and of sodium and chloride ions, as well as of the base secreted in the intestine. Severe diarrhea depletes the body's potassium also.

Disturbances of Kidney Function

Because the kidney is so intimately concerned with the regulation of fluid and electrolyte balance, any impairment in renal function may disturb this balance. Damage to the kidney itself may interfere with its ability to reabsorb water and electrolytes in the tubules. An imbalance in the antidiuretic hormone (caused by pituitary gland dysfunction, for example) affects kidney functioning, particularly the reabsorption of water. Similarly, an imbalance in aldosterone (which may result from steroid therapy, for example) affects sodium retention and potassium excretion by the kidneys. The kidneys are also affected by disturbances in cardiovascular function. An insufficient flow of blood through the kidneys due to a poorly functioning heart, for example, hampers the efficiency of the kidneys in that there may not be enough blood circulating through the kidneys to produce an adequate amount of glomerular filtrate. Retention of fluid in body tissues may then occur. This is evidenced by edema, which is a frequent accompaniment of many cardiac conditions.

Excessive Perspiration or Evaporation

One of the largest variables in the amount of water lost from the body daily is the volume of perspiration. This may range from zero to several liters per day, depending on the amount of physical activity of the individual, the temperature of the environment, the presence of fever, or the like. When there is excessive perspiration, two protective mechanisms are brought into play: thirst, which increases the amount of fluid intake, and adjustment of the water output by the kidneys.[7]

When fluids are lost through sweating, there is a loss of sodium chloride as well. Hence, people who live in hot climates, and those who must work in temperatures above normal, are frequently advised to take salt tablets to replace that lost through perspiration. As a person becomes acclimatized to higher environmental temperatures, however, the body usually adjusts by lessening the salt content of sweat so that the loss of sodium and chloride ions by this route is minimized.

Hemorrhage, Burns, and Body Trauma

In hemorrhage, not only fluid but also a percentage of all the blood elements is lost. The total circulatory volume is decreased and, in a large hemorrhage, the body's adaptive mechanisms may collapse and shock may ensue.

In burns, as well as in some trauma to the body (including surgical trauma), fluids and electrolytes are lost from the general circulation as these tend to accumulate in the interstitial spaces. Fluids are removed from the plasma, sodium is depleted throughout the body generally, and potassium is released in excessive amounts from the damaged cells. Proteins are also depleted. Therefore, there is a need to replace not only fluids but also sodium, potassium, and proteins in order to restore a balance.

COMMON PROBLEMS

A great many problems may result from disturbances in fluid and electrolyte imbalance. All other systems in the body are dependent on the effective functioning of the fluid system. It serves not only as the transport mechanism for moving nutrients and removing wastes, but also provides an optimal environment for the efficient functioning of body cells.

As a result of fluid and electrolyte imbalance, then, problems may arise in any of the body's functional areas. These problems often require medical or nursing intervention. The type of problem and the intervention required depend to a large extent on the specific nature of the imbalance and the extent of the disturbance. The most common problems that the nurse will encounter are those associated with dehydration and edema.

Dehydration is a general term used to designate a condition in which the body or tissues are deprived of water. It may result from a number of causes, such as an insufficient intake of fluids, an excessive loss of fluids, or other disease conditions, as discussed earlier in the section on factors affecting fluid and electrolyte balance.

Edema is a condition in which there is excessive fluid retained in the tissues; it may be either generalized or localized. It may result from disturbances in kidney function, disturbances in circulatory function (as, for example, in people with cardiac conditions), inflammation, increased permeability of the cell membranes, or a number of other health problems.

---

[7]MacBryde and Blacklow, op. cit., p. 770

ASSESSING FLUID AND ELECTROLYTE PROBLEMS

In order to assess the patient's fluid and electrolyte status, the nurse should be aware of factors in the patient's history which could cause an imbalance. She should be alert to signs and symptoms in the patient which could be indicative of fluid and electrolyte imbalance, and she should be able to identify significant laboratory findings. In addition, the nurse should know the physician's plan of therapy for the patient and understand the rationale on which this plan is based.

The patient's medical history provides the nurse with much valuable information about existing or potential fluid and electrolyte problems. The person who has had a history of nausea and vomiting over several days, for example, is likely to show disturbances resulting from the loss of fluids generally, the loss of acid from gastric secretions, and possibly a depletion of the sodium ions as well. The patient who is admitted for surgery may develop fluid and electrolyte imbalance postoperatively and will need careful observation on the part of the nurse to detect signs and symptoms of impending imbalance. The baseline data entered by the physician and other members of the health team on the patient's record can alert the nurse to the presence of any of the health problems discussed in the section on factors affecting fluid and electrolyte balance.

Subjective Observations

Significant factors in the patient's history which alert the nurse to the possibility of fluid and electrolyte imbalance include recent changes in the individual's usual patterns of intake and output or the presence of any one of the health problems already mentioned. When taking the nursing history, the nurse should obtain information about the patient's normal habits of food and fluid intake and output. How many glasses of water does he usually drink per day, for example? How many cups of tea or coffee? What types of fluids does he like? What foods does he usually eat? This type of information not only provides baseline data with which to compare but also helps the nurse to plan the patient's care to prevent fluid and electrolyte imbalances from developing or to assist in correcting those that have occurred.

In addition to obtaining information about usual habits, the nurse should ascertain if there have been any recent alterations in the individual's pattern of intake and output. For example, has the patient been suffering from anorexia, and not taking the usual amount of food and fluid? Has he noticed that he is not voiding as much as usual or, conversely, has been voiding more than usual? Is he taking any medications which could affect fluid and electrolyte balance, as, for example, steroids? Has he experienced any changes in his food intake or fluid output as a result of illness recently? Has he noticed that he is particularly thirsty lately? Is he aware of any recent rapid gain or loss in weight, or gradually increasing obesity? Has he noticed any weakness in his muscle strength, or signs of muscular irritability, such as tremors or twitching of the muscles?

Objective Observations

Although fluid and electrolyte disturbances are usually the result of other disorders in the body, they may in themselves give rise to specific problems.

Of particular importance to the nurse is an awareness of the early signs of dehydration in a patient. His tongue is often dry and furry. He may complain of thirst, his skin tissues usually appear to be loose and flabby (loss of tissue turgor), and the mucous membranes appear dry. The patient frequently also complains of fatigue. The nurse will note that the patient's urine is scanty in amount and darker in color than normal urine. If the dehydration progresses, evidence of a greater degree of imbalance may be noted. Fluid is first drawn from the interstitial spaces and then from within the cells in order to maintain an adequate blood volume. However, as dehydration advances, the blood volume may also be lessened, and the patient's pulse may then become

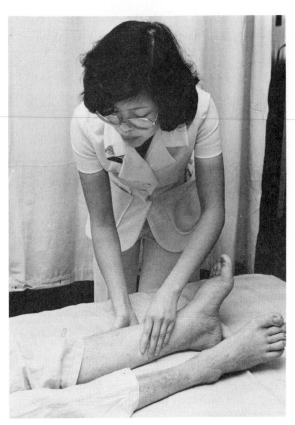

The nurse checks for signs of edema in this patient.

weak and his blood pressure low. He may experience a feeling of faintness, and sometimes signs of mental confusion are evident. With moderately advanced dehydration, the individual's temperature is usually elevated and there is a marked weight loss as well. In the most extreme cases of dehydration, the patient may go into shock, which progresses to a comatose state.

Also important to the nurse is the early recognition of retention of fluid in the body tissues. Edema may be localized or generalized. Generalized edema can usually be observed first in the soft tissues around the eyes and in dependent areas of the body. If the individual is up and walking around, the edema may be noted first in the feet and ankles. With bed patients, the nurse may notice edema particularly around the sacral area. The patient's skin appears puffy and soft to the touch. The edematous patient usually

shows a gain in weight, which is due to the extra fluid he is retaining. When there is marked edema, the blood volume becomes increased, with a resultant rise in blood pressure. The lungs may be affected since the lungs are a low pressure area in the circulatory system and extra fluids tend to accumulate there. Thus, the patient may show symptoms of dyspnea, with moist and noisy breathing. When there is a retention of fluids, there is usually a lessened volume of urine output.

Diagnostic Tests

Diagnostic tests for patients who have fluid and electrolyte problems usually involve the laboratory examination of specimens of blood and urine. Electrolyte levels in the blood serum can be determined after the collection of approximately 5 ml. of venous blood. Potassium, sodium, calcium, and magnesium concentrations are frequently measured.

A blood gas analysis is often carried out to assess the acid-base balance. For this, 5 ml. of arterial blood is withdrawn. Measurement of the pH, PCO_2, and standard PCO_3 is usually ordered. The pH indicates the overall acid-base balance of the body (normal, 7.35–7.45). PCO_2 is the pressure of carbon dioxide dissolved in the plasma and indicates carbonic acid retention (normal, 35–40 mm. Hg). Standard PCO_3 measures the amount of bicarbonate buffer (normal, 25–29 mEq./liter). Often a PO_2 reading is requested; it measures the oxygen tension, normally 95 to 100 mm. Hg.

Diagnostic tests of the urine are done to measure the fluid and electrolyte balance. Tests for acetone and diacetic acid may indicate a disturbance in the metabolism that results in a type of acidosis. Urine is examined to test for the excretion of chlorides and sometimes potassium. The specific gravity of urine indicates the concentration of dissolved materials, such as waste products, and can reflect the degree of hydration of the patient. Other urine and kidney tests are more likely to assess kidney functioning, which may or may not be a contributing factor to fluid and electrolyte imbalance.

PRIORITIES FOR NURSING ACTION

Disturbances in fluid and electrolyte balance can have serious effects on body functioning. The nurse must be particularly alert in noting early indications of *imbalance*. These should be drawn to the attention of the attending physician promptly so that appropriate therapy can be instituted to correct the situation before it becomes too advanced. The consequences of marked imbalance of fluids and the major electrolytes in the body have been documented throughout this chapter. It should be stressed, therefore, that all measures to maintain or restore fluid and electrolyte balance should receive priority from the nurse.

The individual with an elevated temperature is especially vulnerable to disturbances in his fluid and electrolyte balance. His fluid requirements are higher than normal (at least 3000 cc. of fluid is believed to be required by the person with pyrexia), and his fluid losses are usually also in excess of the normal (see Chapter 25).

Children, in particular, show signs of dehydration with accompanying electrolyte balance very rapidly in acute illnesses. A child who has been running a temperature, or who has had diarrhea for even a few days, may be brought into hospital in a state of acute dehydration. He will need immediate medical and nursing intervention.

The nurse should also always be alert to the possibility of circulatory collapse, or shock, which occurs when the body's fluid system is not able to cope with major disturbances. Shock is always considered a medical emergency and requires prompt intervention. It may be caused by a sudden, extensive loss of fluids from the body, such as occurs in hemorrhage or in severe burns, or by prolonged dehydration. It may also result from severe trauma of any kind, surgery, heart conditions, infections, allergic reactions, or toxicity from drugs. Shock may occur immediately after an injury, or its appearance may be delayed.

It should be noted that in the case of a sudden hemorrhage, there is no time for the development of early symptoms and the patient may show signs of circulatory collapse very suddenly. Again, prompt intervention is essential to save the person's life. It is important to remember that any injury produces shock, which may range from mild to severe—so severe, in fact, that the patient may die from the effects of shock itself rather than from the disturbance that caused it.

Shock is frequently present in persons admitted to the emergency unit of a health agency; it is also a possible complication in many conditions for which people are hospitalized as, for example, surgery or cardiac conditions. It may, however, just as easily occur in people on the street, at home, or in a physician's or dentist's office. The subject of shock will be treated in much more detail in courses you will take later in your nursing program; however, as a first-year student you should:

1. Be able to recognize the existence of shock in a patient, and indications of impending or worsening shock
2. Be aware when prompt intervention is needed and summon assistance
3. Be able to take steps to facilitate the institution of emergency measures

The signs of shock evident in a patient may vary somewhat, depending on its cause, its severity, and the length of time the patient has been in shock. However, there are some classic signs and symptoms with which the student should be familiar. These may be divided into those which the patient may be aware of (subjective data) and those which the nurse may observe (objective data). The patient may complain of a feeling of faintness, dizziness, and a blurring of vision; he may be thirsty and he may become apprehensive. The nurse may observe that he is very pale, his skin is cold and clammy, and he may be sweating profusely. His pulse rate usually becomes rapid, weak, and thready, his blood pressure is low, and his breathing becomes rapid and shallow (this may progress to air hunger). Nausea and vomiting may occur. The patient may become drowsy and lapse into unconsciousness.[8] Any or all of these signs and symptoms may be present.

If you suspect that a patient is going

---

[8]Thomas Flint and Harvey D. Cain: *Emergency Treatment and Management.* 5th edition. Philadelphia, W. B. Saunders Company, 1975, pp. 585–586.

PRINCIPLES RELEVANT TO FLUID AND ELECTROLYTE BALANCE

1. The average adult requires 2100 to 2900 ml. of fluid in a 24 hour period.
2. Normally, fluid intake is balanced against fluid loss.
3. When fluids are lost or retained in excessive amounts, there is an accompanying loss or gain of electrolytes.
4. The signs and symptoms accompanying electrolyte imbalance vary according to the excess or deficiency of the specific electrolyte.
5. The specific electrolytes lost from the body in any fluid loss depend on the route of the loss.

into shock, you should alert the nurse in charge so that prompt action can be taken to obtain emergency intervention. Most health agencies have a standard routine for such emergencies and a well-stocked cart available for treatment needs.

The recommended treatment for patients in shock has undergone considerable revision in recent years and opinions vary with regard to the use of different drugs to aid in the restoration of blood pressure. There has also been controversy over the positioning of the patient. It is, therefore, a good idea to acquaint yourself with the specific routine of the agency in which you are having experience and also with the contents of the emergency cart. It is generally recommended at present that the patient be placed flat in bed (dorsal recumbent position) with the feet and legs slightly elevated, unless there are contraindications to this position, as in the case of the cardiac patient, for example. You are usually safe in assuming that intravenous therapy will be started (to raise the volume of circulating fluids) and the necessary equipment should be gathered. Oxygen equipment and intubation equipment may also be required, so these should be available.

The patient is usually very apprehensive and frightened; therefore, he needs to be reassured. A calm, unhurried manner and competent actions on the part of the nurse can help to prevent the patient from becoming anxious and also help to reassure worried family members who may be present. The key to appearing calm and competent lies in knowing what to do in an emergency. It is important then to learn the procedures and policies

of the agency in which the nurse is working.

GOALS FOR NURSING ACTION

The basic goals of care for the patient with actual or potential fluid and electrolyte problems are to assist the patient to maintain a homeostatic balance insofar as this is possible or to restore a balance that has been disturbed.

SPECIFIC NURSING INTERVENTIONS

Measures to Maintain Fluid and Electrolyte Balance

Ensuring Adequate Food and Fluid Intake. Of primary importance in the nursing care of the patient with fluid and electrolyte problems is the maintenance of a therapeutic fluid intake. In many instances the physician orders the exact amount of oral fluid for a patient. Sometimes, however, it is a nursing function to judge the oral fluid needs of the patient; for example, the nurse determines that the patient with a fever or an infection requires large amounts of fluid (at least 3000 ml. per day).

Generally speaking, if the patient is dehydrated, or has lost an excessive amount of fluids, he should be encouraged to take extra fluids. Additional fluid intake may be contraindicated in some cases, however. If the patient is nauseated or vomiting, for example, it is not reasonable to expect that he can toler-

2-8738	RIVERSIDE HOSPITAL OF OTTAWA	NORTH JANE SP 1249 223 TREE RD OTT 234-7566-600 NORTH RICHARD HUS SAME

TOTAL 24 hr Intake _4090cc_ Date _Sept 1/77_ | 1.9.77 1PM F 30 M SURG RC
420 1

2330 – 0730			0715 – 1545			1545 – 2345		
Time	Type	Amount	Time	Type	Amount	Time	Type	Amount
2400	I/v 5% D/w I/v 5% D/s 1000cc put up.	200cc —	0800	Juice Coffee H2O	100 130 150	1700	I/v 5% D/w absorbed & discontinued	200cc
			0830	I/v D/s 5% I/v D/w 1000cc put up.	150cc	1730	Soup Tea Milk	170 130 200
0015	H2O	100 cc	1000	Milk	100cc	2030	Tea Gingerale	130 200
0700	I/v D/s	850 cc	1200	Soup Tea	170 130			
0715	Tea	130 cc	1530	H2O I/v D/w 5%	50 800			
Total		1280cc	Total		1780 cc	Total		1030 cc
Oral		230	Oral		830	Oral		830
I.V.		1050	I.V.		950	I.V.		200
T.B.A.		150cc	T.B.A.		200cc	T.B.A.		/

Total 24 Hr Output

Time	Type	Amount	Time	Type	Amount	Time	Type	Amount
2400	Urine	300	0900	Urine	200	1800	Urine	300
0700	Urine	700	1200	Urine	600	2200	Urine	600
			1500	Urine	500			
Total	1000cc		Total	1300cc		Total	900 cc	
Urine	1000		Urine	1300		Urine	900	
Other	/		Other	/		Other	/	

Large Glass = 200 cc   Soup Bowl = 170 cc
Small Glass = 100 cc   Cup = 130 cc

A sample fluid balance work sheet. (Courtesy of the Riverside Hospital of Ottawa.)

ate oral fluids. Patients with kidney or heart conditions may require restriction of their fluid intake. The nurse should be aware of the physician's objectives in medical therapy and never push or force fluids beyond the limit prescribed.

People normally get electrolytes from the food and fluids they ingest. Therefore, to maintain good electrolyte balance, adequate nutrition is essential. When the patient is deficient in certain electrolytes or extra are needed in the body these may be administered by medication. For example, calcium tablets are frequently ordered for pregnant women because of the heavy demands for additional calcium to promote growth of the fetus.

In addition, it is not unusual for restricted electrolyte intake to be prescribed; for example, the physician might order a salt-free diet for a patient. The usual purpose here is to restrict the oral intake of sodium (Na^+). It is frequently the nurse's responsibility to help the patient to understand the necessity for the restriction and to help him plan meals with this in mind. Most people are able to assume the responsibility for restricting their diets. Nevertheless, in hospitals it is not unknown for a helpful roommate to lend his salt shaker to a person on a restricted salt diet.

Monitoring Fluid Intake and Output. With patients who have existing or potential fluid and electrolyte problems, it is essential to monitor fluid intake and output accurately. When the physician wishes to know the fluid intake of a particular patient, accurate measurements are made of all the fluids he is given. This includes fluid given orally, intravenously, interstitially, and rectally. Most hospitals provide chart forms for recording fluid balance.

Body fluids are normally excreted through the kidneys, the intestine, the lungs, and the skin. In recording the amount of fluid output, the nurse measures the amount of the patient's urine accurately. In addition, she measures any drainage, such as bile drainage and suction returns. In some instances, significant amounts of fluid lost in the feces, from wounds, or by perspiration are also recorded.

It is difficult to obtain an exact record of fluid intake and output in all cases. Most hospitals have charts or written material which show the estimated fluid content of the drinking glasses, cups, soup bowls, and other utensils usually used in the agency. However, it requires the cooperation of all personnel to maintain an accurate record of the patient's total fluid intake. The patient can often help to keep his own record, particularly if he understands the need for doing this.

An accurate recording of output is usually more difficult. For example, the amount of fluid loss from perspiration may be considerable in the patient with a fever, yet measuring this is not easy. The nurse should, however, record the fact that the patient is perspiring profusely and draw this to the attention of the physician. Often the amount of fluid lost from wounds can only be estimated. Sometimes, the number of dressing pads that are soaked through is helpful in assessing the extent of wound drainage.

When drainage tubing is irrigated, or such procedures as gastric washings or bladder irrigation are done, the amount of fluid inserted must always be included in the calculations of fluid intake and output.

Keeping an accurate record of urine output can also present some problems. When patients have bathroom privileges, it is necessary to place a measured container in the bathroom and to enlist the patient's cooperation in collecting urine and, if feasible, measuring the amount voided. Patients who are incontinent of urine and feces present additional problems in the assessment of fluid losses. The nurse must watch these patients carefully for fluid retention or excessive fluid loss.

The urine output of the average adult is 1100 to 1700 ml. in a 24 hour period. When urine output is less than 25 ml. or more than 500 ml. per hour, it generally is abnormal. Abnormalities of either excess or inadequate urine output should be drawn to the attention of the patient's physician so that appropriate therapy can be instituted.

Observing for Signs and Symptoms of Imbalance. In assisting in the maintenance of fluid and electrolyte balance, the nurse must be alert to early indications of imbalance. Observations of the degree of hydration of the patient are noted and recorded. The nurse should watch particularly for early signs of dehydration or fluid retention, as these were outlined in the section on assessment of the patient.

When observing for indications of electrolyte imbalance, the nurse should have an understanding of the patient's medical condition and the potential problems that may occur. If she is aware, for example, that the patient has a condition involving dysfunction of the adrenal cortex or impairment of renal function, she should observe him carefully for signs of sodium and potassium imbalance. Most of the body potassium is normally in the fluid within the cells, yet the potassium in the blood plasma is maintained at a fairly constant volume even when there is a significant loss of the ion from the cells. Thus the body may be seriously depleted of potassium before significant changes can be noted in the blood plasma level, which is the only tabulated measurement. Therefore, the nurse should be alert to the early signs and symptoms of potassium deficiency such as muscular weakness, irregularities of the pulse, or nervous irritability.

When the nurse is aware of potential problems, her observations are more directed and purposeful. She knows what to look for, and her observations can be of inestimable assistance to the physician in diagnosing the patient's condition and planning therapy.

Assisting in the Restoration of Fluid and Electrolyte Balance

General Considerations. Whenever a disturbance in fluid or electrolyte balance occurs, steps must be taken to restore homeostasis. Since the principal sources of fluid and electrolytes are the foods and fluids a person takes in, adjustments in diet or fluid intake or both may be sufficient to rectify a mild imbalance. In the case of deficiencies of specific electrolytes, supplements may be given in the form of medications. Often, however, fluid loss is too extensive and the accompanying loss of electrolytes too great to be corrected by oral intake alone, or this method of replacement may be contraindicated. Fluids and electrolytes may then be administered by other routes, by intravenous infusion, by blood transfusion, or by interstitial or rectal infusion. The decisions of route to be used and the type of solution to be administered are made by the physician. His decisions are based on his knowledge of the patient's condition and the particular factors causing the imbalance. The patient's intake and output record is of considerable assistance to the physician in assessing the extent of fluid loss and in calculating the balance between intake and output. The nurse's observations of the patient's state of hydration, of his nutritional status, and of signs and symptoms of impending fluid and electrolyte imbalance also contribute significantly to the physician's assessment of the need for replacement or corrective therapy.

The care of the patient with fluid and electrolyte problems includes good supportive nursing measures as well as assistance with curative measures. Hygiene is of particular importance for patients with these problems. The patient's physical comfort is largely dependent upon his feeling of cleanliness and freshness. Profuse diaphoresis may necessitate frequent changes and baths; dry, scaly skin and mucous membranes are lubricated with emollient creams. One of the dangers of cracked lips and dry mouth is the increased risk of secondary infections.

The overhydrated patient, in particular, should turn in bed regularly to promote circulation and adequate nourishment to all tissues. The presence of edema or even the weight of the patient can restrict circulation to particular areas, thus predisposing the area to tissue death and the formation of decubitus ulcers.

Intravenous Infusion. The infusion of fluids directly into the peripheral veins is often indicated when a patient is unable to take fluids orally. Infusion permits the patient to obtain many fluids, electrolytes, and nutrients that are necessary to life. In addition, it has the advantage of rapid absorption, which is particularly important in the administration of some medications.

Many kinds of intravenous fluid are

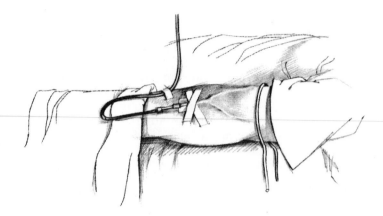

The site of an intravenous infusion.

available for infusion. The physician decides which kind of fluid the patient needs. For example, a patient may require 5 per cent dextrose in water, normal saline, or 10 per cent dextrose in normal saline. Usually intravenous fluid is provided in 250, 500, or 1000 ml. (cc.) containers.

In some agencies, only the physician is permitted to start an intravenous infusion; in others it is a responsibility of the graduate nurse. Often hospitals have policies regarding the kinds of infusions which nurses can initiate. Sometimes the physician orders the addition of drugs such as norepinephrine, vitamin C, potassium chloride, Neo-Synephrine, or nitrogen mustard to an intravenous solution. It is the responsibility of the nurse to know which she is permitted to add and which drugs the physician must administer.

The choice of site for an intravenous infusion is dependent upon a number of factors. The condition of the patient's veins as well as his comfort must be considered. The *cephalic* and *basilic* veins in the inner aspect of the elbow are used most frequently. These sites may require extension of the patient's arm, which can be uncomfortable after a prolonged period. If, however, these veins are entered along the shaft of radius and ulna (bones of the forearm), the bones provide a natural splint and make extension of the elbow unnecessary.

Prior to starting an intravenous infusion, the tubing is attached to the intravenous flask. Sterile precautions are taken throughout this procedure in order to protect the patient from infection. In addition to the flask and the intravenous tubing, the nurse requires a tourniquet, an antiseptic swab, a sterile syringe, a standard to hold the flask, and a receptacle for the discarded fluid.

After the tubing has been attached to the intravenous flask, the flask is hung upon the standard and the fluid is then run through the tubing before the tubing is clamped. By running the fluid through the tubing, air is removed so that it will not be introduced into the patient's vein. Air injected into a vein can result in an air embolus. An embolus is a clot or plug in a blood vessel which has been transported from another place by the blood and which can result in the blocking of blood flow.

A tourniquet is applied to the patient's arm above the intravenous site. At the same time, the patient clenches and unclenches his fist. These measures distend the veins in his arm to make them more accessible for venipuncture. The injection site is cleansed with antiseptic and a sterile needle (No. 18, 19, 20, or 21) is then attached to the syringe and inserted at a 45 degree angle, bevel up, into the vein. Some resistance to the needle is encountered at the skin, but the subcutaneous tissues and veins offer very little resistance. The patient perceives pain when the needle goes through the skin but little discomfort thereafter. The

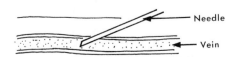

plunger of the syringe is drawn back to ascertain that the needle is in the vein (indicated by obtaining blood). The syringe is disconnected, and the tubing is attached to the needle. The rate of flow is then established. Depending upon the patient's condition, the rate of flow may range from 40 to 100 drops per minute. The usual rate is 80 drops per minute. The rate of flow for an intravenous infusion is often ordered by the physician.

The tubing and the needle are then attached to the arm by adhesive tape. The patient can be provided with an armboard to immobilize his arm if this is necessary. Whenever the site of the needle insertion is near a joint, as, for example, the elbow or the wrist, it is wise to use an armboard to prevent the needle from being dislodged with the patient's movement. It is very difficult to maintain immobility of a part without support such as a board provides. To be effective the armboard should reach from above the elbow joint to the end of the fingertips. The board should always be padded for the patient's comfort and safety.

If intravenous fluids are to be administered over a prolonged period of time, polyethylene tubing (Intra-cath) may be used instead of a needle for an infusion; the tubing fits through the needle, which is removed after the tubing has been inserted into the vein. Tubing is more flexible than a needle, but it must be checked to make certain that it does not become dislodged and move down the patient's vein, particularly when it is being removed.

Often with children, and sometimes with adults whose surface veins are inaccessible or unsuitable for infusion, it is necessary to make a small incision in order to locate an appropriate site for the needle insertion. In these cases, a "cutdown" will be used by the physician. This technique is not carried out by nursing personnel, although the nurse should have the equipment ready and assist the physician as needed.

It may be necessary to vary the height of the intravenous flask according to the pressure with which one wishes the fluid to enter the vein. The higher the flask, the stronger is the gravitational pull on the fluid, and the greater the pressure it exerts. Usually 1 meter (3 feet) above bed level is an adequate height for most intravenous infusions.

Frequently it is the nurse's responsibility to adjust the rate of flow of the intravenous solution. Various methods of deriving the number of cubic centimeters per minute are used, the objective being to divide the total amount of solution equally over the time period prescribed for the infusion. For example, if 250 ml. of fluid is to be given over a two hour period, the rate of flow should be approximately 2 ml. per minute to allow all of the fluid to run through in two hours.

During an intravenous infusion, the patient is observed for any untoward effects. Specifically, the nurse should note the entry site of the intravenous needle or catheter for swelling, redness, or pain. These reactions can indicate that the needle has slipped out of the patient's vein, with the result that the fluid is flowing into the surrounding tissues. Patients are also observed for signs of overhydration or cardiac overload. A faster pulse rate, an increase in blood pressure, or dyspnea can indicate cardiac overload and consequently are reported to the physician immediately.

The nurse records on the patient's chart the amount and the kind of intravenous fluid being administered, as well as the name of the person who initiated the procedure. The site of the intravenous puncture and the rate of flow are also recorded. In this way another site can be chosen for the next infusion. Generally the sites are chosen by starting from the lower part of the arm and working upward so that previous infusion sites will not impede the flow of solution in the veins.

Several problems may be encountered in the administration of intravenous fluids. If the fluid stops running or flows spasmodically, the needle may have become dislodged, or the bevel of the needle (or the end of the plastic tubing) may be resting against the wall of the patient's vein. Slight alteration of the position of the needle or tubing can often correct this. If the intravenous solution flows into the interstitial spaces, the infusion must be restarted with another sterile needle. The nurse can tell if the infusion has gone into the interstitial spaces by the

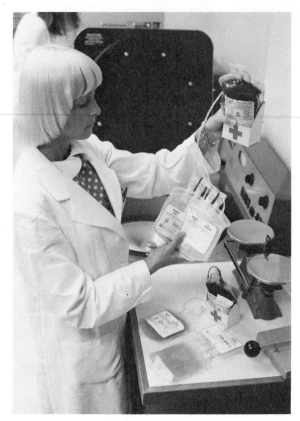

Proper identification of blood for transfusion is essential.

edema which forms around the injection site when fluid infiltrates the subcutaneous tissues. Another problem is the appearance of air bubbles in the tubing. When this happens the tubing can be disconnected at the needle and the fluid allowed to run through the tubing until the bubbles are expelled.

DISCONTINUING AN INTRAVENOUS INFUSION. To discontinue an intravenous infusion, an antiseptic swab for cleansing the open area is needed. The intravenous tubing is clamped, and then the adhesive tape on the patient's arm is loosened. The needle is removed quickly from the patient's vein, the antiseptic swab is placed over the puncture wound, and digital pressure is applied until the bleeding stops. If plastic tubing has been used instead of a needle, it is withdrawn carefully and checked to make sure that none of the tube remains in the patient's vein.

Since the length of the tube that was inserted is often recorded in the patient's chart, the length of the removed tube can be checked against this record.

Whenever bleeding persists from the intravenous site, pressure is prolonged by means of a small dressing in order to prevent bleeding into the tissues and resultant bruise. Subsequently, the kind and amount of fluid that was infused is recorded, as is the time the intravenous infusion was terminated.

Blood Transfusion. Prior to a blood transfusion, the patient's blood is typed. There are many blood groups besides the basic A, AB, B, and O types. The Rh factor is determined along with the blood group. Usually 5 ml. of blood is taken for typing.

Blood transfusions are usually started by a physician or a specially qualified nurse. Initiating a transfusion is similar to starting an intravenous infusion. A careful check is always made to be certain that the patient is getting the right blood. Usually this means that two nurses check the number on the blood bottle against the number on the duplicate request form on the patient's record, and the name on the requisition against the name on the patient's record and identification band. In some hospitals it is also necessary to check the patient's hospital identity number on the blood bottle, the blood requisition, the chart, and the identification band.

A No. 18 needle is usually used for a blood transfusion, and the rate of flow of the blood is normally 40 drops per minute. Special note is made of the patient's reaction and condition; at any sign of urticaria, chills, backache, or respiratory or circulatory distress, the transfusion is terminated and the physician notified. The patient's temperature and blood pressure are taken and a sample of urine obtained for laboratory analysis. Because most reactions to a blood transfusion occur within a short time after it has been started, the nurse should stay with the patient for the first 15 minutes.

Recording the initiation of a blood transfusion should include the time it was started, the amount of blood, the number on the bottle of blood, and the name of the person who initiated the transfusion.

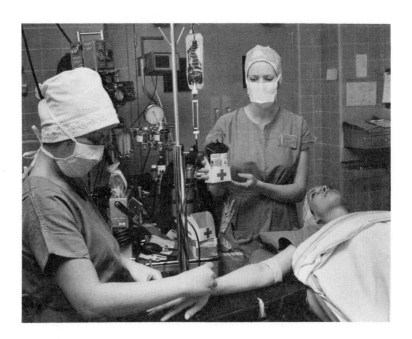

Ready reserves of blood must be available during surgical procedures.

Termination of the blood transfusion is similar to the termination of the intravenous infusion.

On occasion a patient requires a phlebotomy, that is, an opening into a vein in order to remove blood. This measure is carried out by the physician, usually to decrease blood volume (in order to relieve dyspnea caused by congestion of blood in the lungs, for example). For this procedure, empty bottles to receive the blood are required, in addition to the equipment that is needed to enter a vein.

Interstitial Infusion. Interstitial infusion, hypodermoclysis, and subcutaneous infusion are synonymous terms referring to the administration of large amounts of fluid into subcutaneous tissue. This measure is not used often; it is utilized when a patient is unable to take fluids orally, rectally, or intravenously. Its purpose is to supply the patient with fluids, electrolytes, and occasionally nourishment. Hyaluronidase (Wydase) is often added to the fluid to hasten its absorption. This enzyme breaks down the hyaluronic acid of the connective tissue.

Whether the initiation of an interstitial infusion is the responsibility of the nurse or the physician depends on the policy of the specific agency. The usual sites for the administration of an interstitial infu-

sion are just below the scapula, the abdominal wall above the crest of the ilium, the lower aspect of the breast, and the anterior aspect of the thigh.

The equipment that is used is similar to that used in intravenous infusions. A No. 19, 20, 21, or 22 needle is used. Usually, two sites are used simultaneously. After the equipment has been set up (see Intravenous Infusion), the needle is inserted into the skin at a 20 degree angle. It is then taped in place and the flow of the fluid is adjusted in accordance with the physician's order. The usual rate of flow for an interstitial infusion is 60 to 120 drops per minute. The rate is dependent upon the ability of the individual to absorb the fluid. Thin people usually absorb fluid more easily than obese people, because they have fewer fat cells.

The nurse assists the patient to assume a comfortable position, since this treatment is often lengthy. Observations are indicated to detect untoward symptoms, particularly those related to circulatory collapse (for example, an accelerated, weak pulse). The patient should also be watched for signs of respiratory difficulty that could indicate overhydration, such as dyspnea or moist and noisy breathing. Sometimes the infusion is poorly absorbed and the nurse may notice that tissues at the site of injection are becoming edematous. If untoward symptoms develop, the infusion should be stopped and the physician notified promptly. Because of the site of interstitial infusions, adequate draping is necessary for the patient's comfort.

At the termination of an infusion the needle is removed and a small antiseptic dressing is taped over the wound with slight pressure to prevent leakage of the fluid. The nurse records the time of initiation and termination of the infusion, as well as the type of fluid, the amount of fluid absorbed, the addition of any medications, the rate of flow, and the patient's reaction to the treatment. Again it is wise to record the site of the infusion so that the injection sites can be changed for subsequent infusions.

GUIDE TO
ASSESSING FLUID
AND ELECTROLYTE
STATUS

1. What is the patient's usual pattern of fluid intake and output?
2. Have there been any recent changes in this pattern? Has the patient been anorectic, for example, and not taking the usual amount of food and fluid? Has he noticed that he has a lessened amount of urine output? an increased amount?
3. Has he noticed any loss or gain in weight recently?
4. Does he have a health problem which could cause fluid and electrolyte imbalance? For example, has he been nauseated or vomiting, has he had diarrhea? Does he have a kidney problem? a cardiac condition? Has he lost large amounts of fluid from any cause?
5. Is he taking any medication which could affect fluid and electrolyte balance?
6. Does he show signs or symptoms of dehydration? of fluid retention?
7. Do laboratory tests show findings indicative of fluid or electrolyte imbalance?
8. Has measurement of intake and output been ordered for this patient? If so, are the totals of intake and output normal for a 24 hour period?
9. Are there restrictions on the patient's fluid or electrolyte intake? Does he need help to plan a diet to meet these restrictions?
10. Is the patient receiving medications to supplement or replace electrolytes?
11. Have parenteral fluids been prescribed? If so, why have they been ordered? What are the nurse's responsibilities in their administration? Are there special precautions to be observed with any of these?

GUIDE TO
EVALUATING THE
EFFECTIVENESS OF
NURSING
INTERVENTION

1. Is the patient taking adequate food and fluids to meet his fluid and electrolyte needs?
2. Is his urine output compatible with his fluid intake?
3. If there are restrictions on the patient's fluid or electrolyte intake, are these being observed?
4. If parenteral fluids have been prescribed, have they been given at the correct time? Have sterile precautions been observed in their administration? Is the infusion flowing at the proper rate?

5. Is his skin in good condition? his mouth?
6. What does this patient need to know about maintaining or restoring his fluid and electrolyte balance?

STUDY VOCABULARY

Active transport
Anion
Cation

Diffusion
Electrolyte
Embolus

Osmosis
Tissue turgor

STUDY SITUATION

Mr. R. Miller is admitted to a medical nursing unit of a large city hospital late one evening. His diagnosis was tentatively given as dehydration and emaciation. The physician has directed that the patient be given food and fluids as tolerated. He has ordered various laboratory tests. He also ordered an intravenous infusion of 1000 ml. of 5 per cent dextrose in normal saline to be started at midnight and to be run at 80 drops per minute. Mr. Miller is 70 years old and is on Social Security. He has no family and lives alone in a rooming house where he cooks on a small hot plate. A friend accompanied him to the hospital. Mr. Miller is very thin and says he has not eaten well in many months. He appears frightened; this is his first admission to a hospital.

1. What are dehydration and emaciation?
2. What subjective and objective observations might you anticipate? Why?
3. How long can you expect this patient's intravenous infusion to run?
4. What factor should be taken into consideration in explaining the intravenous infusion to this patient?
5. What observations should you make regarding his intravenous infusion?
6. Outline a nursing care plan for this patient.
7. How can you evaluate the results of your planned nursing interventions for this patient?

SUGGESTED READINGS

Andrews, I. D.: Physiological Response Following Trauma. *Nursing Times,* 70:387–390, March 14, 1974.

Begley, L. A.: External Counter-Pulsation for Cardiogenic Shock. *American Journal of Nursing,* 75:967, June 1975.

Colley, R., et al.: Helping With Hyperalimentation. *Nursing '73,* 3:6–17, July 1973.

Daly, J. M., et al.: Central Venous Catheterization. *American Journal of Nursing,* 75:820, May 1975.

Deitel, M.: Intravenous Hyperalimentation. *Canadian Nurse,* 69:38–43, January 1973.

Durham, N.: Looking Out for Complications of Abdominal Surgery. *Nursing '75,* 5:24–31, February 1975.

Freshwater, M. F.: "Dutch Boy" Technique Helps During I.V. Insertion. *RN,* 39:7, March 1976.

Grant, M. M., et al.: Assessing a Patient's Hydration Status. *American Journal of Nursing,* 75:1306–1311, August 1975.

Kee, J. L.: Fluid Imbalance in Elderly Patients. *Nursing '73,* 3:49, April 1973.

Lee, C. A., et al.: Extracellular Volume Imbalance. *American Journal of Nursing,* 74:888–891, May 1974.

Lee, C. A., et al.: What to Do When Acid-Base Problems Hang in the Balance. *Nursing '75,* 5:32–37, August 1975.

Metheny, N. A.: Water and Electrolyte Balance in the Postoperative Patient. *Nursing Clinics of North America,* 10:49–57, March 1975.

Moyer, J. H., and L. C. Mills: Vasopressor Agents in Shock. *American Journal of Nursing,* 75:620, April 1975.

Reed, G. M.: Confused About Potassium? Here's a Clear Concise Guide. *Nursing '74,* 4:20–28, March 1974.

Reed, G. M., and V. F. Sheppard: *Regulation of Fluid and Electrolyte Balance.* 2nd edition. Philadelphia, W. B. Saunders Company, 1977.

Sharer, J. E.: Reviewing Acid-Base Balance. *American Journal of Nursing,* 75:980, June 1975.

Tharp, G. D.: Shock: The Overall Mechanisms. *American Journal of Nursing,* 75:2208–2211, December 1974.

Wiley, L.: The Threat of Thrombophlebitis. *Nursing '73,* 3:38–43, November 1973.

CHAPTER 30

Dyspnea

30 DYSPNEA

The nurse should be able to:

Define dyspnea
Use appropriate terminology in recording and reporting
  observations about the patient with dyspnea
Describe the physiology of respiration, including the five basic
  processes involved
Discuss factors which may interfere with the normal functioning
  of these processes
Identify symptoms of oxygen deficiency which may be present in
  the patient with dyspnea
Identify priorities for nursing action in the care of patients with
  dyspnea, and take appropriate action
Apply relevant principles in the planning and implementation of
  nursing interventions to:
  1. Maintain patency of the patient's airway
  2. Increase ventilatory efficiency
  3. Ensure adequate oxygen intake
  4. Decrease bodily needs for oxygen
  5. Minimize the patient's anxiety
Evaluate the effectiveness of nursing intervention

INTRODUCTION

Respiration is one of the body's vital functions. Normal breathing (eupnea) is silent and effortless. A person who is breathing normally is usually not conscious of his respirations. The respiratory rate and its depth can, however, be altered voluntarily. Eating and drinking, for example, may involve voluntary changes in the breathing pattern. Similarly, speaking and singing require a certain amount of control over respirations. Some people develop considerable skill in adjusting their breathing patterns to produce specific effects with the voice. Singers and actors are usually particularly adept at this. Under normal circumstances, however, most people are not aware of the regular pattern of breathing in (inspiration) and breathing out (expiration) which occurs rhythmically 12 to 18 times per minute in the normal adult.

When a person has difficulty in breathing (dyspnea), he usually becomes acutely aware of his respirations and attempts to control their rate and depth. Dyspnea is a subjective symptom. It is something which the individual feels, and he frequently expresses his distress by such complaints as "I can't breathe" or "I feel as if I am suffocating." Generally, the patient with respiratory problems is an anxious patient. The inability to obtain oxygen and to control a function that is essential to life can be terrifying. Prompt attention to the patient's needs is imperative, not only because of the vital role of oxygen in sustaining life, but also because the anxiety induced by difficulty in breathing can in itself affect a person's respirations and further aggravate the situation. The competence of the nurse in handling inhalation equipment and in helping the patient to feel that he has some control over the situation are important supportive measures in caring for the patient with respiratory problems.

THE PHYSIOLOGY OF RESPIRATION

The physiology of respiration can be divided into five logical sections:

1. The provision of oxygen from the atmosphere (or from inhalation equipment)
2. The mechanisms which regulate the respiratory process
3. The passage of air from the atmosphere to the alveoli of the lungs and from the alveoli to the atmosphere
4. The diffusion of oxygen and carbon dioxide between the alveoli and the blood and between the blood and the tissue cells
5. The transportation of oxygen to the cells and carbon dioxide away from the cells by the blood stream.

1. Basic to the respiratory process is the availability of oxygen. Normally, the atmosphere supplies all the oxygen an individual requires. The air at sea level contains approximately 20 per cent oxygen and 0.04 per cent carbon dioxide. The provision of oxygen is essential to life. Tissues of the body are differentially sensitive to a lack of oxygen. Nerve cells are particularly vulnerable; a few minutes of severe oxygen deprivation may cause irreversible damage to brain cells. Longer periods of less severe degrees of oxygen deprivation can lead to death or to permanent damage of brain tissue.[1]

2. A number of factors regulate the res-

---

[1]Donald F. Egan: *Fundamentals of Respiratory Therapy.* 2nd edition. St. Louis, C. V. Mosby Company, 1973, p. 166.

piratory process. The principal mechanism of control is the respiratory center located in the medulla. The respiratory center contains both inspiratory and expiratory centers. Generally speaking, these operate as an "alternating circuit" type of mechanism; when one is active, the other is inactive.

Impulses from a number of specialized receptors in the body are transmitted to the respiratory center to effect changes in respiration. The well-known Hering-Breuer reflex is initiated by impulses from *stretch receptors* located principally in the visceral pleura around the lungs. At a specific point in inspiration, these receptors transmit impulses to the respiratory center, which promptly inhibits inspiration and triggers the expiratory phase of respiration. The reverse takes place during expiration. Chemical receptors in the respiratory center, aorta, and carotid sinuses are called *chemoreceptors*. These receptors are sensitive to changes in the chemical composition of blood and tissue fluid. A lowered concentration of oxygen, a higher concentration of carbon dioxide, a lowered blood pH, and an elevation in blood temperature will all stimulate increased respirations. An alteration in the arterial blood pressure affects *pressoreceptors* in the aorta and carotid sinuses, and these receptors then transmit impulses to the respiratory center. A sudden rise in arterial blood pressure inhibits respirations. Respiration may also be affected by impulses arising from *proprioceptors* located in the muscles and tendons of movable joints. These receptors are stimulated by movements of the body. Active exercise is a powerful stimulant to respiration.

Emotions also have an effect on the character of respirations. Anxiety, for example, can cause a prolonged state of respiratory stimulation. Pain, fear, and anger usually cause an increase in the rate and depth of respirations.

3. The passage of air from the atmosphere to the alveoli of the lungs, the exchange of gases there, and the subsequent return of air to the atmosphere are collectively referred to as *ventilation*. During ventilation, the air passes through the nasal passages, pharynx, larynx, trachea, bronchi, and bronchioles to the al-

veoli and then back. In its passage to the lungs the air is humidified, cleansed of foreign materials, and warmed. The respiratory tract is lined with mucous membrane, part of which contains cilia and excretes mucus to trap organisms and other foreign material.

4. Once oxygen enters the alveoli of the lungs, it passes into the blood as a result of the difference in the pressures of the gases on either side of the alveolar membrane. Since the partial pressure of oxygen in the inspired air is higher than the pressure of the oxygen in the venous blood, the oxygen passes from the area of higher pressure to the area of lower pressure. The same principle holds for the passage of carbon dioxide from the blood to the alveoli.

5. Once the oxygen enters the blood, it combines with hemoglobin to form oxyhemoglobin and is carried by the arteries to the capillaries throughout the body. From there it is transported via the interstitial fluid to the tissue cells, again because of the difference in the pressures. It is apparent that the delivery of oxygen to the cells depends on the hemoglobin level in the blood plasma and the adequacy of the blood circulation.

FACTORS AFFECTING RESPIRATORY FUNCTIONING

A decrease in the availability of oxygen from the atmosphere can cause serious respiratory problems. The term "ambient anoxia" is used to describe this condition. For example, at high altitudes, where the pressure of oxygen in the air is low, a person will experience considerable difficulty in breathing until he becomes acclimatized to the rarefied atmosphere. Once acclimatized, his breathing rate may be seven times as fast as at sea level in order to provide him with sufficient oxygen.

The presence of noxious gases in the air will displace the oxygen normally present and lessen the amount available for respiration. In most fires, for instance, suffocation from smoke is usually as great a hazard as bodily injury from the flames. In heavily industrialized areas, a combination of gaseous wastes from industrial plants and the exhaust fumes from automobiles may pollute the atmosphere to a level that it is dangerous to health. Many cities now have a pollution monitoring system. When the pollution level reaches a point that is considered dangerous, industries in the area may be restricted in their operations until the pollution level is relatively safe again.

Respiratory problems may also be caused by anything that interferes with the control mechanisms for breathing. A number of different factors may depress or totally inactivate the respiratory center in the medulla. Depressed respirations almost invariably accompany a head injury and are believed to be due to cerebral edema. The edema causes increased pressure within the cranial cavity, which depresses the activity of the respiratory center. Drugs and anesthetics which act as depressants on the central nervous system will also depress respirations and may, when administered in large dosage, cause respiratory arrest. Morphine is usually cited as an example of a drug which depresses respirations, although any central nervous system depressant will decrease respirations as well as depress other parts of the central nervous system.

As discussed earlier in the section on the physiology of respiration, the respiratory center is sensitive to chemical stimuli resulting from changes in the composition of blood or tissue fluids. If a person faints, or voluntarily holds his breath until he faints, the accumulation of carbon dioxide in the blood quickly triggers the mechanism for inspiration and the patient automatically begins to breathe again. A lessened quantity of oxygen in the blood acts more slowly than an increased amount of carbon dioxide as a respiratory stimulant. This is because the blood normally carries an amount of oxygen greater than that which is needed for immediate use. It takes a longer period of time for the body to feel the need for more oxygen and to respond to the oxygen lack. Increased acidity of the blood (a lowered pH) will increase both the rate and depth of respirations as the body attempts to "blow off" acid through the expired carbon dioxide. In patients with a fever, the accelerated rate of metabolism caused by the higher than normal body temperature leads to an increase in the amount of end products of metabolism, which are acid in character. The respiratory response is an increase in the rate and depth of respirations.

The passage of oxygen from the atmosphere to the alveoli and the passage of carbon dioxide from the alveoli to the air require an unobstructed airway. Anything which interferes with the patency of any part of the respiratory tract can interfere with the efficiency of respirations. Normally the cough is a mechanism by which the respiratory tract is cleared of foreign materials. Obstructions in the pharynx, larynx, trachea, and bronchi can stimulate the cough reflex.

Some patients have difficulty in clearing mucus from the bronchial tree, perhaps because it is painful to cough, because of lack of strength, or because of unconsciousness. At any rate, fluids can accumulate and require nursing intervention for their removal. Continual bed rest and maintaining a prone or supine position can contribute to this difficulty by limiting chest expansion and alveolar ventilation. Also, certain drugs and diseases of the nervous system interfere with muscle control and the normal methods of clearing the respiratory system.

Under certain circumstances, oxygen and carbon dioxide are impeded from crossing through membranes of the alveoli, the capillaries, or red blood cells. This impediment is referred to as "alveolocapillary block." For example, the distance the gases have to travel may be increased owing to pulmonary edema or inflammation. The successful exchange of gases depends on the efficient functioning of the two major pump systems in the body, the lungs and the heart.

Any malfunctioning of the lungs or the muscles of respiration because of injury or disease will interfere with the transfer of oxygen and carbon dioxide. For example, conditions which disturb the balance of the partial pressures of these gases can result from disturbed passage through the airway, such as in occurs in asthma, in which expired air is obstructed in the bronchioles. In addition, any decrease in the elasticity of the lung tissue can impair respiration. For example, in emphysema (a condition common among chronic smokers) extra effort must be made to deflate the lungs because of the inelastic tissue.

The principal muscles concerned with respiration are the muscles of the chest wall and the diaphragm. These include the internal and external intercostals, the sternocleidomastoid, the scalenes, the thoracohumeral, and the thorascapular muscles. In addition, in forced breathing, the abdominal muscles may be brought into use. Trauma to any of these muscles, as may result from accidental injury or from surgery, will impair respiration. Similarly, any disease process which weakens or paralyzes these muscles (such as poliomyelitis) will affect the individual's ability to breathe normally.

A great many factors may affect the efficient functioning of the heart. In some conditions there may be inadequate force to pump the blood through the lungs, or there may be an impediment in the return flow of blood from the lungs to the heart, causing a slowing up (stasis) of blood in the small vessels which surround the alveoli. Such conditions will interfere with respiration by disturbing the balance of partial pressures of oxygen and carbon dioxide within the blood circulating through the lungs.

Similarly, any condition affecting the circulation of blood to the tissues can interfere with the transportation of oxygen from the lungs to the cells. This would include all types of heart disease and arterial or venous disorders, as well as blood dyscrasias. Since hemoglobin carries the oxygen in the blood stream, a reduction in the amount of hemoglobin, such as in anemia, lessens the amount of oxygen carried to the cells.

ASSESSING THE PATIENT WITH DYSPNEA

Subjective Data

One of the prominent indications of respiratory distress is the feeling of difficulty in breathing experienced by the patient. This is termed *dyspnea*. The patient's breathing efforts become obvious, and he attempts to control his breathing to overcome the difficulty. In all probability, a change in the rate and character (for example, in depth) of the patient's respirations and a general restlessness can be observed. *Orthopnea,* the inability to breathe except when in a sitting position, often accompanies dyspnea.

Difficulty in breathing is a subjective symptom. It is therefore difficult to assess objectively. The nurse can supplement her observations with information the patient can tell her about his condition. Pertinent information includes how long the patient has had the problem, the nature and extent of the respiratory distress, and whether it is brought on or relieved by specific factors. Often the patient's family can give assistance in providing background information about the patient's condition prior to his seeking medical care.

Dyspnea must be evaluated in relation to the patient's age, sex, normal pattern of breathing, position, physical activity, emotional state, and disease condition. Any medications which the patient is receiving should also be taken into consideration.

Many patients with respiratory problems complain of pain in the chest. The pain may or may not be associated with the act of breathing. Pain may be caused by a number of different factors, such as inflammation, the presence of space-occupying lesions, or increased muscular activity as the patient works harder to breathe. The presence or absence of chest pain should be noted. A description of the pain (for example, sharp, dull, intermittent, or steady) should be reported, as should its location and its relationship to breathing.

Objective Data

The nurse's alert and astute observations play a very important role in gathering data for assessment of the patient's condition and his needs for medical and nursing intervention. Continuing observations are important for evaluating the effectiveness of therapy and nursing care measures.

Observations should be directed and purposeful. They are based on the nurse's knowledge of the physiological mechanisms involved in respiration, her ability to identify deviations from the normal, and her understanding of the disease process affecting the patient.

Pertinent observations include an assessment of the character of the patient's respirations, his color, his behavior, and the presence of pain, cough, or sputum, as well as observations related to his general physical status.

In observing the character of the patient's respirations, the nurse should note the rate and rhythm of breathing. The normal rate for adults is 12 to 18 per minute, and normal breathing is silent and effortless. Labored breathing may be observed in the use of accessory muscles for inspiration or expiration and in the flaring of the nostrils on inspiration. Distention of the neck veins may also be present. Difficult breathing is often accompanied by abnormal sounds. For example, *wheezing* is frequently observed in patients with asthma or chronic bronchitis and indicates that the air is passing through a narrowed lumen. *Rales*, short bubbling sounds, are indicative of fluid in the respiratory tract. An obstruction of the upper airway may result in *laryngeal stridor*, a coarse, high-pitched sound which accompanies inspiration.

The nurse should also note the movements of the patient's chest on breathing. Normal respiration results in deep and even movements. Labored respirations may be persistently shallow, or there may be alterations in rhythm and depth. For example, in Cheyne-Stokes breathing there is a regular pattern of gradually decreasing depth to the respirations followed by a cycle of increasing depth. The pattern of inspiration-expiration may be varied also. Normally, the inspiratory phase is shorter than the time for expiration (1.0 to 1.5 seconds for inspiration, 2 to 3 seconds for the expiratory phase). A prolonged expiratory pause is seen in many types of lung conditions.[2]

Air hunger is one of the symptoms associated with *hypoxia,* a condition in which there is a reduced oxygen content of the tissues. In air hunger the respiratory rate and the depth of respirations are markedly increased as the body attempts to obtain more oxygen to augment the depleted reserves in the tissues.

The patient's color is frequently an important indication of respiratory distress. *Cyanosis*, a bluish tinge in the skin and mucous membranes, is frequently associated with respiratory distress. Cyanosis may appear as a general duskiness of the skin surface, but more frequently it is observed as a bluish tinge in the lips, or around them (circumoral cyanosis), in the earlobes, and in the beds of the nails. It is not, however, considered a very reliable sign of respiratory distress, since its presence depends on a number of factors, including the tissue blood flow and volume, tissue oxygen uptake, the hemoglobin content of the blood, and skin color.

Cyanosis is not always present in respiratory insufficiency. There are some conditions in which the patient's skin may show an increased reddish tint. This may occur as a result of prolonged anoxia in which there is an increased renal output of *erythropoietin* and a secondary polycythemia develops.[3]

When an obstruction occurs in the respiratory tract, coughing is usually stimulated. The cough is a protective mechanism of the body. To *expectorate* is to bring up mucus from the lungs. *Hemoptysis* is the expectoration of blood-streaked sputum. *Sputum* consists mostly of mucus which is brought up from the lungs. It usually also contains leukocytes, epithelial cells, secretions from the nasopharynx, bacteria, and dirt. Patients with respiratory diseases frequently expectorate sputum. Sputum should be observed for amount, color, consistency, odor, and the presence of foreign material, such as blood or pus. The character of the sputum is often specific to the type of disease the patient has. For example, the sputum of patients with emphysema or chronic bronchitis is usually thick and tenacious, whereas that from patients with pulmonary edema is usually pink in color and frothy in appearance.[4]

---

[2]Marie Kurihara: Assessment and Maintenance of Adequate Respiration. *Nursing Clinics of North America*, 3:69–70, March 1968.

[3]Ibid., p. 72.

[4]Jane Secor: *Patient Care in Respiratory Problems.* Saunders Monographs in Clinical Nursing, Vol. 1. Philadelphia, W. B. Saunders Company, 1969, pp. 40–41.

If the patient has a cough, the nurse's observations should include its frequency and time of occurrence, its relationship to activity (that is, if it is present on exertion or under some other condition), whether it is productive of sputum, and whether there are specific factors which induce cough or effectively relieve it.

Because nervous tissue is very sensitive to oxygen deficiency, the patient with respiratory problems may show signs of impaired brain functioning. An early sign is faulty judgment, which may progress to confusion and disorientation. Safety precautions such as using siderails on the bed should be taken to protect the patient. Other signs that the brain is suffering from oxygen lack include headache, vertigo (dizziness), and drowsiness. The nurse should be alert for signs of mental confusion, drowsiness, or abnormal behavior in the patient. It is important to remember that these symptoms are reversible.

Additional observations the nurse may note that may be present are tachycardia, as the heart beats faster in an attempt to keep up with the body's demands for oxygen, and increased blood pressure. Because of the vital role of respiration in total body functioning, other systems may also be affected, and signs and symptoms indicative of their impaired functioning may be present. Because muscular activity, for example, demands increased oxygen consumption, the patient tires easily, particularly with any extra exertion.

Diagnostic Tests

Numerous diagnostic tests are performed in examinations of the respiratory tract. X-ray, fluoroscopy, bronchography, and bronchoscopy are all means by which the lungs may be visualized. In fluoroscopy the chest movements can also be observed.

In *bronchography*, an iodized oil is instilled into the bronchial tree as a contrast medium so that, when a chest x-ray is made, the structures of the lung are visualized. For a bronchogram the patient usually has a local anesthetic sprayed on his pharynx to prevent gagging and coughing. After the procedure the patient

should not take any food or fluids until the anesthetic has worn off, because of the danger of aspiration.

Bronchoscopy is the examination of the bronchial tree with a lighted instrument. A local anesthetic is sprayed on the patient's pharynx and he is usually sedated before the examination. In preparation for bronchoscopy, the patient does not take food or fluids for at least six hours beforehand. If he wears dentures, they are removed before the examination.

The *examination of sputum* is a common diagnostic test. Normally a sterile wide-mouth vial or Petri dish is used to collect the sputum. Sputum is best collected early in the morning, when it is most easily expectorated. The sputum should be coughed up from the lungs, not from the back of the throat. Sometimes a 24 hour specimen of sputum is ordered. If this is the case, the quantity is usually to be measured. The sputum should be collected in a graduated container. If an ungraduated one is used, the nurse can put into the container a measured amount of saline solution. The specimen when collected can then be poured into a graduated container and the quantity of saline subtracted from the total to give an accurate estimate of the amount of sputum in the 24 hour period.

For *nose and throat cultures*, a sterile, cotton-tipped applicator is touched to the inside of the nose or throat and then returned to a sterile test tube. Separate swabs and containers are used for the nose and throat.

An important laboratory test that is performed frequently is the measurement of *partial pressures of blood gases*. For this test, a sample of arterial blood is drawn and sent to the laboratory for analysis. The analyses of blood gases reflect the efficiency of ventilation and of the transport system for oxygen and carbon dioxide, and the rate of metabolism in the cells, as well as the state of the buffer systems. Normal values for PO_2 are 95 to 100 mm. Hg and for PCO_2 are 35 to 40 mm. Hg.[5] The P stands for partial pressure—that is, the pressure of the gas dissolved in the blood. (The particular gas is only a part of

---

[5] Ibid., pp. 26–27.

the total volume of gases in the blood, hence the term "partial pressures.") It is important that the sample be taken to the laboratory immediately. The container is usually surrounded by ice to ensure that the gases remain in solution.

There are a number of *tests of pulmonary function* which may also be ordered for the patient. Among those that are commonly done are *maximum voluntary ventilation* (MVV) and *forced vital capacity* (FVC).

The measurement of maximum voluntary ventilation is a good indication of a person's ability to take air into his lungs. It measures the maximal amount of air a person can breathe in one minute. The normal for adult males is 125 to 150 liters per minute; for females, 100 liters per minute.[6]

Forced vital capacity (often referred to simply as vital capacity) measures the volume of expired air which the patient exhales following deep inspiration. This test requires the expenditure of less effort on the patient's part and yields essentially the same information as the MVV. Sometimes the results are given as a ratio of vital capacity (VC) to maximum voluntary ventilation (MVV). A ratio below 75 per cent indicates obstruction in the airway.

---

[6]Ibid., pp. 23–24.

For additional information on these tests and other tests of pulmonary function, the nurse is referred to Secor's *Patient Care in Respiratory Problems.*

Nursing responsibilities with regard to diagnostic tests ordered for the patient include explaining the purpose of the test to the patient, giving him a description of the procedure, and telling him what is expected of him. Many anxieties and fears can be allayed by a simple explanation in nontechnical terms which the patient can understand. The nurse may also be asked to assist in carrying out these tests. She should know the purpose of the test and the significance of the results. The laboratory findings are important not only for assessing the patient's nursing problems, but also as an aid in evaluating the effectiveness of therapy.

PRIORITIES FOR NURSING ACTION

Difficulty in breathing is a distressing symptom. It always requires immediate attention by nursing and medical personnel. Early and prompt intervention can often minimize attacks and prevent the need for radical measures. The nurse should therefore observe the patient closely for any changes in his condition that indicate increasing difficulty with respira-

---

PRINCIPLES RELEVANT TO DYSPNEA

1. Oxygen is essential to life.
2. A patent airway is essential to normal respiratory function.
3. The respiratory tract is lined with mucus-secreting epithelium.
4. Coughing, swallowing, and sneezing are mechanisms by which the respiratory tract is cleared of foreign materials.
5. The average respiratory rate for an adult is 12 to 18 respirations per minute. Respiratory rates under 8 per minute may lead to hypoxemia.
6. Carbon dioxide concentrations between 3 and 10 per cent increase the rate and depth of respirations.
7. An individual can survive only a few minutes without oxygen. Cells in the cerebral cortex begin to die as soon as they are deprived of oxygen; it is believed that irreparable damage may follow only a few minutes of oxygen deprivation.
8. Difficulty in breathing provokes anxiety.
9. An insufficient supply of oxygen impairs functioning of all body systems.
10. Air at sea level contains approximately 20 per cent oxygen; prolonged exposure to high oxygen tension can result in oxygen poisoning.

tion. These should be reported immediately, and appropriate measures instituted. Severe distress in breathing is a medical emergency. Signs of impending respiratory failure include rapid, shallow breathing; rapid, thready pulse; fear and apprehension; restlessness; and confusion. Restlessness often occurs early and is an important sign to watch for in patients. Cyanosis may or may not be present.

If respiratory failure seems imminent, the nurse should make certain that the patient's airway is clear; institute ventilation by mechanical means; and obtain assistance. Measures for the resuscitation of patients with respiratory failure are detailed in a later section.

GOALS FOR NURSING ACTION

Principal goals of nursing action in the care of patients who are having difficulty in breathing include the following:

1. Maintaining the patency of the airway
2. Increasing ventilatory efficiency
3. Ensuring that the patient has an adequate supply of oxygen
4. Decreasing the demands of the body for oxygen
5. Minimizing the patient's anxiety

SPECIFIC NURSING INTERVENTIONS

Measures to Maintain the Patency of the Airway

The maintenance of the patency of the patient's airway is essential to adequate respirations. The conscious, rational patient can tell the nurse when fluids have accumulated in his pharynx and trachea; however, when a patient is unconscious the nurse must rely upon her own observations, and to intervene when necessary—for example, with suctioning to clear the patient's air passages. One of the surest indications of partial blockage of air passages by mucus is the sound of "wet breathing"; as the air passes through the secretions it creates a typical gurgling sound.

Suctioning, positioning (for example, the Sims position), and coughing are measures used to maintain the patency of the air passages. The frequency with which a patient needs suctioning is variable, but if the patient tends to accumulate fluids, a suction catheter should always be near him for immediate use. Suctioning is discussed later in this chapter.

For the conscious patient, medications such as nose drops and aerosol sprays help to liquefy secretions and facilitate their removal from the air passages.

The body position also affects respirations. For the unconscious patient, a semiprone (Sims) position, without a pillow for his head and with the mandible extended forward and up, prevents the tongue from falling back and permits the drainage of fluids from the mouth. For the conscious patient, Fowler's position allows maximum chest expansion and ease of expectoration of sputum. One reason for helping the patient to change his position every four hours while he is in bed is to permit expansion of all areas of the lungs. Obviously, while a patient is lying on his left side he is not likely to be able to expand his left lung to its maximum capacity.

Coughing is a means by which a person clears his respiratory tract of secretions and foreign material. For the patient who finds it painful to cough, the pain will be eased if the nurse supports the painful area, such as an operative incision, firmly while he coughs.

Throat Suctioning. Oxygen reaches the alveoli of the lungs by passing through the mouth, the nose, the pharynx, the larynx, and the bronchi and bronchioles. A patent airway is essential to the passage of air through this route. The purpose of throat suctioning is to help a patient clear his airway by removing secretions and foreign materials from his nose, mouth, and pharynx. In most instances, the patient needs an explanation of the procedure. He can be reassured that this is a painless measure that will relieve his breathing so that he will be more comfortable. If the patient can cough while the suction is applied, it will facilitate the removal of mucus.

The equipment required includes a

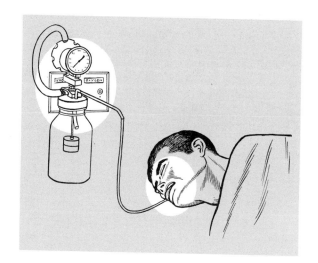

Suctioning a patient's throat to remove
mucus that is obstructing the airway.

throat suction, a container for cold water, and a clean catheter. In hospitals, catheters are sterilized after each use. The catheter has a narrow lumen with a fine tip and several openings along the sides. The openings prevent irritation of the mucous membrane in any one area by distributing the negative pressure of the suction over several areas. Whenever there is any indication that a person might require emergency suctioning, this equipment is kept nearby.

The respiratory tract is lined with mucous membrane which can easily be injured by mechanical means; therefore the catheter is never forced against an obstruction. Normally the catheter is inserted by the nurse as far as the pharynx for suctioning; deeper suctioning is generally a physician's procedure.

The catheter is attached to the suction machine and then lubricated with water. Water is drawn through the catheter in order to ensure the patency of the lumen. The patient assumes a position with his head turned to one side, facing the nurse. In this position his tongue falls forward and does not obstruct the entry of the catheter. The catheter is then gently inserted through the nose or mouth into the pharynx, rotated gently and withdrawn. Suctioning is begun when the catheter is

in place. This procedure is repeated until the airway is clear. If the patient coughs while the catheter is in place, it helps to remove the mucus accumulations and foreign materials.

A Y tube is sometimes used with suction equipment. One stem of the Y is closed off with a finger to apply suction through the catheter. When this stem is left open, the suction is stopped in the catheter. This method does away with the repeated insertion and removal of the catheter, and thus minimizes trauma to

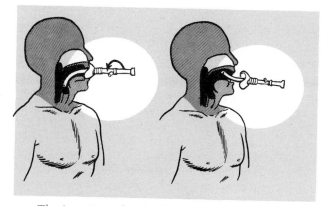

The insertion of a shallow airway.

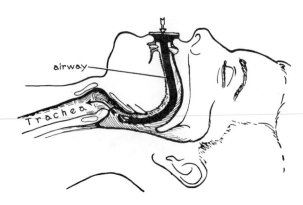

airway

Trachea

An airway in place.

the mucous membranes of the air passages.

Measures to Increase Ventilatory Efficiency

The principal factors that impede ventilation are obstruction of the airway and inadequate expansion of the chest. Measures to ensure patency of the airway, as just discussed, are therefore essential to increasing ventilatory efficiency.

Measures which assist in optimal expansion of the chest include positioning of the patient (as already noted) and the alleviation of pain or discomfort associated with breathing. The chest is sometimes splinted to relieve painful respirations, or the physician may leave orders for analgesics to be given. Usually these are given at the nurse's discretion. Coughing may also interfere with respirations. The administration of cough mixtures will usually provide relief from this discomfort. Frequently cough mixtures are left at the patient's bedside to be taken as needed.

Deep breathing at frequent intervals should be encouraged. Exercise helps to improve ventilatory functioning, and active or passive exercise within the patient's level of tolerance should be promoted. Abdominal distention should be prevented by giving the patient small, frequent meals of easily digestible food. Foods that are gas-forming (see Chapter 16) should be avoided. The patient's garments should be loose-fitting and bed coverings should not be tucked in tightly.

Artificial Airways. An artificial airway is inserted into a patient's throat in order to keep his tongue forward and the airway patent. Artificial airways are usually made of plastic or rubber. There are long and short airways for deep and shallow intubation. In deep intubation the airway extends through the pharynx into the trachea. This type of airway is usually inserted by a doctor. In shallow intubation the airway extends behind the tongue and terminates in the pharynx. This type of airway is often inserted by the nurse.

In shallow intubation the patient's tongue is brought forward and the airway is placed in his mouth with the base of the curve against his tongue. The airway is then turned so that the base of the curve is against the soft palate. It is then in position in the pharynx.

After the lungs of an unconscious patient have been suctioned, the patient should remain in a semiprone (Sims) position to facilitate drainage of secretions from his mouth and prevent their accumulation in his pharynx. The approximate amount and the nature of the secretions that were suctioned are recorded on the patient's chart. The appearance of any blood should also be reported.

Measures to Ensure Adequate Oxygen Intake

General measures to ensure an adequate supply of oxygen include the provision of fresh air. The patient's room should be kept well ventilated. Many patients with respiratory problems like to have the bed placed beside a window so that they can get fresh air. These patients are often particularly sensitive to alterations in the temperature and humidity of the environment. Atmospheric oxygen may need to be supplemented by inhalation aids, such as oxygen tents, oxygen masks, nasal cannulae, and nasal catheters. The use of these aids is discussed later in this chapter.

Inhalation Therapy

HUMIDITY THERAPY. The provision of air that has a high water content is a form of therapy that has been used for people with respiratory problems for many generations. Traditionally used in the form of steam inhalations, there are now many techniques available to provide a high humidity environment for those who require this form of therapy. The purpose of humidity therapy is to provide extra moisture to the mucous membranes lining the respiratory tract. The moisture helps to soothe irritated mucous membranes, and also helps to dilute thick secretions and to loosen the crusts that frequently form on the mucous membranes as a result of respiratory infection. The secretions and crusts can then be coughed up or aspirated more easily. The moisture may also be used as a vehicle for administering a medication directly to the respiratory tract. In this case, the water vapor is passed over the medication from which it picks up molecules that are then inhaled with the vapor.

A high humidity environment may be established in oxygen tents, in specially constructed plastic hoods, and in entire rooms; however, the most common method of increasing the humidity in the atmosphere immediately surrounding the patient is by means of a humidifier (steam kettle). Many types of humidifiers are manufactured commercially, and both hot and cold humidifiers are available. In the home, a small commercially bought humidifier or an electric kettle may be used to supply steam. Whatever type of equipment is used in the home or in the hospital, most patients require some help with it.

The physician may order continuous *humidity therapy* (or steam inhalations), or he may order it for one-half hour every four hours (humidity therapy, 1/2 hour q4h).

Nursing care measures relevant to *humidity therapy* include:

1. Explaining the equipment to the patient and advising him to breathe in the water vapor (steam) deeply

2. Taking safety precautions to protect the patient from burns if heated humidity (hot steam inhalations) is used; the patient should be warned not to touch any of the equipment that may become hot, and the humidifier (kettle) should be kept well out of reach if the patient shows any signs of mental confusion

3. Arranging the humidifier so that the water vapor surrounds the patient's head

4. Preventing drafts which could be chilling

5. Changing linen when it becomes damp

6. Encouraging the patient to expectorate mucus during the inhalations and providing him with a container for the sputum

OXYGEN INHALATION THERAPY. It is necessary under some circumstances to provide the patient with a concentration of oxygen that is higher than that found in the air. The physician orders the method of administration of the oxygen, the concentration, and the length of time that the patient is to receive the oxygen. The latter factor is sometimes left to the nurse's judgment, the order simply stating "oxygen as necessary."

Oxygen is generally supplied in two ways, from tanks or from wall outlets (piped-in oxygen). Oxygen from the latter source is stored in a central storage area. Many newer hospitals employ the piped-in method of supply. In the home, oxygen is supplied in portable tanks.

Oxygen tanks are steel cylinders in which the oxygen is stored under a pressure of 2200 pounds per square inch at 21° C. (70° F.). There are different sizes of oxygen tanks: the larger ones store 244 cubic feet of oxygen; the smaller tanks store less oxygen but are readily portable. Each tank has a pressure reduction valve which enables the oxygen to be released at a pressure lower than that within the tank. An oxygen tank normally has two gauges: one indicates the amount of oxygen in the tank (the pressure) and the other indicates the amount of oxygen being released (in liters per minute).

The oxygen gauges are generally attached to the tank before it is brought to the patient. In most hospitals respiratory

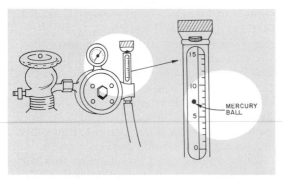

An attachment for an oxygen tank showing the pressure gauge and the liter flow gauge (mercury-ball type).

(inhalation) technologists usually supply and service the oxygen equipment. The following steps are followed in order to attach the gauges to the tank.

1. Open the cylinder valve slightly and then close it quickly to remove any dust in the outlet ("cracking the tank"; this produces a loud hissing sound which can be frightening when not explained beforehand)

2. Connect the regulator valve to the cylinder outlet and tighten the nut with a wrench

3. Make sure that the liter flow valve is in the "off" position

4. Open the cylinder valve slowly until the pressure gauge registers the pressure in the cylinder

5. Adjust the liter flow valve to the desired rate of flow

There are a variety of liter flow indicators. The gauge type and the ball float type are two that are commonly seen.

Piped-in oxygen is usually under low pressure, between 50 to 60 pounds per square inch. Usually only a liter flow valve is needed. To attach the equipment for piped-in oxygen:

1. Make sure that the liter flow valve is in the "off" position

2. Attach the valve to the outlet—some valves are attached by a screw nut; others are inserted directly into the wall outlet

3. Slowly turn the liter flow valve to the desired liter flow

FEARS AND PRECAUTIONS IN THE USE OF OXYGEN EQUIPMENT. When nursing a patient who is receiving oxygen inhalations, there are certain precautions, practices, and facts with which the nurse needs to be familiar. The administration of oxygen is often a frightening experience for the patient and his family. To many patients, it denotes a serious illness; a surprising number of patients remember a relative or a friend who died while receiving oxygen. Oxygen is essential to life and to have to depend upon equipment in order to live is in itself anxiety-producing. This is a situation over which the patient often has little control, and because he is so completely dependent upon others even for the air he breathes, he feels helpless.

Such fears can often be allayed. Explanations about the oxygen equipment are geared to the patient's needs. Some people want to understand in great detail; others are satisfied with a simple explanation. If the patient is well enough to help with his therapy, the nurse can teach him to administer the oxygen himself and thus help him to feel that he has some control over the situation.

Some patients fear suffocation when using inhalation equipment; many dislike the feeling of being enclosed within a tent. Other patients feel isolated from their fellow patients when they are inside a tent. In addition, the necessity of depriving the patient of everyday pleasures such as the use of cigarettes, facial creams, and perfumes adds to his feelings of helplessness. Cigarettes are never permitted because a spark could readily start a fire in the presence of concentrated oxygen. Creams and perfumes with an alco-

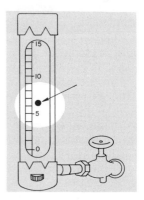

An attachment for an oxygen wall outlet with a mercury-ball liter flow gauge.

hol base are not used because they can contribute to a fire.

When handling oxygen equipment the operator's hands should be free of oils and alcohol, which are highly flammable. Normally the use of electrical equipment around oxygen is restricted to appliances that have been checked and found safe—that is, appliances that will not spark or start a fire.

Lotions and liquids for the patient's use should have a water rather than oil or alcohol base. Special mouth care solutions and back rub lotions that are not flammable must be used in the presence of oxygen equipment.

PRINCIPLES RELEVANT TO THE ADMINISTRATION OF OXYGEN

Oxygen is a colorless, odorless, and tasteless gas that is essential to life. Because oxygen can be neither seen, tasted, nor smelled, the equipment gauges are relied upon to indicate that oxygen is being supplied. The concentration of oxygen in a tent can be tested by an analyzer. The patient who is receiving oxygen is interrupted as little as possible in order to decrease oxygen loss and promote rest.

Oxygen dries and irritates mucous membranes. Most patients who are receiving oxygen require special mouth care in order to maintain good oral hygiene. The provision of fluids for the patient is also important; often the patient is dependent upon the nurse for the administration of fluids. Oxygen is often humidified before it is supplied to the patient.

Oxygen supports combustion. It is essential to the patient's safety that there be no smoking within 4 meters (12 feet) of oxygen equipment. This applies to patients and visitors and usually requires continual explanation and enforcement. Oxygen is not explosive, but a spark created in the presence of a high concentration of oxygen can ignite a fire quickly.

METHODS OF ADMINISTERING OXYGEN. There are four basic methods of administering oxygen: tent, nasal catheter, face mask, and nasal cannulae (nasal prongs).

The Oxygen Tent. Tents were at one time the most common method of administering oxygen. Today they are seldom used for adults except in instances where the patient requires a high humidity environment in addition to supplemental oxygen. The tents are still used frequently with children; in this case they are referred to as *croupettes.*

Oxygen tents are usually made of a clear plastic material that does not permit the diffusion of oxygen or air through it. The motor unit of the tent is usually electrically driven; it circulates the air in the tent and cools it to the desired temperature.

The oxygen concentration in a tent can generally be kept between 50 and 60 per cent, although each time the tent is opened oxygen is lost. Oxygen analyzers are instruments which measure the concentration of oxygen inside the tent. These measurements should be done regularly—for example, every four hours.

A temperature between 20° and 21° C (68° to 70° F) in the tent is comfortable for most people. The ventilation fan can be set at a moderate speed in order to provide sufficient circulation of air. The minimum liter flow of oxygen for the tent is generally 12 liters per minute; however, some patients require a higher liter flow to meet their oxygen needs.

To set up an oxygen tent, the following steps are performed:

1. Turn on the motor and set the liter flow to the desired level

2. Arrange the canopy over the patient's head so that most of the space in the tent is in front of the patient's face.

3. Tuck the canopy under the mattress and secure the canopy over the patient's thighs with a drawsheet folded lengthwise and tucked in on each side of the bed

4. Flush the tent for 20 minutes to bring the concentration of oxygen up quickly to 50 per cent; warn the patient that this makes a hissing noise

5. Provide the patient with a mechanical bell for calling nursing personnel

Because oxygen supports combustion, precautions are taken to prevent fires. Patients do not smoke in an oxygen tent, nor are any electrical devices used inside the tent, such as electrically controlled signal lights, hearing aids, transistor radios, and electric shavers. "No smoking" signs should be placed on the door of the patient's room and visitors should be counseled not to smoke. The patient in the tent may feel cold because of the circulat-

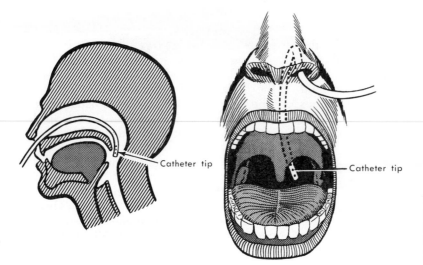

Catheter tip

Catheter tip

The position of the nasal catheter for oxygen administration. Note that the tip of catheter is opposite the uvula.

ing air. The temperature can often be raised and extra covers provided. Patients should be discouraged from plugging the oxygen outlet of the tent with towels in order to close off drafts.

Nursing measures for the patient in an oxygen tent are planned so that the tent is opened as infrequently as possible. Each time the tent is opened oxygen is lost, and the patient consequently receives less than the desired concentration of oxygen.

Patients in oxygen tents often feel isolated from fellow patients; however, they have the same needs to communicate and feel a part of a group. Tent motors today are usually so quiet that patients can hear reasonably well inside them. People can normally be heard by the patient if they speak distinctly.

The Nasal Catheter. Oxygen catheters are made of plastic and are disposable. They have a series of six or eight holes on the sides and are about 45.7 cm. (18 inches) long. A No. 14 French catheter is usually used for an adult patient. Because oxygen dries and irritates mucous membranes, the oxygen is passed through water (humidified) before it is administered by catheter.

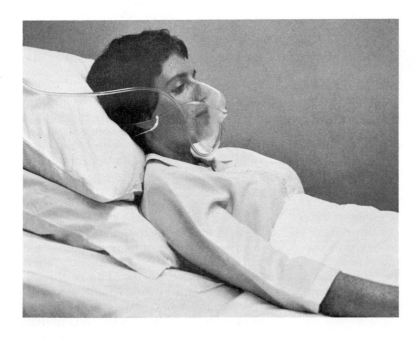

A plastic oxygen mask.

The advantage of the administration of oxygen by catheter is the freedom of movement that it affords the patient. Patients receiving oxygen by this method can obtain about a 50 per cent concentration of oxygen. The minimum liter flow of oxygen by catheter is generally 6 to 7 liters per minute.

The catheter is lubricated before insertion, preferably with water. An oil base lubricant is dangerous because it can be aspirated and subsequently irritate the lungs. The catheter is inserted to a distance about equal to the distance from the patient's nose to his earlobe. It is inserted until the tip is opposite the uvula in the oropharynx (seen through the mouth) and is then taped in place as illustrated. It is never forced against an obstruction. In another technique of shallow insertion, a nasal catheter is inserted approximately 3 inches—that is, into the nasopharynx.

Oxygen catheters are removed every eight hours, and a clean catheter is inserted into the other naris. Patients receiving oxygen by catheter require special mouth and nose care. The catheters tend to irritate the mucous membranes, thereby stimulating secretions, which must be removed. Water base lubricants will soothe irritated nares.

The Face Mask. A variety of inhalation masks are available for use. The lightweight plastic mask which covers the patient's nose and mouth is used extensively today. It provides a concentration of oxygen of about 50 per cent with a minimum liter flow of 8 liters per minute. There are also several non-rebreathing masks in use which can provide an oxygen concentration as high as 95 per cent.

After the liter flow valve is turned on, the mask is applied to the patient's face. Oxygen masks come in different sizes; the mask selected should rest comfortably on the patient's face. Patients who are receiving oxygen by mask are assisted in taking fluids and performing hygienic measures to protect the skin and mucous membrane of the face and mouth from irritation.

Positive-pressure masks are used when oxygen is administered under pressure. These masks apply pressure on exhalation only. A variety of positive-pressure masks are available. With the meter mask, the concentration of oxygen is regulated by a dial on the flow meter. The rebreathing mask has a bag below the mask which permits the partial rebreathing of exhaled air along with the oxygen.

Nasal Cannulae (Nasal Prongs). Nasal cannulae provide a convenient and comfortable method of administering oxygen. Usually made of a soft plastic material, they consist of two tubes approximately one-half inch in length which are fitted into the patient's nostrils and are held in place with a light elastic halter. A concentration of approximately 37 per cent oxygen in the alveolar air may be achieved with a liter flow rate of 5 liters per minute; approximately 40 per cent is achieved with a flow rate of 8 liters per minute. Oxygen applied in this way is always humidified; the cannulae are changed frequently and nasal care is provided as needed.[7]

CARBON DIOXIDE INHALATION. The administration of carbon dioxide is sometimes used to increase the rate and depth of respirations. It is also administered as a treatment for singultus (hiccups).

Carbon dioxide is usually supplied in cylinders in combination with oxygen; this mixture is called carbogen. It is usually administered by mask as a 5 per cent concentration in 95 per cent oxygen. Today in many hospitals CO_2 is given by means of an Adler Rebreather which eliminates the use of the heavy cylinders.

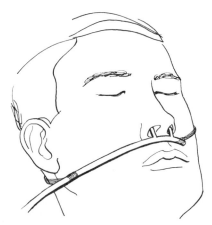

Oxygen nasal cannulae (nasal prongs).

[7]*Merck Manual.* Twelfth edition. David N. Holvey (ed.), Merck & Co. Inc., Rahway, N.J., 1972, p. 174.

The treatment is generally ordered by the physician for 10 to 15 minute periods several times a day, repeated no oftener than q1h.

In carrying out this treatment, the nurse alternates the application of the mask with periods of normal atmospheric breathing during the 10 or 15 minute intervals. That is, the nurse applies the mask for a few minutes, then removes it and lets the patient breathe without it for several respirations, then reapplies the mask. This procedure is repeated during the interval designated for the treatment.

In administering carbon dioxide, the nurse must watch for the signs and symptoms of CO_2 toxicity. At the first indication of vertigo, dyspnea, nausea, or disorientation, the treatment is stopped and the condition reported to the physician.

AEROSOL THERAPY. Aerosol inhalation (nebulization) is a method by which a nonvolatile drug is inhaled into the respiratory tract. A stream of oxygen or compressed air is passed over a solution of the drug and picks up small particles to form a spray. The patient breathes in the spray deeply to force the tiny particles to travel deep into the respiratory tract. Different kinds of aerosols are marketed for use, some of which attach to a face mask which the patient wears during the treatment.

Most aerosol treatments are given by IPPB (intermittent positive-pressure breathing), but a similar spray can be formed by means of a hand atomizer for use in the home. When the bulb of the atomizer is squeezed, air passes over the medicine and picks up small particles to form the spray which the patient inhales. The particles formed by the hand atomizer are usually larger than the particles formed in a nebulizer.

When the physician orders aerosol inhalation, he also orders the type of drug to be administered, the quantity of the drug, and the frequency of the treatment. The liter flow of oxygen that is necessary for aerosol therapy is usually 6 to 8 liters per minute. The exact flow is determined by the density of the spray. A treatment usually lasts 15 to 20 minutes; more exactly, it lasts until all the medicine has been inhaled.

When intermittent aerosol therapy is ordered, the treatment is usually carried out by a respiratory technologist, but in some instances it may be a nursing responsibility. The nurse should then be familiar with the equipment and its use. The most commonly used machines for this type of therapy are the Bird and the Bennett respirators.[8]

HELIUM INHALATION. Helium in combination with oxygen (80:20) is sometimes required for dyspneic patients. Because helium is lighter than the nitrogen it replaces, it eases dyspneic breathing by lessening the work expenditure required of the patient.

Helium is supplied by mask, often a partial rebreathing mask. It may be administered at intervals or, if well tolerated by the patient, for prolonged periods.

Mechanical Ventilation of the Lungs. When an individual's own respiratory apparatus is not functioning normally, it is sometimes necessary to use mechanical aids to ventilate the lungs. Depending on the extent of respiratory dysfunction, either "assisted" or "controlled" ventilation may be used. "Assisted" ventilation is the term used to describe a mechanically generated airflow that is initiated by the patient's own efforts at inspiration and serves to increase his inadequate breathing. In "controlled" ventilation, the airflow is delivered according to a preset cycling pattern without influence of the patient's own breathing.

Basically, ventilators can be divided into two groups, those operating on the principle of negative pressure and those employing positive pressure. The negative-pressure machines generate a suction (negative pressure) on the outside of the chest. This creates within the thorax a pressure gradient with the atmosphere and air flows into the lungs. The positive-pressure ventilators, on the other hand, force air into the lungs by means of a power-driven source, thereby creating intrathoracic pressure (positive) that causes the lungs and chest to expand.

A variety of ventilators are now available on the market. The Bird and Bennett respirators mentioned previously are ex-

[8]A comprehensive description of these machines and their use may be found in Audrey L. Sutton: *Bedside Nursing Techniques in Medicine and Surgery.* 2nd edition. Philadelphia, W. B. Saunders Company, 1969, pp. 56–63.

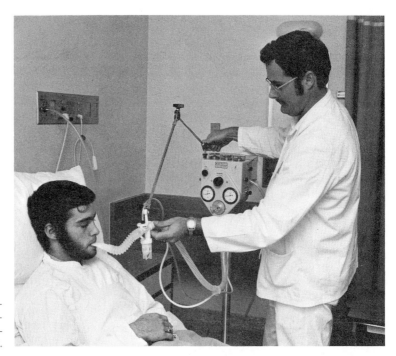

A patient receiving a treatment with a Bennett respirator. The respiratory technologist is assisting the patient.

amples of positive-pressure machines; the Emerson Cuirass, which is a shield-like appliance that fits over the body, is now more commonly used for negative pressure than the Drinker (iron lung) respirator used formerly.[9]

Postural Drainage. Postural drainage is done to facilitate the drainage of secretions from the respiratory tract. The position of the patient for postural drainage depends on the areas of the lung to be drained. For drainage from the lower lobes, the patient assumes a position in which his chest is lower than his hips so that gravity will assist the movement of the mucus. Several special postural drainage beds are now available. If a special bed is not available, one way of assuming this position is for the patient to lie in a prone position across the bed with the waist at the edge of the bed. The upper part of the body is supported by the arms, which rest on a chair at the side of the bed. A receptacle for sputum is put on the chair in front of the patient.

Another position assumed by hospital patients who require postural drainage is a prone position over the knee break of the bed. The patient lies facing the bottom of the bed so that his waist is at the

knee break and his head and chest incline downward.

Postural drainage is carried out to drain sputum from the lungs and to obtain a specimen of sputum. It is ordered by the physician, usually for 10 to 15 minutes, three to four times daily, for therapeutic purposes.

Percussion of the chest helps to dislodge mucus and is frequently done prior to the treatment. For more detailed instructions on techniques used in postural drainage, the nurse is referred to Secor's *Patient Care in Respiratory Problems* (pp. 147–152).

Measures to Decrease Bodily Needs for Oxygen

The need for oxygen by the body is related to the rate of metabolism of the tissue cells. Factors affecting metabolic rate include physical activity, disease processes, and emotional reactions. Although a certain amount of activity is essential to promote optimum ventilation of the lungs, excessive activity should be avoided. The patient's level of tolerance must be carefully assessed and care taken that the patient does not overexert himself.

---

[9]Egan, op. cit., pp. 305–352.

An elevated body temperature increases the basal metabolic rate and contributes to respiratory distress. Care should be taken then to prevent the patient from developing an infection, and measures taken to keep body temperatures within normal limits.

Emotional tension is also a factor to be considered in patients with respiratory problems. Anxiety, for example, may be mediated through the parasympathetic nervous system and result in constriction of the smooth muscles of the bronchioles. The expression of other emotions, such as fear, anger and grief, is also closely related to respiration. Strong emotions such as anger and fear initiate responses to prepare the body for action, and respirations become faster and deeper.

Measures to Minimize Anxiety

Anxiety almost invariably accompanies dyspnea. To be unable to breathe easily and normally is a frightening experience. The person with chronic respiratory problems may live in constant fear that his next breath may be his last one.

The patient's anxiety contributes to his respiratory problems, as noted in several places throughout this chapter. A vicious circle may develop: that is, the patient becomes dyspneic; his dyspnea produces anxiety; the anxiety results in more dyspnea. It is essential that this circle be broken.

Helping to establish the patient's confidence in the care he is receiving is a nursing responsibility and an important factor in alleviating anxiety. Prompt attention to the patient's needs, such as answering his call-light immediately and attending to his wants without delay, can often prevent or minimize an attack of dyspnea. It is important in this regard to remember that anxiety is not always expressed openly. The patient may not necessarily say "I am frightened," but his actions can convey this meaning to the astute and observant nurse. Often, the anxious patient may make a seemingly excessive number of requests, or attempt to keep the nurse engaged in conversation. The physical presence of someone competent who can assist him if need be is reassuring to the patient.

Efficient handling of equipment and skillful execution of procedures contributes to the patient's feeling that he is in good hands. The nurse should be familiar with the equipment used in the care of patients with respiratory problems and should have confidence in her own ability to perform the necessary procedures.

Caring for the patient who has difficulty in breathing can be anxiety-provoking for the nurse. Knowing what measures to take and how to use equipment contributes to her feelings of confidence in giving care.

Measures to ensure the patient's comfort and improve his sense of well-being are also valuable adjuncts in the care of patients with respiratory problems. Good personal hygiene is important, and the patient who experiences dyspnea on exertion may need assistance from the nurse in this regard. Many patients with respiratory disorders are "mouth-breathers" and good oral hygiene is needed. Because of the drying effects of oxygen, patients who are receiving oxygen therapy require special mouth care to maintain hydration of the tissues in the oral cavity and prevent the development of infection or other complications.

Dyspnea is often related to emotional problems. Distressing situations may provoke attacks of difficulty in breathing. The nurse should be alert to conditions which appear to precipitate such attacks and should report these to the physician.

Emergency Situations

Among the several methods of resuscitation for respiratory failure, the most widely used are: (1) the oral method (mouth-to-mouth or mouth-to-nose), (2) the revised Sylvester method, and (3) the self-inflating bag-mask method. The oral method is the simplest to use and is generally considered the most effective in first aid situations. It can be used by and with almost all age groups and in most situations. As an alternative method when physical, religious, or esthetic reasons preclude use of the oral method, the revised Sylvester method (Brosch modification) is internationally advocated for first aid situations when mechanical aids are not available. When available (as, for example, in hospitals or first aid stations) the self-inflating bag-mask method is generally preferred.

Oral Method

1. Place the patient in a supine position if possible

2. Ensure an open airway — lift the patient's neck and press his forehead so that head is tilted backward; lift the chin upwards

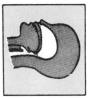

3. Remove any foreign material from mouth and throat

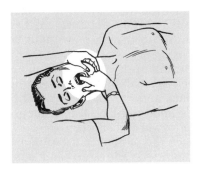

AIRWAY CLOSED   AIRWAY OPEN
(HEAD HYPEREXTENDED)

4. If an airway such as the Brook airway is available, insert it in the patient's mouth over his tongue (see section on artificial airways)

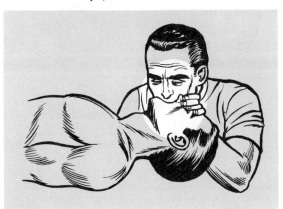

5. Occlude the patient's nostrils (by pinching them together) and blow into his mouth by placing your mouth directly over the patient's; observe the rise of the patient's chest

6. After each inflation, raise your mouth from the patient's and allow the patient to exhale

7. Repeat this procedure approximately 12 to 15 times each minute; continue until normal breathing is restored

If it is not possible to achieve an airtight seal between your mouth and that of the patient, the mouth-to-nose method may be used. Bring your hand which is holding the patient's chin up over his mouth to seal it off. Blow directly into the patient's nostrils. When using the oral method with infants and small children, bring your mouth over the nose *and* mouth of the child. Repeat the procedure 20 to 30 times per minute, using gentle puffs of air to avoid undue pressure which could damage the lungs.[10]

Revised Sylvester Method. The procedure recommended by the St. John Ambulance Association is as follows:

Quickly place the casualty on his back, elevating the shoulders with a folded coat or other suitable padding. Extend the neck and tilt the head straight back as far as possible in order to raise the tongue off the back of the throat, thus *opening the airway.* Make sure his airway is not obstructed.

Compression Phase: Kneel at the casualty's head, grasp his wrists, and cross them over the lower half of the sternum (breastbone). Rock forward, pressing firmly downward upon the casualty's chest, thus forcing the air out of his

---

[10]*First Aid.* Third Canadian edition. Ottawa, St. John Priory of Canada Properties, 1974.

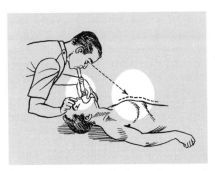

Mouth-to-mouth resuscitation using an airway.

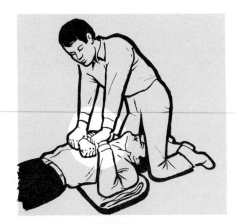

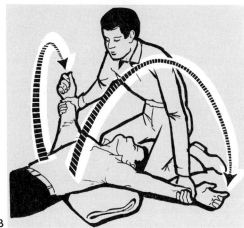

A, Compression phase. B, Expansion phase.[10]

obstruction, such as stomach contents, in the mouth. He may relieve the First Aider since this method of Artificial Respiration is physically demanding.[11]

Self-Inflating Bag-Mask Method. The self-inflating bag-mask unit consists of a mask, system of valves, self-inflating bag, and oxygen tube-connector. The mask is designed to form an air-tight seal around the patient's mouth and nose. When squeezed and released, the bag reinflates itself rapidly. The valves permit air to enter the mask when the bag is squeezed; an exhaust valve carries the exhaled air away so that it does not enter the bag. The unit can be used with or without supplemental oxygen.

To use this unit effectively, an air tight seal must be maintained between the patient's face and the mask. In addition, the patient's head must be tilted, keeping the jaw in a forward position.

1. Place the patient in a supine position with shoulders elevated and neck extended

2. Stand at the head of the patient and apply mask over his nose and mouth; hold the mask with the thumb and index finger on the top of the mask and the third, fourth, and fifth fingers on the patient's jaw (the pointed end of the mask goes over the nose)

---

[11]Ibid.

lungs. This phase should take about two seconds. . . . Count *one and two and.* . . .

Expansion Phase: Release the downward pressure and draw the casualty's arms upward, outward, and backward. This pulls the chest wall into the expanded position and sucks air into the lungs. Count *three and four and.* . . .

Now return the wrists to their original position across the sternum. . . . Count *five.*

Timing: In order to simulate normal breathing, movements should be repeated in a rhythmic manner—about 12 times each minute for an adult, somewhat faster for a child. The First Aider should watch for signs of obstruction in the airway or change in the color of the face of the casualty and adjust his movements when the casualty shows signs of voluntary breathing. Care should be taken to use a reasonable amount of pressure in relation to the age and physical build of the casualty.

If an assistant is available, have him maintain the position of the casualty's head—tilted well back—and watch for the presence of any

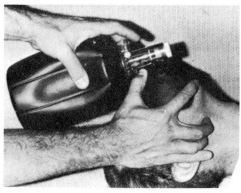

The basic position of the hands in holding a bag mask in place is demonstrated. A tight seal should be maintained between the mask and the patient's face with one hand while the bag is squeezed with the other hand. The patient's airway must be kept open by keeping the neck extended as shown.[12]

3. With the other hand, squeeze the bag firmly and continue squeezing until you see the patient's chest rise, then release your grip on the bag and allow it to expand on its own; do not remove the mask from the patient's face; repeat the procedure 12 to 15 times per minute

With this method, you must be particularly alert to signs of vomiting or regurgitation. If the patient vomits or regurgitates food, quickly remove the mask, turn the patient's head to the side, and use your finger or a suction unit to clean out the mouth. Then resume the ventilation.[12]

---

[12]*Emergency Care and Transportation of the Sick and Injured.* Committee on Injuries. American Academy of Orthopaedic Surgeons, 430 N. Michigan Avenue, Chicago, Illinois 60611.

GUIDE TO ASSESSING DYSPNEA

1. Does the patient complain of difficulty in breathing? How long has he had this condition?
2. Is he anxious about his ability to breathe? What can the nurse do to alleviate his anxiety?
3. What are his respirations like in rate, depth, regularity, and sound? Is he using accessory muscles of respiration in breathing?
4. Does he show signs of cyanosis?
5. Does his condition require immediate medical or nursing intervention? What measures should the nurse institute first?
6. Has the specific causal factor for the dyspnea been identified? Which of the five processes involved in respiration have been impaired in function?
7. Is the patient's airway clear? Does he need suctioning or other measures to clear the airway?
8. Is the patient receiving an adequate supply of oxygen? Has oxygen therapy been ordered? If so, by what method of administration?
9. What position is best for this patient to promote maximal ventilatory efficiency?
10. Is the patient distressed by coughing?
11. Is he bringing up sputum?
12. Is the patient showing signs of restlessness? of mental confusion?
13. Have diagnostic tests and examinations been ordered for this patient? What are the patient's learning needs relative to these? What are the nurses's responsibilities?
14. Has the patient or his family other learning needs (for example, needs relating to the patient's activities, measures to prevent dyspnea, or the use of equipment for his treatment)?

GUIDE TO EVALUATING THE EFFECTIVENESS OF NURSING INTERVENTION

1. Is the patient breathing more easily?
2. Has his anxiety been relieved?
3. Is his airway patent?
4. Has his ventilatory efficiency been improved?
5. Have distressing symptoms such as coughing been relieved?
6. Has cyanosis been lessened?
7. Is the patient able to bring up sputum sufficiently to clear the bronchial tree?

8. Are his activities commensurate with his level of tolerance?
9. Has he (or his family) gained the knowledge and skills necessary to prevent further attacks of dyspnea or to continue his treatment at home?

STUDY VOCABULARY

Acapnia	Expectorate	Laryngeal stridor
Ambient oxygen	Hemoptysis	Orthopnea
Asphyxia	Humidity	Sputum
Cheyne-Stokes respirations	Hyperpnea	Syncope
Dyspnea	Hypoxemia	Transudation
Eupnea	Hypoxia	Vertigo

STUDY SITUATION

Mr. R. S. Rowlands is a 38 year old patient who has been in the hospital for three weeks. His medical diagnosis is acute bronchial asthma. When he was admitted his breathing was dyspneic, he appeared cyanotic, and his respiratory rate varied from 28 to 34 respirations per minute.

Mr. Rowlands did not want his bed to be flat; he demanded five pillows from the nurse and spent most of his time bent forward in bed. He was thin and appeared anxious. The physician ordered an oxygen mask for Mr. Rowlands, who liked to use the oxygen and to turn it on and off himself.

1. What factors should be taken into consideration in explaining to this patient how to use the oxygen equipment?
2. By what means can the patient's need for oxygen be assessed?
3. For what reason might the patient demand five pillows, and why would he like to handle the oxygen himself?
4. What nursing interventions might ease this patient's breathing?
5. How can the effectiveness of these measures be evaluated?
6. What objectives could help to guide the nursing care of this patient?
7. What observations should you make about this patient?
8. What are his nursing problems? How would you resolve these problems?

SUGGESTED READINGS

Beaumont, E.: Portable I.P.P.B. Machines. *Nursing '73*, 3:26–31, January 1973.

Brennemann, F. C.: Special Therapeutic Measures. In: *Practice of Paediatrics*. Vol. I. New York, Harper & Row, 1973, pp. 24–26.

Brennemann, F. C.: Oxygen. In: *Practice of Paediatrics*, Vol. III. New York, Harper & Row, 1973, p. 23.

Bushnell, S., et al.: *Respiratory Intensive Care Nursing*. Boston, Little, Brown & Company, 1973.

Chrisman, M.: Dyspnea. *American Journal of Nursing*, 74:643–646, April 1974.

Codd, J., et al.: Postoperative Pulmonary Complications. *Nursing Clinics of North America, 10*:5–15, March 1975.

Drain, C. B.: A Vigilant You Can Reverse Respiratory Distress. RN, 39:1–2, December 1975.

Foss, G.: Postural Drainage. *American Journal of Nursing*, 73:666–669, April 1973.

Fuhs, M. F., et al.: Better Ways to Cope With C.O.P.D. *Nursing '76*, 6:28–38, February 1976.

Garvey, J.: Infant Respiratory Distress Syndrome. *American Journal of Nursing*, 75:614–617, April 1975.

Kudla, M. S.: The Care of the Patient With Respiratory Insufficiency. *Nursing Clinics of North America*, 8:183–190, March 1973.

Libman, R. H., and J. Keithley: Relieving Airway Obstruction in the Recovery Room. *American Journal of Nursing*, 75:603, April 1975.

Nett, L., et al.: Oxygen Toxicity. *American Journal of Nursing*, 73:1556–1558, September 1973.

Patterson, A.: Keeping in Trim for "Code Blue." *Supervisor Nurse*, 7:12, May 1976.

Tinker, J. H., and R. Wehner: The Nurse and the Ventilator. *American Journal of Nursing*, 74:1276, July 1974.

Traver, G. A. (Guest Editor): Symposium on Care in Respiratory Disease. *Nursing Clinics of North America*, 8:97–110, March 1974.

Ungvarski, P. J., et al.: CPR: Current Practice Revised. *American Journal of Nursing*, 75:236, February 1975.

31 PAIN

The nurse should be able to:

Describe the physiological mechanisms for receiving, transmitting,
    and interpreting pain sensations
Explain present thinking regarding the cause of pain by various
    types of stimuli
List major types of pain
Differentiate between pain perception and pain reaction
List factors which affect pain perception
Describe physiological manifestations of the pain reaction
List factors influencing an individual's behavioral response to pain
Assess the nursing needs of patients who have pain
List principles relevant to the care of patients in pain
Establish goals for nursing action
Determine priorities for care
Describe appropriate nursing intervention including measures to
    eliminate or minimize painful stimuli, measures to alleviate
    pain, and measures to assist patients to handle pain
Evaluate the effectiveness of nursing intervention

INTRODUCTION

Of all of the signs and symptoms of illness, pain is perhaps the most common and the most important. Pain is a sensation that is caused by the action of stimuli of a harmful nature. People who have pain experience varying degrees of distress, from a mild feeling of discomfort to an acute feeling of agony that obliterates all other sensations.

Although distressing, pain is in most instances a protective mechanism that warns the individual that body tissues are being damaged or are about to be damaged. The point at which pain is first felt is called the *pain perception threshold.* In controlled laboratory experiments, it has been found that this threshold is remarkably similar in most individuals under normal circumstances; that is, people subjected to an increasing amount of a painful stimulus, such as an increasing degree of heat applied to an area of the body, report feeling pain at almost exactly the same point of intensity of the stimulus. However, this threshold may be altered by a person's physical condition or by his emotional state at the time the pain is experienced.

Then, too, each person's reaction to pain is highly individualistic. Some people accept pain with stoical indifference; others react to similar pain with weeping or other outward displays of suffering. Also, the same individual may react to pain differently under different circumstances. The way in which an individual reacts to pain at any given time appears to be influenced by a number of factors: physical, emotional, and cultural.

The reasons for the anomalies in both the perception of pain and the reaction of people to it has intrigued physiologists, psychologists, and sociologists for many years. Although pain is such a common symptom of illness, there are still large gaps in our knowledge concerning the mechanisms for receiving, transmitting, interpreting, and reacting to pain sensations. Recent research in the fields of neurophysiology, experimental psychology, sociology, and nursing has increased our understanding of the phenomenon of pain and contributed to our ability to help people in pain. However, there are still many unanswered questions for which different theories have been proposed.

THE PHYSIOLOGY OF PAIN

It is generally agreed that pain begins with the stimulation of sensory nerve endings located on the body's surface or in the deeper structures. Although it has been traditionally assumed that there were specific receptors for pain, as for touch and temperature, there seems to be evidence that pain is not a pure sensation. Rather, it may be caused by intense stimulation of all types of sensory receptors. Thus, a hot water bottle may feel comfortably warm in one instance but in another—if the temperature of the water it contains is too high—the heat may be painful. Similarly, stroking or patting of the skin with a light pressure may be soothing, whereas rough massage can hurt.

The sensory nerve endings appear to be differentially sensitive to painful stimuli; that is, some are more sensitive to pain than others. Also, some areas of the body are richly supplied with free sensory nerve endings which are sensitive to painful stimuli, while other areas are not. The skin has an abundant supply, as have 609 some of the internal organs, such as the arterial walls, the joints, and the periosteum. Other organs have fewer receptors that are sensitive to pain; the brain and the alveoli of the lungs have none.

Once a pain impulse is initiated by the stimulation of a sensory receptor, the impulse is transmitted rapidly via first-level neurons to the lateral portion of filaments in the spinothalamic tracts of the spinal cord and thence to the thalamus. In the thalamus, there is a crude sorting-out and evaluation of the pain impulses, which are then transmitted via third-level neurons to higher centers in the brain. Between the thalamus and the sensory areas of the cerebral cortex where pain is perceived, it is believed that there is a further sorting-out and evaluation of the sensory impressions. Not all impressions reach the cortex; a person can only focus his attention on a limited number of stimuli at any one time. It is believed that the reticular system of the brain performs the function of evaluating the sensory impressions received in the thalamus and forwarding on to the cortex those of sufficient importance to merit attention.[1] Once the impression reaches the cortex, the person becomes aware of the pain. Action is then set in motion to counteract the noxious stimulus which has caused the pain.

In some instances, the stimulus is of sufficient intensity for a response to be initiated at the cord level. For example, the slightest touch of a hot stove causes a reflex reaction, and the individual withdraws his hand immediately.

Sometimes pain is perceived in one area of the body although the stimulus for its origin was in another area. Pain that is initiated in a deep visceral organ, for example, may be perceived by the individual on a surface area, or sometimes pain appears to be transferred from one surface area to another. This is called *referred pain*. The pain of myocardial infarction (a blockage in one of the blood vessels supplying the heart muscle) typically gives rise to feelings of pain in the left shoulder and down the left arm of the afflicted individual, in addition to the pain felt in the region of the heart.

The physiological mechanism of referred pain is more complicated than the mechanism just described for the perception of pain. In referred pain, the fibers carrying pain impulses from the viscera are believed to synapse (join together) with other neurons in the spinal cord. If the pain stimulus from the visceral organs is sufficiently intense, the sensation tends to spread over into some areas that normally receive stimuli only from the skin. Thus the individual has the sensation of pain coming from the skin rather than, or as well as, from the viscera.

THE SPINAL-GATING HYPOTHESIS

An interesting theory about pain which has received a considerable amount of attention in recent years is the spinal-gating hypothesis. The proponents of this theory, Ronald Melzack and Patrick Wall, contend that the mechanism of pain is not so simple as the explanation given above would indicate. In Melzack and Wall's "gate control theory,"[2] they propose that a neural mechanism, located in the "substantia gelatinosa" of the dorsal horns of the spinal cord, acts like a gate which can increase or decrease the flow of nerve impulses from peripheral fibers to higher centers in the brain.

Pain impulses are carried by two types of fibers in the spinal cord—one large in diameter, the other small. The large fibers conduct rapidly and adapt quickly; they become inactive in the absence of stimulus change. Input from these fibers has an excitatory effect on the spinal gating mechanism, causing it to close. Sharp, immediate pain is thought to travel via the large fibers and, since it travels quickly, some input will pass through the gate before the mechanism is activated to close. The small fibers conduct more slowly than the large fibers, and are slower to adapt; they are tonically active.

[1]Ronald Melzack: *The Puzzle of Pain.* New York, Basic Books, Inc., 1973, pp. 153–190.

[2]Ibid.

Prolonged pain, it is thought, travels through the smaller fibers (because the larger ones adapt quickly when there is no change in stimulus); input from these fibers has an inhibiting effect on the gating mechanism, causing the gate to open (or remain open).

Additional factors in the operation of the gate controlling mechanism are the motivational and cognitive influences from the higher centers of the brain. These influences, which include such factors as attention, anxiety, expectations, suggestion, and memory of previous experiences (including cultural and social background), descend from the brain and modulate the pain impulses traveling upward from peripheral sites. Through a process of comparison of the input from the sensory systems and from the central control (the brain), the spinal-gating mechanism will be excited and close, or be inhibited and open.

Beyond the gating mechanism are transmission cells. When the amount of information passing through the gate to the transmission cells reaches a critical level, these cells fire, thus activating the neural areas responsible for pain perception and response.

The gate-control theory helps to explain some of the puzzling features of pain. For example, rubbing or otherwise stimulating a painful area, according to this theory, reduces the perception of pain because the change in stimulus activates the large fibers (which had adapted), causing the gate to close. In pathological pain syndromes, where, in some cases, the larger fibers have been destroyed, more input is carried through the smaller fibers, which have an inhibitory effect on the spinal-gating mechanism. With regard to spontaneous pain or delayed pain, this theory indicates that a summation of input from the smaller fibers (which conduct more slowly) occurs in the transmission cells, causing a latent response.

Although the gate-control theory is considered by many to be the most advanced and complete explanation of pain thus far proposed, there still remain many unresolved mysteries concerning the process of pain perception and response.

COMMON CAUSES OF PAIN

Generally speaking, any stimulus that causes tissue damage, or is perceived by the individual as potentially causing injury to body tissues, causes pain. Thus, pain may result from a number of different kinds of damaging stimuli, including irritating chemical substances, mechanical trauma, thermal extremes, or ischemia (lack of blood flow to a part), as well as from psychogenic factors.

Chemical Irritants

Direct stimulation of free sensory nerve endings by irritating chemical substances will cause pain. A common example of this is the pain that occurs when one spills a drop of acid on the skin. Also, it is now believed that whenever tissues are damaged, certain chemical substances are liberated by the injured cells. Some of these substances trigger the inflammatory response (see Chapter 21). Others, it is thought, excite pain receptors in the damaged area. These substances are believed to include *histamine* and peptides of the *bradykinin* group. They are sometimes referred to simply as *kinins*.[3] Thus, in the case of the acid burn, there is usually an initial sharp, stinging pain, caused by the chemical irritation of the nerve endings by the acid, followed by a longer-lasting pain that is due to the action of substances released by cells that have been damaged by the acid.

Ischemia

Other chemical irritants that are believed to cause pain are the acidic waste products of cellular metabolism. When these substances accumulate, as, for example, in areas of the body where blood supply to a part is not sufficient to carry them away, pain is believed to result from

---

[3]Cyril M. MacBryde and Robert S. Blacklow (eds.): *Signs and Symptoms: Applied Pathologic Physiology and Clinical Interpretation.* 5th edition. Philadelphia, J. B. Lippincott Company, 1970, p. 47.

the irritating effect of these substances on free nerve endings. This helps to explain the pain in ischemic areas where blood supply has been cut off or impaired and metabolic waste products accumulate. Another factor in the pain of ischemia is the death of tissue cells in the area, resulting from the loss of blood supply. The decaying cells also liberate irritating chemical substances, as already discussed, and this would contribute to the pain.

Mechanical Trauma

Pain may be incurred by physical force or other mechanical means. When an individual is driving a nail into the wall, for example, the hammer may accidentally hit the thumb instead of the nailhead. The resulting bruise and painful thumb are familiar to most of us. The pain is felt to be caused in this instance by pressure on the nerve endings initially, with chemical irritation from the kinins released by damaged cells as a factor in the continued pain of the bruised tissues.

Pain may also result from *stretching or contraction* of body tissues, or from prolonged pressure on the tissues. Distention of a hollow organ such as the stomach is a common example of stretching of the tissues. If a person eats a very big meal (as at Thanksgiving or Christmas), he may develop considerable discomfort in the region of his stomach. It is believed that stretching of the tissues causes pain because of two possible factors: stretching of the nerve endings in the sensory receptors and the occlusion of small blood vessels in the stretched tissue, which results in localized ischemia.

When *tissues are contracted* (as, for example, in a muscle spasm), there is constriction of small blood vessels in the area with, again, localized ischemia resulting. There may also be stretching of the nerve endings. In addition, in prolonged muscular contraction, cellular metabolism is greatly increased, with a resultant buildup in metabolic waste products, which the constricted blood vessels cannot carry away. As already stated, these metabolic waste products are believed to be chemi-

cally irritating to sensory nerve endings and therefore to cause pain.

Continued pressure on any body structure causes tissue damage and concomitant pain. The pain is thought to be due to pressure on the nerve endings and also to localized ischemia resulting from the occlusion of small blood vessels in the tissues being pressed. Even the prolonged pressure of sitting too long in the classroom may cause pain unless one changes position or stretches occasionally. Normally a person alters his position every few minutes. This is a conditioned response to the perception of pain sensations, which are felt whenever pressure is exerted on any one area for too long. People who have impaired pain perception — for example, unconscious or paralyzed patients — may not feel these pain sensations. The individual does not therefore of his own accord alter his position, and pressure areas can easily develop. For this reason, it is particularly important that the patient be turned frequently and that other measures be taken to prevent prolonged pressure on any part of the body (see Chapter 20).

Heat and Cold

Extremes of heat and cold cause pain. These also damage body tissues. Everyone is familiar with the burn which is caused by excessive heat, and with the pain that results from even a small burn on the tip of the finger. Here, the initial burning pain probably results from the intensity of the thermal stimulus. The lingering after-pain is believed to be due to the destruction of tissue and the release of irritating chemical substances from the injured cells. Because burns are one of the most frequent causes of accidental injury to patients, the nurse must be ever alert to protect patients from the danger of solutions that are too hot, heating pads that are set at too high a temperature, and the like (see Chapter 25). Again, these precautions are especially important when the patient's pain perception is impaired.

Extreme cold, particularly if there is freezing of body tissues, as in frostbite, also causes tissue damage and accompanying pain. Cold constricts the blood vessels in the affected tissue and may completely cut off the blood supply. The pain in a frostbitten nose or fingers is most severe when the blood flow is returning and the constricted vessels are being dilated.

Psychogenic Pain

Pain may be experienced by an individual in the absence of any physiological basis for it. This occurs in a *conversion reaction,* for example, in which emotional disorders are experienced by the patient as bodily symptoms rather than as mental ones. Pain may also arise from the physiological accompaniments of psychogenic disorders, as in the tension headache caused by contraction of the muscles in the back of the neck and vasodilatation of blood vessels in the head.

TYPES OF PAIN

Pain can be classified as superficial, deep, or visceral. *Superficial pain* is usually described as having either a burning or a pricking quality. It arises from stimulation of receptors in the skin or the mucous membranes of the body. As a rule, an individual is able to localize surface pain fairly accurately because of the large number of free sensory nerve endings on the surface of the body.

Deep pain arises from the deeper structures of the body, such as the muscles, tendons, joints, and fasciae. It is usually described as dull, aching, cramping, gnawing, or boring. Muscles and tendons are particularly sensitive to pain and may give rise to pain of considerable intensity.

Visceral pain may be perceived as originating in the organ itself, or pain may be felt at a site far removed from the affected viscera through the mechanism of referred pain. It is usually more difficult to localize visceral pain because there are fewer sensory nerve endings in the viscera than on the skin or mucous membranes. The nature of the pain experienced is sometimes highly specific to the particular organ involved and the patho-

logical process that is taking place. In myocardial infarction, for example, the pain is often described as constricting, viselike, or compressing. Pain in hollow muscular organs frequently gives rise to sensations of gripping, cramping, or twisting. In the case of a peptic ulcer, the patient often describes pain as having a gnawing, burning, or sometimes knifelike quality. An accurate description of the nature of the pain as reported by the patient often helps the physician to diagnose the cause of the patient's condition. The nurse should be careful, however, not to put her own interpretation on the patient's description nor to suggest words for the patient to use. It is far better to record and report the patient's pain as he describes it in his own words.

The nurse may also hear the term *"central pain"* used. This type of pain arises from injury to sensory nerves, the neural pathways, or the areas in the brain which are concerned with pain perception. It is often very difficult for the patient to describe this type of pain since it is usually unlike anything he has experienced before. Some people have, however, described it as gnawing, burning, or crushing.[4]

There are also cases of *phantom pain* such as the pain that a patient feels in his toes after the limb has been amputated. This is thought to be due to the persistence of the pain sensation or a "pain memory" after the cause for it is removed.

PAIN PERCEPTION AND PAIN REACTION

There are always two aspects to pain: pain perception and pain reaction. The pain perception threshold, although remarkably the same in most individuals under normal circumstances, may be altered by certain physical and emotional factors. Pain reaction, or the way in which a person reacts to pain, varies considerably from one individual to another and within the same individual under different circumstances. The two aspects of

---

[4]Ibid., p. 57.

pain can be dissociated. For example, in certain conditions a physician may not be able to do anything about a person's perception of pain, but he may be able to treat the reaction to pain.

Pain Perception

The ability to perceive pain is dependent upon the integrity of the nerve fibers which receive, transmit, and interpret pain impulses. Thus, injury to sensory nerves, the sensory tracts in the spinal cord, the thalamus, or sensory areas in the cerebral cortex will interfere with pain perception. A patient who has had a spinal cord injury, for example, and is paralyzed from the waist down does not feel pain in the lower half of his body. This patient must then be protected from harmful stimuli to which a person with normal pain perception would respond by taking suitable action to prevent injury to body tissues. For example, paraplegic patients must be taught to alter their position frequently when they are sitting in a wheelchair, or they soon develop decubitus ulcers. The nurse must also take special precautions to protect paralyzed or unconscious patients from the pressure of tight bed coverings, which may cause foot drop, among other distressing effects.

Sometimes pain perception seems to be facilitated. In some disease conditions affecting the central nervous system (for example, in a neuritis in which the nervous tissue is inflamed), the individual often becomes hypersensitive to painful stimuli. Also, with the prolonged application of painful stimuli, the neural pathways appear to become worn and the pain perception centers hypersensitive. Thus, a person who suffers from continuous pain becomes more, rather than less, sensitive to it.

Areas of the body adjacent to injured areas are usually more sensitive to pain than normal tissue is. The skin adjacent to a wound area, for example, is usually very tender. It is thought that in these cases there is a spillover of pain impulses into neighboring pathways, much the same as in the case of referred pain. There is also the factor of engorgement of the tissues in the wounded area owing to the inflammatory process, and this may cause pressure on sensory nerve endings in the surrounding tissue.

Tissues that are already damaged react to additional painful stimuli, even of minimal intensity, much more readily than does normal intact tissue. The sensitivity of the sunburned skin is usually cited as an example of this phenomenon, which might be considered as a case of stimulus overload.

On the other hand, intense pain in one part of the body may raise the pain threshold in other areas. A person who is suffering considerable pain from a broken leg, for example, may not be aware of pain from an abrasion on his elbow. This is probably due to selective perception, the stimulus of greater priority (or intensity) taking precedence in attention over the less intense, or less significant, stimulus.

The pain perception threshold is also altered by an individual's level of consciousness. The unconscious person—for example, the patient under a general anesthetic—does not feel pain. The ability to perceive pain, as tested by a person's reaction to a pinprick or to supraorbital pressure, is frequently used to determine a patient's level of consciousness. Both pain perception and pain reaction may be altered by the emotional state of the individual and by the amount of attention that is focused on the pain. These points are discussed later.

Pain Reaction

There are both physiological and behavioral manifestations in the reaction to pain. The *physiological manifestations* are those of the "alarm reaction" of the body to the threat of danger from any harmful stimulus (see Chapter 2). Among the signs and symptoms that the nurse can observe are pallor, elevated blood pressure, and increased tension of the skeletal muscles. Gastrointestinal functioning may also be impaired. The person in pain usually does not want to eat, and nausea and vomiting are not uncommon accompaniments of pain. Restlessness and irritability are frequently seen. The patient who is in pain cannot rest and he cannot sleep.

With severe pain of any sort, the body's defenses may collapse. In such an event, the nurse may observe signs of weakness and prostration in the patient. His blood pressure may drop and his pulse become weak and slow. There may be increased pallor, and the patient is often described as being "white as a ghost." Collapse and loss of consciousness may ensue.

The *behavioral responses to pain* differ much more widely from one individual to another than do the physiological manifestations. Everyone has observed the individual who "never flinches" even though the pain he experiences is intense. Such behavior is usually much admired in our Western society. On the other hand, some people react to pain with loud groans, weeping, screaming, thrashing about, or violent attempts to remove themselves from the source of pain.

A person's reaction to pain is influenced by a number of factors. The individual's physical condition, his emotional state, and the way in which he has been conditioned to respond to pain will all affect his reaction to pain in a particular situation.

If a person is tired, or weakened physically, his resistance and control over his reactions are lessened. He may then react to a minimal stimulus with an exaggerated response that is all out of proportion to the intensity of the stimulus. When one is tired, even a small cut on the finger may seem too much to endure, and tears or profanity may be evoked. Thus, the harassed mother who is attempting to cook dinner and, at the same time, look after small children may suffer a slight burn at the stove and promptly burst into tears.

Conversely, in extreme exhaustion, the individual's attention span is markedly reduced and he may not be able to concentrate his attention on any one stimulus for a sufficient length of time to react to it. Thus, the severely sunburned sailor who has been adrift in an open boat may not complain of pain at all, or, if he does, his mind soon wanders from it to other things.

The emotional state of the individual also modifies his reaction to pain. Anxiety and fear aggravate it. This is understanda-ble, since anxiety, fear, and pain all provoke the same physiological "alarm reaction" in the body in response to stimuli that threaten the individual's safety. Certainly, if anxiety is relieved, the patient's reaction to pain is considerably lessened. If there is a strong emotional response to stimuli other than the pain-producing one, however, this emotional state may block out the awareness of pain. A football player injured during a game may not notice that he has been hurt until the game is over. In this case, excitement and the desire to win may be so intense as to demand the individual's full attention so that the sensory impressions of pain from the injury become of lesser priority and he does not perceive them. A similar explanation could account for the numerous reports of soldiers wounded in battle who state that they did not feel pain even though they had injuries of considerable extent. The overriding fear during the battle and the necessity for self-preservation at all costs may take precedence over impressions from any other sensory stimulation so that pain is not perceived. Pleasurable emotions tend to nullify pain perception so that the person who is in a happy or contented mood does not usually seem to feel pain to the same extent as the worried patient.

Then, too, an individual's emotional makeup, his cultural and social background, and his early home and school training have a great deal to do with his behavior in response to painful stimuli. There has been much study by sociologists, for example, of the differing reactions of various cultural groups to pain.[5] The North American Indian is often cited as an example of a member of a cultural group in which stoical indifference to pain is a highly valued characteristic. Among people of Latin origin, on the other hand, an open display of suffering is usually permitted as the socially approved response to pain.

In our Western society, very strong values are placed on bravery, endurance, and the ability to bear pain with silent fortitude. Children in our culture are taught

---

[5]Mark Zborowski: *People in Pain*. San Francisco, Jossey-Bass Inc., 1969.

very early that they are expected not to cry when they are hurt. "Be brave," "Don't be a sissy," and "Only babies cry," are the frequent admonishments of mothers to young children. Even children from differing ethnic groups, in which the open display of suffering is permitted, soon learn from their teachers and from their peer groups in school and on the playground that they must react to pain in the accepted North American manner or be scorned by their fellows.

The nurse who has been raised in this framework of "only babies cry" may find herself reacting negatively to the patient who does not handle his pain in the "approved" manner. If she realizes that her reaction is normal and a reflection of her social values, which are different from those of the patient, she is in a better position to analyze and accept her own feelings. These feelings then need not interfere with her acceptance and support of the patient.

ASSESSING PAIN

Pain is probably the most personal and the most distressing of all the symptoms of disease. Only the individual who is experiencing the pain really knows what it is like. The primary source of information about the pain he is having, then, is always the patient. Other sources the nurse can use include her own observations of the patient and those of other members of the health team.

Subjective Data

In gathering information about the patient's pain, the nurse should ascertain, whenever possible, the following aspects of the pain experience:

1. The quality of the pain
2. The location of the pain
3. The intensity of the pain
4. The time the pain occurs and its duration
5. Any factors which appear to precipitate the pain
6. Any measures which relieve it or measures with which the patient has tried to relieve it

Quality. Patients use many descriptive terms when talking about pain. A number of the terms commonly used have been mentioned earlier in the chapter in the section on classification of pain. Frequently patients describe pain in terms of something that is familiar to them. Thus, pain may be likened to the cutting action of a knife, if it is a sharp, piercing pain; or to "hammers pounding inside the head" in certain types of headache. In recording and reporting pain, the nurse should use the exact words the patient has used in order to convey an accurate description of the pain as the patient perceives it.

Location. The patient is usually able to localize superficial pain fairly accurately and also pain arising from bones, muscles, joints, and blood vessels. Visceral pain is more difficult to localize. Often, the patient complains of pain generally in the epigastric region, or in the lower part of the abdomen, in the chest, or the lower back when a visceral organ is affected. Often, too, the pain from viscera is referred to a surface area. An exact description of the location of the pain is of considerable assistance to the physician in diagnosing the patient's condition, and to the nurse in planning her care.

Intensity. The degree of pain felt by the patient is also important in assessing his nursing needs and the need for medical or nursing intervention. Certain tissues are more sensitive to pain than others; for example, muscle tissue appears to be highly responsive to painful stimuli, and the pain from bruised or ischemic muscles may be excruciating. Hence, it is necessary to use great care in moving patients who have disorders involving the musculoskeletal system.

When the intensity of the patient's pain changes abruptly, it is usually an indication that the nature of his condition has altered. For example, when an inflamed appendix ruptures, or a peptic ulcer perforates, the patient usually experiences very sharp and severe pain, which persists and is quite different both in quality and intensity from the pain felt previously.

Time and Duration. An accurate description of the patient's pain should include when it occurs, how long it lasts, and whether it is an intermittent pain that recurs or a steady pain that continues. Pain is often most severe at night, when a person is alone. A possible explanation for this is that, in the absence of other people or activities to distract him, the individual's full attention is then focused on his discomfort. The duration of the pain is very important. An example of this may be found in obstetrics, in which the length of the interval between pains and the time each pain lasts are significant in assessing the patient's progress in labor, the muscular contractions of the uterus becoming stronger and closer together as delivery becomes imminent.

Precipitating Factors. Pain is often related to the patient's activities. In some cardiac conditions, pain may be brought on by exertion, and in planning the patient's care, it is important to know how much activity the patient can tolerate. Sometimes it is necessary to space nursing measures to allow the patient to rest between activities. For example, it may be wise in some cases to leave the patient's bath until an hour or so after breakfast in order to give him time to rest after the exertion of eating a meal. With patients who have musculoskeletal problems, pain is frequently associated with movement of the affected structure. Again, it is important to know exactly what movement precipitates pain, both for medical assessment of the patient's condition and for planning care to minimize the patient's discomfort. Pain in the gastrointestinal tract may be precipitated by eating certain foods. Again, pain may be related to an intolerance of factors in the environment. Noise may bring on a headache, for example. Very often the patient is able to identify the specific factor or factors which cause pain, and these should be recorded and reported, again using the patient's own words in preference to an interpretation of what he says.

Measures Which Relieve Pain. Frequently, the patient has tried a number of measures to relieve his pain before he seeks medical help. The nurse should ascertain the measures he has tried and the effectiveness of these in relieving his pain. For example, does rest relieve the pain that is brought on by exertion? Does holding the limb in a certain

way prevent pain on movement? This type of information is of value both to the physician in assessing the patient's condition and developing a plan of therapy, and to the nurse in her determination of nursing measures which will help to alleviate pain.

Objective Data

The nurse can supplement the information she obtains from the patient with her observations of his reaction to the pain. She should be alert to the physiological manifestations of pain as these have just been described. Very often the patient's facial expression and posture will indicate that he is having pain. The patient in pain often has a typical facial grimace: his brows are knotted, his facial muscles are tense and drawn, and his mouth is often drawn downward. In addition, he may assume a characteristic position to minimize the pain. With abdominal pain, the patient may draw up his knees and curl into a ball; for a sore arm he may hold the affected part. In severe pain patients sometimes lie rigidly because any movement intensifies the discomfort. Some patients, because of their training to bear pain in stoical silence, do not like to complain of pain. As a result, the nurse may find it difficult to identify even the existence of pain. Pallor, muscular tension (as in the drawn facial muscles or a clenching of the fists), posture, inactivity, and profuse perspiration may be the only outward evidences of pain in these people.

The nurse may, however, often note other behavior in patients who are having pain. Restlessness and increased sensitivity to stimuli in the environment, such as noise and bright lights, are frequently indicative of pain. The patient in pain often shows evidence of increased emotional tension as well; he may react with irritability and bad humor to people or things that disturb him. Pain usually prevents people from sleeping or resting comfortably, and, because pain is usually worse at night, insomnia may be a problem. Nursing measures to ensure that the patient is relieved of pain are important in order to enable him to rest.

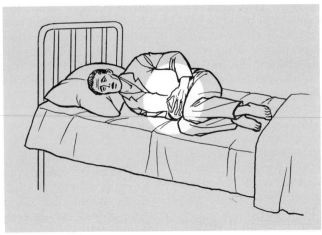

A person who is experiencing pain may assume a position indicative of the site of the pain.

Information from Other Sources

Frequently pain is the principal symptom which prompts people to seek medical help. The physician then has usually investigated the nature of the patient's pain, and the nurse can often obtain much information from the patient's physician or from the notes made on the patient's record. Of particular importance are notations made regarding factors which precipitate pain, since the nurse may be able to institute measures to eliminate or minimize these factors.

The observations made by all members of the nursing team who are caring for the patient contribute to the total picture of the patient's pain. These observations should be accurately reported and recorded so that all staff members are aware of measures that prevent, minimize, or alleviate the patient's pain, as well as factors that aggravate it.

In addition, other members of the health team, such as the physical therapist, can often contribute information about the patient's pain. The physical therapist usually assists in assessing the patient's mobility and functional ability and can provide guidance to nursing personnel on activities which the patient can tolerate without pain. The patient's family too can be helpful in regard to the nature of the patient's pain, factors that precipitate it, and measures which help to alleviate it. Some people are reluctant to admit that they have pain, or may try to minimize its severity when talking to medical personnel, usually again because of their cultural background; yet they have often confided the extent of their suffering to their wife or husband. Or, the wife may be aware of such evidences of her husband's discomfort as his inability to sleep or his restlessness and increased irritability.

PRIORITIES FOR NURSING ACTION

The relief of pain is always a matter of priority for nursing action. However, there are some circumstances in which it is more urgent than in others, when the prompt treatment of pain is essential to save a person's life or to prevent damage to body structures. Severe pain can cause a collapse of the body's adaptive mechanisms. Hence, the presence of severe pain in a patient requires immediate intervention. The nurse's judgment of the patient's condition is extremely important. If she observes signs of weakness and prostration, such as markedly increased pallor, a lowered blood pressure, and weakened pulse in a patient who is having pain, the physician should be notified immediately so that his (or her) guidance can be obtained on the measures to be taken. He may wish the administration of analgesics discontinued and other measures such as intravenous infusion with suppor-

PRINCIPLES RELEVANT TO PAIN

1. Pain has a protective function in warning a person of present or potential damage to body tissues.
2. Pain may be caused by a number of different kinds of stimuli.
3. Tissues of the body differ in their sensitivity to painful stimuli.
4. Severe pain can cause collapse of the body's adaptive mechanisms.
5. The ability to perceive pain is dependent upon the integrity of the neural structures which receive, transmit, and interpret pain impulses.
6. Pain perception may be altered by certain physical and emotional factors. A person's reaction to pain is highly individualized and depends on a number of factors — physical, emotional, and cultural.

tive drug therapy instituted. Or he may feel that the patient's condition warrants immediate surgical intervention.

The action of pain-relieving drugs is more effective if these are administered before the pain reaches a peak. Early intervention at the beginning of pain, then, can often prevent a serious attack. This is important in such conditions as myocardial infarction, or biliary or renal colic (stones in the bile duct or the ureter of the kidney), in which the pain can mount to agonizing proportions. The patient's request for pain relief should be answered without delay.

Another situation in which the prompt relief of pain is imperative is in the care of the surgical patient. The restlessness that accompanies increasing pain can sometimes cause damage to newly sutured tissues. The patient should therefore be kept comfortable at all times during the immediate postoperative period. Analgesics for the relief of pain are usually prescribed every three to four hours as needed (p.r.n.) for the first 48 hours following surgery. The nurse's judicious administration of these medications can make the patient's recovery from surgery much easier.

The relief of pain is not always, of course, a matter of administering a medication. Many times nursing measures such as changing the patient's position, straightening his bed, or helping him to overcome his anxiety are equally effective in alleviating pain. In exercising judgment as to the appropriate measures to be taken, the nurse utilizes her knowledge about the patient's medical condition and also her knowledge of each individual patient and his reaction to pain.

GOALS FOR NURSING ACTION

Nursing action for the patient who is having pain is directed primarily toward three goals:
1. Eliminating or minimizing the stimuli that are causing pain
2. Alleviating pain
3. Assisting the patient to handle pain

SPECIFIC NURSING INTERVENTIONS

Measures to Eliminate or Minimize Painful Stimuli

Whenever possible, it is always better to prevent pain than to treat it. One cannot always do this, of course. Many times pain is the chief reason a person has sought medical help. Investigation of the cause of pain and elimination of its source frequently constitute a major part of the patient's total care. The nurse can often help to control the extent of suffering, however, through eliminating or minimizing known causes of pain and discomfort.

Pain is usually a warning signal that body tissues are being damaged or are about to be damaged. When exertion brings on pain, the patient's activities may need to be curtailed to prevent further injury to body cells. The patient with a heart condition, for example, must learn to moderate his activities to prevent further damage to the heart and concomitant pain. The activities of the surgical patient, to use another example, are usually restricted until the wounded tissues have healed sufficiently that normal movement will not disturb the healing process.

It is not possible to curtail all movement that is painful, though, nor is it always wise. The dangers of immobility in people who are sick have been well documented and referred to many times throughout this text. The postoperative patient, for example, must move about and must breathe deeply and cough to prevent respiratory complications, even though these activities cause him some pain. The nurse's actions are then directed toward minimizing the patient's discomfort. Supporting the patient's incision can lessen pain when he coughs or breathes deeply. The nurse may use her hands to support the incision, or sometimes a pillow held firmly against the operative area will accomplish the same purpose. A binder may be needed to provide support to the operative area when the patient is up and walking around.

Whenever it is necessary to lift or turn a patient for whom movement is painful, the utmost gentleness should be used. The nurse should always make certain that she has sufficient help in moving the patient so that he is not subjected to unnecessary pain or discomfort. Supporting a painful limb while turning the patient can help to minimize his discomfort. In addition, devices such as a "turning sheet," which is placed under the patient, can sometimes be used to advantage to prevent excessive handling of painful limbs.

All the comfort measures which have been discussed in earlier chapters are important in eliminating sources of pain for the patient. For example, helping a patient to change his position relieves muscle strain and also prevents pressure on any particular part of the body for too long a period of time. Positioning to maintain good body alignment aids in preventing painful muscular contractures. A soothing back rub will often help to relax a patient and ease muscular tension. Also, helping the patient to stay dry and comfortable and relieving any sources of irritation can aid in eliminating stimuli that can cause pain.

The nurse should remember too that helping the patient to meet his basic

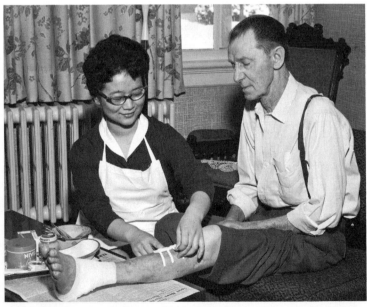

Changing a patient's dressing helps to eliminate irritating stimuli that can cause pain.

physiological needs can eliminate many existing or potential sources of pain. For example, food can prevent or relieve the uncomfortable muscular contractions of an empty stomach. Seeing that the patient is taking sufficient fluids helps to prevent the distressing effects of dehydration (see Chapter 29). The pain caused by a distended bladder and the discomfort of constipation are both preventable by nursing action and may be relieved by specific nursing techniques (see Chapters 27 and 28). Ensuring that the patient gets sufficient rest and sleep is an important consideration also, since fatigue lowers a person's resistance and control, thereby increasing his reaction to painful stimuli.

Measures to Alleviate Pain

In determining the most appropriate action to alleviate pain, the nurse must take into consideration both the physical pain the patient is experiencing and the emotional distress that accompanies it. It is often difficult to assess how much of the pain is caused by psychological factors and how much is due to physical factors. Measures that focus on relieving the emotional component can often dispel pain in themselves, or can enhance the effectiveness of physical measures.

Psychological Measures. In some instances, dramatic results have been obtained in pain relief with the use of purely psychological measures. Hypnosis, for example, has been a successful form of treatment for some patients, and sometimes "placebos" (which contain no drugs) are as effective as the administration of analgesics. In both hypnosis and placebo administration, *suggestion* is the key factor in relieving the patient's pain.

Distraction is helpful sometimes in lessening an individual's awareness of painful stimuli. Pain is accentuated when attention is focused on it. The individual who is engaged in activities such as reading, watching an interesting television program, or talking with other people has a number of sensory impressions competing for his attention, and his awareness of pain sensations may thus be lessened. It should be remembered that, if a patient does not have diversional activities, he becomes much preoccupied with his own self. Mild discomforts which might otherwise not be noted assume major importance. In planning situations or activities that are diversional, though, the nurse must assess them carefully to ensure that they are neither irritating to the patient nor fatiguing. Visitors are sometimes helpful in distracting patients from their discomfort. However, the nurse should be aware of the individual patient's preference in this regard; some prefer not to have visitors because they find them tiring or irritating.

Changing a person's attitude toward a potentially painful experience can alter his reaction to pain. The success of "natural childbirth" methods in obstetrics illustrates this point. These methods are based largely on the preparation of the expectant mother to anticipate childbirth as a joyful event rather than as a cause of pain and suffering. It should be noted that this approach does much to eliminate the fear of childbirth.

The extent to which anxiety and fear are contributing factors in pain is difficult to determine. Both anxiety and fear intensify the reaction to pain so that, if these can be successfully reduced, the individual is often relieved of much of his distress. Measures to assist in relieving anxiety were discussed in Chapter 12, and it is suggested that, at this point, the student may find it helpful to review that chapter.

A number of studies in recent years have demonstrated that the nurse's interaction with the patient is a significant factor in the relief of pain. Such actions as talking with the patient, using comfort measures, or positive suggestion coupled with a comfort measure, have all been used with success in various situations. To be effective, however, these actions must be based on a feeling of trust and confidence that has been established between the patient and the nurse. The student may find it helpful in this regard to read the reports of some of the studies which have been done on nursing approaches to the patient in pain. A number of these reports are listed in the bibliography at the end of this chapter.

Physical Measures. Psychological measures will not, of course, relieve all pain. In some cases, the physiological cause of pain can be ameliorated by using physical agents. The pain-relieving actions of *heat* and *cold*, for example, are well known (see Chapter 25). In general, heat tends to relieve pain through increasing circulation in the part of the body to which it is applied. Hence, heat is often effective in the relief of muscular aches and pains, since the increased circulation helps to carry away metabolic waste products, which are thought to be a factor in causing muscular pain. A warm bath, for example, often helps to relieve aching muscles after a person has engaged in strenuous exercise. Cold has the opposite effect of heat—that is, it decreases peripheral circulation. In doing so, it helps to reduce swelling and therefore pressure on sensory nerve endings. An ice collar is frequently used to relieve pain following operations on the throat when the tissues are swollen and painful. Cold is also used sometimes as a local anesthetic agent. The intense cold in this case serves to deaden sensory nerve endings, thus preventing the transmission of pain impulses.

Therapeutic baths are also used to relieve pain. Sometimes the bath is a means of applying heat or cold to the body. Sometimes it is a vehicle for other agents, as, for example, the colloid baths that are frequently used for people with irritating skin conditions (see Chapter 20).

Massage has had a long history of use in the treatment of pain of muscular origin. The effect of massage is similar to that of heat in that it increases circulation to a part, thereby accelerating removal of the waste products of cellular metabolism.

Medications. Then, too, there are the numerous *pharmacological agents* that are used for pain relief. These tend to fall into two groups: those that are "specifics" for certain conditions and those which have a general analgesic effect. Among the specifics are the muscle relaxants, such as meprobamate, which is used in conditions such as spastic paralysis, and phenylbutazone, which is a central nervous system depressant frequently prescribed for patients with arthritic conditions.

The principal drugs used as general analgesics include the narcotics, such as morphine, codeine, and their derivatives; synthetic compounds such as Demerol and Darvon; and the analgesic-antipyretic group of drugs, of which aspirin is by far the most widely used. Considerable con-

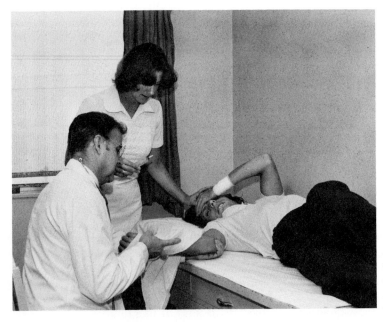

Despite the warm hand and comforting manner of the nurse, this young man's pain persists anyway. Perhaps the medication will help.

troversy still exists over the physiological reason for the effectiveness of these drugs in pain relief. The narcotics, we know, have a depressant action on the central nervous system. Some experts believe that these drugs act on the corticothalamic pathways and the perceptive areas of the brain to cause a reduction in pain sensations. Others feel that the action of morphine and the other narcotics is principally that of mood alteration, so that the person remains aware of the pain, but his reaction to it is diminished. Morphine, its derivatives, and some of the stronger synthetic compounds, such as Demerol, are used in cases of severe pain; codeine is used for pain of lesser intensity. Tranquilizing drugs, such as Phenergan and chlorpromazine, are sometimes given at the same time as a narcotic. Their action appears to enhance the pain-relieving properties of the narcotic so that a smaller dosage of the analgesic may be used.

With regard to the analgesic-antipyretic group of drugs, most experts seem to agree that these agents in some way block the transmission of pain impulses, probably in the thalamic pathways, thus decreasing the perception of pain. Aspirin and other drugs of this group are used extensively for the relief of minor aches and pains.[6]

The nurse's responsibility in the administration of analgesics is a crucial one. Sometimes prescriptions are written for analgesics to be given every four hours, or at other specified times (as, for example, is frequently the case with patients who have arthritic and rheumatoid disorders). In most instances, however, the orders are written as *p.r.n.*, and the nurse must use her judgment as to the time of administration and the interval between medications. Many times the nurse is faced too with the decision of which of two or three analgesic orders to use for a patient. He may, for example, have morphine sulphate, Darvon, and aspirin all prescribed for pain relief. If the patient is having

pain, the nurse must then decide on the medication to be used in this particular situation or whether, in fact, the patient may be made comfortable by measures other than drugs. In making this decision, the nurse is guided by her knowledge of the disease process the patient has, her understanding of the factors causing his pain, and her knowledge of the individual patient. A patient who is suffering from incurable cancer and is in the terminal stages of illness may require a strong narcotic to effectively relieve his pain. For the person who has a simple headache, aspirin may be sufficient to bring relief. Sometimes, changing the patient's position is all that is needed to make him more comfortable.

Acupuncture. Acupuncture has been used for centuries in China for the treatment of various disorders, for the relief of pain, and, more recently, for surgical analgesia. During the past few years it has attracted the attention of Western medicine, and is beginning to be utilized in some parts of North America as an alternative method of treating pain.

The technique of acupuncture consists of inserting long, fine needles into particular areas of the skin. Sometimes an electrical current is passed between two needles, but more commonly the needles are twirled continuously by hand. Traditional sites on the skin are used for the insertion of the needles; these sites are said to be associated with specific internal organs of the body, as indicated on the example of a typical acupuncture chart shown here.

The physiological mechanisms involved in the relief of pain by acupuncture are not fully understood. However, the gate-control theory (see page 610) offers a possible explanation. Melzack, in his book *The Puzzle of Pain*, suggests that acupuncture may be a special case of hyperstimulation analgesia.[7] In other words, the stimulation of particular nerves or tissues by the acupuncture needles results in increased input to the gate-control mechanism, causing the gate to close to pain impulses from selected areas of the body.

---

[6]For a more extensive coverage of analgesics, the nurse is referred to *The Drug, The Nurse, The Patient* by Mary W. Falconer, Annette Schram Ezell, H. Robert Patterson, and Edward A. Gustafson. 5th edition. Philadelphia, W. B. Saunders Company, 1974, pp. 118–128.

[7]Melzack, op. cit., pp. 185–190.

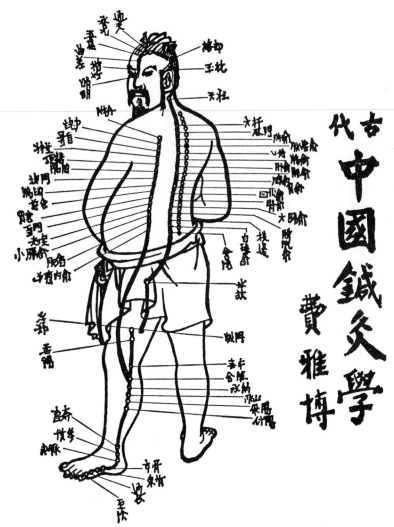

The acupuncture charts here and on the next page show the traditional sites for insertion of acupuncture needles.

Measures to Help the Patient to Handle Pain

One of the nurse's most important functions is the provision of psychological support for the patient in pain. Discussing the meaning pain holds for the patient is one way of doing this. Sometimes the nurse will find that it is not really pain which is bothering the patient but something else. He may be concerned with the results of his surgery, for instance, and view anything that he thinks is unusual as indicative that he has an incurable condition. Possibly the patient may be worried about his ability to tolerate pain, particu-

larly if he has been raised with the Western ethic of stoicism.

Knowing what to expect in the way of pain often enables a person to prepare himself to cope with the situation; it also removes much of the fear of the unknown so that anxiety is lessened. Many diagnostic and therapeutic procedures which patients have to undergo are uncomfortable or even painful. If it is known that a patient is scheduled for an examination or treatment that is potentially painful, it is usually better to explain to the patient exactly what is going to be done, the nature of the pain he may experience, and what he can do to assist. If the individual un-

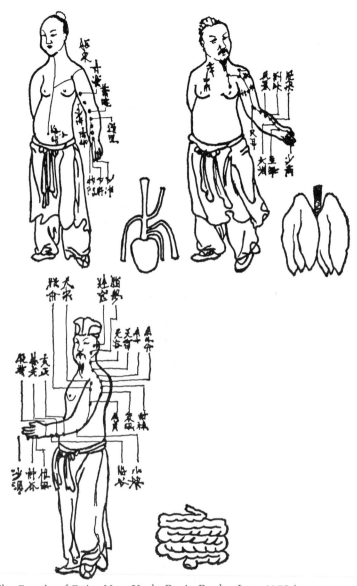

(From Melzack, R.: The Puzzle of Pain. New York, Basic Books, Inc., 1973.)

derstands also why the procedure is necessary, he is usually much better able to cooperate. Explanations of this sort can often help to change the individual's attitude toward the painful experience, since pain that is viewed as an aid in getting better is usually more tolerable than pain that is thought inflicted for reasons a person does not understand.

Even with children, telling them that a procedure is going to hurt a little, and what the hurt will be like, is much preferable to telling them that it is not going to hurt and then proceeding to inflict pain. The latter course of action can destroy a child's trust in health personnel. A factual explanation of exactly what is going to happen to them can usually eliminate much fear for both adults and children.

Reassuring the patient that pain will not be beyond his level of tolerance is sometimes advisable. "If it hurts too much, we will give you something to relieve the pain" is an example of words that can sometimes be used. Touch, for instance, placing a hand on the patient's arm, is often helpful when a patient is undergoing a painful procedure. The nurse should be careful in the use of touch, however. Some patients dislike it, particularly if they are striving to maintain their independence. Many, however, are grateful for a hand to hold when pain seems too much to bear alone.

Enabling the patient to retain a measure of control over the situation can also be helpful in minimizing the reaction to pain. "Tell me when it hurts and we will stop for a minute" is one way of doing this. Involving the patient in some part of the activity, such as holding a piece of the equipment, can help to make him feel a participating member of the health team rather than an object of its actions. Again, distraction can sometimes be used. If the patient is concentrating on taking deep breaths, for example, his attention will not be entirely focused on his pain.

After a painful experience is over, the nurse should make certain that the patient is settled comfortably. Evidence of the painful procedure, such as the dressing tray, should be removed as soon as possible. Some nurses have found that staying with the patient and allowing him to talk over the experience helps him to put it into perspective.

Helping the patient who suffers pain over a long period of time—for instance, the patient with a chronic disease condition—is frequently a challenge to nursing personnel. The nurse can often help to minimize his pain, if not always to completely alleviate it, by some of the measures discussed in previous sections. The nurse can also make certain that in her care of the patient she does not aggravate his pain. She can, for example, use gentleness when handling painful limbs and remove potential sources of pain and discomfort. It has been suggested, too, that helping the patient to find a meaning for his suffering can be of assistance to the patient in handling chronic pain. In this regard, many patients have found their spiritual counselor of considerable help and some have benefited from psychiatric counseling.

GUIDE TO ASSESSING PAIN	1. What words does the patient use to describe his pain?

1. What words does the patient use to describe his pain?
2. Where does the patient feel pain? Can he describe its exact location?
3. How severe is the pain? Does its intensity vary?
4. When does the pain occur? How long does it last? Is it intermittent or steady?
5. Has the cause of the patient's pain been identified?
6. Is the patient aware of any factors which precipitate the pain? which aggravate it or relieve it?
7. Are there observable signs of pain—for example, evidence of muscular tension, protective posture, pallor, diaphoresis?
8. Are there signs that would lead you to suspect that the patient's pain has been sufficiently intense to cause a collapse of the body's adaptive mechanisms, such as a lowered blood pressure or weakened pulse?
9. Is the patient restless, irritable? Does he have difficulty in getting to sleep?
10. Are the patient's basic physiological needs being met?
11. Are there factors which might cause the patient to be anxious or fearful?
12. How much exertion can the patient tolerate without pain? Are there certain movements or activities which are painful?
13. Does he have to undergo any procedures which may be painful?
14. What measures have been prescribed for relief of the patient's pain?

GUIDE TO
EVALUATING THE
EFFECTIVENESS OF
NURSING
INTERVENTION

1. Does the patient state that he is more comfortable? Has the pain gone or lessened in intensity?
2. Does the patient appear more comfortable—that is, is he more relaxed or less restless and irritable?
3. Has the patient been able to get to sleep without difficulty? or to rest quietly?
4. Is he able to enjoy his usual activities?

STUDY
VOCABULARY

Acupuncture	Deep pain	Pain reaction
Analgesic	Histamine	Phantom pain
Bradykinin	Ischemia	Referred pain
Central pain	Pain perception	Superficial pain
Conversion reaction	Pain perception threshold	Visceral pain

STUDY SITUATION

Mrs. Jean Roberts is admitted to the hospital after an automobile accident in which she has possibly fractured her ribs. Mrs. Roberts' husband was also injured at the same time, and he is admitted to a nearby nursing unit. He has a fractured pelvis. Mrs. Roberts is 33 years old, has three small children at home and is in a great deal of pain upon admission. Her physician does not wish to bind her chest at this time. His orders include:

Demerol, 100 mg. I.M. q4h p.r.n.
Seconal, gr. 1½ q.h.s.
Up and about as desired
Food and fluids as desired
Chest x-rays as soon as possible

1. Describe the physiology of this patient's pain.
2. What factors would enter into this patient's perception of and reaction to pain?
3. How might this patient describe her pain?
4. What observation would indicate to the nurse that the patient has pain?
5. What should the nurse include in her recording about this patient's pain? Give an example of the recording, including subjective data, objective data, assessment, and plan.
6. What are the goals of nursing care for this patient?
7. What specific nursing intervention might help alleviate pain?
8. By what criteria can the nurse evaluate the success of the nursing care?

SUGGESTED READINGS

Cady, J. W.: Dear Pain. . . . *American Journal of Nursing,* 76:960–961, June 1976.

Collins, J., et al.: Acupuncture and Pain. *American Association of Nurse Anesthetists Journal,* 44:62–64, February 1976.

Davitz, L. J., et al.: Suffering as Viewed in Six Different Cultures. *American Journal of Nursing,* 76:1296–1297, August 1976.

Johnson, J. E., et al.: Sensory and Distress Components of Pain. *Nursing Research,* 23:203–209, May-June 1974.

Johnson, M.: Pain: How Do You Know It's There and What Do You Do? *Nursing '76,* 6:48–50, September 1976.

McCaffery, M.: Intelligent Approach to Intractable Pain. *Nursing '73,* 3:26–32, November 1973.

Pain and Suffering. *American Journal of Nursing,* 74:489–520, March 1974.

Strauss, A., et al.: Pain: An Organizational-Work-Interactional Perspective. *Nursing Outlook,* 22:560–566, September 1974.

Wiener, C. L.: Pain Assessment on an Orthopedic Ward. *Nursing Outlook,* 23:508–516, August 1975.

Wiley, L. (ed.): Intractable Pain. How Nursing Care Can Help. *Nursing '74,* 4:54–59, September 1974.

CHAPTER 32

The Terminally Ill Patient

32 THE TERMINALLY ILL PATIENT

The nurse should be able to:

List and describe the five stages of dying

Discuss a nursing approach for each stage experienced by a patient

Explain the spiritual needs of the terminally ill patient and his family

Assess the physical needs of the terminally ill patient

List the signs of imminent death

List the signs of death

Identify the components of caring for the patient after death

Discuss the nurse's possible reactions to death and dying

THE TERMINALLY ILL 32
PATIENT

INTRODUCTION

Inextricably involved in nursing is the preservation of life, the alleviation of suffering, and the restoration of health. Our society exalts health, life, and youth. Death is a subject which generally is avoided; even when it is imminent, it is frequently denied. Yet death is a not infrequent occurrence on hospital wards or among the sick in the community. Nurses and physicians, by the very nature of their work, encounter the presence of death more often than most people do in the normal course of their lives.

The frequency of the encounter does not, however, make it easier. The care of the terminally ill patient and the comforting and consoling of the patient's family, whether death is sudden or follows a lengthy illness, presents one of the most difficult situations in nursing practice. It is particularly distressing for the young student who has possibly never been face to face with the realities of death before in her life. However, the five stages of dying (described below) are typical stages of individual or group adjustment to any calamity. Flunking a test, auto accidents, divorce, breaking up with a loved one, environmental disasters, and loss of a limb or a vital body part are a few examples of common occurrences "handled" in the same way as physical death. Thus, the student's own natural feelings of grief over the loss of the patient are something she has to work through in much the same way as the patient and his family do. It is helpful, then, if she understands the nature of the process of grieving so that she is better able to handle her own reactions and to help the patient and his family to meet their needs.

THE STAGES OF DYING

In her book, *On Death and Dying,* Dr. Elisabeth Kubler-Ross suggests that there are five stages that most people go through when they learn that they are going to die. These are: denial, anger, bargaining, depression, and acceptance.[1]

The first stage is one of nonacceptance. This is not happening to them! Surely, there must be some mistake. Often the patient seeks reassurance from the nurse and questions her regarding what the doctor has said. While the decision of what to tell the patient belongs to the physician, and the nurse accepts his guidance in this area, she should know what the patient and his family have been told so that she can provide support. Throughout the denial state, the nurse must accept the fact that the patient is not yet ready to acknowledge the seriousness of his illness. Some patients maintain this denial up to the point of impending death, and continue to talk optimistically of future plans and of what they are going to do when they get better. Nursing personnel often mistakenly admire this type of behavior, considering that the patient is being "very brave," although in fact, it is usually more difficult for this patient when the time comes when he can no longer deny that death is near. Many patients, however, are aware of their prognosis, even though they have never been told in words, and yet they may pretend not to know. Often, they maintain a façade of cheerfulness for the benefit of their families, whom they sense are uncomfortable talking about death, or because they feel that

---

[1] Elisabeth Kubler-Ross: *On Death and Dying.* New York, Macmillan Company, 1969.

they are expected to behave in this manner by the hospital staff. For these patients, it is frequently a relief to drop the façade in the presence of someone who understands what they are going through. It should be pointed out, however, that most patients appear to prefer to hold onto some hope—that a new cure may be found or a miracle happen—even though they do not rationally expect one.

Once the person has passed the stage of denial, he usually goes through an understandable period of anger and hostility. Why should this be happening to him? What did he do to deserve this punishment? At this point, the patient often lashes out at those nearest to him—the physicians, the nurses, the hospital, his family. He may be highly critical of the care he is receiving. If the nurse is aware that there is nothing personal in his attack, that he is in reality angry at God and whatever fates there be rather than at those who are caring for him, it is easier for her to have patience and tolerance with his behavior. The patient's family will usually go through this stage of anger and hostility also, and may take out their feelings on the staff. It is helpful to remember that this too is a normal reaction and one which the nurse should not counter with defensiveness or hostility on her part.

The third stage of dying is often one of bargaining. From early childhood, one is taught that good behavior is rewarded and bad actions are punished. Therefore, promising to be very good may bring about a reversal of the decision that death is due. The nurse may hear the patient say that he would do anything—repent his sins, make up for previous errors—if he can just live a little longer or, perhaps, have a day free of pain. The nurse is probably personally familiar with the bargaining process; she has perhaps stated to herself or prayed that if she could just pass this exam she would faithfully study every night in the future. The nurse cannot change the patient's prognosis, of course, but the relief of pain is usually something which she can do something about. The patient should be kept as comfortable as possible. The effectiveness of analgesic drugs is generally considered to be better if these are given regularly every three to four hours rather than waiting for the patient to request them when pain becomes unbearable.[2] Some analgesics have the unfortunate side effect of clouding the consciousness. Consequently the patient may ask that they be withheld near the time of death so that he can think and talk clearly. The nurse is guided by the physician's orders, but in most instances, the physician and the nurse follow the patient's wishes in this respect.

When the patient realizes that his bargaining efforts are of no avail, he usually enters into a depressed phase. This again is a normal reaction, as the individual contemplates all that he has held dear in life and mourns its loss. During this stage the patient may be very concerned about how his family is going to manage when he is gone, and he may be anxious to "put his affairs in order." Sometimes it is difficult for him to discuss these matters with members of his family, who frequently react very emotionally to any talk of death. In this case, a third party such as the chaplain, a social worker, or a close friend of the patient may be the best person to deal with these practical concerns. During this stage of depression, the patient may not want to talk a great deal. He may wish to see only those nearest and dearest to him. Because of his withdrawal, however, the nurse should not take it for granted that he wishes to be left entirely alone. The presence of someone who sympathetically cares for him is reassuring. Many hospitals permit a member of the family to stay with a patient who is seriously ill, or family members to visit as often as they wish. A terminally ill patient is often placed in a single room so that the patient and his family may have privacy. Yet often this contributes to the patient's sense of isolation. By stopping in to see the patient at frequent intervals, if he has no family members with him, or spending time with him as her schedule permits, the nurse can help to overcome the patient's feelings of isolation.

---

[2]Eleanor E. Drummond: Communication and Comfort for the Dying Patient. *Nursing Clinics of North America*, 5:55–63, March 1970.

The final stage of the dying process comes when the patient has accepted that he is going to die soon and he is prepared for it. By this time, the patient is usually tired but at peace. At this stage, it is the patient's family who usually require the most support. Patients' families react to death and dying in a variety of ways. They too go through the same stages as the patient does, but not always at the same time. When relatives are with a terminally ill person, they are often at a loss as to what to say and how to act. It is not uncommon to see even imminent death denied by a family. The nurse can often help the family by such actions as ensuring them privacy, permitting them access to the patient, and showing them small kindnesses in ministering to their comfort as well as to the patient's.

It is important to the family that they feel the patient is receiving the best care possible. Helping the patient to die in a dignified and peaceful manner is perhaps one of the most valuable contributions the nurse can make to the comfort of both the patient and the members of his family.

At times, it is up to the nurse to tell the family that a patient has died. It is best told to the family group in privacy. The nurse should anticipate that they will be upset and will look to her for supportive understanding. Many agencies have a small prayer room or a chapel where the nurse may take grieving families so that they can be alone for a while. With all cultural groups, there are certain rituals that are performed at the time of death, and these help the family to work through their grief. The nurse should be aware of these rituals and make provisions to ensure that they can be carried out. Often, family members will want to go in and pay their last respects to the dead person, and this should be permitted. Some ethnic groups expect that the members of the immediate family will be very vocal in their outpouring of grief. With others, a more stoical behavior is expected. Regardless of the cultural background, however, the death of an immediate family member is one situation in which crying is considered not only permissible but helpful in the grieving process.

THE SPIRITUAL NEEDS OF THE TERMINALLY ILL PATIENT

Terminally ill patients have many needs: emotional, spiritual, and physical. Perhaps the need which can best guide the nurse is the need of a patient to die gracefully. In describing a way to acquire a positive approach to death, Saunders advises us "to look continually at the patients, not at their need but at their courage, not at their dependence but at their dignity."[3]

In gaining the strength and courage to face death with dignity many people find their religious beliefs of inestimable assistance. Often patients and their families seek support from representatives of their religious faith. Even patients who profess not to believe in a Superior Being may find the visits of a chaplain comforting. The nurse is frequently the person who first identifies the spiritual needs of the patient and she may be called upon to act as a liaison between the patient and the chaplain. Many hospitals maintain a list of clergymen of the different faiths who may be called if the patient does not have his own spiritual counselor, or the hospital may have its own chaplain. Nurses too may feel the need to talk over their feelings about death and the dying patient with someone and often find the chaplain a helpful person in this regard.

THE PHYSICAL NEEDS OF THE TERMINALLY ILL PATIENT

The physical needs of the dying person are similar to the needs of any seriously ill patient. Unless death occurs suddenly, there is usually a progressive failure of the body's homeostatic mechanisms as the individual becomes weaker. The following changes take place:
1. Loss of muscle tone
2. Progressive cessation of peristalsis
3. Slowing of blood circulation
4. Labored respirations
5. Loss of the senses

[3]Cicely Saunders: The Last Stages of Life. *American Journal of Nursing*, 65:70, March 1965.

Loss of muscle tone is usually manifested in the patient's inability to control defecation and urination. The sphincter muscles of the rectum and bladder relax, and as a result there is involuntary micturition and defecation. A retention catheter may be required, and absorbent pads can be used to help the patient keep dry and comfortable. Since patients are often embarrassed about their inability to control these functions, it is important that the nurse be discrete and understanding in her care. Deodorants are frequently used to keep the air in the patient's room fresh and free from unpleasant odors.

Involuntary micturition and defecation predispose the patient to decubitus ulcers. By helping the patient to keep dry and clean and to change his position regularly, the nurse can usually prevent these complications.

Because of the progressive loss of muscle tone the dying patient finds it increasingly difficult to maintain his position in bed without support. If the patient is conscious, Fowler's position is usually indicated in order to increase the depth of ventilation of the lungs. If he is unconscious, a semiprone position promotes the drainage of mucus from his mouth. Family members may become anxious when they see the patient positioned in this manner, and it is wise to explain to them the reasons for it. Regardless of the position that the nurse judges to be most beneficial, the patient will need supportive measures, such as pillows, to maintain it (see Chapter 18). If possible, the various parts of the body should be kept out of dependent positions to prevent the pooling of blood.

The inability to swallow (dysphagia) is also characteristic of the loss of muscle tone in the dying patient. Mucus tends to accumulate in the patient's throat, and as a result the air passing through it causes a typical gurgling sound, "the death rattle." Throat suctioning usually helps to keep his airway patent.

There is a *progressive diminution in peristalsis* of the gastrointestinal tract of the dying patient. His desire for food is usually minimal, but he may want frequent sips of water. His mouth may be dry, owing to dehydration and perhaps to a slight fever, which sometimes precedes death. Good oral hygiene is essential. Because of the reduced peristalsis, flatus accumulates in the stomach and intestines, often distending the patient's abdomen and causing nausea. More than a few sips of water at a time can, as a consequence, cause vomiting. Dying patients are often given nourishment and fluids parenterally but rarely are sips of fluid contraindicated.

As *blood circulation slows,* the patient's extremities appear cyanosed or mottled and feel cold and clammy to the touch, although he probably perceives warmth and his temperature is above normal. When circulation is considerably decreased, the effectiveness of the administration of analgesics, intramuscularly or hypodermically, is decreased. As a consequence, the patient may require analgesics in an intravenous solution.

Respiratory embarrassment is alleviated by throat suctioning, by positioning (such as Fowler's position), and by the administration of oxygen. Aside from its effect on the patient, respiratory difficulty is one of the most distressing signs that his family has to witness.

There are also *alterations in the senses* of the dying patient. His vision frequently becomes blurred, and as a result the patient prefers a lighted room, rather than the darkened room that so often comes to mind. His eyes may need special attention also. Frequently secretions tend to gather, and these should be removed with absorbent cotton dipped in normal saline to prevent crusting. Sometimes, however, the eyes become dry and it may be necessary to instill some sterile ophthalmic ointment onto the lower conjunctivae to keep them lubricated.

Hearing is considered to be the last sense to leave the body; hence the patient who cannot respond verbally often understands what people are saying. When people talk to a dying person, they should take care to speak distinctly in a normal voice. Whispering is to be avoided, because it may disturb the patient to realize that people are talking and yet he is unable to understand what they are saying.

Varying degrees of consciousness precede death: Drowsiness is a state of sleepiness, stupor is a state of unconsciousness from which one can be aroused, and coma is an unconscious state from which one cannot be aroused. The patient may remain conscious and rational until the moment of death, or he may become unconscious or confused several days or even weeks prior to death.

For the comfort of the dying patient and his family, the patient's room is kept clear and tidy. As mentioned, frequently the dying patient is given a private room on the nursing unit of the hospital so that he and his family may have privacy.

Some patients experience pain while they are critically ill. Generally in such cases the physician orders an analgesic to prevent discomfort.

SIGNS OF IMMINENT DEATH

Certain signs are indicative of the imminence of death. The patient's reflexes gradually disappear and he is unable to move. His respirations become increasingly difficult; Cheyne-Stokes respirations may occur. Typically his face assumes a pinched expression, and often a faint cyanotic pattern becomes discernible in the skin of his face. The patient's skin feels cold and clammy and his pulse accelerates and becomes weaker. With increasing anoxia, the pupils become dilated and fixed. Low blood pressure, an elevated temperature, and a rapid respiration rate are often seen.

SIGNS OF DEATH

Death is considered to have occurred when the patient's respirations and heart have ceased to function for several minutes. Usually breathing stops first; the heart stops beating a few minutes later.

In this day of cardiac massage and mouth-to-mouth resuscitation, it is not unusual for a patient to "die" only to revive and walk out of the hospital.

Nursing personnel should note for the medical record the exact time that respirations cease and the heart stops beating. A physician pronounces the patient dead.

For the purpose of human transplants, it has become necessary to have a more precise definition than the cessation of respiration and heart beat as the absolute signs of death. The absence of brain wave activity as measured by the electroencephalogram is usually used to confirm that death has occurred.

CARE AFTER DEATH

In caring for the body of the patient after death, whatever procedures are carried out are performed with dignity and respect. In some religious faiths, only family members are permitted to care for the body of the deceased. Generally, however, this is a nursing responsibility. Although each agency usually has its own specific procedures, there are some general guidelines for the care of the body after death which are fairly universal.

The body is generally placed in a supine position in bed with one pillow under the head. The head is slightly elevated to prevent postmortem hypostasis of blood, which could discolor the face. The body is positioned immediately after death and before rigor mortis sets in.

Rigor mortis, a stiffening of the body after death, is a result of a chemical action within the muscles in which glycogen is coagulated and lactic acid is produced. It generally occurs shortly after death, progressing from the jaw down the trunk to the extremities. Once rigor mortis has set in, the body remains rigid for one to six days.

When relatives wish to see the body, the nurse first tidies the room and removes extraneous equipment. The body should appear clean, comfortable, and peaceful. A slightly shaded room affords a comforting effect.

In some hospitals it is the policy to insert dentures immediately after death; other institutions send the dentures with the body to the morgue, where they are inserted later by the mortician. In most institutions, rings are removed; if a ring cannot be removed it is taped in place and a notation is made on the patient's chart and on the form which goes with the body to the morgue.

The preparation of the body by the

nurse involves the application of pads to the perineal area or the insertion of packing into the rectum and vagina. Rarely is it necessary to bathe the body; this procedure is carried out by the mortician. It is, however, necessary to cleanse the body of any blood or drainage which may have accumulated after death.

At most hospitals bodies are labeled twice: one label is attached to the ankles, the other to the shroud in which the body is wrapped. If the ankles and wrists are to be tied together, they should be well padded in order to prevent bruising. In some areas it is the practice to treat the body as if the patient were still living, and no shroud is used. When the preparation of the body is complete it is taken to the hospital morgue. If the hospital does not have a morgue, the mortician should be notified to come for the body.

The patient's valuables and clothes should, whenever possible, be sent home with the relatives. If there is no one present who can assume responsibility for these, valuables should be placed in the hospital safe and the clothes labeled and stored until such time as the family collects them.

The family of the deceased may be asked by the physician to sign a permission for an *autopsy* (postmortem examination). Under some circumstances an autopsy is required by law. For example, when a patient dies within 24 hours of admission to a hospital or when he dies as a result of injury or accident, some states require an autopsy. It is usually not the nurse's responsibility to secure permission for an autopsy. She may, however, be called upon to explain to the family the reasons for the autopsy.

The death certificate is signed by the physician and then sent to the local health department. If the deceased has a communicable disease, special regulations are observed regarding the care and disposition of the body.

GUIDE TO ASSESSING NURSING PROBLEMS OF THE TERMINALLY ILL	1. Is the patient aware of his prognosis? 2. What have the patient and his family been told about his prognosis? 3. Does the patient have any special requests? 4. Does the patient wish to have a chaplain visit him? 5. Is the patient in pain? 6. Is he lonely? 7. What problems do the family have which the nurse can help to resolve?

STUDY VOCABULARY	Autopsy Coma	Drowsiness Dysphagia	Rigor mortis Stupor

STUDY SITUATION	Mr. John Edwards is in a hospital with a malignancy which the doctors consider terminal. He is 93 years old and has three sons and seven grandchildren. Mr. Edwards has been in a stuporous state and upon waking he complains of pain. 1. What are some of the nursing needs of this patient? 2. What is stupor? 3. What needs of the family could be met by the nurse? 4. Which other members of the health team might be able to assist Mr. Edwards and his family? 5. How can you evaluate Mr. Edwards' nursing care?

SUGGESTED READINGS

Annas, G. J.: Rights of the Terminally Ill Patient. *Journal of Nursing Administration,* 4:40–44, March-April 1974.

Fletcher, J.: Ethics and Euthanasia. *American Journal of Nursing,* 73:670–675, April 1973.

French, J., et al.: Terminal Care at Home in Two Cultures. *American Journal of Nursing,* 73:502–506, March 1973.

Griffin, J. J.: Family Decision: A Crucial Factor in Terminating Life. *American Journal of Nursing,* 75:794–796, May 1975.

Gyulay, J. E.: Care of the Dying Child. *Nursing Clinics of North America, 11:*95–108, March 1976.

Halachi, S.: A Lesson You Won't Learn in School. *RN,* 39:47–51, May 1976.

Hampe, S. O.: Needs of the Grieving Spouse in a Hospital Setting. *Nursing Research,* 24:113–120, March-April 1975.

Hendrickson, S.: A Philosophy of Death Made Personal. *American Journal of Nursing, 76:*90, January 1976.

Kavanaugh, R. E.: Dealing Naturally With Dying. *Nursing '76,* 6:22–29, October 1976.

Kobryzcki, P.: Dying with Dignity at Home. *America Journal of Nursing,* 75:1312–1313, August 1975.

Lacasse, C. M.: A Dying Adolescent. *American Journal of Nursing,* 75:433–434, March 1975.

Popoff, D., et al.: What Are Your Feelings About Death and Dying? *Nursing '75,* 5:15–24, August 1975.

Rinear, E. E.: Helping the Survivors of Expected Death. *Nursing '75,* 5:60–65, March 1975.

Rogers, J., et al.: Nurses Can Help the Bereaved. *Canadian Nurse,* 71:16–19, June 1975.

Ufema, J. K.: Dare to Care for the Dying. *American Journal of Nursing,* 76:88–90, January 1976.

Weber, L. J.: Ethics and Euthanasia—Another View. *American Journal of Nursing,* 73:1228–1231, July 1973.

White, J. F.: Yes, I Hear You, Mr. H. *American Journal of Nursing,* 75:411–413, March 1975.

Wise, D. J.: Learning About Dying. *Nursing Outlook,* 22:42–44, January 1974.

Yeaworth, R. C., et al.: Attitudes of Nursing Students Toward the Dying Patient. *Nursing Research,* 23:20–24, January-February 1974.

Zopf, D.: The Dying Patient: Meeting His Needs Could Be Easier Than You Think. *Nursing '75,* 5:16–20, March 1975.

GLOSSARY

abduction. movement away from the central axis of the body.

abrasion. an area of the body rubbed bare of skin or mucous membrane.

abscess. a localized collection of pus in a cavity formed by the disintegration of tissue.

acapnia. a condition of decreased carbon dioxide in the blood.

acceptance. the ability to be nonjudgmental, understanding, and respecting of another's point of view.

acetone. a colorless liquid with a pleasant ethereal odor. It is found in small quantities in normal urine and is used as a solvent for fats, resins, rubber, and plastics.

acidosis. a condition in which there is an excessive proportion of acid in the blood and a reduced reserve of alkali (bicarbonate).

acne. an inflammatory disease of the sebaceous glands.

acromion process. the outward extension of the spine of the scapula, forming the point of the shoulder.

active exercise. exercise in which the muscles actively contract.

active transport. mechanism which transfers electrolytes from the cells to the extra-cellular fluid to achieve balance.

actual problem. a problem which is causing the patient to have difficulty at the present time.

acupuncture. the practice of inserting long, fine needles into particular sites of the skin in order to cure disorders, relieve pain, or anesthetize an area of the body for surgery.

acute. having a short and relatively severe course.

adaptation. condition in which the brain no longer perceives the available stimuli because the receptors are not picking up enough stimuli or too much of the same stimulus.

addiction. the state of being given to some habit, as a drug habit.

adduction. movement toward the central axis of the body.

adhesion. a fibrous band or structure by which parts may abnormally adhere.

adipose. of a fatty nature.

adrenal gland. endocrine gland located atop the kidney.

adrenocortical hormone. a hormone secreted by the cortex of the adrenal gland.

agitate. to excite the mind or feelings; to move with irregular, rapid, or violent action.

air-fluidized bed. a bed which uses the flotation principle to provide uniform support to all parts of the body.

air hunger. respirations that are abnormally deep and accompanied by an increased respiratory rate.

alarm reaction. mobilization of the body's defense forces in response to physiological or psychological stress.

albuminuria. the presence of protein in the urine, in the form of white blood cells. 639

aldosterone. a hormone secreted by the cortex of the adrenal glands; a mineralocorticoid.

alkalosis. a condition in which there is an excess of alkali, such as bicarbonate, in the blood.

alternating pressure mattress. an air- or water-filled mattress, areas of which are alternately deflated and inflated with a resultant continual change of pressure upon the various parts of the body.

alveolus (i). an air sac of the lungs formed by the terminal dilatations of a bronchiole.

ambulate. to move about; to walk from place to place.

ameba. a minute one-celled animal organism of the phylum Protozoa.

amino acid. the structural unit of protein.

ampule. a sealed glass container.

anabolism. the synthesis of compounds by the cells.

anaerobe. a microorganism that grows in the absence or near absence of oxygen.

analgesic. relieving pain; a pain-relieving agent.

anatomical position. the position of the human body standing erect, with all body parts in good alignment.

anemia. a condition in which the blood is deficient in hemoglobin or red blood cells.

aneroid. containing no liquid.

anesthesia. loss of feeling or sensation.

anesthetic bed. a bed prepared to receive a patient immediately after surgery.

anion. a negatively charged ion.

anogenital. pertaining to the area around the anus and genitalia.

anorexia. loss of appetite.

anoxemia. a decrease in the amount of oxygen in the blood below physiological levels.

anoxia. a decrease in the amount of oxygen in the tissues below physiological levels.

antecubital. situated in front of the cubitus or forearm.

anthelmintic. destructive to worms.

antibiotic. a chemical substance produced by microorganisms which has the capacity to destroy or inhibit the growth of other microorganisms.

antibody. a substance formed in the body in response to an antigen.

antidiuretic hormone. a hormone produced by the posterior pituitary gland which inhibits the secretion of urine.

antigen. a substance which stimulates the production of antibodies within the body.

antipyretic. an agent which reduces fever.

antisepsis. the prevention of sepsis by inhibiting the growth of microorganisms.

anuria. the absence of urinary excretion from the body.

anus. the distal orifice of the alimentary canal.

anxiety. an emotional response to danger of unknown origin.

aortic receptor. a nerve ending in the aortic arch which is sensitive to changes in blood pressure.

apathy. lack of feeling or emotion.

aphasia. the state of being unable to speak at all.

apical beat. the beat of the heart as it is felt over the apex.

apical-radial pulse. the results of taking the apical and the radial pulses at the same time on the same watch.

apnea. a period of cessation of breathing.

apomorphine. an alkaloid which is a powerful emetic and relaxant.

appendicitis. inflammation of the vermiform appendix.

appetite. desire for food.

arachnoidal granulations. the capillary-like projections of the arachnoid membrane.

arachnoid membrane. a membrane between the pia mater and dura mater surrounding the brain and spinal cord.

areolar connective tissue. loose connective tissue widely distributed in the body.

Aschheim-Zondek test. a pregnancy test in which urine from a female is injected into mice.

ascites. abnormal accumulation of fluid in the peritoneal cavity.

asepsis. freedom from infection—that is, from pathogenic organisms.

asphyxia. suffocation; a condition in which there are anoxia and an increase in carbon dioxide tension in the blood and tissues.

aspiration. the act of breathing or drawing in; the removal of fluids or gases from a cavity by suction.

assault. a threat to do bodily harm to another.

assessment. the collection and analysis of information leading to the identification of problems.

asthma. a condition marked by periodic attacks of dyspnea, with wheezing and a sense of constriction.

astringent. an agent which causes contraction and arrests discharges.

asymmetric. not symmetrical; lack of correspondence in paired organs.

atelectasis. incomplete expansion of the lungs at birth or collapse of the adult lung.

atrioventricular valve. the valve between the atrium and the ventricle of the heart.

atrophy. a wasting away or diminution in the size of a cell, tissue, organ or other part.

attendant. a person who assists with care, such as dressing and feeding patients and looking after their personal hygiene.

auditory. pertaining to the sense of hearing.

auscultation. observation by listening for body sounds.

autonomic. self-functioning; independent.

autonomy. the condition of being functionally independent.

autopsy. a postmortem examination.

bactericidal. capable of destroying bacteria.

bacteriostatic. capable of inhibiting the growth or multiplication of bacteria.

bacterium(a). any microorganism of the order Eubacteriales.

Balkan frame. a frame made of wood or metal which extends lengthwise over the bed and is supported at either end by a pole.

barbiturate. a salt or derivative of barbituric acid used as a sedative.

barrier technique. medical aseptic practices to control the spread of pathogenic bacteria and contribute to their destruction.

basal metabolism. the rate of energy expenditure of the body at rest.

basic need. a need that is necessary for survival, such as the need for air.

basilic vein. superficial vein of the arm.

battery. the unlawful beating of another or the carrying out of threatened physical harm.

behavior. deportment or conduct.

Bence-Jones protein test. examination of urine to detect bone tumors.

binder. a type of bandage.

biological clock. the physiologic mechanism that governs the rhythmic occurrence of certain biochemical, physiological, and behavioral phenomena in plants and animals.

biopsy. the removal and examination of tissue or other material from the living body.

Biot's respirations. irregular respirations as to speed and depth; pauses may be associated with a sigh.

bleb. a skin vesicle filled with fluid.

blister. a collection of fluid in the epidermis causing an elevation of the outer layer (stratum corneum).

body temperature. the internal temperature of the human body.

boil. furuncle; a painful nodule in the skin caused by bacteria and often having a central core.

bolus. a mass of food ready to be swallowed or a mass passing along the intestines.

brachial pulse. the pulse located on the anterior surface of the arm, just below the elbow, where the brachial artery passes over the ulna.

Bradford frame. a canvas, stretcher-like device supported by blocks on the foundation of the bed. It is used to immobilize patients who have injured spines.

bradycardia. a very slow heart beat, reflected in a pulse of under 60 beats per minute.

bradykinin. chemical substance released by damaged cells which excites pain receptors.

bradypnea. an abnormal decrease in the respiratory rate.

bronchoscopy. inspection of the bronchi with a lighted instrument (bronchoscope).

bronchus(i). one of the two main branches of the trachea; also the divisions of the main bronchi within the lungs.

burette. a graduated glass tube.

cachexia. a general physical wasting, often associated with chronic disease.

calculus(i). a stone formed in various parts of the body, such as the gallbladder or kidney.

calorie. a unit of heat. One small calorie is the amount of heat required to raise the temperature of 1 gm. of water 1°C. A large calorie is the amount of heat required to raise the temperature of 1 kg. of water 1° C.

calyx(ices). a cup-shaped organ or cavity; in the kidney, one of the recesses in the pelvis.

cannula. a tube for insertion into the body, often made of a hard substance, and the lumen of which contains a trochar during the insertion.

canthus. the angle formed at either end of the eye by the upper and lower eyelids.

carbohydrate. an organic chemical compound composed of carbon, hydrogen, and oxygen, found in most plants, fruit sugars, and natural starches.

cardiac sphincter. the band of circular fibers stituated at the opening of the esophagus into the stomach.

carminative. a medicine which relieves flatulence.

carotid receptors. nerve endings located in the carotid sinuses and carotid bodies that are sensitive to changes in blood pressure, excess blood CO_2, and blood pH.

carrier. an individual who harbors disease organisms in his body and yet does not manifest symptoms but who can pass on the infection.

cast. coagulated protein in the urine, passed from the lumen of the kidney tubules.

catabolism. a destructive process within the cells in which complex substances are converted into simpler substances.

cathartic. a medicine that hastens bowel evacuation.

catheter. a tube used to withdraw fluid from body cavities (such as urine from the bladder or blood samples from major vessels or heart chambers) or to introduce fluids (as in intravenous feedings or in injecting radiopaque material for angiocardiography).

cation. a positively charged ion.

cementum. true bone that protects root of a tooth.

central pain. pain arising from injury to sensory nerves, neural pathways, or areas in the brain concerned with pain perception.

cephalic vein. a superficial vein on the thumb side of the arm.

cerebral cortex. the outer layer (gray matter) of the largest part of the brain (cerebrum).

cerebrospinal fluid. the fluid which surrounds the brain and spinal cord.

certification. a mechanism for ensuring the quality of a practitioner's competence in a specialized area at a level higher than licensure.

ceruminous. secreting wax.

cervix. a necklike structure; the lower narrow portion of the uterus.

Cheyne-Stokes respirations. respirations with rhythmical variations in intensity occurring in cycles, often with periods of apnea.

chill. involuntary contractions of the voluntary muscles, with shivering and shaking.

chordotomy. surgical division of the anterolateral tracts of the spinal cord.

choroid plexus. a network of capillaries found in the ventricles of the brain which produce the cerebrospinal fluid.

chronic. persisting over a long period of time.

cicatrization. a healing process which leaves a scar.

cilium(a). a minute hairlike process attached to the free surface of a cell, as in the nose.

cinefluorography. the production of a motion picture record of a sequence of fluoroscopic images.

circadian rhythm. a rhythmic repetition of certain things in living organisms at approximately the same time each 24 hours.

circumcision. removal of all or part of the foreskin of the penis.

circumduction. circular movement, as of a limb or an eye.

cisterna. a closed sapce serving as a reservoir.

cisterna magna. an extension of the subarachnoid space below and behind the corpus callosum.

cisternal puncture. the insertion of a needle into the cisterna magna.

clarification. the act of making clear one's impressions on a particular point.

clavicle. the collar bone. It articulates with the sternum and the scapula.

clinic. a community or hospital agency providing services for promotion of health, prevention of illness, and care and treatment of sick on an ambulatory basis.

clinical nursing specialist. A nurse who has expanded her nursing knowledge and skills in one particular branch of nursing.

clean. denoting the absence of disease-producing microorganisms.

closed bed. an empty bed, to which no patient has as yet been assigned.

cognition. the process by which we become aware through thought or perception, including reasoning and understanding.

cohesion. a force which unites particles.

collagen. an albuminoid supportive protein found in connective tissue.

colostomy. the surgical creation of an opening between the colon and the surface of the body.

coma. a state of unconsciousness from which an individual cannot be aroused.

combustible. inflammable; liable to take fire.

comfort. ease of body or mind.

commode. a portable toilet-like structure.

communicable disease. a disease capable of being transmitted from one person to another.

Community Health Center. a center providing comprehensive health care for residents in a community.

compensation. attempting to make up for real or imagined inferiorities by becoming highly competent in a sphere of endeavor.

compress. a pad or cloth that is folded and applied to press upon a body part.

concave. rounded inward or hollowed.

concurrent disinfection. ongoing measures to control the spread of infection during the time the patient is considered infectious.

conditioned. learned through repetition of a stimulus, as in Pavlov's experiment.

conductive heat. heat transmitted to the body by contact with a heated object, such as a hot water bottle.

confused. mental state of appearing bewildered and perplexed, and/or making inappropriate answers to questions.

congenital. health problems present at birth.

congestion. an abnormal accumulation of blood in a part.

consciousness. the normal state of awareness.

constant data. information that is not expected to change during the period of care.

constipation. abnormal delay in the passage of feces.

contact. a person who is known to have been sufficiently near an infected person to be exposed to the transfer of infectious organisms.

contaminate. to soil or make unclean.

context. the environment; the portions of a discourse that precede or follow a word or words.

contracture. a shortening or distortion of muscle tissue.

convalescence. the stage of transition from illness to health.

convection. transmission of heat in liquids or gases.

conversion reaction. a condition in which emotional disorders are experienced as physical symptoms.

conversive. pertaining to a change in the state of energy, as from electricity to heat.

conversive heat. heat developed in the tissues by a current of electricity or by some form of radiant energy.

corneal reflex. closing of the eyelids as a result of irritation of the cornea.

counterirritant. an agent applied to the skin to produce a reaction which relieves irritation.

covert. hidden; covered.

cradle. a frame placed over the body of a bed patient for protecting the injured parts from contact with the bedclothes.

creatinine. nitrogenous waste excreted in the urine.

crime. a legal wrong, generally committed against the public.

cultural shock. stress caused by exposure to customs and social values at variance with one's own.

culture. those aspects of society which include knowledge, beliefs, art, morals, laws, and customs.

curative aspects. pertaining to diagnostic, therapeutic, and rehabilitative measures in health care.

custom. a practice that is common to many or to a place or class or that is habitual to an individual.

cyst. a sac, usually containing a liquid or semisolid material.

cystitis. inflammation of the urinary bladder.

cystoscopy. examination of the urinary bladder with a lighted instrument.

dandruff. dry, scaly material shed from skin of the scalp.

data base. the sum total of information gathered in the admission work-up of a patient.

debilitated. enfeebled; lacking strength.

deceleration. the state of moving at decreasing speed.

decubitus ulcer. a bedsore.

deep pain. pain arising from deeper structures of the body, such as muscles, tendons, joints.

defamation of character. the damaging of an individual's reputation by written or spoken statements.

defecation. the evacuation of feces.

defense mechanism. an individual's reaction to disturbances in psychosocial equilibrium, manifested by changes in intellectual behavior.

dehydration. removal of water from the body or tissues.

delirious. suffering from mental confusion, incoherence, and physical restlessness.

denial. refusing to acknowledge a problem or forbidden motive.

dependency. having to rely on others for the satisfaction of basic needs.

dependent nursing function. the carrying out by the nurse of a decision made by another health professional.

depression. a feeling of sadness or melancholy.

deprivational stress. stress produced by a lack of some factor essential for the well-being of an organism.

dermis. the inner, thicker layer of the skin.

detergent. an agent which purifies or cleanses.

detrusor muscle. the three layers of smooth muscle of the urinary bladder.

developmental crises. major changes in an individual's life as he reaches certain stages in his physical and/or psychosocial development.

diabetes. a hereditary disease in which the body is unable to burn up its intake of sugars, starches, and other carbohydrates because of the deficiency of insulin.

diacetic acid. acetoacetic acid; an acid excreted in the urine.

diagnoal toe bed. a bed made up to expose the leg or foot of the patient, at the same time providing warmth and adequate covering for the rest of the body.

diagnosis. the determination of the nature of a disease.

diaphoresis. profuse perspiration.

diarrhea. undue frequency of the passage of feces, with the discharge of loose stools.

diastolic blood pressure. the pressure in the arteries when the ventricles of the heart are relaxed.

diathermy. the generation of heat in the tissues by the application of high frequency electric currents.

dietitian. a person educated in the use of diet in health and disease.

differentiation. distinguishing of one thing or disease from another on the basis of differences.

diffusion. process whereby nolecules and ions distribute themselves equally within a given space.

digital. pertaining to the fingers.

diplopia. double vision; seeing two objects when there is only one.

disassociate. to separate; to detach from association.

discipline. a field of study.

disease. a cluster of abnormalities in functioning, producing recognizable signs and symptoms.

disinfection. the destruction of disease-producing microorganisms.

disorientation. a state of mental confusion; a lack of awareness of time, place, or person.

displacement. redirecting aggressive feelings and actions toward a substitute.

distal. farther from a point of reference or point of attachment.

distention. the enlargement of the abdomen due to the internal pressure of gas or liquid or other causes.

diuresis. the abnormal secretion of urine.

diuretic. a substance which increases the secretion of urine in the kidneys.

doctor's order sheet. a written record of the orders given by the physician for the patient's treatment.

dorsal. pertaining to the back; posterior.

dorsal recumbent. supine; lying on one's back.

dorsalis pedis pulse. the pulse felt on the dorsum of the foot in a line between the first and second toes, just above the longitudinal arch.

drowsiness. readiness to fall asleep.

drug. a chemical compound used for diagnosis or therapy or as a preventive measure.

duodenum. the first part of the small intestine.

dysphagia. difficulty in swallowing.

dysphasia. difficulty in speaking.

dyspnea. difficult breathing.

dysuria. difficulty in voiding or pain on voiding.

ecchymosis. extravasation of blood into the tissues.

ecology. the study of man's relationship with the environment.

edema. the presence of excessive amounts of fluid in the intercellular spaces.

edentulous. without teeth.

efferent. carrying outward from the center.

electrocardiogram. a graphic tracing of the electrical current produced by the contraction of the heart muscle.

electroencephalogram. a record of the electrical impulses produced by the brain.

electrolyte. a compound which in an aqueous solution is able to conduct an electrical current.

elopement. the act of running away clandestinely.

emaciated. excessively lean.

embolus. a clot in a blood vessel which has been transported from another vessel.

emesis. vomiting.

emollient. softening or soothing.

emphysema. a condition in which the pulmonary alveoli are distended or rupture as a result of air pressure.

emulsion. a liquid which is distributed throughout another liquid in small globules.

enamel. the hard, inorganic substance covering the crown of a tooth.

endemic. present at all times among a particular people or within a particular country.

endogenous. developing from within.

endogenous spread. the transfer of microorganisms from one area of a person's body to another.

endothelium. the layer of squamous cells which lines the blood vessels.

enema. a liquid to be injected into the rectum.

enteric coated. medications with a coating that prevents them from dissolving until reaching the intestines.

enteroclysis. the injection of a nutrient or medicine into the bowel.

enuresis. incontinence of urine during sleep.

environment. the sum total of the external surroundings and influences.

environmental equilibrium. the balance achieved by an organism in its interactions with the surrounding environment.

environmental technologist. a worker primarily concerned with the improvement, control, and management of man's environment.

epidemic. attacking many people in a region at the same time; widely diffused and rapidly spreading.

epidermis. the outer, thinner layer of the skin.

epididymitis. inflammation of the epididymis, the oblong body containing a duct, attached to the testicle.

epinephrine. a hormone produced by the medulla of the adrenal gland or prepared synthetically; a vasopressor.

epistaxis. nosebleed.

equilibrium. a static or dynamic state of balance between opposing forces or actions.

erythema. redness of the skin due to congestion of the capillaries.

esophagus. the canal extending from the pharynx to the stomach.

etiology. the study of the causes of disease.

eupnea. normal, regular, or effortless breathing.

evaluation. determining whether the expected outcomes have been attained or not.

evaluative response. reacting to statements by imposing one's own values on another individual.

eversion. a turning outward.

excoriation. the loss of superficial layers of skin.

excreta. waste materials excreted by the body.

exogenous. developing from outside.

expectorate. to bring mucus up from the lungs or trachea.

expiration. the act of expelling air from the lungs (breathing out).

explicit policy. a written governmental plan of action on which health programs are based.

extended care facility. an agency whose primary purpose is the care of people with long-term illnesses.

extension. the act of straightening a limb.

extracellular. situated outside the cells.

extravasation. the escape of blood from a vessel into the tissues.

exudate. a substance produced and deposited on or in a tissue by disease or a vital process.

false imprisonment. the unjustifiable detention of an individual without a legal warrant.

family nutritionist. a member of a community health agency who is primarily concerned with matters of food and its relationship to health.

fantasy. the use of daydreaming to temporarily escape from reality.

fastigium (stadium). the high point of a fever.

fats. organic compounds composed of carbon, hydrogen, and oxygen, found in nature, in animals, and in plant seeds.

fear. an emotional response to a known and identifiable danger.

feces. excreta discharged from the intestines.

femoral pulse. pulse which may be taken at the point in the middle of the groin, where the temporal artery passes over the pelvic bone.

femur. the leg bone extending from the pelvis to the knee.

fever. an elevated temperature.

fibrin. a protein substance which forms an essential part of a blood clot.

fibroplasia. the formation of fibrous tissue.

Fishberg concentration test. a special urine test to determine specific gravity.

fissure. a deep cleft or groove.

fistula. an abnormal passage leading from an abscess or hollow organ to the body surface or from one hollow organ to another.

flatulence. distention of the stomach or the intestines with air or gases.

flatus. gas in the intestines or stomach.

flexion. the act of bending.

flight-fight reaction. the body's response to immediate (real or imagined) danger.

flowsheet. a special form which details a specific intervention or group of related interventions to be done on a regular basis and which documents the results thereof.

fluoroscopy. examination of structures of the body such as the stomach by means of roentgen rays and a fluorescent screen.

flushing. a redness of the skin, particularly noticeable in the face and neck.

fomite. a substance other than food which can harbor microorganisms.

footboard. a device placed toward the foot of the patient's bed as a support for his feet.

forgetful. suffering from a temporary loss of memory.

fossa navicularis. a widened area of the lumen of the male urethra just superior to the meatus; a depression on the internal pterygoid process of the sphenoid bone.

Fowler's position. the sitting position in which the head gatch of the patient's bed is raised to at least a 45 degree angle.

fracture board. a support placed under the patient's mattress to give it added rigidity.

free clinic. a clinic providing readily accessible health services on a free or nominal charge basis for people living in poor neighborhoods.

frequency. in reference to voiding, abnormally short intervals between times of voiding.

friction. the force which opposes motion.

Friedman test. a test for pregnancy which involves the injection of urine into rabbits.

frontal plane. the plane that divides the body into dorsal and ventral sections.

fulcrum. the fixed point of a lever.

functional pathology. referring to diseases which have no apparent physical basis.

gastrocolic reflex. mass peristalsis of the colon stimulated from the stomach.

gastroenteritis. inflammation of the stomach and intestines.

gastroscopy. the examination of the stomach with a lighted instrument.

gavage. feeding through a stomach tube.

general adaptation syndrome. the generalized response of the body to any agent that causes physiological stress.

genitalia. the reproductive organs; generally, the external reproductive organs.

geriatric nursing. the nursing care of older people.

gingivae. the gums in the mouth.

glaucoma. a condition in which there is increased tension within the eyeball.

gliding. movement in one plane, as in sliding.

glomerulus. a tuft of capillaries such as that of the nephron of the kidney.

glossopharyngeal nerve. the ninth cranial nerve; the nerve serving the tongue and pharynx.

glottis. the vocal apparatus of the larynx.

glycerol. glycerin; a byproduct of the breakdown of fats.

glycogen. a polysaccharide stored in cells after the breakdown of carbohydrate.

glycosuria. the presence of glucose in the urine.

Good Samaritan Law. a law designed to protect a person from malpractice suits arising from care given at the scene of an emergency.

granulation. fleshy projections formed on the surface of a wound that is not healing by first intention.

gravity. the force which pulls all objects toward the center of the earth.

Guérin's fold. a fold of mucous membrane occasionally seen in the fossa navicularis of the urethra.

gustatory. pertaining to the sense of taste.

gynecology. the branch of medicine which deals with diseases of the female reproductive tract.

halitosis. foul odor of the breath.

hallucination. distortion in sensory perception.

hallucinogens. drugs which cause distortions in sensory perception.

health. a positive state of being which includes physical fitness, mental (or emotional) stability, and social ease.

health educator. person primarily responsible for the development of health education programs in the community.

Health Maintenance Organization. organization of private physicians providing a comprehensive range of health services on a fixed contract basis.

health status indicators. statistical information about illness and death, usually compiled on an annual basis by national governments.

health team. all those who participate in providing health care services.

hectic (septic) fever. an intermittent fever with wide variations in temperature elevation but in which the temperature falls to normal during each 24 hour period.

hematemesis. the vomiting of blood.

hematuria. the discharge of blood in the urine.

hemiplegia. the loss of motor functions on one side of the body.

hemoglobin. the red pigment of the red blood cell which carries oxygen.

hemoglobinuria. hemoglobin in the urine.

hemophilia. a hereditary blood disease in which the blood lacks elements necessary for normal clotting.

hemoptysis. the spitting up of blood or of blood-tinged sputum.

hemorrhage. bleeding; the escape of a large amount of blood from the blood vessels.

hemorrhoid. enlarged, often infected veins and sinuses at or near the anus.

hemothorax. a collection of blood in the thoracic cavity.

herbalist. a nonmedical practitioner of the healing arts who makes use of herbs (plants) to treat disease.

Hering-Breuer reflex. the reflex which limits respiratory inspirations and expirations.

hierarchy. an arrangement in a graded series.

histamine. a chemical substance found in all animal and vegetable tissues, liberated when cells are injured.

holism. the concept of the individual as a whole, including physical, social, and emotional components.

homeostasis. tendency to uniformity or stability in body states; dynamic equilibrium.

hospital. an institution whose chief purpose is to provide inpatient services for the care of people with health problems.

host. an animal or plant which harbors or nourishes another organism.

human biology. the science of human life.

humidity. the degree of moisture in the air.

hunger. an uncomfortable feeling which indicates a need for nourishment.

Huntington's chorea. a hereditary disease characterized by progressive degeneration of the nervous system.

hyaluronidase. an enzyme which initiates the hydrolysis of the cement material (hyaluronic acid) of the tissues.

hydration. the act of combining with water; the state of having adequate body fluids.

hydraulic. pertaining to the action of liquids.

hydrostatic. pertaining to fluids in a state of equilibrium.

hydrostatic pressure. the pressure of liquids.

hygiene. the science of health and its preservation; practices conducive to good health.

hyperalgesia. excessive sensitivity to pain.

hypercalcemia. an excessive amount of calcium in the blood.

hyperemia. excessive blood in any part of the body.

hyperextension. extending beyond the normal range of motion.

hyperglycemia. an increased concentration of glucose in the blood.

hyperkalemia. an excessive amount of potassium in the blood.

hypernatremia. an excessive amount of sodium in the blood.

hyperplasia. an abnormal increase in the number of cells in a tissue or organ.

hyperpnea. an abnormal increase in the rate and depth of respirations.

hypersomnia. uncontrollable drowsiness.

hypertension. persistently high arterial blood pressure.

hyperthermia. an abnormally high body temperature; fever.

hypertonicity. a state characterized by excessive tone or activity.

hypertrophy. an abnormal increase in the size of an organ or tissue as a result of an increase in the size of the cells.

hypervolemia. an abnormal increase in blood volume.

hypnotic. a drug that acts to induce sleep.

hypocalcemia. a decrease in the amount of serum calcium.

hypochloremia. a reduced concentration of chlorides in the blood.

hypodermoclysis. the introduction of fluids into the subcutaneous tissues.

hypogastric nerve. the nerve trunk of the autonomic nervous system which serves the abdominal viscera.

hypoglycemia. a reduction in the amount of glucose in the blood.

hypokalemia. a reduction in the amount of potassium in the blood.

hyponatremia. a decrease in the amount of sodium in the blood.

hypotension. an abnormally low arterial blood pressure.

hypothalamus. part of the diencephalon of the brain, from which fibers of the autonomic nervous system extend to the thalamus, neurohypophysis, and so forth.

hypothermia. an abnormally low body temperature.

hypoxemia. a reduction in the oxygen content of the blood.

hypoxia. a reduction in the oxygen content of the tissues.

identification. modeling oneself upon the image of another person.

immunity. the condition of being protected against a particular disease.

impacted bowel. the condition in which there is an accumulation of feces in the rectum, pressed firmly together so as to be immovable.

impaction. the condition of being firmly lodged or wedged.

implementation. the carrying out of the specified measures outlined in a plan.

implicit policy. a health plan demonstrated by the actions of a health department, though not formally expressed.

inattentive. unable to focus the mind on an idea or some aspect of the surroundings.

incoherent speech. speaking in such a way that one's meaning is not clear (to people speaking the same language).

incontinent. unable to control urination and/or defecation.

independent nursing function. the carrying out, or delegation by the nurse, of a decision made by herself in respect of the care of a patient.

industrial hygienist. a person whose main concern is the detection and control of environmental hazards in the work situation.

infant mortality. the death of infants under one year of age.

infection. the invasion of the body by disease-producing microorganisms and the body's reaction to their presence.

infestation. invasion of the body by arthropods, including insects, mites, and ticks.

inflammation. a condition of the tissues in reaction to injury.

infusion. the therapeutic introduction of a fluid into a vein or part of the body.

inguinal hernia. the protrusion of an organ or tissue through an abnormal opening into the inguinal canal.

inhalation. the drawing of air or other substances into the lungs.

inhalation therapist. a technician who is skilled in the performance of diagnostic procedures and therapeutic measures dealing with the respiratory tract.

insertion (of a muscle). the place of attachment of a muscle to the bone that it moves.

insomnia. the inability to sleep.

inspection. observation by use of the sense of sight.

inspiration. the act of taking air into the lungs.

instillation. the dropping of a liquid into a cavity such as the ear.

insulator. a material or substance which prevents or inhibits conduction, as of heat.

intercostal. located between the ribs.

interdependent nursing function. the carrying out by the nurse of a decision made by herself in consultation with other health professionals.

intermittent (quotidian) fever. fever which falls to normal at some time during a 24 hour period.

intern. a graduate of a basic professional program (medicine, nursing, and so forth) who is receiving a planned program of clinical experience, usually in order to complete requirements for licensure.

interstitial. located between the cells of tissue.

interview. a talk with a purpose.

intracellular. located within the cells.

intradermal. located within the dermis.

intramuscular. located within the muscle tissue.

intraosseous. located within the bone.

intravascular. located within a vessel.

intravenous. located within a vein.

intravertebral. intraspinal.

intrathecal. located within the spinal canal.

intubation. the insertion of a tube.

invasion of privacy. the exposing of an individual or his property to public scrutiny without his consent.

inversion. a turning inward.

inward rotation. a turning of a bone upon its axis toward the midline.

irradiation. exposure to x-rays or radioactive matter such as radium and ultraviolet rays.

irrational. confused as to time, place, or person; not possessing normal judgment.

irritant. an agent applied to the skin to produce a reaction.

ischemia. localized anemia due to an obstruction to the inflow of blood.

isolation. the separation of one person, material, or object from others.

isometric exercise. exercise in which muscle tension is increased but the muscles are not shortened and the body parts are not moved.

isotonic. pertaining to equal tone or pressure; pertaining to solutions having equal osmotic pressure.

isotonic exercise. exercise in which the muscle is shortened and body parts are moved.

jargon. technical terms used in a particular line of work which are not in common use outside the field.

jaundice. a condition in which yellowish pigment is deposited in the skin, tissues, and body fluid.

keratin. a scleroprotein substance in hair, nails, and horny tissue.

ketone. a compound containing the carbonyl group.

17-ketosteroid. a type of hormone classed as an androgen and excreted in the urine. It is partially produced in the adrenal cortex and partially derived from testosterone.

kilogram. a unit of weight equal to 1000 grams or approximately 2.2 pounds.

kinesiology. the science of motion.

Kussmaul's breathing. air hunger; dyspnea occurring periodically without cyanosis.

labored breathing. breathing that involves the active participation of accessory inspiratory and expiratory muscles.

languor. listlessness; lassitude.

laryngeal stridor. a coarse high-pitched sound which accompanies inspiration.

lassitude. weariness; fatigue; languor.

lateral. relating to the side; situated away from the midline.

lavage. therapeutic washing out of an organ such as the stomach.

lesion. an open area or break in the skin surface.

lethargy. abnormal drowsiness; state of being lazy or indifferent.

leukocyte. white blood cell.

lever. a rigid bar which revolves around a fixed point.

liability. responsibility.

libel. the damaging of an individual's reputation by a written statement.

licensed practical nurse. one who is licensed to perform standardized nursing procedures and treatments, working under the direction of a registered nurse or physician.

licensed vocational nurse. the designation given to licensed practical nurses in some states of the United States.

licensure. approval by an appropriate authority that permits a person to offer to the public his skills and knowledge in a particular jurisdiction.

life expectancy. the average number of years that a person of a given age may be expected to live.

lifestyle. the way of life of an individual, dictated in part by circumstances and in part by active decision.

ligament. a band of connective tissue that connects bones or supports organs.

local. restricted to one spot or part.

local adaptation syndrome. the body's localized reaction to stress affecting a specific part or organ.

lumbar puncture. the introduction of a needle into the subarachnoid space in the lumbar section of the spinal cord for diagnostic or therapeutic purposes.

lumen. the cavity of a tubular organ.

lymph nodes. an accumulation of densely packed lymphatic tissue.

lymphatic. pertaining to or containing lymph.

lysis. the gradual fall of an elevated temperature.

malaise. a vague sense of debility or lack of health.

malignancy. a tendency to progress in virulence.

malnutrition. a disorder of nutrition.

malpractice. improper or injurious action on the part of a professional practitioner.

mandatory licensure. legislation requiring a professional nurse to hold a valid, current license in the state (province) in which she is employed in order to be able to practice.

manometer. an instrument for measuring the pressure of liquids or gases.

massage. systematic stroking and kneading of the tissues.

mastication. the process of chewing food in preparation for swallowing and digestion.

meatus. an opening.

medial. pertaining to the middle; situated toward the midline.

medical asepsis. practices which are carried out in order to keep microorganisms within a given area.

medical diagnosis. the physician's opinion as to the nature of a patient's illness.

medical laboratory technologist. a person responsible for collecting, treating, and analyzing many of the specimens needed for laboratory tests used in the detection and treatment of illness.

medicament. an agent used in therapy; medicine; drug.

medicine. any drug or remedy.

medulla oblongata. the part of the rhombencephalon which attaches to the spinal cord and contains a number of the vital centers.

meniscus. a crescent-shaped structure; the surface of a liquid column.

menstruation. the monthly flow of blood from the female genital tract.

metabolism. the sum of all physical and chemical processes by which living substance is produced and maintained.

microorganism. an organism which can be seen only by means of a microscope.

microwave. an electromagnetic wave of high frequency and short wavelength.

micturition. voiding.

minerals. inorganic elements or compounds occurring in nature.

minim. a unit of volume equal to 1/60 part of a fluid dram.

miter. to square a sheet at a corner when making a bed

mold. a type of fungus.

morbid. pertaining to disease.

morbidity data. information relating to the frequency of illness within specific population.

mortality. the quality of being subject to death.

mortality rate. the death rate.

Mosaic Law. writings attributed to Moses.

mucoid. a moist viscid protein substance.

mucous membrane. the membrane that lines passages and cavities of the body which communicate with the air.

myelography. the x-ray examination of the spinal cord by using a contrast medium.

myocardium. heart muscle.

narcolepsy. a condition marked by an uncontrollable desire for sleep or by sudden attacks of sleep occurring at intervals.

narcotic. a drug which relieves pain or induces sleep or stupor.

nasopharynx. the upper part of the pharynx continuous with the nasal passage.

naturopath. a nonmedical practitioner of the healing arts who makes use of physical forces such as heat and massage to cure disease.

nausea. stomach distress accompanied by an urge to vomit.

necrosis. localized death of tissue.

need. something an individual perceives as being useful or necessary.

negligence. failure to take appropriate action to protect the safety of the patient.

Neighborhood Health Center. a center providing comprehensive health services for the residents of a given community in their own neighborhood.

neonatal mortality. the death of infants within 28 days of birth.

neoplasm. any new and abnormal growth.

Neo-Synephrine. phenylephrine hydrochloride, an adrenergic drug which produces vasoconstriction.

nephron. functional unit of the kidney.

nervousness. state of being easily excited, irritated, jumpy, uneasy, or disturbed.

neurogenous. arising in the nervous system.

neuron. functional unit of the nervous system.

nitrogen mustard. an agent used therapeutically to inhibit the growth of abnormal new cells, such as white blood cells in leukemia. It is very irritating to tissues.

nocturia. excessive urination at night.

nonverbal communication. the conveying of feelings or attitudes by such behavior as facial expressions, gestures, and so forth, rather than with words.

norepinephrine. a hormone produced by the adrenal medulla.

norm. a fixed or ideal standard.

nurse practitioner. a nurse functioning in an expanded role by providing primary health care in the community.

nurse's aide. person who is usually trained on the job to perform tasks ranging from those principally of a housekeeping nature to assisting in the care of patients.

nursing action. those measures which nurses carry out to help patients in the achievement of health goals.

nursing assistant. the designation given to practical nurses in some provinces in Canada.

nursing audit. the examination of a nurse's charts for redundancy, evidence of poor judgment, and lack of explicitness in the definition of problems, and/or the failure to carry out appropriate nursing interventions.

nursing care plan. a plan of care for a patient.

nursing diagnosis. an assessment of those needs of patients which a nurse can help to meet through nursing action.

nursing history. a written record of information about a patient obtained by the nurse through interview and observation.

nursing intervention. action taken by the nurse as a result of the identification of specific problems.

nursing orderly. a member of the nursing team who assists in the personal care of male patients and who may perform simple nursing tasks.

nursing process. the series of steps the nurse takes in planning and giving nursing care.

nutrient. nourishing; a substance affording nourishment.

obese. corpulent; excessively fat.

objective symptom. evidence of a disease process or dysfunction of the body which can be observed and described by other people.

obstetrics. that branch of medical science which deals with birth and its antecedents and sequelae.

occult. hidden.

occupational health nursing. the employment of nurses in various work settings to provide care, health counseling, maintenance, and protection services for employees.

occupational therapist. a member of the health team who assists patients to develop new skills or to regain skills lessened or lost through illness.

official health agency. a government agency concerned with the prevention of disease, the promotion of health, and the detection and treatment of illness.

olfactory. pertaining to the sense of smell.

oliguria. secretion of a diminished amount of urine.

open bed.   a bed that has been prepared for an incoming patient.

ophthalmoscope.   an instrument used to examine the interior of the eye.

optimal health.   the highest level of functioning attainable by an individual.

oral.   concerning the mouth.

organic.   of, relating to, or containing living organisms.

organic pathology.   pertaining to disease processes which can be identified physically, as, for example, tumors or communicable diseases.

oriented.   aware of time, place, and person.

orifice.   entrance or outlet of any body cavity.

origin (of muscle).   the fixed end or attachment of a muscle.

oropharynx.   that division of the pharynx between the soft palate and the epiglottis.

orthopnea.   the inability to breathe except when in a sitting position.

osmosis.   passage of a solvent through a membrane from a lesser to a greater concentration of two solutions.

osmotic pressure.   the pressure exerted by particles, which tends to draw a solvent towards it.

otoscope.   an instrument used to inspect the ear.

outward rotation.   a circular motion directed away from the midline.

overbed cradle.   see cradle.

ovulation.   the discharge of an ovum from the ovary.

pain.   unpleasant sensation resulting from the stimulation of specialized nerve endings.

pain perception.   the ability to perceive pain.

pain reaction.   the behavioral response to pain.

palliative.   affording relief but not cure.

pallor.   a lack of color.

palpation.   examination by using one's fingers (sense of touch).

pandemic.   widespread epidemic disease.

panic.   a severe state of anxiety in which the individual is unable to say or do anything meaningful.

Papanicolaou smear.   a cytologic test in which cells are taken from the cervix for examination, chiefly to detect malignancy.

papillary reflex.   tactile response of the skin.

paracentesis.   the removal of fluid from the peritoneal cavity.

paralysis.   loss or impairment of motor or sensory function due to neural or muscular disease.

paraplegic.   paralyzed from the waist down.

parasite.   a plant or animal which lives upon or within another living organism.

parasympathetic nervous system.   the craniosacral part of the autonomic nervous system.

parenteral.   occurring outside the alimentary tract.

paresthesia.   an abnormal sensation without objective cause; for example, numbness or tingling in any or all parts of the limb or other body parts.

Parkinson's disease.   a chronic condition marked by muscular rigidity and tremor.

parotid glands.   salivary glands situated near the ear.

parotitis.   inflammation of the parotid glands; mumps.

passive exercise.   exercise in which the muscles do not actively contract.

patent.   open; unobstructed.

pathogen.   a disease-producing microorganism or material.

pathogenic.   capable of producing disease.

pathology. the branch of medicine which deals with the nature of disease.

patient. a person who seeks professional help or advice concerning his health.

patient advocate. someone who speaks on the patient's behalf and who can intercede in his interest.

patient profile. a brief account of the patient's assets and liabilities in relation to health.

patient's record. a written record of a person's medical history, examinations, tests, diagnosis, prognosis, therapy, and response to therapy while he is a patient.

pediculosis. infestation with lice.

peer. one of equal standing.

peer review. an examination by a third party of equal standing of the health care process.

pelvis (of kidney). funnel-shaped cavity of the kidney.

perception. the conscious, mental registration of a sensory stimulus.

percussion. examination by tapping the body.

perineum. the area between the anus and the posterior part of the genitalia; entire ano-genital area.

periosteum. fibrous membrane surrounding bone.

peripheral. outward or toward the surface.

peristalsis. wormlike movement by which the alimentary tract propels its contents along.

peritoneal cavity. the potential space between the layers of the peritoneum.

peritoneum. the serous membrane lining the abdominal cavity.

peritonitis. inflammation of the peritoneum.

permissive licensure. the situation in which a professional nurse is free to choose whether or not to register for a license.

personal information. information of a specific nature about a person's feelings, attitudes, behaviors, or details of his personal life.

perspiration. the secretion of fluid by sweat glands of the skin.

petechia. a pinpoint spot of blood in the skin or mucous membrane.

Petri dish. a shallow glass receptacle for growing bacterial cultures.

phantom pain. pain believed to be caused by a pain "memory," after the cause of the pain has been removed, as pain in amputated limbs.

pharmacist. a person responsible for the preparation and dispensing of drugs and other substances used in the detection, prevention, and treatment of illness.

phenolsulfonphthalein. a chemical used to test the function of the kidneys.

phlebotomy. an opening into a vein made in order to remove blood.

physical therapist. a member of the health team who assists in assessment of patients' functional ability and carries out therapeutic and rehabilitative measures dealing particularly with the musculoskeletal system.

physician. a person who has successfully completed a basic course of medical studies, concerned with preventing, diagnosing, and treating human illnesses, and is authorized to practice medicine in a given jurisdiction (state, province, or country).

physician's assistant. a trained person, usually employed by a physician, who performs, under the physician's supervision, many tasks considered a part of medical practice.

physiological. concerning body function.

physiology. the science which deals with the function of living organisms and their parts.

placenta. the "afterbirth"; the tissue attached to the uterus wall by which the fetus is nourished by its mother's blood.

planning. developing a course of action to help the patient.

plantar flexion. a reflex in which an irritation of the sole of the foot contracts the toes; extension of the foot away from the body.

plaque. film of mucus and bacteria that forms on the teeth.

plasma. the fluid portion of blood.

pleura. the serous membrane lining the thoracic cavity.

pleural cavity. the potential space between the plurae.

pneumothorax. the accumulation of gas or air in the pleural cavity.

poliomyelitis. a virus disease which when serious can involve the central nervous system, with resultant paralysis.

polydipsia. excessive thirst.

polyethylene. a lightweight plastic resistant to chemicals and moisture and having insulating properties.

polypnea. an abnormal increase in the respiratory rate.

polyuria. secretion of an increased amount of urine.

POMR. the concept of problem-oriented medical records, which offers health care personnel a set of rules based on the scientific problem-solving process.

popliteal. concerning the posterior surface of the knee.

population density. the number of persons per square mile of a given area.

posterior fornix (of the vagina). a vaultlike space at the back of the vagina.

post-neonatal mortality. the death of infants from 28 days of age up to, but not including, one year of age.

posture. the relationship of the various parts of the body at rest or in any phase of motion.

potential problem. a problem which may arise because of the nature of the patient's health problem, or because of the nature of the diagnostic or therapeutic plan of care.

precordium. the region over the heart or stomach.

preoptic center. the nerve center anterior to the optic center.

prepubic urethra. the part of the male urethra inferior to the pubis.

preventive. directed at averting the occurrence of.

primary care. the initial health care given to an individual.

primary nursing. the method of allocating nursing responsibility whereby each patient is assigned on admission to a specific nurse, in whose care he remains for the duration of his hospital stay.

principle. a concept, scientific fact, law of science, or generally accepted theory.

private duty nursing. the employment of nurses on a one nurse–one patient basis in cases of acute illness.

problem. anything with which the patient needs help.

problem list. a summary of all the known health problems of the patient.

proctoclysis. Murphy drip; the slow injection of a large amount of liquid into the rectum.

proctoscopy. examination of the rectum and the anus by means of a lighted instrument.

progesterone. a hormone produced by the corpus luteum of the ovary.

prognosis. medical opinion as to the outcome of a disease process.

progress notes. information concerning the monitoring, plan modification, and follow-up phases of the problem-oriented process.

projection. ascribing one's own unacceptable feelings or attitudes to other people.

proliferation. growth by rapid reproduction.

pronation. turning down towards the ground.

prone. lying on the stomach (face down).

prophylactic. preventive.

prostate. a gland which surrounds the male urethra just below the bladder.

prostration. extreme exhaustion.

protein. a complex organic compound containing carbon, hydrogen, oxygen and nitrogen found in nature, in animals and plants.

proteinuria. the presence of protein in the urine.

protoplasm. the living substance of cells.

proximal. closer to the point of reference or to the point of attachment.

prudence. the habit of acting after careful deliberation.

pruritus. intense itching.

psychiatry. the branch of medicine which deals with disorders that are mental, emotional, or behavioral.

psychology. the science of mind and mental processes.

psychosomatic. concerning the mind and the body.

public health inspector. a worker concerned with the elimination or control of factors in the environment that may endanger health.

pulse. the throbbing of an artery as it is felt over a bony prominence.

pulse deficit. the difference between the apical rate and the pulse rate.

pulse pressure. the difference between the systolic and diastolic blood pressures.

pulse rate. the number of pulse beats per minute.

pupil. the opening in the center of the iris of the eye.

purulent. containing pus.

pus. the thick liquid product of inflammation, composed of leukocytes, liquid, tissue debris, and microorganisms.

pyemia. a general septicemia in which there is pus in the blood.

pyloric sphincter. the thickened layer of circular fibers which surrounds the opening between the stomach and the duodenum.

pyrexia. fever.

pyrogen. a fever-producing substance.

pyuria. pus in the urine.

quadriplegic. paralyzed from the neck down.

Queckenstedt's sign. in a normal person, when the veins on either side of the neck are compressed, the pressure of the cerebrospinal fluid rises.

radial pulse. the pulse located on the inner aspect of the wrist on the thumb side, where the radial artery passes over the radius.

radiation. treatment with x-rays, radium, or other radioactive matter.

radiologic technologist. a person who performs diagnostic or therapeutic measures involving the use of radiant energy.

radiopaque. not permitting the passage of roentgen rays.

rales. the term used when bubbling sounds can be heard in the air cells or bronchial tubes during breathing.

rapport. a relationship marked by accord or affinity.

rationalization. giving socially acceptable reasons for one's behavior.

reaction formation. attempting to remove a subconscious and forbidden motive or desire by vigorously attacking it.

reciprocal. given in return; mutual.

recording. the communication in writing of essential facts in order to maintain a continuous history of events over a period of time.

recreation specialist. a person responsible for developing recreation, sports, or physical fitness programs in the community.

rectum. the distal portion of the large intestine.

referred pain. pain perceived in one area of the body when the stimulus for its origin is in another area.

regimen. a regulated pattern of activity.

registered nurse. a person who has successfully completed a basic program of professional nursing and is authorized to practice in a specific jurisdiction (state, province, or country).

regression. reverting to a previously acceptable, but no longer appropriate, form of behavior.

rehabilitation. the restoration of the ill or injured to function at their full capacity.

relapsing fever. a fever in which there is one or more days of normalcy between febrile periods.

remittent fever. a fever with marked variations but in which the temperature does not reach normal.

REM sleep. the stage of sleep in which dreaming is associated with mild, involuntary muscle jerks, and rapid eye movements.

renal. relating to the kidney.

renal dialysis. the process whereby blood is continually removed from an artery and allowed to circulate through a channel with a thin membrane, which removes the impurities from the blood before it is returned to the patient through a vein.

repression. unconsciously forgetting problems or experiences.

resident. a qualified medical practitioner who is in residency in a hospital, usually while preparing for practice in a medical specialty.

residual volume. the amount of air remaining in the lungs after a forceful expiration.

respiration. the means by which the individual's lungs exchange gases with the atmosphere.

respiratory technologist. a person who performs diagnostic procedures and therapeutic measures used in the care of patients with respiratory problems.

rest. repose after exertion.

resuscitation. restoration to life or consciousness.

retching. an unproductive attempt at vomiting.

retention (of urine). a condition in which urine is accumulated in the bladder and not excreted.

rickettsiae. minute rod-shaped micoorganisms of the family Rickettsiaceae.

rigor mortis. the stiffening of a dead body.

roentgen. the unit of measurement of x-radiation.

role. the pattern of behavior that is expected of an individual in a particular group or situation.

rotation. turning in a circular motion around a fixed axis.

rubefacient. reddening of the skin; an agent that reddens the skin.

ruga(e). a ridge, wrinkle or fold.

sacrament. a formal religious act.

sagittal plane. the plane which divides the body into right and left sections.

sanguineous. pertaining to blood.

saphenous veins. superficial veins of the legs.

scab. the crust of a sore, wound, ulcer, or pustule.

scapegoating. directing feelings or actions of hostility towards one particular person or group of persons.

sclerosis. an induration or hardening.

scored. marked with significant notches, lines or grooves.

sebaceous. secreting oil.

sebum. the secretion of the sebaceous glands.

secretion. a product of a gland.

secularism. indifference to religion.

sedative. tending to calm or tranquilize; a sedative agent.

self-esteem. an individual's feeling that he is a worthwhile human being.

semantics. the study of meaning in language.

semicircular canal. an organ within the temporal bone which functions to give the sense of equilibrium.

semilunar valves. pulmonary and aortic valves of the heart.

senility. the feebleness of body and mind incident to old age.

sensitivity. responsiveness to various stimuli; frequently used to refer to the responsiveness of bacteria to specific antibiotic agents.

sensory deficit. a partial or total impairment of any of the sensory organs.

sensory deprivation. a lack or alteration of impulses conveyed from the sense organs to the reflex or higher centers of the brain.

sensory overload. an overabundance of sensory stimulation.

septic. due to or produced by putrefaction.

septic fever. hectic fever.

serum. the clear portion of an animal liquid; the liquid part of blood as distinct from the solid particles.

shock. a condition of acute peripheral circulatory failure.

sigmoidoscopy. examination of the sigmoid colon with a lighted instrument.

sign. an objective symptom which can be detected through special examination.

Sims's position. a lateral position in which the patient is placed in a semiprone (sometimes called ¾ prone) position.

slander. the damaging of an individual's reputation by a spoken statement.

sleep. a period for the body and mind during which volition and consciousness are in partial or complete cessation, and the bodily functions are partially suspended.

sleep deprivation. loss of sleep.

slipper pan. a bedpan with one end flattened for ease of slipping under the patient.

slurring. sliding or slipping over utterances that would normally be heard and understood.

smear. a specimen for microscopic study prepared by spreading the specimen across a glass slide.

SOAP format. the method of writing the narrative aspect of the patient's progress notes. S stands for subjective (the patient's expression of the problem); O, objective (clinical findings); A, assessment; P, proposed plan of action.

social worker. a member of the health team who assists in evaluating the psychosocial situation of patients and helps them with their social problems.

sociology. the science of the social institutions and relationships.

somnambulism. habitual walking in one's sleep.

sordes. a collection of bacteria, food particles, and epithelial tissue in the mouth.

spasm. involuntary contraction of a muscle or a group of muscles.

speculum. an instrument for opening to view a cavity or canal.

sphincter. a ringlike muscle which closes a natural orifice.

sphygmomanometer. an instrument used to measure blood pressure in the arteries.

spinothalamic tract. the neural pathway along the spinal cord to the thalamus.

split foam rubber mattress. a mattress divided horizontally into three sections, which is generally used for debilitated patients and those unable to move.

spore. the reproductive element of a microorganism which is surrounded by a thick wall.

sprain. the wrenching of a joint resulting in injury to its attachments.

sputum. matter ejected from the respiratory tract, often from the lungs.

stammering. hesitant speech.

stasis. stagnation of fluid such as blood.

stenosis. a narrowing or constriction.

sterile. free from microorganisms.

sterilization. the destruction by heat or chemicals of all forms of bacteria, spores, fungi, and viruses.

sternum. the breastbone.

stertorous. noisy breathing.

stethoscope. an instrument used to transmit sounds, as the heart beat.

stomatitis. inflammation of the oral mucosa.

stool. the fecal discharge from the bowels.

stopcock. a valve for stopping or regulating the flow of fluids or gases.

strain. the overstretching or overexertion of muscles; a group of organisms within a species or variety.

stressor. any factor which disturbs the body's equilibrium.

stricture. an abnormal narrowing of a passage or canal.

stroke volume output. the amount of blood ejected by the heart with each beat.

structured interview. a conversation controlled and directed by the interviewer.

stupor. partial or nearly complete unconsciousness.

stuttering. spasmodic repetition of the same syllable when speaking.

subarachnoid space. the space beneath the arachnoid tissue.

subcutaneous. beneath the skin.

subjective symptom. evidence of disease or bodily dysfunction which can be perceived only by the patient.

sublimation. channeling unacceptable motives into acceptable forms of behavior.

sublingual. situated under the tongue.

subscapular. situated below the scapula.

sulfanilamide. a drug used in infections.

superficial pain. pain arising from stimulation of receptors in the skin or mucous membranes.

supination. turning upwards.

supine. lying on the back.

suppository. a medication which is molded into a firm base so that it can be inserted into a bodily orifice or cavity.

suppression. the sudden stoppage of a secretion, excretion or normal discharge; consciously putting out of one's mind problems or unpleasant experiences.

suppuration. the formation of pus.

supraoptic. pertaining to the area above the eye.

supraorbital. situated above the orbit of the eye.

surgery. that branch of medicine that treats diseases by operative procedures.

surgical asepsis. practices carried out to keep an area free of microorganisms.

suture. a surgical stitch.

sympathetic nervous system. the thoracolumbar branch of the autonomic nervous system.

symptom. evidence of a disease process or a disturbed body function.

synapse. juncture of nerve cells; to form a synapse.

syncope. a faint.

syndrome. a group of symptoms which commonly occur together.

synthesis. the process of putting together parts of a whole.

systemic. pertaining to or affecting the body as a whole.

systolic blood pressure. the pressure of the blood in the arteries at the time of ventricular contraction.

tachycardia. an accelerated heart beat, with a pulse rate of over 100 per minute.

tachypnea. abnormal increase in the respiratory rate.

tactile. pertaining to the sense of touch.

tartar. film formation on the teeth.

temporal pulse. the pulse felt anterior to the ear at the mandibular joint, where the temporal artery passes over the temporal bone.

tenacious. adhesive.

tenesmus. ineffectual and painful straining at stool or urination.

terminal disinfection. measures taken to destroy pathogenic bacteria in an area that has been vacated by a patient with an infection.

testator. a person who makes a will.

tetany. tonic spasm of the muscles.

thalamus. part of the diencephalon of the brain; one of its functions is the relay of sensory impulses.

therapeutic environment. an environment which helps a patient grow, learn, and return to health.

therapy. treatment that is remedial.

thermal trauma. injury involving the presence of harmful levels of heat or cold.

thoracentesis. the insertion of a cannula into the pleural cavity.

thrombosis. the formation or development of a blood clot.

thyroxine. a hormone produced by the thyroid gland.

tidal volume. the amount of air normally inhaled and exhaled.

tinnitus. buzzing or ringing in the ears.

tissue turgor. the condition of normal tissue fullness and resilience.

tolerance. the ability to endure without ill effect.

tonsillectomy. surgical removal of the palatine tonsils.

tonus. the slight continuous contraction of muscle.

topical. pertaining to local external application.

tort. a legal wrong committed by one person against the person or property of another.

tourniquet. an instrument to compress blood vessels in order to control circulation.

toxin. any poisonous substance of microbic, vegetable, or animal origin.

trachea. the windpipe; the tube extending from the larynx to the bronchi.

tracheotomy. a surgical incision into the trachea.

traction. the act of drawing, as in applying a force along the axis of a bone.

transition. a period of change.

transudation. the passage of serum or other fluid through a membrane.

transverse plane. the plane which divides the body into superior and inferior sections.

trauma. injury.

tremors. quivering or involuntary, convulsive muscular contractions.

Trendelenburg's position. the position in which the patient is lying on his back with the foot of the bed elevated.

trocar. a sharp-pointed instrument often used with a cannula.

troche. lozenge.

tumor. an abnormal mass of tissue that arises from cells of preexistent tissue and possesses no physiologic function.

ulcer. a break in the skin or mucous membrane with loss of surface tissue.

ultrasound. those sound waves which have a frequency above that heard by the human ear.

ultraviolet. pertaining to rays whose wavelengths lie between those of the violet rays and the roentgen rays.

umbilicus. the site of attachment of the umbilical cord in the fetus.

unresponsive. making no response to sensory stimulation.

urban. relating to or characteristic of a city.

urea. the final nitrogenous product of the decomposition of protein. It is formed in the liver and carried by the blood to the kidneys, where it is excreted.

urea frost. the appearance on the skin of salt cyrstals left by evaporation of the sweat in cases of acute renal failure.

uremia. a condition in which the urinary constituents are found in the blood.

ureter. the tube that carries the urine from the kidney to the bladder.

urethra. the canal that conveys the urine from the bladder to the body's surface.

urgency. a compelling desire to void.

urinalysis. examination of the urine.

urobilin. a brownish pigment normally found in feces.

urticaria. a temporary condition of raised edematous patches of skin or mucous membrane which are itchy.

uterus. the muscular organ of the female reproductive tract in which the fetus grows and is nourished.

vagina. the canal in the female reproductive system extending from the cervix to the vulva.

variable data. information concerned with the current status of the patient, such as temperature, which is liable to vary with changes in the patient's health status.

vasoconstriction. a narrowing of the lumen of the blood vessels, particularly the arterioles.

vasodilation. an increase in the size of the lumen of the blood vessels, particularly the arterioles.

vector. an organism which transmits a pathogen.

ventral. anterior; situated toward the front when in anatomical position.

ventricle. a cavity, such as those of the brain or heart.

ventriculography. x-ray examination of the ventricles of the brain after the insertion of a radiolucent medium.

vermin. external animal parasites, such as lice.

vertigo. dizziness.

vesicant. an irritant that is used to produce a blister upon the skin.

vestibule. a space or cavity at the entrance to a canal.

vial. a glass container with a rubber stopper.

virulence. the degree of pathogenicity of a microorganism.

virus. a submicroscopic pathogen.

viscera. plural of viscus.

visceral pain. pain arising from the viscera.

viscosity. the quality of being sticky.

viscus (viscera). any large interior organ such as the stomach.

vital capacity. the amount of air which can be expired after an inspiration.

vital signs. indications of basic physiological functioning as evidenced by an individual's temperature, pulse, and respirations.

vitamins. organic chemical substances, widely distributed in natural foodstuffs, which are essential to normal metabolic functioning.

voiding. evacuation of the bowels or bladder.

volatile. tending to evaporate rapidly.

voluntary health agency. a private, nonprofit agency which is established and supported by people in a community.

vomitus. emesis; matter ejected from the stomach via the mouth.

warmth. a genuine liking for people.

wheezing. difficult breathing accompanied by whistling sounds.

xiphoid process. the inferior part of the sternum.

x-rays. the visualization of parts of the body by roentgen rays.

x-ray technologist. See radiologic technologist.

yeast. a minute fungus, particularly *Saccharomyces cerevisiae*.

APPENDIX

Prefix	Meaning	Suffix	Meaning
adeno-	gland	-ectomy	a cutting out or excision
arthro-	joint	-oscopy	examination by means of a lighted instrument
chole-	bile		
chondro-	cartilage	-ostomy	formation of a fistula or opening
colpo-	vagina		
cranio-	skull	-otomy	a cutting or an incision
entero-	intestine	-pexy	fixation
gastro-	stomach	-plasty	molding
hystero-	uterus	-rhaphy	a suturing of
laparo-	loin, flank		
litho-	stone		
masto-	breast		
myo-	muscle		
nephro-	kidney		
neuro-	nerve		
osteo-	bone		
phleb-	vein		
pneumo-	air		
pyelo-	pelvis, basin		
salpingo-	tube		
teno-	tendon		
thoraco-	chest		
trachel-	neck		

INDEX